ATLAS OF PULMONARY SURGICAL PATHOLOGY

ATLASES IN DIAGNOSTIC SURGICAL PATHOLOGY

Consulting Editor
Gerald M. Bordin, M.D.
Department of Pathology
Scripps Clinic and Research Foundation

Published:

WOLD, McCLEOD, SIM AND INNI: **ATLAS OF PATHOLOGY**

Forthcoming Titles:

Kanel and Korula: **Atlas of Liver and Biliary Tract Pathology**

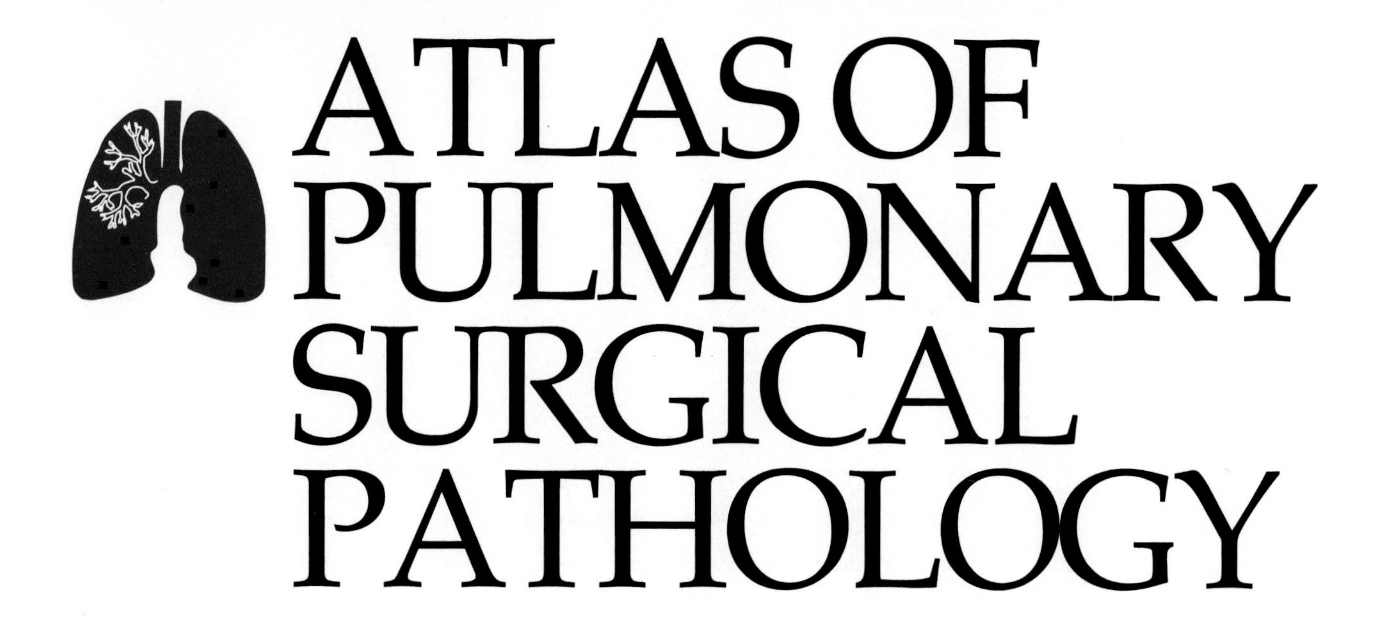

ATLAS OF PULMONARY SURGICAL PATHOLOGY

Thomas V. Colby, M.D.
Consultant in Pathology
Mayo Clinic
Rochester, Minnesota

Charles Lombard, M.D.
Clinical Assistant Professor of Pathology
Stanford Medical Center
Attending Pathologist
El Camino Hospital
Mountain View, California

Samuel A. Yousem, M.D.
Assistant Professor of Pathology
Presbyterian University Hospital
Pittsburg, Pennsylvania

Masanori Kitaichi, M.D.
Pulmonary Pathologist
Department of Medicine
Chest Disease Research Institute
Kyoto University
Kyoto, Japan

1991

W.B. SAUNDERS COMPANY
Harcourt Brace Jovanovich, Inc.
Philadelphia ■ London ■ Toronto ■ Montreal ■ Sydney ■ Tokyo

W. B. Saunders Company
Harcourt Brace Jovanovich, Inc.
The Curtis Center
Independence Square West
Philadelphia, PA 19106

Library of Congress Cataloging-in-Publication Data

Atlas of pulmonary surgical pathology / Thomas V. Colby . . . [et al.].
p. cm.
ISBN 0-7216-2893-1
1. Respiratory organs—Histopathology—Atlases. 2. Pathology, Surgical—Atlases. I. Colby, Thomas V.
[DNLM: 1. Lung Diseases—pathology—atlases. 2. Pathology, Surgical—atlases. WF 17 A881]
RC711.A85 1991
616.2′00471—dc20
DNLM/DLC 90-8652

Editor: Jennifer Mitchell
Designer: W. B. Saunders Staff
Production Manager: Carolyn Naylor
Manuscript Editor: Joan Powers
Illustration Coordinator: Peg Shaw
Indexer: Kathy Garcia

ATLAS OF PULMONARY SURGICAL PATHOLOGY ISBN 0-7216-2893-1

Printed in the United States of America

Last digit is the print number: 9 8 7 6 5 4 3 2 1

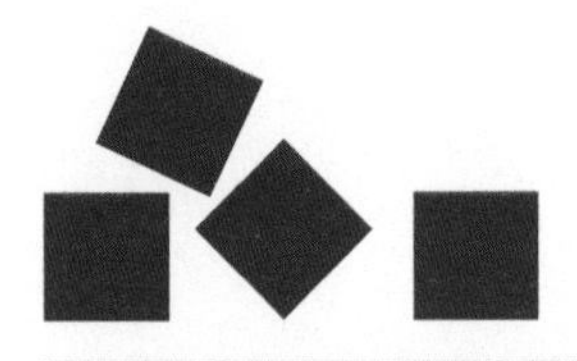

ACKNOWLEDGMENTS

The authors gratefully acknowledge Dr. M. Joseph, Dr. J. Austenfeld, and P. Colby for comments and critique.

IN MEMORIAM

Charles B. Carrington, M.D.

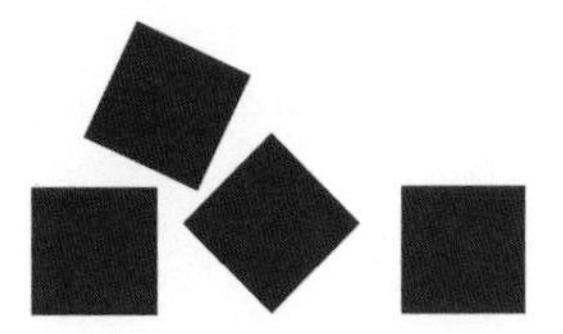

PREFACE

This book is an atlas intended as a practical "cookbook" for the surgical pathologist facing lung diseases and is based primarily on routine histologic interpretation. The accompanying text is abbreviated but is practically oriented. The majority of lung diseases, particularly non-neoplastic ones, can be recognized without special studies, such as electron microscopy and immunoperoxidase staining. This book is by no means encyclopedic, and only a minimal number of references are supplied. It is oriented primarily toward adult pulmonary disease.

Most medical texts are organized on the basis of diagnosis or specific lesions, and readers need to know what they are looking for before they can find it. We have tried to base the approach in this atlas on dominant histologic findings and the differential diagnoses that can be generated from them. The lesions discussed include those encountered by the surgical pathologist.

There are a number of terms used throughout the book that are common in pulmonary pathology. These are defined in the glossary of histologic terms that follows. Common entities, particularly carcinomas, are not extensively illustrated; however, the problem areas, the rarer tumors, and the spectrum of changes seen in various lesions are shown.

How should you use this book? We recommend thumbing through from start to finish to see what is included and then to appreciate the lists of differential diagnoses found in Chapter 1 and in the appendices located at the end of the book. Lesions are approached from several points of view: localized versus diffuse, acute versus subacute or chronic, and by histologic distribution and cellular components. The differential diagnoses listed include those that are "possible" as well as those that are "probable," and there is a deliberate intent to have overlap among the differential diagnosis groupings. Chapters 2 through 9 constitute an atlas of surgical pathology of the lung, including the lesions referred to in the first chapter and the appendices. Once you have narrowed the differential diagnosis, you may choose to follow up with the references listed in Chapters 2 to 9. General references that we think are useful as well as specific references are supplied.

The general references that we find useful include the following:

1. Carter D, Eggleston JC. Tumors of the lower respiratory tract. AFIP Atlas of Tumor Pathology, Second Series. Fascicle 17. Washington, DC, Armed Forces Institute of Pathology, 1980.
2. Churg A, Green FHY. Pathology of Occupational Lung Disease. New York, Igaku-Shoin, 1988.
3. Dail DH, Hammer SP (eds). Pulmonary Pathology. New York, Springer-Verlag, 1988.

4. Flint A, Colby TV. Surgical Pathology of Diffuse Infiltrative Lung Disease. Orlando, Fla., Grune & Stratton, 1987.
5. Katzenstein ALA, Askin FB. Surgical Pathology of Non-Neoplastic Lung Disease. 2nd ed. Philadelphia, WB Saunders Co, 1990.
6. Mark EJ. Lung Biopsy Interpretation. Baltimore, Williams & Wilkins, 1984.
7. Thurlbeck WM (ed). Pathology of the Lung. New York, Thieme, 1988.
8. World Health Organization Monograph: Histologic Typing of Lung Tumors. 2nd ed. WHO, Geneva, 1981.

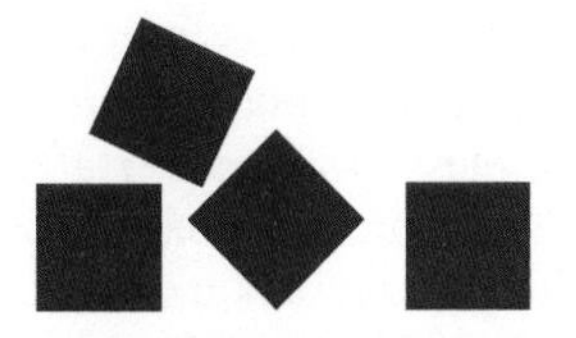

GLOSSARY OF HISTOLOGIC TERMS

The following terms are used widely in this book. In the past, they have been used in a number of different ways, and this glossary offers our functional definitions.

Acinus ■ The functional unit of the lung: a respiratory bronchiole and its supplied alveolar ducts and alveolar sacs. (*Note:* The definition of "acinus" varies somewhat in the literature.)

Angiocentric ■ A descriptive term for lesions that appear to center on vessels. *Angiocentricity* may be appreciated with lesions that are actually centered on vessels (either arteries or veins) or with lesions that are distributed around the vessels and which may or may not secondarily infiltrate the vessels. *Angiocentric* should be distinguished from *angiotropic,* which describes intravascular lymphomatosis (angiotropic lymphoma) as well as any lesion prone to *intraluminal* invasion of a vessel.

Asbestos Body ■ A ferruginous body with an asbestos (thin translucent) core.

Bronchiolitis Obliterans ■ A *histologic* term referring to two broad groups of lesions: *proliferative bronchiolitis obliterans* with granulation tissue polyps filling small airways, and *fibrotic bronchiolitis obliterans* with permanent scarring and stenosis or obliteration of airways. Proliferative bronchiolitis obliterans is often associated with organizing pneumonia in which the same reparative reaction that is present in the bronchiole and extends out into more distal parenchyma. Histologic bronchiolitis obliterans may or may not be associated with clinical evidence of airway obstruction. These two groups of bronchiolitis obliterans are discussed in more detail in the section on small airways disease.

Capillaritis ■ Mural inflammation (vasculitis) of the capillaries analogous to leukocytoclastic vasculitis at other sites.

Cellular Bronchiolitis ■ Cellular infiltrates, either acute or chronic, that involve bronchioles and that are usually mural, although a luminal acute inflammatory exudate is frequently present.

Diffuse Alveolar Damage (DAD) ■ A nonspecific acute response to lung injury, primarily affecting alveoli and alveolar walls. DAD includes both acute injury *and* repair phases and is specifically discussed in the text (p. 227). DAD is the usual histologic correlate of the adult respiratory distress syndrome (ARDS).

Exudate ■ Cells, cellular debris, and/or fibrin (with or without edema fluid) within airspaces.

Ferruginous Body ■ Particulate material covered by hemosiderin, highlighted by iron (Prussian blue) stains. A subset of ferruginous bodies are asbestos bodies that usually have a beaded surface, club-shaped ends, and a central thin translucent core; the last feature is diagnostic of an asbestos body.

Follicular Bronchitis/Bronchiolitis ■ Lymphoid hyperplasia with germinal center formation along airways.

Honeycombing ■ An end-stage lesion seen with many pulmonary injuries, usually chronic interstitial pneumonias. The lung architecture is permanently reorganized into functionally useless tissue (see p. 272).

Hyaline Membranes ■ Dense eosinophilic membranes seen in a number of acute lung diseases, usually diffuse alveolar damage. Hyaline membranes are most prominent in and along the surfaces of alveolar ducts. Hyaline membranes are composed of fibrin, cell debris, hemorrhage, and proteinous material.

Interstitial Fibrosis ■ Interstitial thickening resulting from mature collagen deposition as contrasted to edematous new connective tissue in the interstitium and organization in airspaces.

Interstitial Infiltrate ■ An infiltrate of cells, regardless of type, in the interstitium. Usually the cells are mononuclear; however, interstitial infiltrates of neutrophils and eosinophils are also recognized.

Interstitium ■ Includes alveolar walls, interlobular septa, and connective tissue around bronchovascular structures.

Lambertosis ■ Bronchiolar epithelial metaplasia occurring in peribronchiolar regions of scarred bronchioles, presumably extending through Lambert's canals.

Lobule ■ The pulmonary lobule (sometimes called the secondary lobule) refers to an anatomic unit of lung parenchyma, 0.50 to 2.00 cm in diameter, bounded by interlobular septa. Lobules can be appreciated on cut section of lung tissue and on the pleural surface, and they usually comprise some ten to 30 acini.

Lymphatic Distribution ■ A low-power distribution appreciated in a number of diffuse lung diseases in which the pathologic changes are seen along the lymphatic routes: in the pleura, in the interlobular septa, and along bronchovascular bundles. The lymphatic vessels themselves are often not appreciated as such.

Lymphoid Hyperplasia ■ Lymphoid follicles containing germinal centers, usually found in a lymphatic distribution.

Miliary Distribution ■ Lesions (usually small nodules) appear randomly scattered throughout the lung. Sometimes they may appear perivenular in distribution. Miliary nodules are characteristic of hematogenous granulomatous infections and some viral infections.

Obstructive Pneumonia ■ Changes seen in the lung parenchyma distal to an obstruction, regardless of cause. This disorder typically includes accumulation of foamy macrophages within alveoli, inspissated mucus, prominent type II alveolar lining cells, mononuclear interstitial infiltrates, and, in some cases, organizing pneumonia.

Old Granuloma ■ A term for a nodule with fibrotic rim and necrotic center that is usually, but not always, the result of an old healed infectious granuloma. A palisaded histocytic rim around the necrosis may be present.

Organizing Pneumonia ■ A reparative reaction in the lung with organizing granulation tissue filling alveolar ducts and associated alveoli with only focal attachment to the interstitium where the proliferation originates. Proliferative bronchiolitis obliterans often accompanies this reaction. This type of reaction is associated with modest interstitial infiltrates and prominent type II alveolar lining cells, and it should be distinguished from interstitial fibrosis.

Peribronchiolar ■ A distribution of pathologic changes around small airways including the wall of bronchioles and the immediately adjacent alveoli.

Septal ■ Septal refers to the interlobular septa and structures in them, including veins, lymphatics, and connective tissue.

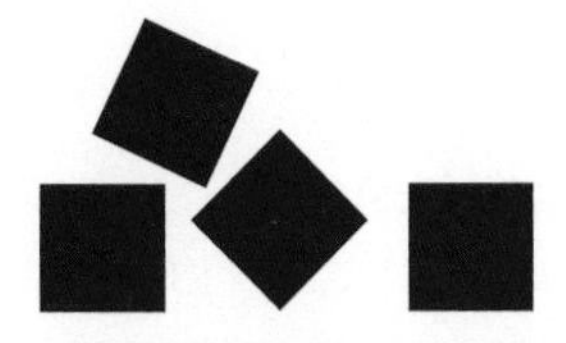

CONTENTS

CHAPTER 1

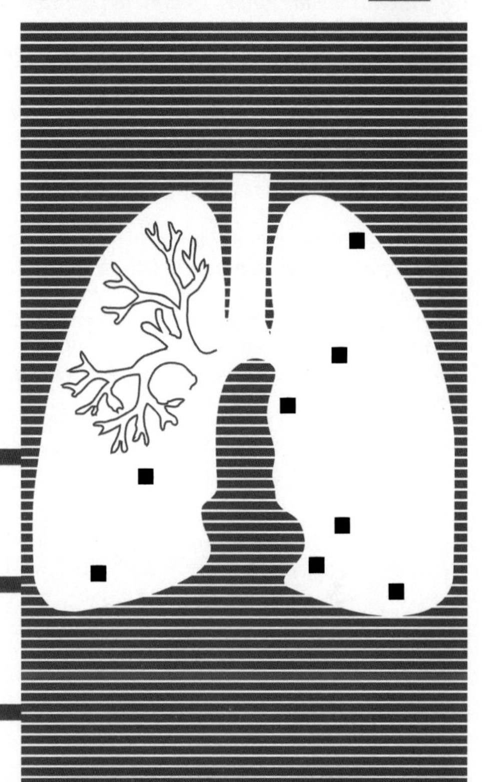

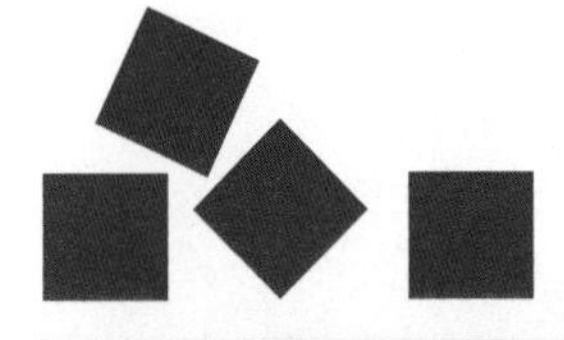

APPROACH TO LUNG BIOPSIES

Pattern recognition
Overview of differential diagnosis based on clinical/radiographic presentation and histologic patterns or components that are recognized
Miscellaneous histologic findings seen in lung biopsies and resection specimens
Considerations for biopsy specimens that appear histologically normal at first inspection
Biopsy in the setting of a normal chest radiograph
Bronchial and transbronchial biopsy
Approach to lung biopsies from immunosuppressed patients (with special reference to patients with AIDS and recipients of organ transplants)
Approach to lung biopsies in patients with collagen-vascular diseases
Histologic findings in pulmonary drug reactions
Histologic findings in patients known to have obstructive lung disease
Pulmonary histologic changes in patients with inflammatory bowel disease
Diagnostic considerations in patients with pulmonary renal syndromes

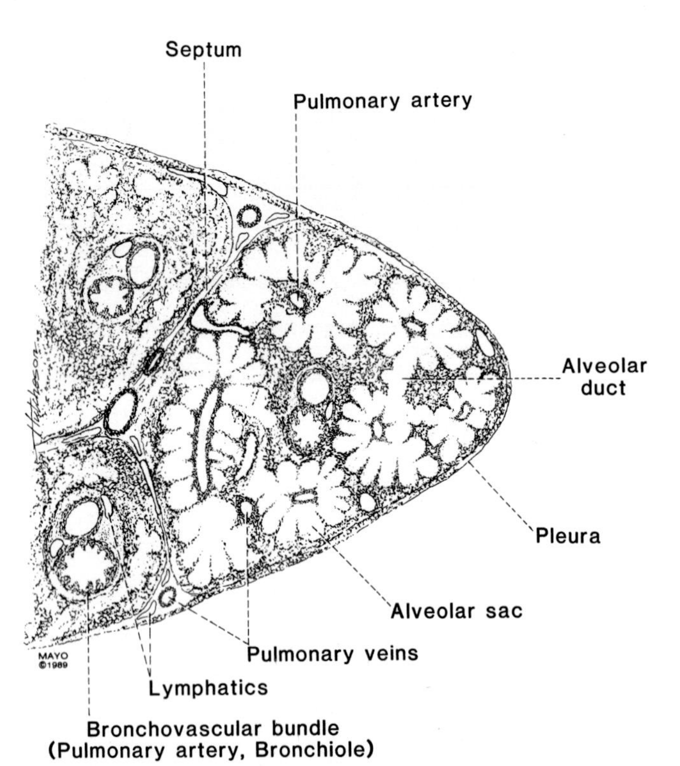

Figure 1–1. Lung biopsy. This schematic illustrates the anatomy of a lung biopsy. Portions of three lobules are bounded by interlobular septa, and within them bronchovascular structures, veins, and (in one) alveolar walls can be discerned. Veins and lymphatics can be seen in the pleura and septa, and a few small lymphatics are present along bronchovascular bundles. Respiratory bronchioles and alveolar ducts are not well shown in this diagram, since longitudinal sections are best suited to illustrate them and only cross sectioning is used in this schematic. Nevertheless, basic patterns of lung disease can all be shown with such a diagram.

■ PATTERN RECOGNITION

It is useful to try to define and categorize a distribution for a lesion (Fig. 1–1). This may not always be possible because the lesion may be obscured in atelectatic tissue or in a traumatized biopsy specimen, but it is worth attempting in virtually every case, particularly in diffuse

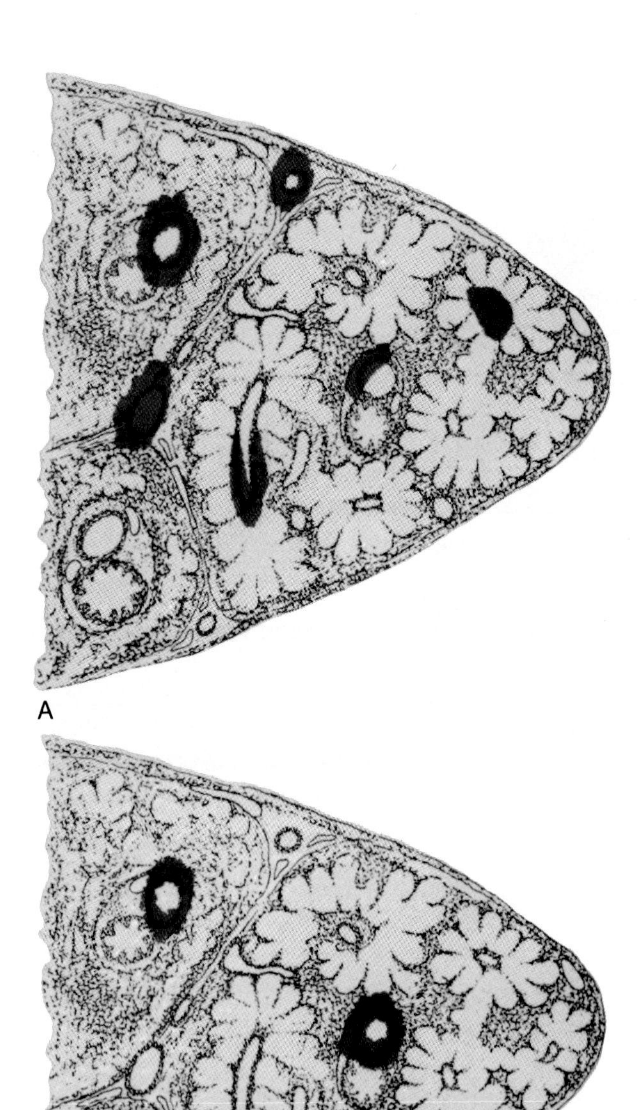

Figure 1–2. Angiocentricity. A lesion with a predisposition for involving vessels may involve (or partially involve) arteries or veins or both, and thus pleural, septal, and centrilobular or centriacinar structures may be affected, as shown in *A*. In some cases, there is a propensity to involve one type of vessel more than others, as illustrated by pulmonary arterial involvement in *B*.

lung disease. It is best accomplished by naked-eye and/or low-power assessment of the tissue sections; recollection of findings from the gross examination may be helpful.

Angiocentric–The lesion appears at low power to center on the vessels. Perivascular changes, vascular infiltration, and/or intraluminal changes are included (Fig. 1–2).

Bronchocentric/bronchiolocentric–The lesions show predilection for involving airways, including peribronchial or peribronchiolar changes, involvement of airway walls, or intraluminal changes (Fig. 1–3).

Pleural/subpleural–Any pleural change may be associated with some subpleural changes as well. Elastic tissue stains may be useful in some instances to define

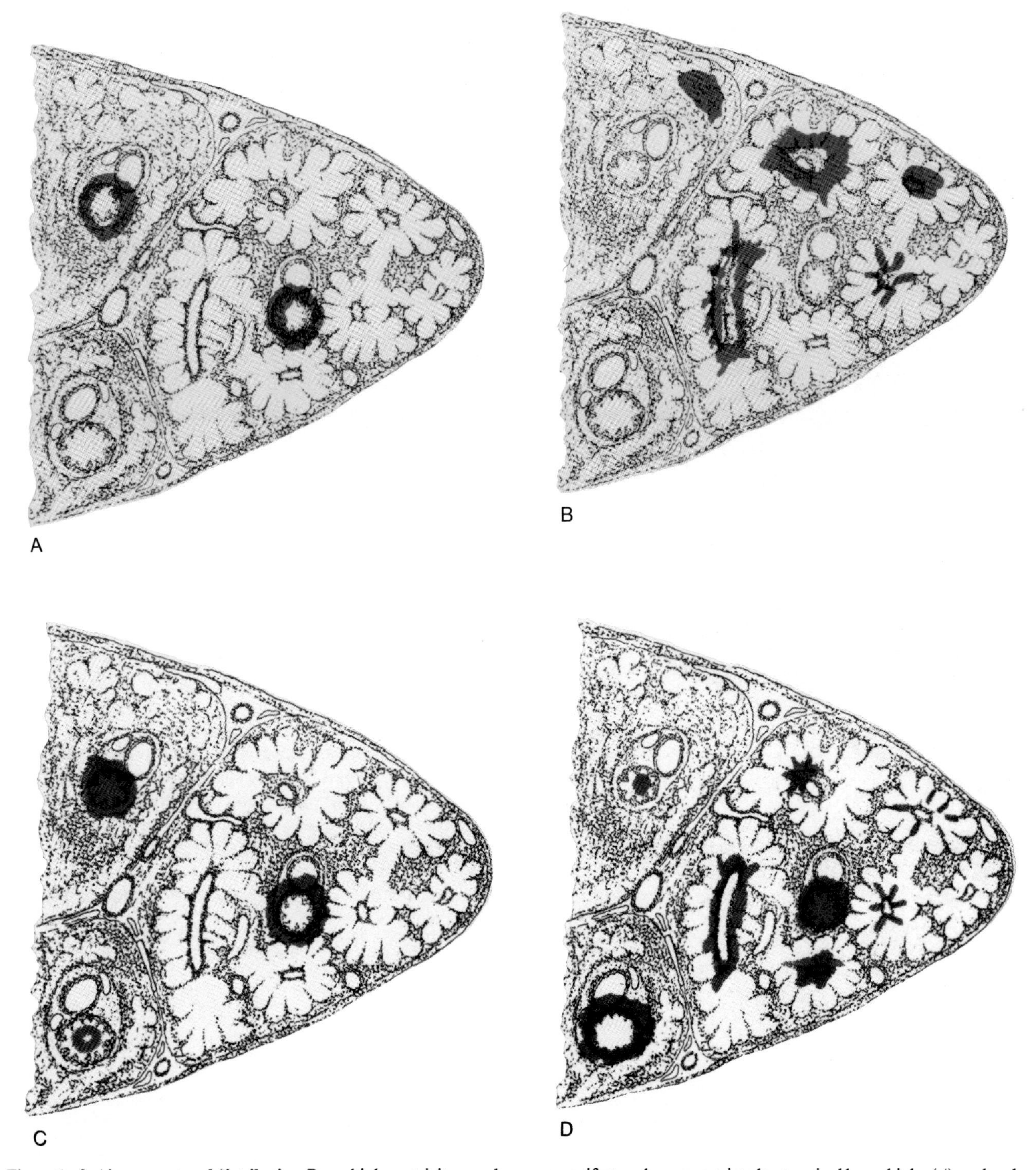

Figure 1–3. Airway-centered distribution. Bronchiolocentricity may become manifest as changes restricted to terminal bronchioles (*A*) or alveolar duct regions (*B*), may show mural and/or luminal changes (*C*), or may show mixtures of the patterns (*D*).

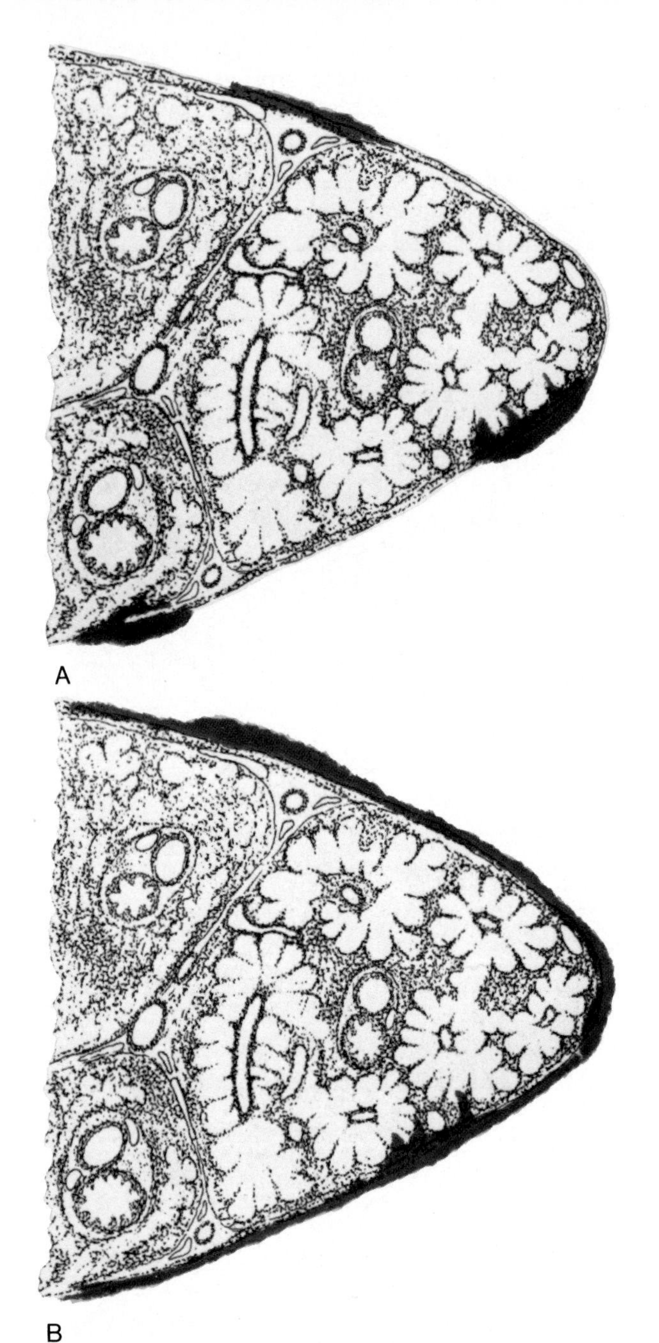

Figure 1–4. Pleural distribution. A lesion showing a pleural distribution may do so in a patchy (*A*) or diffuse (*B*) fashion.

the extent of change relative to the elastica of the visceral pleura. (Fig. 1–4).

Lymphatic distribution–The lymphatics of the lung are found in the pleura and septa and along the bronchovascular bundles (i.e., the lymphatic routes). A lesion showing a lymphatic distribution may show infiltrates and/or changes in any or all of these structures (Fig. 1–5).

Peripheral acinar–This is a somewhat subtle change to appreciate, since the periphery of the acinus includes paraseptal, subpleural, peribronchial, and peribronchiolar (membranous bronchioles and larger bronchioles) regions. Peripheral acinar changes are often the first changes noted in usual interstitial pneumonia (UIP) (idiopathic pulmonary fibrosis) (Fig. 1–6). This pattern correlates with the peripheral opacities apparent in a computed tomographic (CT) scan of the lung.

Septal changes–Lesions of the pulmonary veins and/or interlobular septa themselves may be included among these changes. A septal distribution is not often useful in forming a diagnosis (Fig. 1–7).

Random distribution–None of the previously listed patterns may be discerned, and distribution of lesions appears entirely random (Fig. 1–8).

Airspace consolidation–Diffuse filling of alveoli by cells, fluid, exudate, and/or granulation tissue (Fig. 1–9) may be apparent.

Diffuse interstitial infiltration–Interstitial infiltration is seen in many of the patterns previously listed, and one should try to subclassify this change into a more specific pattern, if possible (Fig. 1–10).

There is considerable overlap among these groups; a lymphatic distribution may appear pleural, angiocentric, bronchiolocentric, or even septal in distribution, since the lymphatics are found in all of these regions. Thus, in some cases of sarcoid, the granulomas may involve only one or two compartments in which the lymphatic routes are found. The peripheral lobular distribution, at first glance, may suggest septal or peribronchiolar distribution until one appreciates that these structures themselves are normal and that the abnormalities are actually in the immediately adjacent alveolar walls.

Text continued on page 9

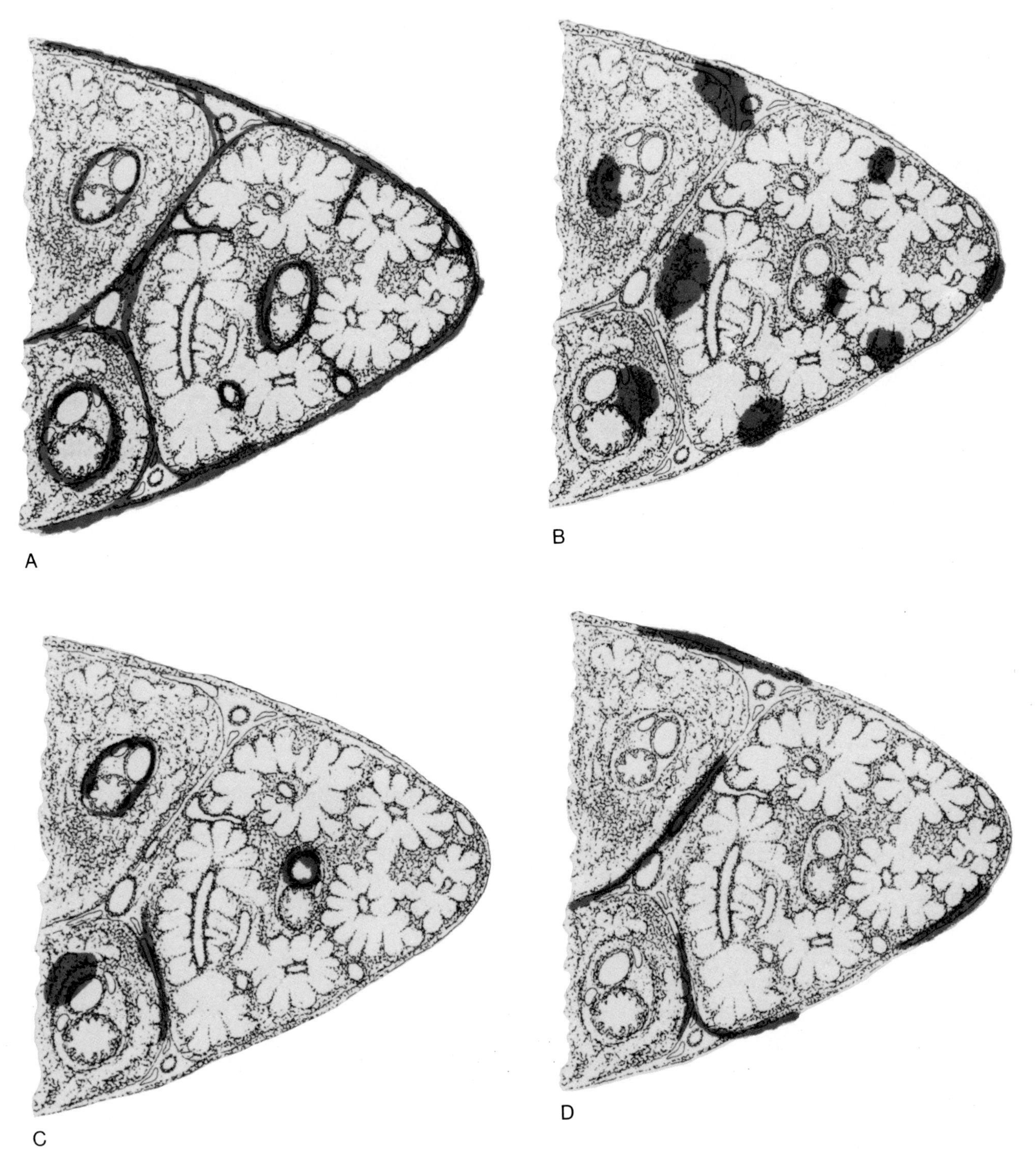

Figure 1–5. Lymphatic distribution. Representative patterns of lymphatic distribution. *A*, Diffuse uniform infiltrates involving the pleura and septa and bronchovascular structures. Such a pattern might be seen in leukemia. *B*, Multiple nodular infiltrates in the pleura and paraseptal regions and along bronchovascular structures. Such a distribution would be typical for sarcoidosis or lymphoma. *C*, A mixture of patterns, including focal septal infiltration, mural vascular involvement, infiltration around a bronchovascular structure, and a micronodular infiltrate adjacent to and involving a pulmonary artery. Such a distribution may be seen with lymphoma. *D*, Patchy infiltration of the pleura and septa. Such a pattern may be seen with lymphoma or leukemia.

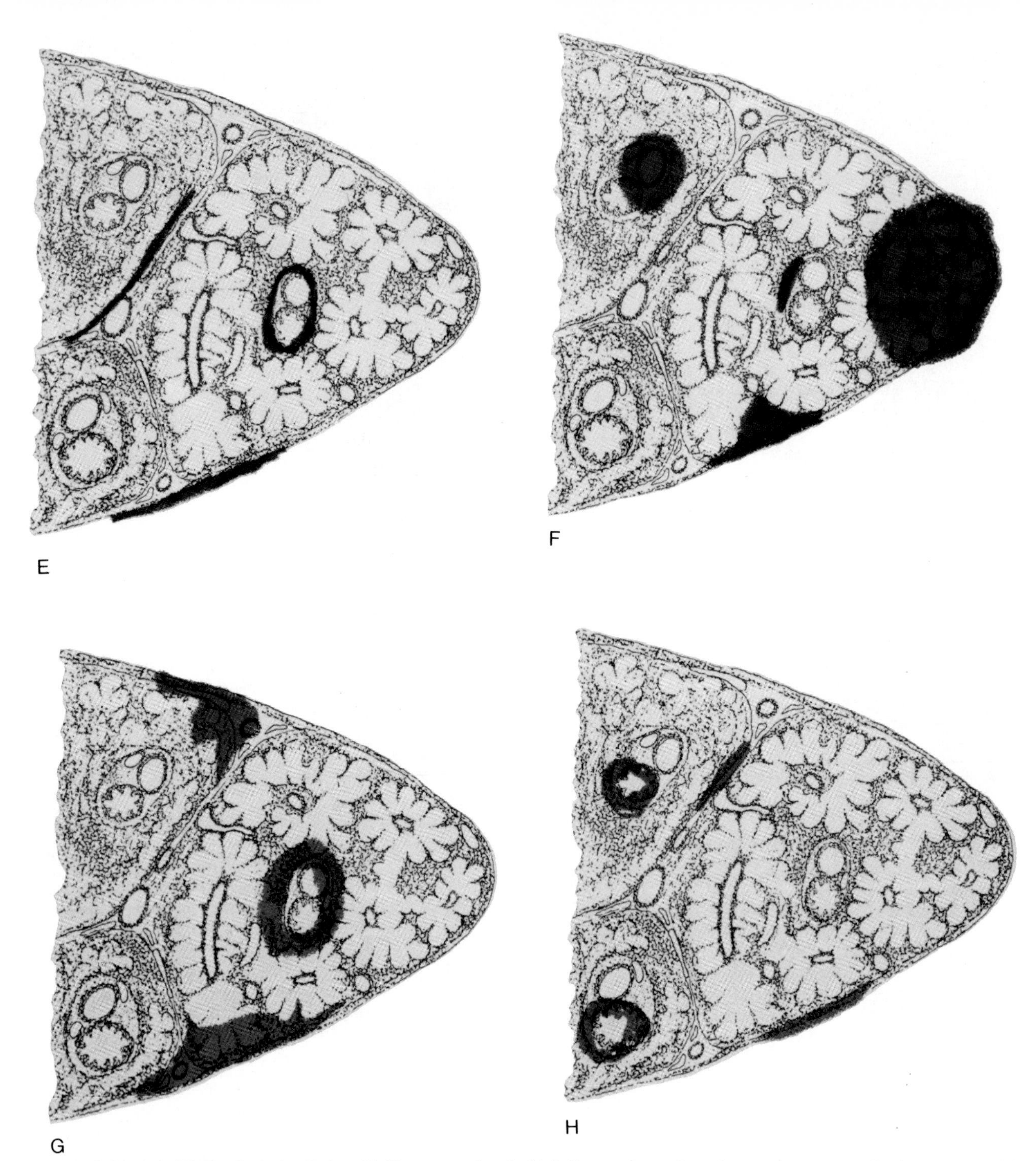

Figure 1–5 *Continued E*, Focal septal and pleural infiltrates associated with infiltrates along a bronchovascular structure. Such a pattern may be seen with lymphoma or leukemia. *F*, Micronodular and focal diffuse infiltrates involving bronchovascular structures and pleura with a large nodule in the pleura. Such a distribution would be typical of lymphoma or sarcoidosis. *G*, Focal dense pleural infiltrates extending along septa associated with an infiltration along one of the bronchovascular structures. Such a pattern is typical of lymphoma and some pneumoconioses. *H*, Peribronchiolar, focal septal, and pleural infiltrates. Such a pattern may be seen with sarcoidosis or lymphoma.

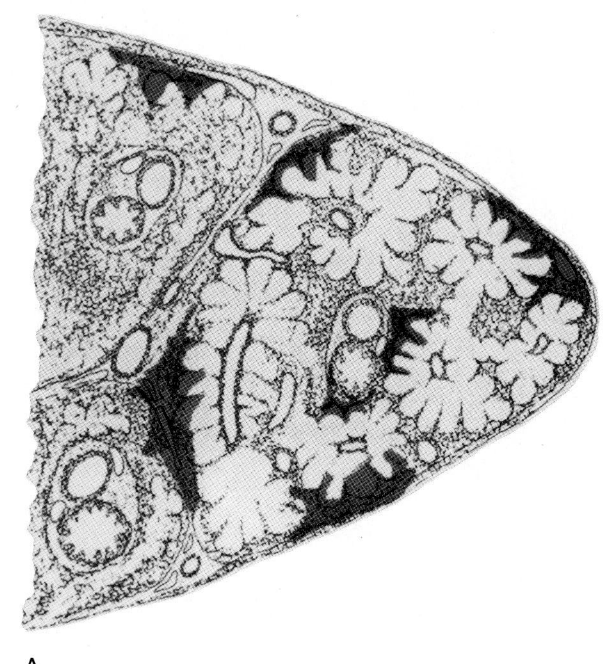

A

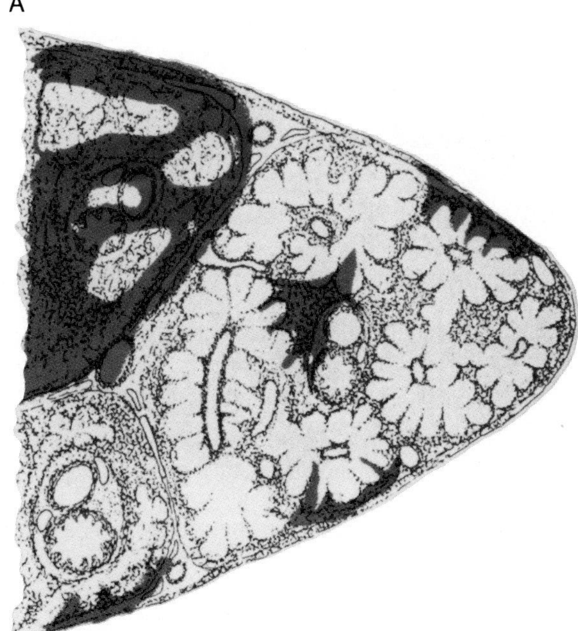

B

Figure 1–6. Peripheral acinar distribution. Irregular involvement of the periphery of acini appears in this diagram as changes in the subpleural, paraseptal, and peribronchiolar zones. The terminal bronchioles illustrated are at the periphery of more distal acini. In *B*, one of the lobules has been replaced by honeycombing. This appearance is characteristic of many cases of usual interstitial pneumonia either early (*A*) or somewhat later with honeycombing (*B*).

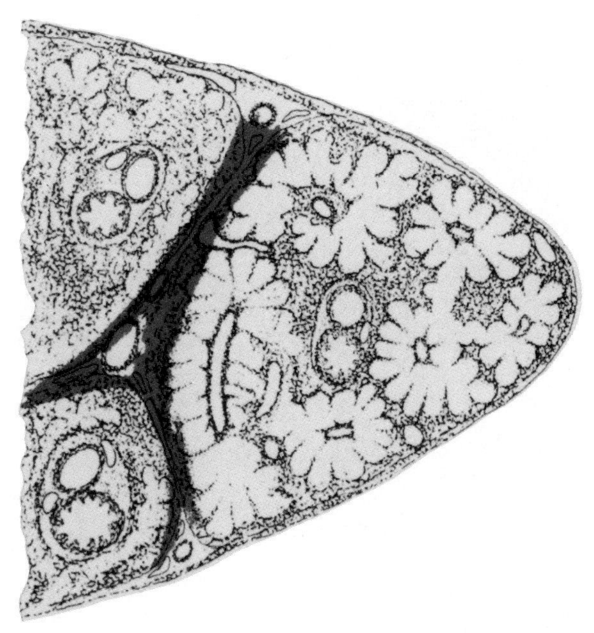

Figure 1–7. Septal distribution. Lesions restricted to the septa are unusual. Vascular changes associated with chronic passive congestion (e.g., heart disease or pulmonary veno-occlusive disease) are examples. Some lesions that are lymphatic in their distribution may mimic septal processes.

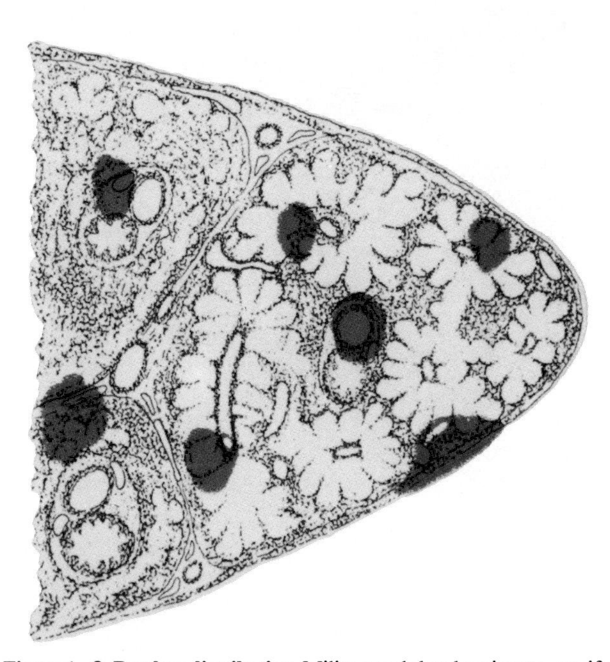

Figure 1–8. Random distribution. Miliary nodules showing no specific affinity for anatomic site are typical of miliary infections. Some miliary infections may show a predisposition for occurring in perivenular regions.

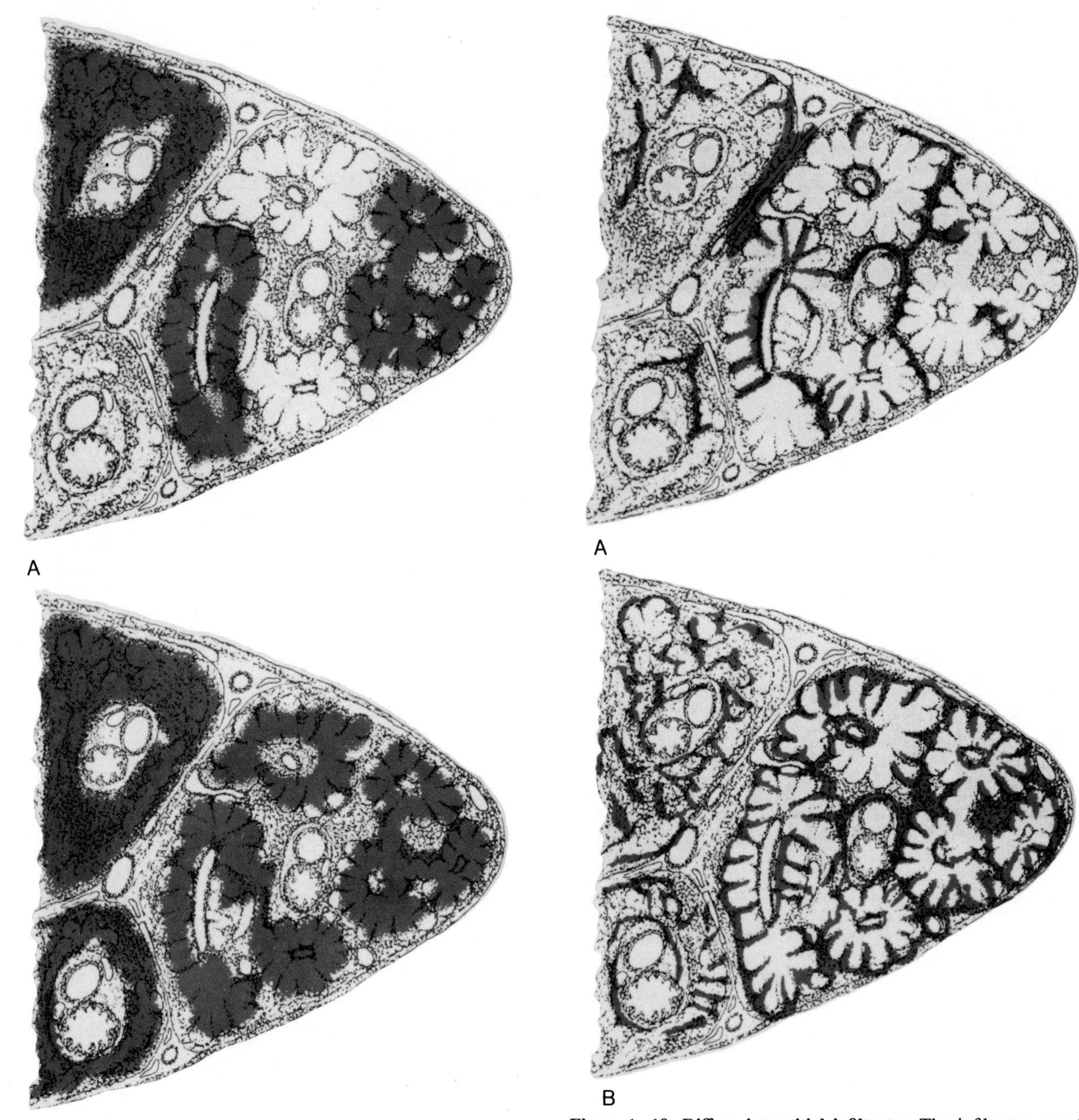

Figure 1–9. Consolidation. Parenchymal consolidation with filling of the airspaces may be patchy in distribution (*A*) or may involve all the alveoli in a given biopsy specimen (*B*). Airspace consolidation often stops abruptly at an interlobular septum.

Figure 1–10. Diffuse interstitial infiltrates. The infiltrates may be patchy (*A*) or diffuse (*B*) without any discernible distribution. When there is little fibrosis and marked infiltration by cells without an apparent distribution, lymphocytic interstitial pneumonia and extrinsic allergic alveolitis should be considered.

■ OVERVIEW OF DIFFERENTIAL DIAGNOSIS BASED ON CLINICAL/RADIOGRAPHIC PRESENTATION AND HISTOLOGIC PATTERNS OR COMPONENTS THAT ARE RECOGNIZED (See appendices for details)

I. Masses and Localized Lesions: Diagnostic Considerations (See Appendix I)
  A. Cysts/anomalies
  B. Lesions with prominent vascular components or vascularity
  C. Distribution
    1. Angiocentric or vasculitic
    2. Airway-centered (bronchocentric and bronchiolocentric)
    3. Pleural and subpleural lesions
  D. Cellular components
    1. Epithelial (epithelioid) masses
    2. Mesenchymal and/or spindle cell lesions
    3. Mixed epithelial and mesenchymal lesions or epithelioid and spindled lesions
    4. Neutrophils and necrosis
    5. Granulomatous inflammation with or without necrosis
    6. Eosinophilic infiltrates
    7. Lymphocytes and/or plasma cells (see also Lymphoid tissue)
    8. Histiocytes (with or without foamy cytoplasm), airspace or interstitial
    9. Lymphoid tissue
      a. Polymorphous in composition
      b. Monomorphous in composition
    10. Fibrosis and organizing pneumonia (with or without necrosis)

II. Diffuse and Multifocal Processes of Acute or Recent Onset: Diagnostic Considerations (See Appendix II)
  A. Distribution
    1. Angiocentric lesions
    2. Airway-centered (bronchocentric and bronchiolocentric) lesions
    3. Lymphatic distribution
    4. Miliary nodules
  B. Cellular or histologic components
    1. Interstitial and/or alveolar edema (with or without hyaline membranes)
    2. Alveolar hemorrhage and/or hemosiderin deposition (see definition of alveolar hemorrhage syndrome) with or without capillaritis
    3. Alveolar fibrinous exudate
    4. Acute neutrophilic inflammation (interstitial, perivascular, and/or within an airspace)
    5. Eosinophils (airspace, vascular, and/or interstitial)
    6. Interstitial chronic inflammatory infiltrate (relatively common, even in some clinically acute reactions; should not lead to a diagnosis of "chronic interstitial pneumonia")
    7. Granulomas and giant cells
    8. Extensive airspace organization or interstitial fibroblast proliferation

III. Diffuse and Multifocal Processes with Subacute or Chronic Clinical History: Diagnostic Considerations (See Appendix III)
  A. Distribution
    1. Angiocentricity, vasculitic
    2. Airway-centered (bronchocentric and bronchiolocentric) lesions
    3. Lymphatic distribution
    4. Pleural fibrosis, pleural inflammation (in patients with interstitial lung disease)
  B. Cellular or histologic components
    1. Fibrinous exudates or eosinophilic intra-alveolar material
    2. Chronic inflammatory infiltrate (lymphocytes and plasma cells with or without other inflammatory cells)
    3. Lymphoid hyperplasia and *dense* interstitial infiltrate
    4. Histiocytes (airspace or interstitial with or without "foamy" change)
    5. Hemosiderin-filled macrophages
    6. Eosinophil infiltrates
    7. Granulomas with or without necrosis
    8. Giant cells (singly or in clusters)
    9. Organizing pneumonia (proliferative bronchiolitis obliterans often present)
    10. Interstitial fibrosis (with or without honeycombing)
    11. Nodular fibrosis
    12. Smooth muscle proliferation

IV. Biopsy Specimens from Immunosuppressed Patients: Selected Diagnostic Considerations (See Appendix IV)
  A. Apparently normal lung biopsy
  B. Diffuse alveolar damage (DAD)
  C. Nodular lesions
  D. Pulmonary alveolar proteinosis-like reactions
  E. Capillaritis
  F. Neutrophilic infiltrates
  G. Histiocytic infiltrates
  H. Pulmonary hemorrhage

■ MISCELLANEOUS HISTOLOGIC FINDINGS SEEN IN LUNG BIOPSIES AND RESECTION SPECIMENS

■ Artifacts

1. Crush, atelectasis, "emphysema" from aggressive specimen inflation, pseudolipoid change with fat-like vacuoles in alveoli
2. Traumatic hemorrhage and neutrophilic margination in vessels
3. Septal edema, dilation of lymphatics from surgical clamping of vessels
4. Postprocedural changes, including airway inflammation, dislodged epithelium, needle tracts
5. Pleural talc, cotton fibers, gelatin sponge (Gelfoam)

■ Normal Variations and Common Nonspecific Findings

1. Intrapulmonary lymph nodes
2. Apical fibrous caps
3. Pleural fat and prominent vessels in areas of visceral pleural scarring
4. Vascular sclerosis, thickening, and obliteration in a scarred lung
5. Focal scarring and inflammation at the tips of lobes (especially right middle lobe)
6. Upper lobe emphysema in smokers and the elderly
7. Age-related changes including: hyaline medial and intimal thickening in arteries and veins, senile vascular amyloid, ossified bronchial cartilages, bronchial submucosal elastosis
8. Anthracosis along lymphatic routes

■ Histologic Changes Seen in Smokers

1. Large airway changes: mucous gland hypertrophy, goblet cell metaplasia, basement membrane thickening, mild submucosal inflammation
2. Small airway changes: goblet cell metaplasia, mucostasis, mural thickening, and smoker's bronchiolitis with inflammation, septal thickening, and accumulations of alveolar macrophages that are often positive with iron stains and contain small dark flecks of debris
3. Emphysema (especially upper lobe centriacinar)
4. Anthracosis

■ Calcification and/or Bone Formation

1. Amyloid with secondary calcification and ossification
2. Tracheobronchopathia osteoplastica
3. Dystrophic calcification and ossification in scarred foci
4. Metastatic calcification
5. Pulmonary alveolar microlithiasis
6. Chronic passive congestion with metaplastic bone in alveolar spaces
7. Calcified structures: Schaumann's bodies, calcium oxalate, blue bodies, psammoma bodies
8. Broncholiths (often as calcified debris within an abscess if aspirated)
9. Ossified bronchial cartilages

Any lesion with metaplastic bone may also develop bone marrow

■ Pulmonary Hemosiderin Deposition

1. Recent and old pulmonary hemorrhage
2. Incidental finding in smokers
3. Asbestosis and other pneumoconioses
4. Vascular disease and chronic passive congestion
5. Infarct
6. Hemorrhagic pneumonias
7. Miscellaneous inflammatory conditions

■ Pulmonary Vascular Thrombi and Emboli

1. Pulmonary emboli and thromboemboli, including incidental bone marrow emboli
2. Pulmonary hypertension with cor pulmonale and secondary emboli and/or thromboses
3. Veno-occlusive disease with pulmonary venous thrombosis
4. Tumor emboli with inconspicuous tumor cells
5. Any severe acute diffuse lung disease with secondary thrombi (a common incidental finding)
6. Postpulmonary causes of passive congestion (cardiac, pericardial)

■ Polarizable Material

1. Incidental silicates and silica associated with anthracotic pigment
2. Pneumoconioses (e.g., talcosis, silicosis, silicatoses)
3. Schaumann's bodies and oxalate crystals associated with granulomatous inflammation
4. Oxalate crystals associated with *Aspergillus* organisms
5. Intravenous talcosis (IV drug abuse)
6. Artifacts: formalin pigment, surgical glove talc
7. Collagen
8. Amyloid
9. Contaminant that is not part of the tissue

Most polarizable material in surgical lung biopsy specimens is incidental and of no clinical significance; some examples include either Schaumann's bodies or oxalate crystals associated with granulomatous conditions or a small amount of silicates associated with anthracotic pigment. Silica is seen as short stubby particles less birefringent than collagen. Silicates are more birefringent than collagen and are commonly confused with silica. Asbestos is not birefringent.

■ Miscellaneous Features That Are Often Incidental Findings

1. Bronchial cartilage ossification (with or without marrow)
2. Carcinoid tumorlets
3. Minute pulmonary chemodectomas
4. Nonspecific old scars and healed granulomas
5. Focal smooth muscle nodules associated with small airways
6. Hamartomas
7. Blue bodies
8. Schaumann's bodies
9. Corpora amylacea
10. Asteroid bodies
11. Ferruginous bodies
12. Cholesterol clefts
13. Calcium oxalate crystals
14. Anthracosis
15. Silicates
16. Silica
17. Hemosiderin encrustation of elastic fibers (chronic congestion)
18. Occasional granuloma or giant cell
19. Hyaline (resembling Mallory's hyaline) in alveolar lining cells
20. Dystrophic calcification
21. Dystrophic ossification and heterotopic bone
22. Megakaryocytes in capillaries
23. Hamazaki-Wesenberg bodies in hilar lymph nodes

References

Colby TV, Yousem SA. Pulmonary histology for the surgical pathologist. Am J Surg Pathol 12:223–239, 1988.

■ CONSIDERATIONS FOR BIOPSY SPECIMENS THAT APPEAR HISTOLOGICALLY NORMAL AT FIRST INSPECTION

Pathologists are occasionally faced with a biopsy specimen that looks normal even though they know that lung disease is supposed to be present; usually careful reinspection and paying particular attention to the lesions listed below reveal pathologic changes.

■ Vascular Disease

1. Pulmonary hypertension
2. Pulmonary emboli, *including* fat emboli
3. Pulmonary edema and congestion
4. Intravascular carcinomatosis

Fat emboli may be exceedingly subtle and, consequently, can be missed unless one looks specifically for them. Edema fluid commonly washes out during processing; one clue is to look for widened interlobular septa containing dilated lymphatics.

■ Small Airway Injury and Inflammation

1. Asthma
2. Chronic obstructive pulmonary disease (emphysema and chronic bronchitis)
3. Bronchiectasis
4. Idiopathic small airways injury
5. Bronchiolitis obliterans with airflow obstruction in collagen-vascular diseases and transplant recipients
6. Mucous plugging
7. Acute aspiration

The changes in airways may be extremely subtle, and in patients with idiopathic small airway injury, there may be no history indicative of the injury, as there often is in patients with asthma or chronic obstructive pulmonary disease. Subtle clues should be sought, including bronchioles that appear smaller than their accompanying artery, mural thickening of bronchioles, mucostasis in bronchioles, ectatic bronchioles, stenotic bronchioles, and frankly obliterated bronchioles. Elastic tissue staining is sometimes helpful in finding and assessing these airway changes.

■ Interstitial Diseases

Some interstitial disease can be quite subtle, especially very early diffuse alveolar damage with only mild interstitial edema and foci of hyaline membranes.

■ Pleural Disease

Severe visceral pleural fibrosis can be as functionally significant as severe interstitial lung disease with honeycombing. Pleural fibrosis, which one might otherwise think was an incidental finding, may sometimes prove significant if no underlying parenchymal lesion is found.

■ Sampling Error

Sampling error may occur with sarcoid and eosinophilic granuloma as well as with other conditions associated with scattered lesions in the lung parenchyma. Bronchioloalveolar carcinomas and other mucinous carcinomas are sometimes missed, even with a large biopsy specimen. Mucus pooling that might otherwise be overlooked may be the only clue to the presence of adjacent carcinoma. In the case of eosinophilic granuloma, sometimes the lesions that are sampled are old and fibrotic, and active lesions are not seen in the specimen. In the right clinical setting, a diagnosis of "patchy scars consistent with healed eosinophilic granuloma" may be appropriate.

References

Colby TV, Yousem SA. Pulmonary histology for the surgical pathologist. Am J Surg Pathol 12:223–239, 1988.

■ BIOPSY IN THE SETTING OF A NORMAL CHEST RADIOGRAPH

■ Localized Lesion(s)

This group includes many benign and malignant tumors, and the lesions are often endobronchial and/or in the hilar region. Endobronchial carcinoids are notorious examples, but metastases, lymphomas, and many other primary tumors may be associated with a normal chest radiograph.

■ Diffuse Pulmonary Conditions that May Present with a Normal Chest Radiograph

Pulmonary Vascular Disease

1. Primary pulmonary hypertension (plexogenic arteriopathy, pulmonary veno-occlusive disease, chronic thromboembolic disease, pulmonary capillary hemangiomatosis)
2. Pulmonary vascular disease secondary to cardiac disease (e.g., silent mitral stenosis)
3. Intravascular carcinomatosis
4. Thromboembolic disease

Diseases of Small Airways

1. Asthma
2. Postinfectious small airways disease with constrictive bronchiolitis
3. Chronic obstructive pulmonary disease with chronic bronchitis, bronchiolitis, and/or emphysema
4. Respiratory bronchiolitis-associated interstitial lung disease
5. Idiopathic small airway injury

Interstitial Lung Disease

A number of interstitial lung diseases may occasionally be associated with a normal chest radiograph. Sarcoidosis is probably the most common, but a normal chest radiograph may also be seen with UIP, desquamative interstitial pneumonia (DIP), eosinophilic granuloma, extrinsic allergic alveolitis, lymphangioleiomyomatosis, and others.

References

Colby TV, Yousem SA. Pulmonary histology for the surgical pathologist. Am J Surg Pathol 12:233–239, 1988.

■ BRONCHIAL AND TRANSBRONCHIAL BIOPSY (Figs. 1–11 to 1–22)

Tissue obtained by bronchoscopic biopsy is small and may include bronchial wall or peribronchial lung parenchyma; crush artifact is often present. Because of the size of the biopsy, there is always an inherent sampling error that must be considered and reckoned with. Tissue obtained in this fashion is sufficient for electron microscopy, immunofluorescence studies, touch preparations, and immunologic marker studies either on fresh, frozen, or paraffin-fixed sections.

One can broadly group the diagnostic categories of tissue from bronchioscopic biopsies into (1) those with specific histologic features such as tumors, infections, and lymphangioleiomyomatosis; (2) those in which the changes are characteristic such as sarcoid and eosinophilic pneumonia; and (3) those in which the findings are entirely nonspecific.

Changes that should be considered nonspecific include interstitial infiltrates of inflammatory cells, fibrosis, prominence of type II alveolar lining cells, airspace organization, obstruction, and inflammation in the bronchial wall. Particularly in smokers, the peribronchial tissue may show a number of nonspecific changes that are totally unrelated to other clinically significant processes that were not sampled.

Transbronchial biopsy is extremely useful in localized lesions, especially tumors, and often yields a specific diagnosis. When crush artifact is a problem, as it often is in small cell undifferentiated carcinoma, correlation with concurrent cytologic preparations may help in rendering a diagnosis.

Specific diagnosis is considerably less frequent in diffuse lung diseases than in localized lesions; nonspecific findings are especially common in chronic diffuse lung disease. In acute diffuse lung disease, particularly in immunosuppressed patients, the diagnostic yield may be quite good for infections and approaches 90 to 95 percent in patients with acquired immunodeficiency syndrome (AIDS). The usefulness of transbronchial lung biopsy in immunosuppressed patients is increased by concomitant bronchoalveolar lavage.

References

Thurlbeck, WM (ed). Pathology of the Lung. New York, Thieme, 1988.

Wall CP, Gaensler EA, Carrington CB, Hayes JA. Comparison of transbronchial and open biopsies in chronic infiltrative lung disease. Am Rev Respir Dis 123:280–285, 1981.

Text continued on page 17

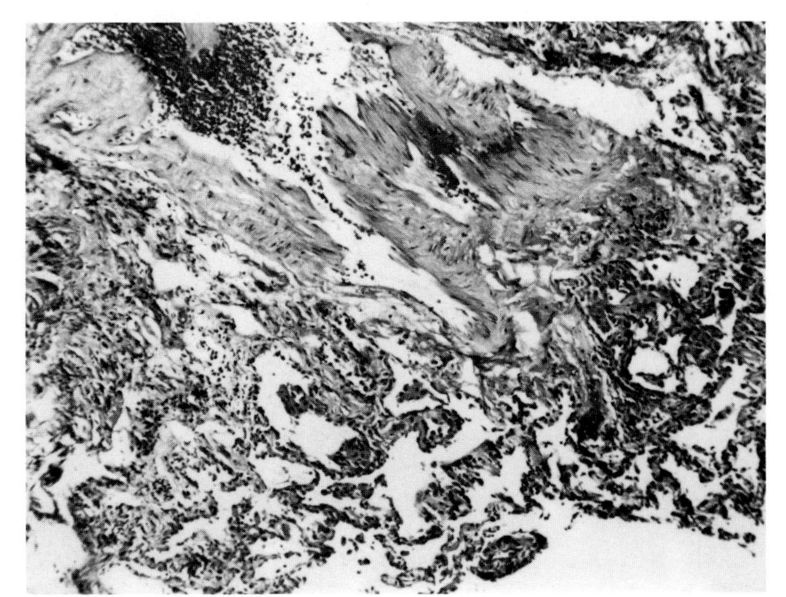

Figure 1 – 11. Nondiagnostic transbronchial biopsy specimen. The lung tissue is clearly abnormal with interstitial inflammation and mild fibrosis. The pattern is entirely nonspecific, and no diagnosis can be made from this biopsy specimen. The patient kept birds and was clinically thought to have hypersensitivity pneumonitis. There is nothing in the biopsy findings to suggest that dignosis.

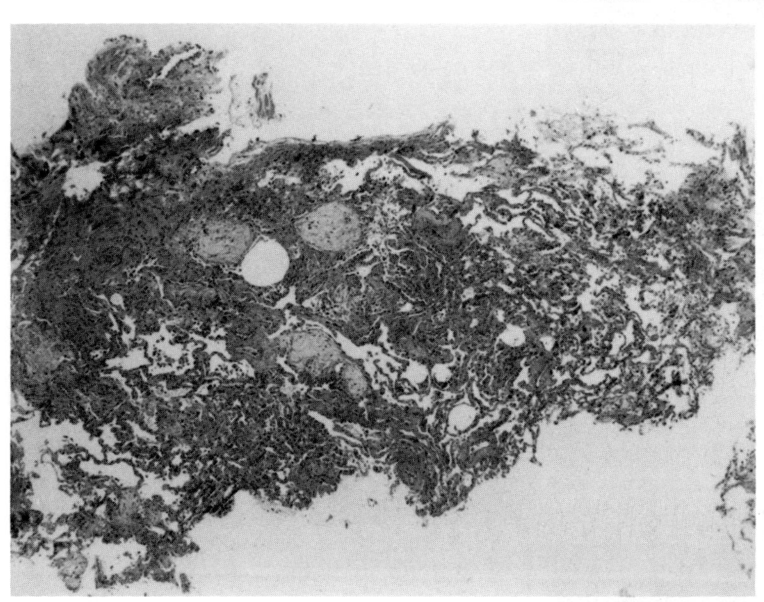

Figure 1 – 12. Nondiagnostic transbronchial biopsy specimen. Findings are consistent with the diagnosis of bronchiolitis obliterans organizing pneumonia (BOOP). The patient had signs, symptoms, and a clinical course typical of BOOP. This generous transbronchial biopsy specimen shows some pale tufts of organizing connective tissue within airspaces, and findings are consistent with the diagnosis of BOOP but not specific for it.

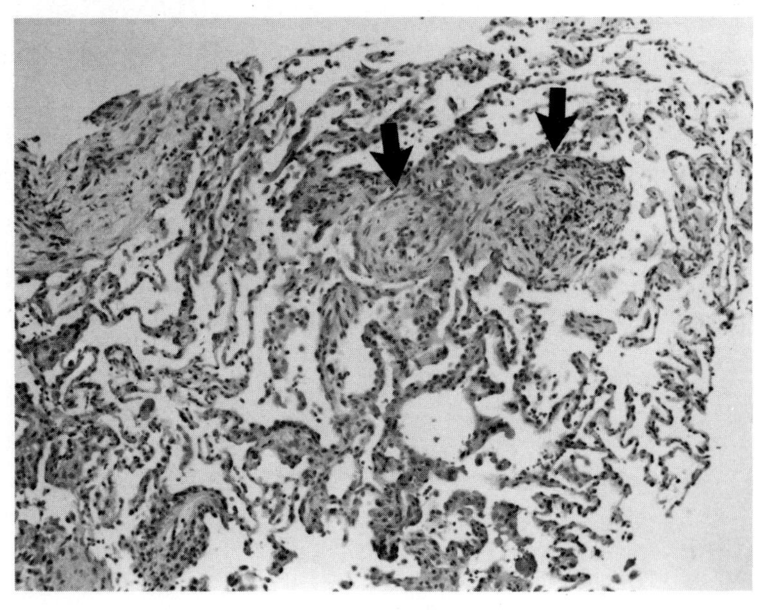

Figure 1 – 13. Nondiagnostic transbronchial biopsy specimen. This biopsy specimen shows considerable similarity to the one in Figure 1 – 12, with mild interstitial inflammation and rounded tufts of organizing connective tissue within airspaces (arrows). In this case, the features are nonspecific. The patient had a fulminant clinical course that was inconsistent with the diagnosis of BOOP. This biopsy should be considered abnormal but nonspecific.

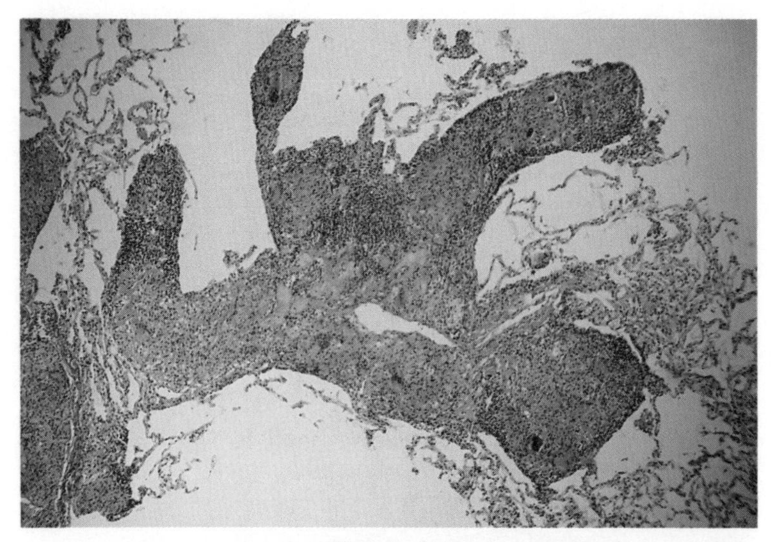

Figure 1-14.

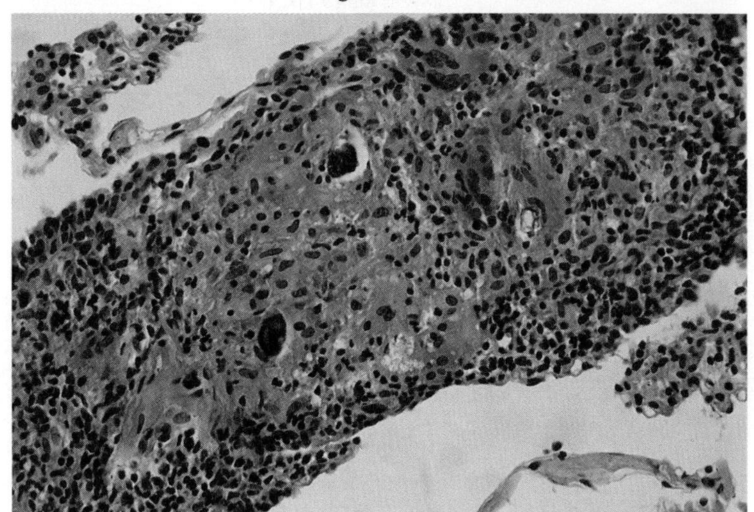

Figure 1-15.

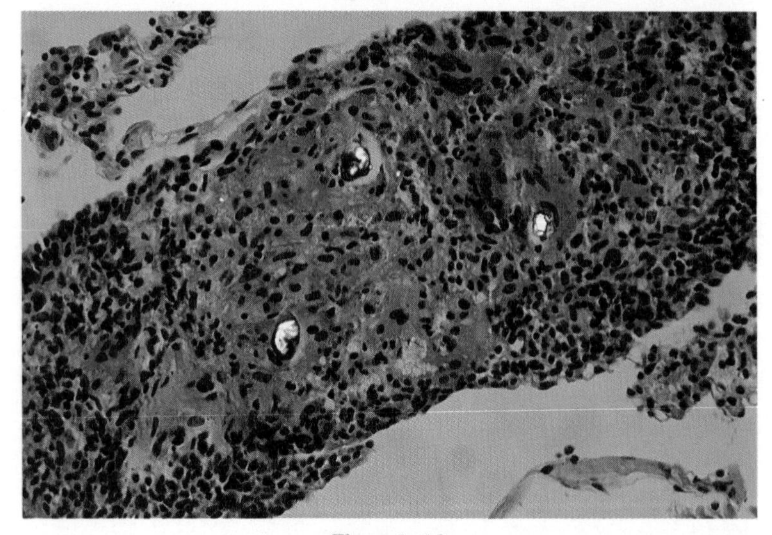

Figure 1-16.

Figures 1-14, 1-15, 1-16. Transbronchial biopsy findings consistent with a clinical diagnosis of sarcoidosis. Clinical and radiographic findings, were consistent with sarcoidosis. The specimen shows confluent non-necrotizing granulomas consistent with that clinical impression. Within some of the granulomas birefringent Schaumann's bodies and oxalate crystals are seen (Fig. 1-16). They should not be considered indicative of a foreign body granuloma.

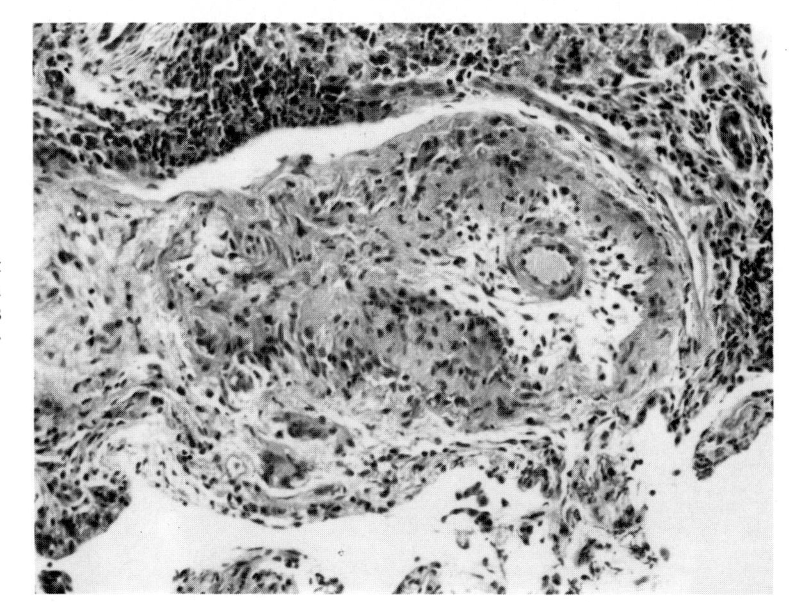

Figure 1–17. Transbronchial biopsy findings consistent with a clinical impression of sarcoidosis. The specimen shows granulomatous inflammation. The granulomatous involvement of the vessel, as illustrated here, is quite characteristic of sarcoidosis.

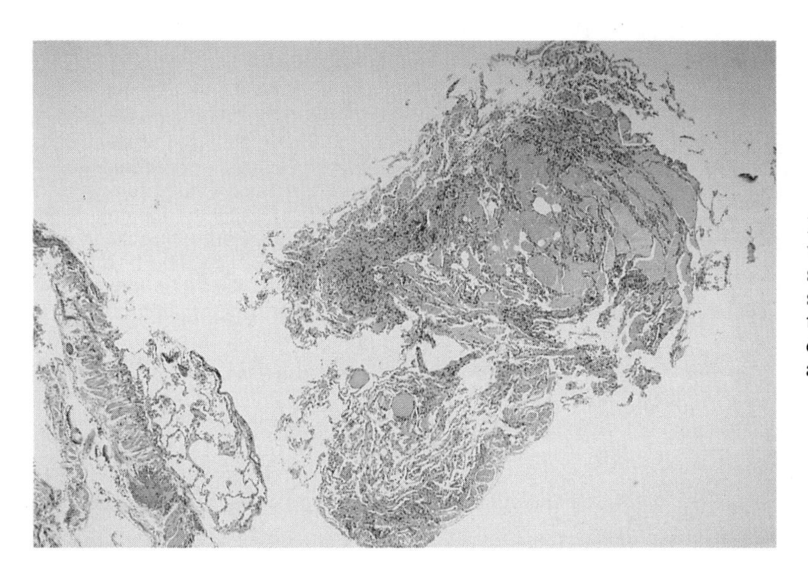

Figure 1–18. Transbronchial biopsy findings consistent with pulmonary alveolar proteinosis. The alveoli are stuffed by eosinophilic material, which on higher power showed the typical features of pulmonary alveolar proteinosis. Clinicopathologic correlation suggested that the diagnosis of pulmonary alveolar proteinosis was appropriate.

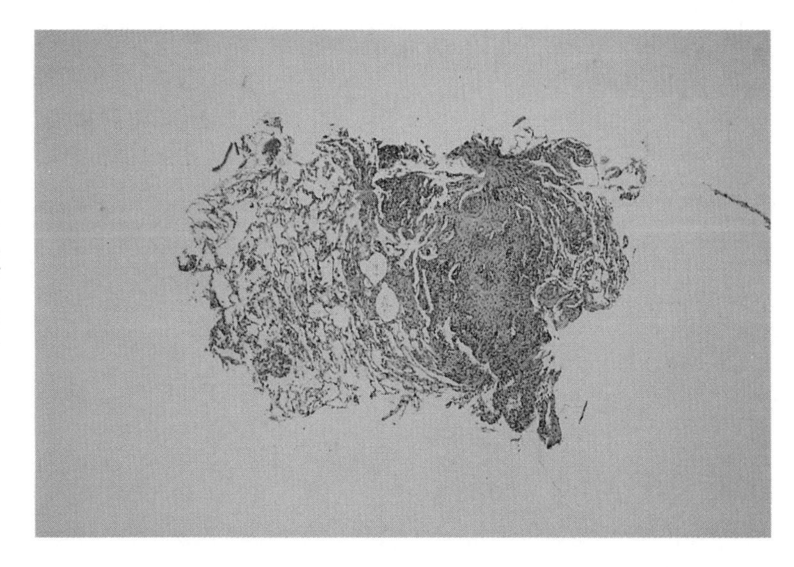

Figure 1–19. Eosinophilic granuloma. Eosinophilic granuloma is identified on a transbronchial biopsy specimen. A portion of a nodular lesion of eosinophilic granuloma is seen in this transbronchial biopsy fragment. Higher power confirmed the presence of Langerhans cells. When carefully sought, the lesions of eosinophilic granuloma can probably be identified in up to 20 percent of transbronchial biopsy specimens from patients with that disease.

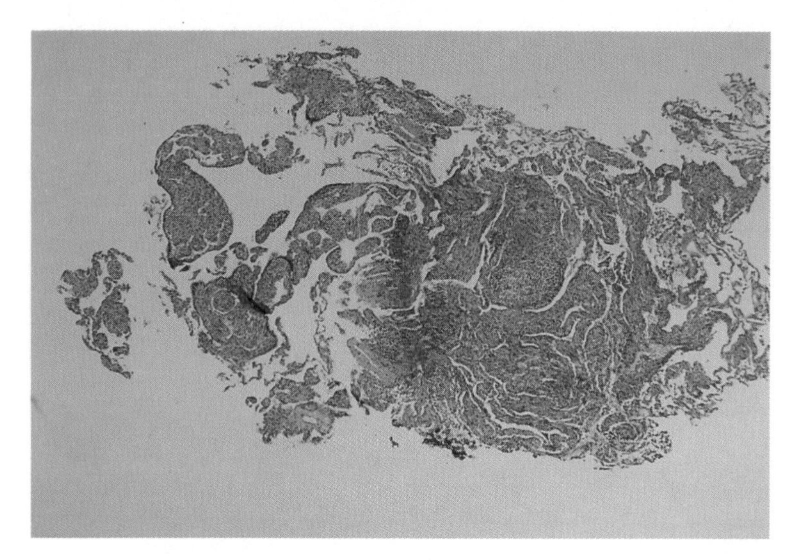

Figure 1–20. Transbronchial biopsy specimen showing lymphangioleiomyomatosis. The smooth muscle–containing septa with rounded fascicles of cells are partially collapsed in this transbronchial biopsy. Without specifically considering lymphangioleiomyomatosis, one could easily mistake these changes for fibrous tissue.

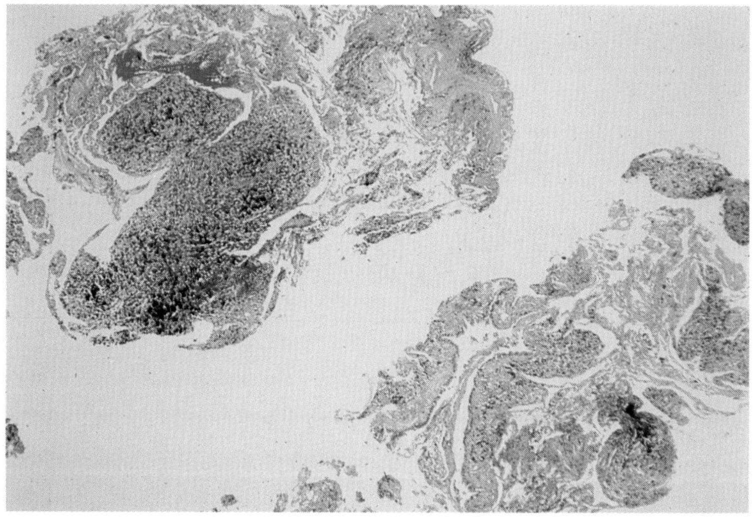

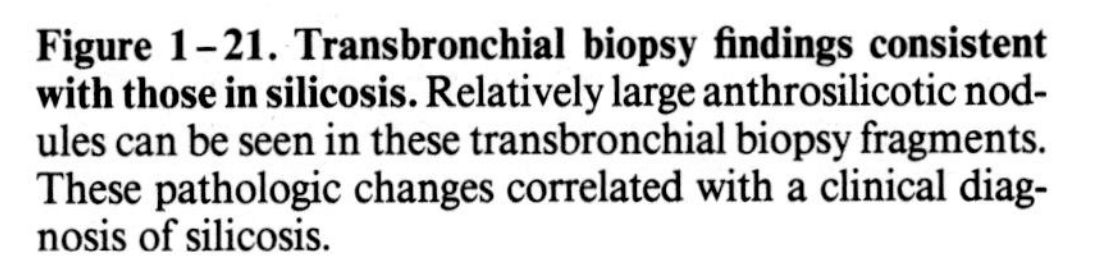

Figure 1–21. Transbronchial biopsy findings consistent with those in silicosis. Relatively large anthrosilicotic nodules can be seen in these transbronchial biopsy fragments. These pathologic changes correlated with a clinical diagnosis of silicosis.

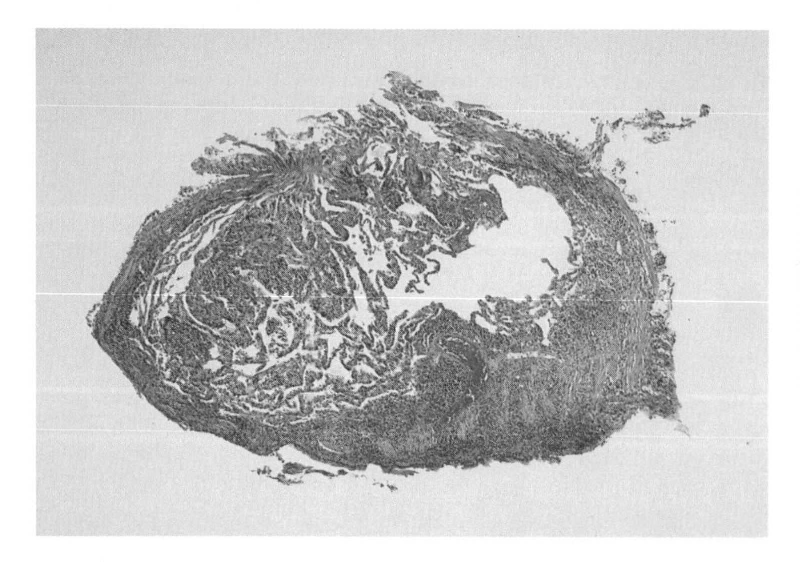

Figure 1–22. Transbronchial biopsy specimen showing lymphoma. The specimen shows well-differentiated (small) lymphocytic lymphoma. There is a dense infiltrate permeating the bronchial wall and splaying apart the smooth muscle fascicles. With clinical correlation and exclusion of infectious agents, a presumptive diagnosis of lymphoma is possible on the basis of transbronchial biopsy findings both at presentation and at the time of pulmonary relapse.

■ APPROACH TO LUNG BIOPSIES FROM IMMUNOSUPPRESSED PATIENTS (WITH SPECIAL REFERENCE TO PATIENTS WITH AIDS AND RECIPIENTS OF ORGAN TRANSPLANTS)

Pulmonary lesions in immunosuppressed patients can be grouped as shown in Table 1 – 1.

The pathologist is usually aware of the immunosuppressed status of the patient and the urgency of the situation; however, the findings at lung biopsy may be the initial suggestion of an immunodeficiency state (such as AIDS).

Patients' defense mechanisms may be altered by a number of mechanisms, both congenital and acquired, and frequently the form of pulmonary disease depends on the type of immunosuppression. Some of the factors

Table 1 – 1
CATEGORIES OF PULMONARY LESIONS IN IMMUNOSUPPRESSED PATIENTS

Extension of Basic Disease Process into Lungs
- Lymphomas, Hodgkin's and non-Hodgkin's
- Leukemias
- Plasma cell neoplasms
- Carcinomatosis, primary and metastatic
- Collagen vascular diseases
- Vasculitides

Opportunistic Infections
- Viruses
  - Herpes simplex
  - Varicella zoster
  - Cytomegalovirus
- Bacteria
  - Gram-positive bacteria
  - Gram-negative bacteria
  - Anaerobes
- Mycobacteria
  - *Mycobacterium tuberculosis*
  - *Mycobacterium avium-intracellulare*
  - *Mycobacterium kansasii*
- Fungi
  - *Aspergillus* species
  - *Candida* species
  - *Zygomycetes (Mucorales)* species
  - *Cryptococcus neoformans*
  - *Histoplasma capsulatum*
  - *Blastomyces dermatitidis*
  - *Coccidioides immitis*
  - *Trichosporon* species
  - *Nocardia asteroides*
- Protozoa
  - *Pneumocystis carinii*
  - *Toxoplasma gondii*
  - *Cryptosporidium* species
- Parasites
  - *Strongyloides stercoralis*

Drug-Induced Pulmonary Disease
- Pulmonary cytotoxic drugs
- Oxygen toxicity
- Radiation pneumonitis and fibrosis
- Transfusion-related acute lung injury

Nonspecific, Noninfectious Interstitial Pneumonitis
- Diffuse alveolar damage
- Nonspecific interstitial pneumonia
- Lymphocytic interstitial pneumonia
- Pulmonary alveolar hemorrhage
- Pulmonary edema

Miscellaneous (Especially Transplant Recipients)
- Graft vs host disease, or host vs graft disease (rejection)
- Bronchiolitis obliterans
- Epstein-Barr virus association lymphoproliferation

Pulmonary Malignancy Associated with Immunosuppression
- Non-Hodgkin's lymphoma
- Kaposi's sarcoma
- Carcinoma of lung

New Pulmonary Process Unrelated to Immunodeficiency
- Pulmonary embolism
- Aspiration pneumonia
- Community-acquired pneumonia
- Nosocomial pneumonia
- Congestive cardiac failure
- Renal failure
- Malignant disease

Combination of Two or More of the Preceding
- More than two thirds of the immune-compromised patients may actually belong in this group.

Modified from Prakash UBS. Pulmonary manifestations of systemic diseases. *In* Baum GL, Wolinsky E (eds). Textbook of Pulmonary Disease. Boston, Little, Brown & Co, 1989.

predisposing to opportunistic infections are shown in Table 1-2.

Table 1-2
FACTORS IN OPPORTUNISTIC INFECTIONS

Congenital and Acquired Immunodeficiency States
Altered Physical Barriers
Indwelling catheters
Nebulizers and ventilators
Local mechanical disruption by tumor, and so forth
Ciliary dysfunction
Bronchospastic disease
Intubation and tracheostomy
Altered Indigenous Microbial Flora
Systemic illnesses (e.g., diabetes mellitus, alcoholism, and so forth)
Surgery
Malnutrition
Aspiration
Broad-spectrum antibiotic therapy
Change in virulence of microbial flora
Intubation and tracheostomy
Leukopenia
Basic disease process
Decreased migration
Defective phagocytosis
Decreased bactericidal activity
Cytotoxic drug therapy
Protein-calorie malnutrition
Impaired Lymphocyte-Mediated Immunity
Corticosteroid therapy
Cytotoxic drug therapy
Radiation
Transplantation
Acquired immunodeficiency syndrome
Protein-calorie malnutrition
Underlying Pulmonary Pathology
Obstructive pulmonary disease
Bronchiectasis
Ancient cavitary disease
Secretory IgA deficiency
Surfactant deficiency

Modified from Prakash UBS, Pulmonary manifestations of systemic diseases. *In* Baum GL, Wolinsky E (eds). Textbook of Pulmonary Disease. Boston, Little, Brown & Co, 1989.

The vast majority of these patients have an acute presentation with localized or, more commonly, diffuse infiltrates, nodules, or both, and many are diagnosed by noninvasive studies.

■ Approach for the Surgical Pathologist to Differential Diagnosis of Pulmonary Lesions in Immunosuppressed Individuals

1. Make a specific diagnosis whenever possible.
   a. Infection: usually the primary concern
   b. Primary disease process: malignancy (e.g., lymphoma), collagen vascular disease
   c. Drug reaction: usually a clinicopathologic diagnosis of exclusion
   d. New pulmonary disease unrelated to primary disease process, immunosuppression, or therapy
   e. Combinations of the above.
2. Exclusion of specific lesions, mainly infections, by all available techniques
   a. Perform a routine battery of special stains for bacteria, fungi, mycobacteria, *Pneumocystis.*
   b. Perform a routine battery of cultures: viral, fungal, bacterial, mycobacterial.
   c. Provide for special studies: such as gene probes, immunoperoxidase stains, chloroacetate esterase staining in cases of myeloid leukemia. Have a protocol to follow to allow for these studies, just to be on the safe side.
   d. *Plan ahead.* Save a little frozen tissue.
3. Negative information is clinically useful
   a. Up to 50 percent of lung biopsy specimens yield a nonspecific diagnosis (usually diffuse alveolar damage).
   b. This negative information (at least for exclusion of an infection) is very useful to the clinican.
4. General principles to keep in mind
   a. Multiple lesions are common.
   b. Necrosis (regardless of type), acute inflamation, and proteinosis-like reaction mean infection until proven otherwise.
   c. Classic histopathologic findings for a given organism may be lacking (e.g., tuberculosis without granulomas).
   d. No specific diagnosis is apparent for a significant percentage of cases.
   e. Expect unusual opportunistic organisms.
   f. The burden of organisms may be overwhelming with little inflammatory reaction.

References

Colby TV, Weiss RL. Current concepts in the surgical pathology of pulmonary infections. Am J Surg Pathol 11(Suppl 1):25-38, 1987.
Rosenow EC, Wilson WR, Cockerill FR. Pulmonary disease in the immunocompromised host (Part 1). Mayo Clin Proc 60:473-487, 1985.
Wilson WR, Cockerill FR, Rosenow EC. Pulmonary disease in the immunocompromised host (Part 2). Mayo Clin Proc 60:610-631, 1985.

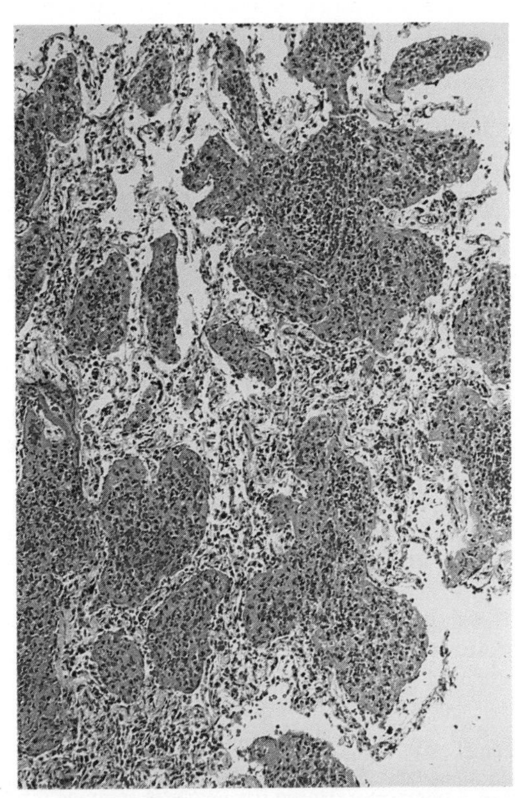

Figure 1-23. Staphylococcal pneumonia in acquired immunodeficiency syndrome (AIDS). An acute hemcrrhagic fulminant pneumonia with consolidation of airspaces is present. Cultures were positive, and the organisms were seen on Gram stain of the tissue.

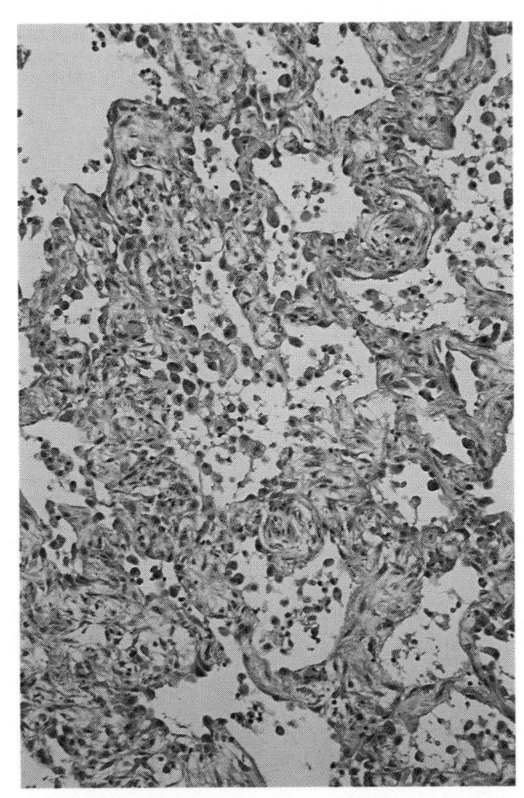

Figure 1-24. Nonspecific interstitial pneumonitis in acquired immunodeficiency syndrome (AIDS). There is a pattern of diffuse alveolar damage. There is edema of alveolar walls and prominent type II cells with a modest interstitial infiltrate. A rigorous search failed to identify an infectious agent in this case.

■ **Acquired Immunodeficiency Syndrome** (Figs. 1-23 to 1-26; see also Figs. 3-185 to 3-189, 5-22 and 5-23)

Infections

1. Viruses
   a. Herpes simplex virus and herpes zoster
   b. Cytomegalovirus
2. Bacteria
   a. *Streptococcus pneumoniae*
   b. *Haemophilus influenzae*
3. Mycobacteria
   a. *Mycobacterium tuberculosis*
   b. *Mycobacterium avium-intracellulare*
   c. *Mycobacterium kansaii*
4. Fungi
   a. *Candida albicans*
   b. *Cryptococcus neoformans*
   c. *Histoplasma capsulatum*
   d. *Nocardia asteroides*
   e. *Aspergillus fumigatus*
5. Protozoa
   a. *Pneumocystis carinii*
   b. *Cryptosporidium* species
   c. *Toxoplasma gondii*
6. Parasites
   a. *Strongyloides stercoralis*

Diffuse Nonmalignant and Noninfectious Pulmonary Disease

1. Idiopathic interstitial pneumonia
2. Lymphoid (lymphocytic) interstitial pneumonia, lymphoid hyperplasia, atypical lymphoid infiltrates
3. Pulmonary alveolar proteinosis
4. Drug reactions

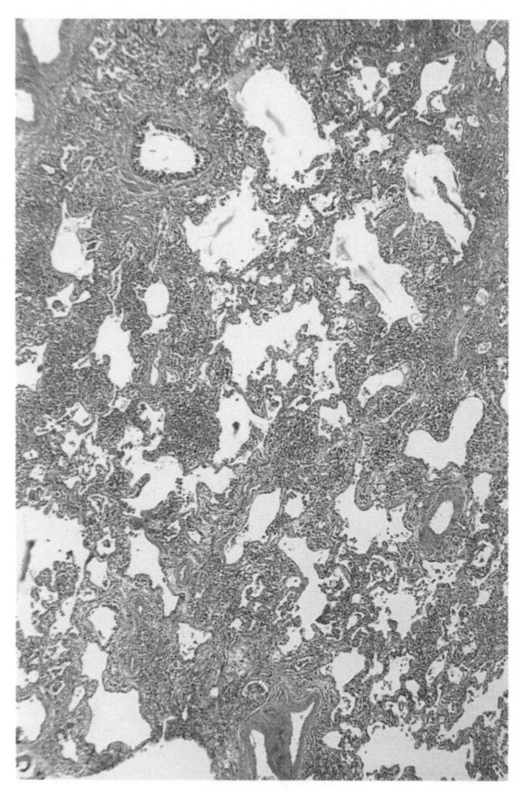

Figure 1–25.

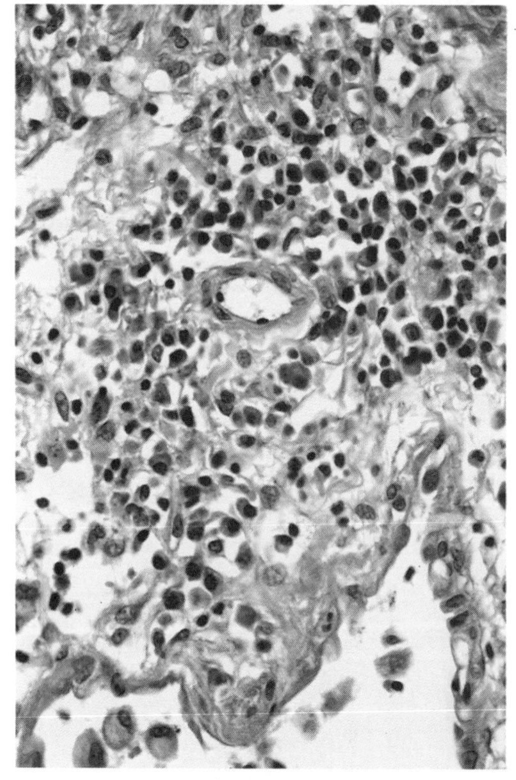

Figure 1–26.

Figures 1–25, 1–26. Lymphocytic interstitial pneumonia in acquired immunodeficiency syndrome (AIDS). There is a dense, diffuse interstitial infiltrate of mononuclear cells. Cytologically, lymphocytes and plasma cells are prominent.

AIDS-Related Pulmonary Malignancies

1. Kaposi's sarcoma
2. Non-Hodgkin's lymphoma

Incidental and Unrelated Pulmonary Lesions

The list of infections in AIDS continues to grow. Pulmonary infections in AIDS are primarily diagnosed on the basis of bronchoalveolar lavage with culture, immunologic studies, or transbronchial biopsy; open lung biopsy is becoming rare. The most common infections are *P. carinii* and cytomegalovirus (CMV) pneumonias.

Idiopathic interstitial pneumonia may be a mild, nearly subclinical lesion or may present as an acute fulminant interstitial lung disease. The histology varies from mild cellular interstitial infiltrates to fullblown diffuse alveolar damage. Alveolar proteinosis is a rare reaction pattern and should lead to rigorous exclusion of infection.

AIDS-related malignancies are probably the most frequent lesions leading to open lung biopsy, although in many cases a transbronchial biopsy might suffice.

References

Rankin JA, Collman R, Daniele RB. Acquired immune deficiency syndrome and the lung. Chest 94:155–164, 1988.

Rosenow EC, Wilson WR, Cockerill FR. Pulmonary disease in the immunocompromised host (Part 1). Mayo Clin Proc 60:473–487, 1985.

Solal-Celigny P, Couderc LJ, Herman D, et al. Lymphoid interstitial pneumonitis in acquired immunodeficiency syndrome-related complex. Am Rev Respir Dis 131:956–960, 1985.

Suffredini AF, Ognibene FP, Lack EE, et al. Nonspecific interstitial pneumonitis: a common cause of pulmonary disease in the acquired immunodeficiency syndrome. Ann Intern Med 107:7–13, 1987.

Wilson WR, Cockerill FR, Rosenow EC. Pulmonary disease in the immunocompromised host (Part 2). Mayo Clin Proc 60:610–631, 1985.

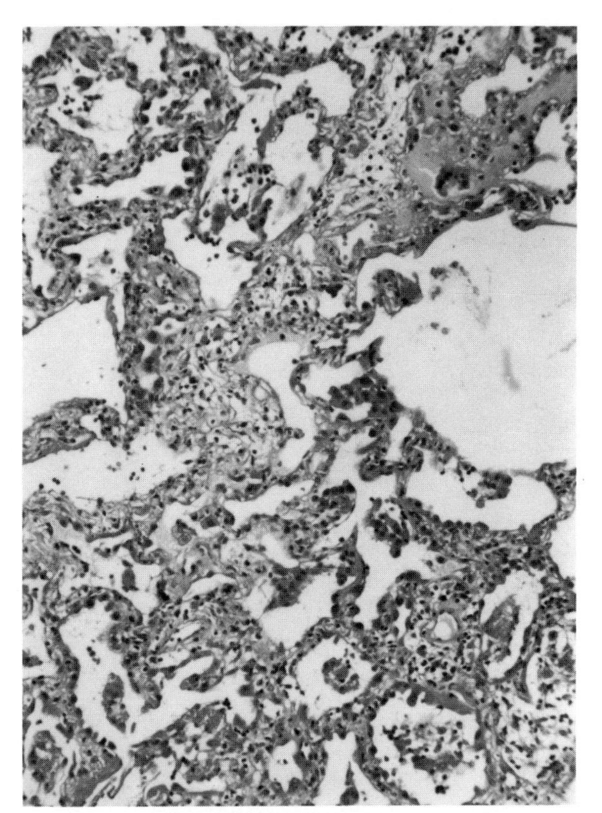

Figure 1-27. Idiopathic interstitial pneumonia. Idiopathic interstitial pneumonia in a bone marrow transplant. Several weeks after transplantation, shortness of breath and diffuse bilateral infiltrates developed. The biopsy findings show the features of organizing diffuse alveolar damage with edema of alveolar walls, mild chronic inflammatory infiltrate, and prominent reactive type II alveolar lining cells. No infection could be identified.

■ Bone Marrow and Heart-Lung Transplant Recipients (Figs. 1-27 to 1-33; see also Fig. 6-18)

In addition to the lesions already listed, other lesions that are unique to or especially common in this setting include the following.

Progressive Bronchiolitis Obliterans with Clinically Progressive Obstructive Lung Disease

The histologic features are usually those of proliferative bronchiolitis obliterans evolving to constrictive bronchiolitis with relatively little associated alveolar parenchymal reaction and little or no organizing pneumonia. Mild cellular bronchiolitis may also be present.

Idiopathic Diffuse Alveolar Damage (Idiopathic Interstitial Pneumonia in Bone Marrow Transplants)

Progressive diffuse alveolar damage develops; no cause can be found, and the prognosis is poor. This may be a multifactorial reaction related to the chemoradiotherapy given prior to bone marrow transplantation. This lesion tends to occur earlier (first month) in the post-transplant period than infection (especially CMV) although there is considerable overlap.

Lung Transplant Rejection (Heart-Lung Transplants, Lung Transplants)

Perivascular (especially perivenular) mononuclear cell infiltrates are seen. As rejection becomes more severe, there are interstitial infiltrates, bronchiolar infiltrates, alveolar exudation and hemorrhage, and finally parenchymal necrosis. Rigorous exclusion of infection is mandatory.

Lymphoproliferative Diseases

These include malignant lymphomas and Epstein-Barr virus-associated lymphoproliferative diseases.

References

Cordonnier C, Bernaudin JF, Bierling P, et al. Pulmonary complications occurring after allogeneic bone marrow transplantation. A study of 130 consecutive transplanted patients. Cancer 58:1047-1054, 1986.

Crawford SW, Hackman RC, Clark JG. Open lung biopsy diagnosis of diffuse pulmonary infiltrates after marrow transplantation. Chest 94:949-953, 1988.

Sale GE, Shulman HM. The Pathology of Bone Marrow Transplantation. New York, Masson, 1984.

Tazelaar HD, Yousem SA. The pathology of combined heart-lung transplantation. Hum Pathol 19:1403-1416, 1988.

Urbanski SJ, Kossakowska AE, Curtis J, et al. Idiopathic small airways pathology in patients with graft-versus-host disease following allogeneic bone marrow transplantation. Am J Surg Pathol 11:965-971, 1987.

Wingard JR, Mellits ED, Sostrin MB, et al. Interstitial pneumonitis after allogeneic bone marrow transplantation. Nine-year experience at a single institution. Medicine 67:175-186, 1988.

Yousem SA, Randhawa P, Nabesuik MA, et al. Post-transplant lymphoproliferative disorders in heart-lung transplant recipients: Primary presentation in the allograft. Hum Pathol 20:361-369, 1989.

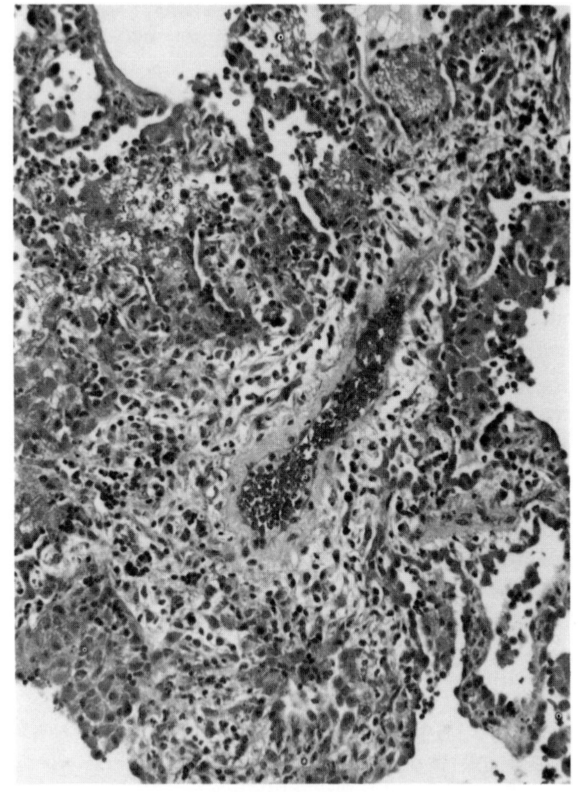

Figure 1-28.

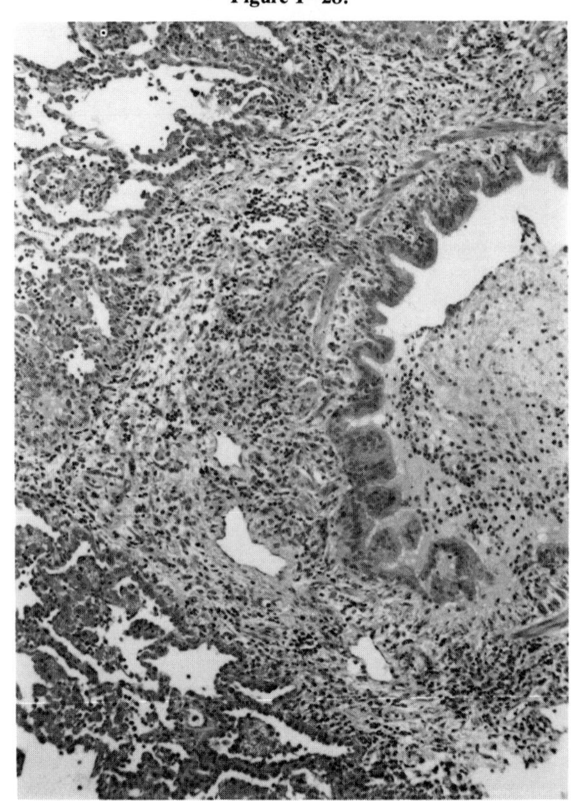

Figure 1-29.

Figures 1-28, 1-29. Heart-lung transplantation with lung allograft rejection. Edematous perivascular and peribronchiolar lymphoid infiltrates are associated with congestion and cellular infiltration of the vascular and bronchiolar walls.

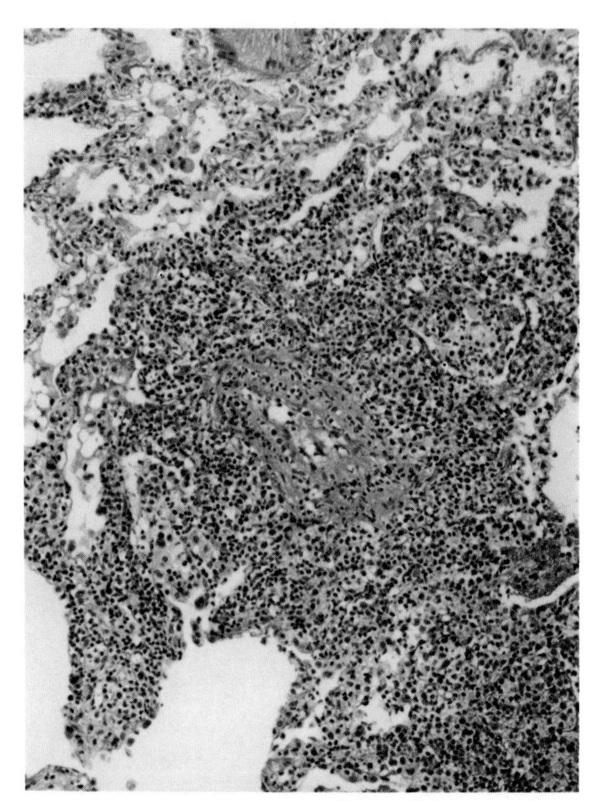

Figure 1-30.

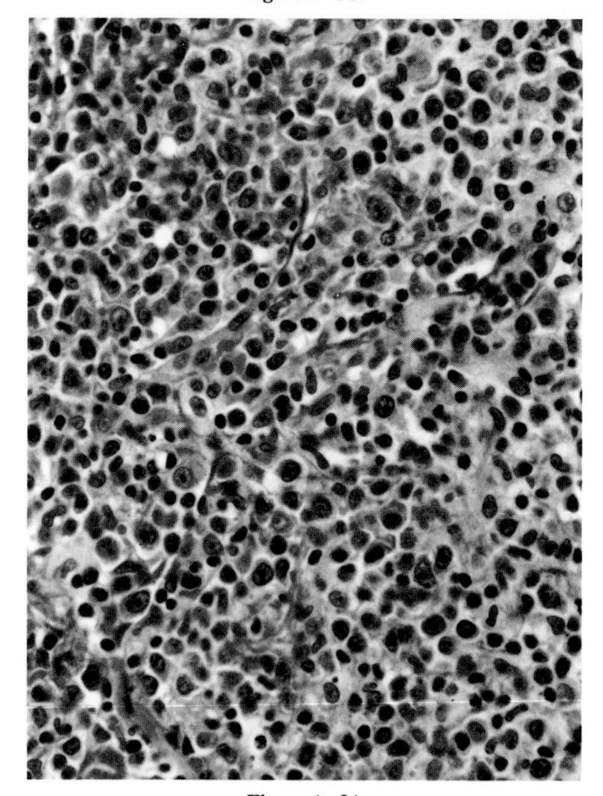

Figure 1-31.

Figures 1-30, 1-31. Epstein-Barr virus (EBV)-associated lymphoproliferative disorder. Polymorphous perivascular infiltrates suggest a mixed cell lymphoma. Some vascular infiltration is present. The lymphoproliferative disease in this case cleared when immunosuppression was decreased. EBV genome was identified in the cells.

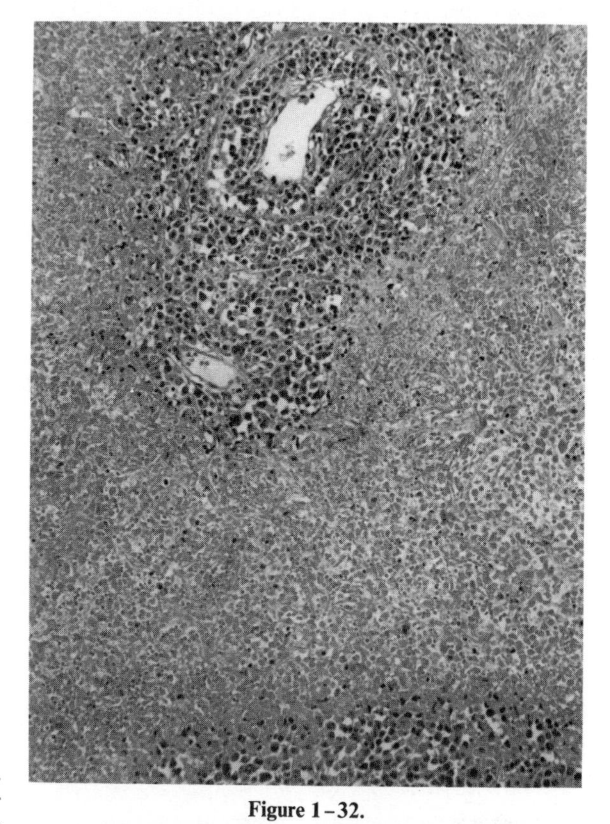

Figure 1–32.

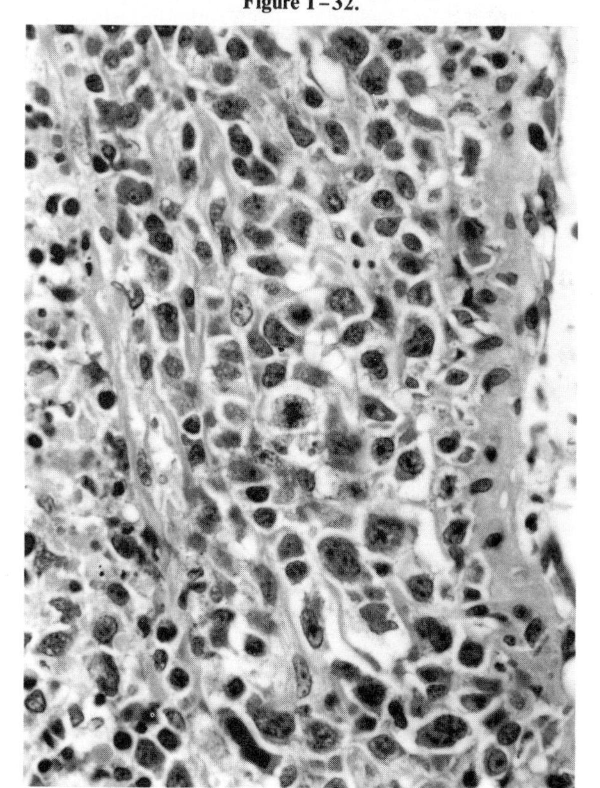

Figure 1–33.

Figures 1–32, 1–33. Epstein-Barr virus (EBV)–associated lymphoproliferative disorder. There are large nodules with extensive necrosis and vascular infiltration, and the cytologic features suggest a large cell lymphoma. In this case the lymphoid proliferation in this case remitted when immunosuppression was decreased. EBV genome was found in the proliferating cells.

■ APPROACH TO LUNG BIOPSIES IN PATIENTS WITH COLLAGEN-VASCULAR DISEASES (Figs. 1-34 to 1-68; see also Fig. 8-49)

Pulmonary involvement is extremely common in many collagen-vascular diseases, with rheumatoid arthritis leading the list. A variety of histologic changes may be observed, and these are summarized in Table 1-3.

Pleural reactions are probably the most common intrathoracic manifestations of collagen-vascular diseases, but only rarely are the histologic findings specific. In the occasional case of systemic lupus erythematosus (SLE), one may find hematoxylin bodies in pleural fluid cell blocks. Rheumatoid arthritis may be associated with an exudative pleuritis (pleurisy) that clinically is a sterile empyema. There is a dense fibrinous exudate lining the pleural space with underlying palisaded histiocyte reaction resembling a rheumatoid nodule that has marsupialized over the pleural surface.

Airway disease as measured by pulmonary function tests is also frequent in collagen-vascular diseases, but morphologic lesions seen in biopsies are considerably less common. Cellular bronchiolitis with or without germinal centers may be seen. Pure bronchiolitis obliterans with airflow obstructive and constrictive bronchiolitis is an uncommon but devastating lesion most often seen in rheumatoid arthritis, either as a primary condition or secondary to penicillamine therapy.

The *interstitial diseases* associated with collagen-vascular diseases are varied. Multiple patterns, which are difficult to classify, often coexist, and they require descriptive tabulation, such as usual interstitial pneumonia-like patterns with marked reactive follicular hyperplasia of germinal centers and follicular bronchitis or bronchiolitis associated with a patchy organizing pneumonia in Sjögren's syndrome. Diffuse alveolar damage with or without hemorrhage is typical of SLE and is the most common histologic correlate of "lupus pneumonitis." Smoldering subacute cellular interstitial pneumonias can be seen in SLE and rheumatoid arthritis and should be descriptively labeled. The major factor in the assessment of interstitial lung diseases in collagen-vascular diseases is to evaluate the presence and degree of permanent interstitial fibrosis and honeycombing, since these features carry an unfavorable prognosis.

The *vascular changes* seen in collagen-vascular diseases are usually associated with pulmonary hypertension, and a true inflammatory necrotizing vasculitis of medium-sized and large pulmonary vessels is rarely seen. Commonly, vasculitis is in the form of a small vessel angiitis (venulitis or capillaritis), which is a common finding in acute pulmonary hemorrhage in SLE. Accelerated atherosclerosis may be seen in the large vessels in patients with pulmonary hypertension.

Apical fibrobullous disease in ankylosing spondylitis is something that rarely comes to the attention of the surgical pathologist.

Because the lymphoid proliferations in Sjögren's syndrome may sometimes be difficult to classify, provision of tissue for immunologic marker studies is recommended whenever possible.

References

Colby TV. Pathology of the lung in collagen vascular diseases. *In* Lenfant C (ed). The Lung Rheumatic Diseases. New York, Marcel Dekker. pp. 145-178, 1990.

Eisenberg H. The interstitial lung disease associated with the collagen-vascular disorders. Clin Chest Med 3:565-578, 1988.

Hunninghake GW, Fauci AS. State of the art—pulmonary involvement in the collagen-vascular diseases. Am Rev Respir Dis 119:471-503, 1979.

Nozawa Y. Histopathological findings of the lung in collagen diseases—especially on their differential diagnosis. Acta Pathol Jpn 22:843-858, 1972.

Yousem S, Colby TV, Carrington CB. Lung biopsy in rheumatoid arthritis. Am Rev Respir Dis 131:770-777, 1985.

Text continued on page 36

Table 1-3
CLINICOPATHOLOGIC PATTERNS IN COLLAGEN-VASCULAR DISEASES

	Rheumatoid Arthritis	Juvenile Rheumatoid Arthritis	Systemic Lupus Erythematosus	Scleroderma	Polymyositis/ Dermatomyositis	Mixed Connective Tissue Disease	Sjögren's Syndrome	Ankylosing Spondylitis	Behçet's Syndrome
Pleural inflammation, fibrosis, effusions	X	X	X	X					
Airway disease, inflammation, obstruction, lymphoid hyperplasia (follicular bronchiolitis)	X	X	X	X			X		
Interstitial disease	X	X	X	X	X	X	X		
Acute (with or without hemorrhage)	X	X	X	X	X				
Subacute/organizing (BOOP pattern)	X		X	X	X		X		
Chronic cellular	X		X				X		
Chronic cellular and fibrosing	X	X	X	X	X	X	X		
Eosinophilic infiltrates	X								
Vascular disease									
Hypertension/vasculitis	X	X	X	X		X	X		X
Parenchymal nodules	X	X							
Apical fibrobullous disease	X							X	
Lymphoid proliferations (reactive, neoplastic)							X		

Abbreviation: BOOP, bronchiolitis obliterans organizing pneumonia.

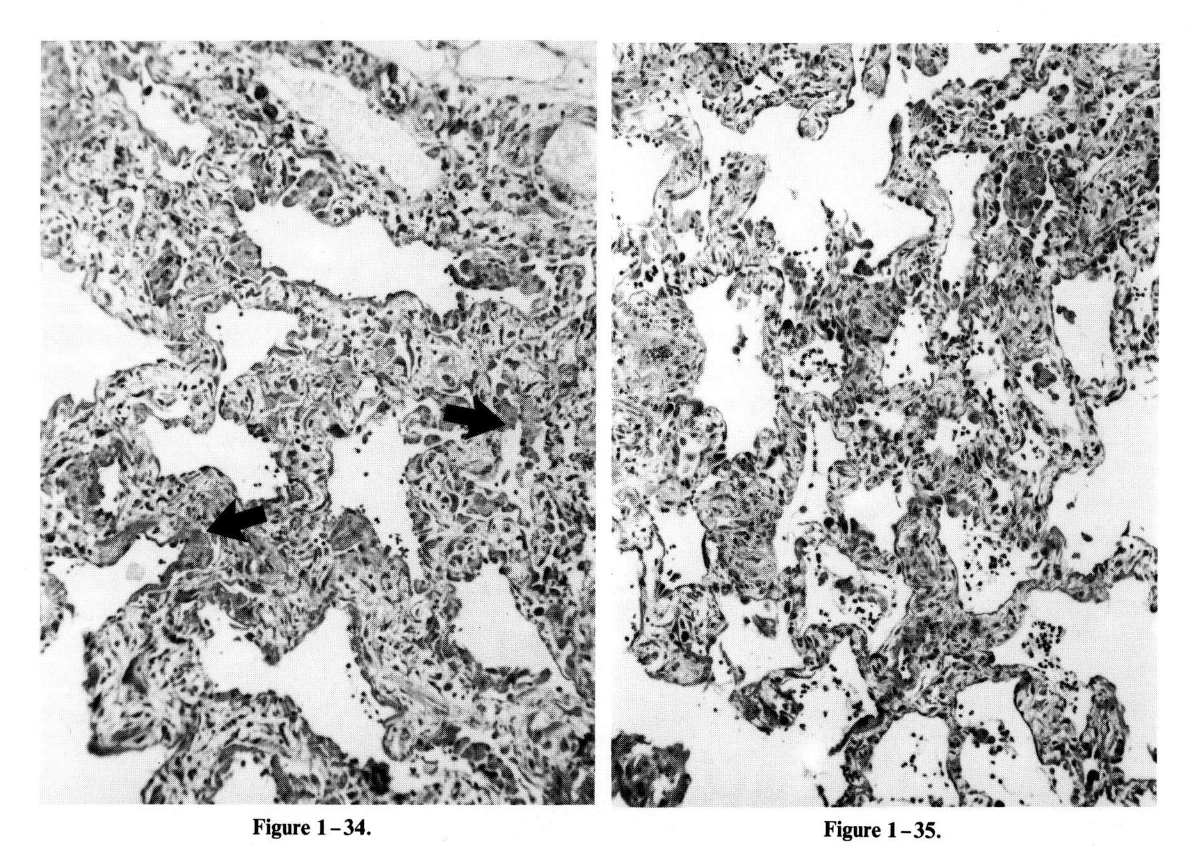

Figure 1-34. **Figure 1-35.**

Figures 1-34, 1-35. Diffuse alveolar damage in rheumatoid arthritis (RA). The alveolar walls are thickened and edematous and in some foci are lined by hyaline membranes that are undergoing organization (arrows), whereas in other foci the alveoli are lined by regenerative type II cells.

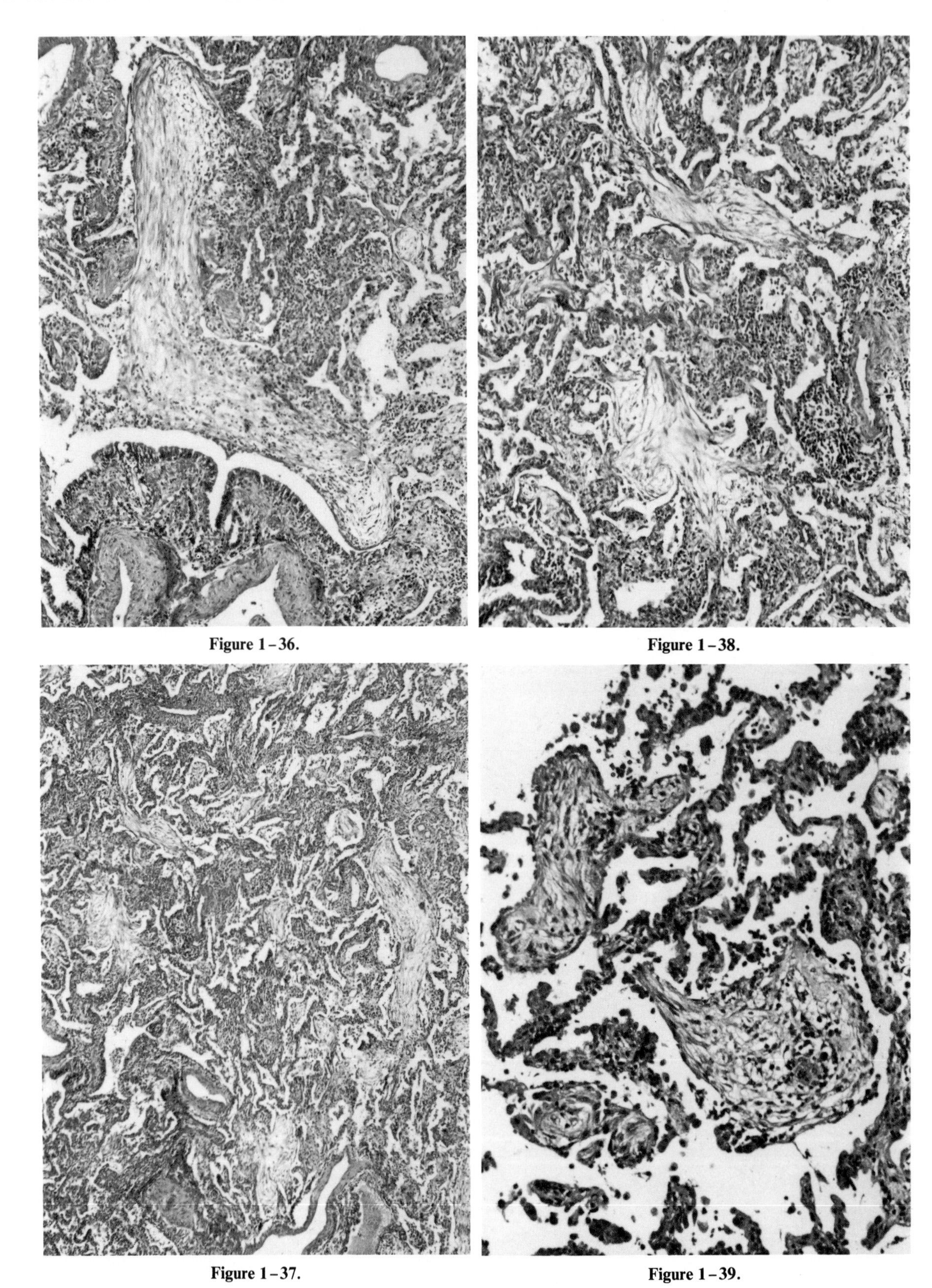

Figure 1-36.

Figure 1-38.

Figure 1-37.

Figure 1-39.

Figures 1-36, 1-37, 1-38, 1-39. Bronchiolitis obliterans organizing pneumonia (BOOP) pattern in rheumatoid arthritis (RA). There is relative architectural preservation with edematous tufts of organizing connective tissue in terminal bronchioles (Fig. 1-36) and alveolar ducts (Figs. 1-37, 1-38) and extending into alveoli (Fig. 1-39).

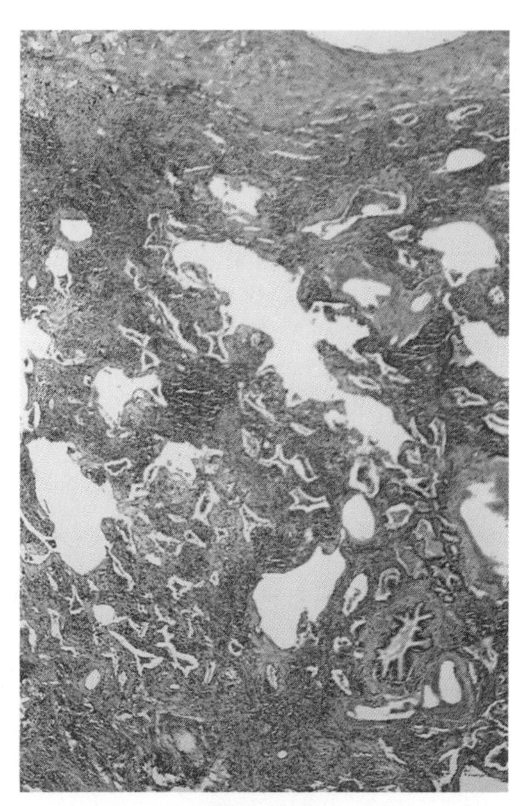

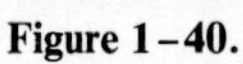

Figure 1–40.

Figures 1–40, 1–41. Lymphocytic interstitial pneumonia in rheumatoid arthritis (RA). There is a dense diffuse interstitial infiltrate of chronic inflammatory cells.

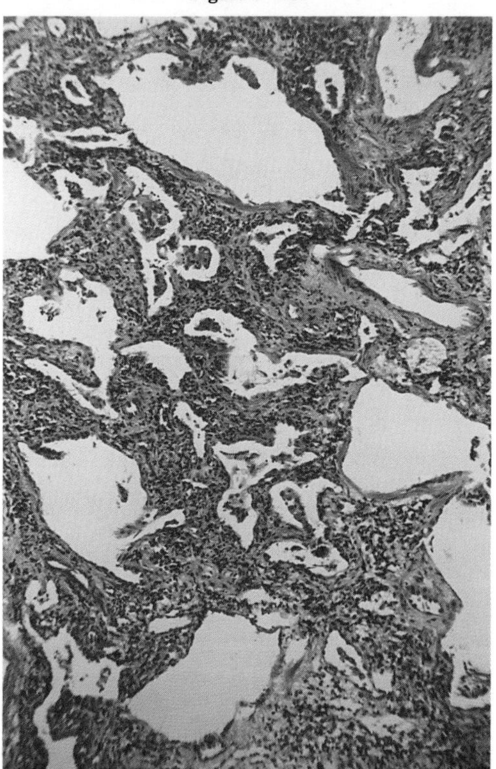

Figure 1–41.

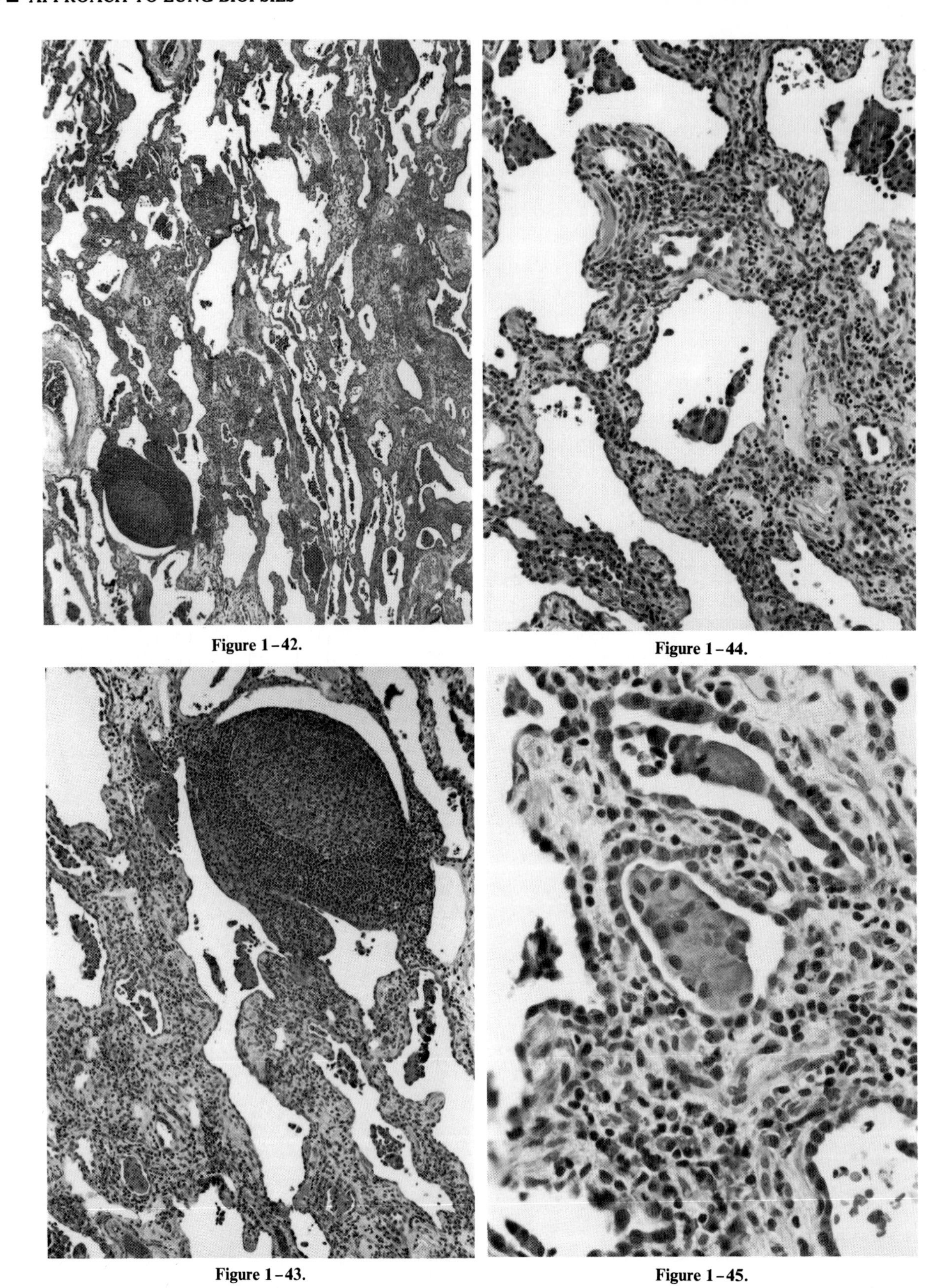

Figure 1-42.

Figure 1-44.

Figure 1-43.

Figure 1-45.

Figures 1-42, 1-43, 1-44, 1-45. Fibrosing interstitial pneumonia in rheumatoid arthritis (RA). There is interstitial thickening and foci of micro-honeycombing with lymphoid hyperplasia. In some foci, the number of macrophages in the airspaces is suggestive of desquamative interstitial pneumonia. The interstitial infiltrate is rich in plasma cells. Overall, the histologic appearance is consistent with that of lymphocytic interstitial pneumonia.

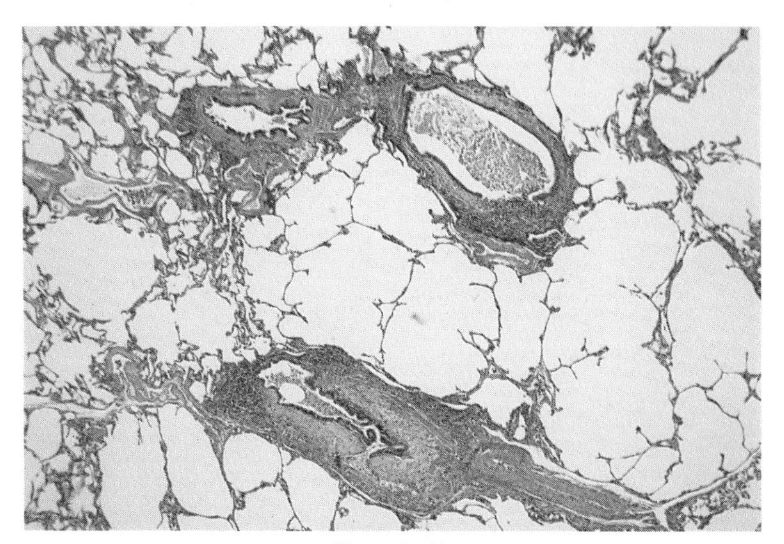

Figure 1–46.

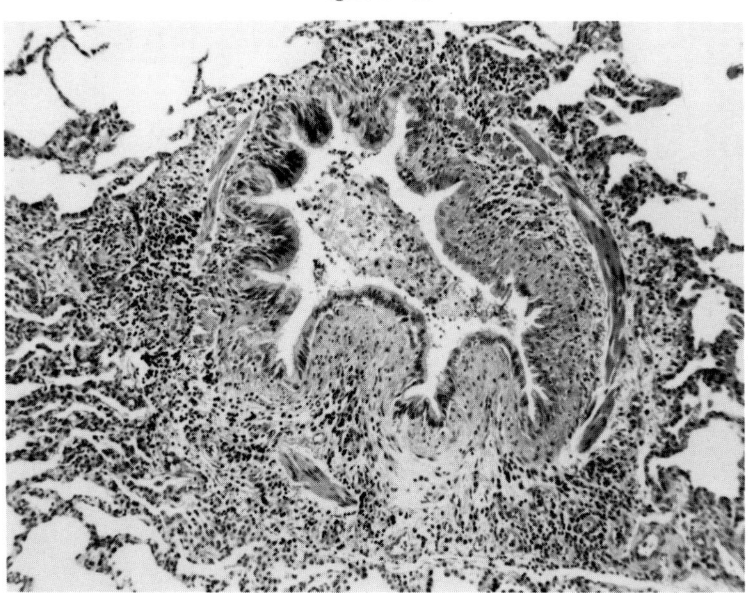

Figure 1–47.

Figures 1–46, 1–47, 1–48. Bronchiolitis obliterans in rheumatoid arthritis (RA). The patient was not receiving drug therapy and was experiencing rapidly progressive shortness of breath. Open lung biopsy findings show constrictive bronchiolitis obliterans with varying degrees of stenosis of small airways caused by inflammation and proliferation of fibrous tissue within the submucosa. Some of the airways are entirely obliterated (Fig. 1–48).

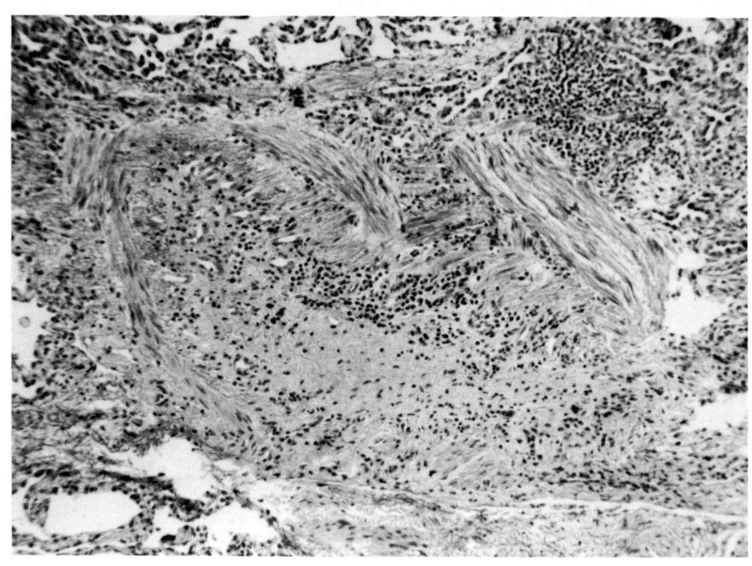

Figure 1–48.

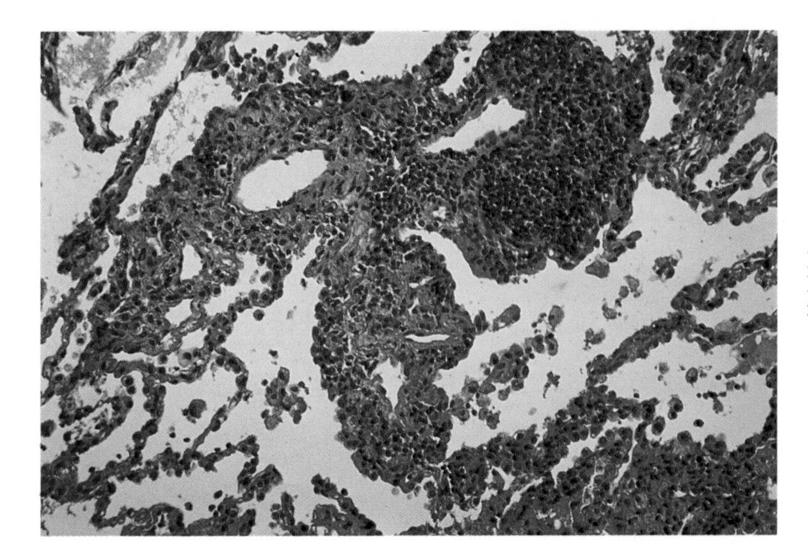

Figure 1–49. Vasculitis in rheumatoid arthritis (RA). Lymphocytic vascular and perivascular infiltrates are seen in the lung in RA.

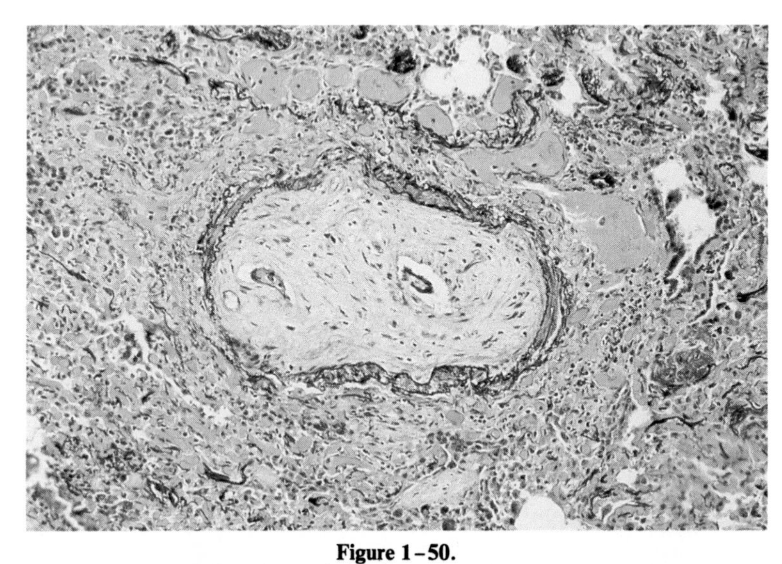

Figure 1–50.

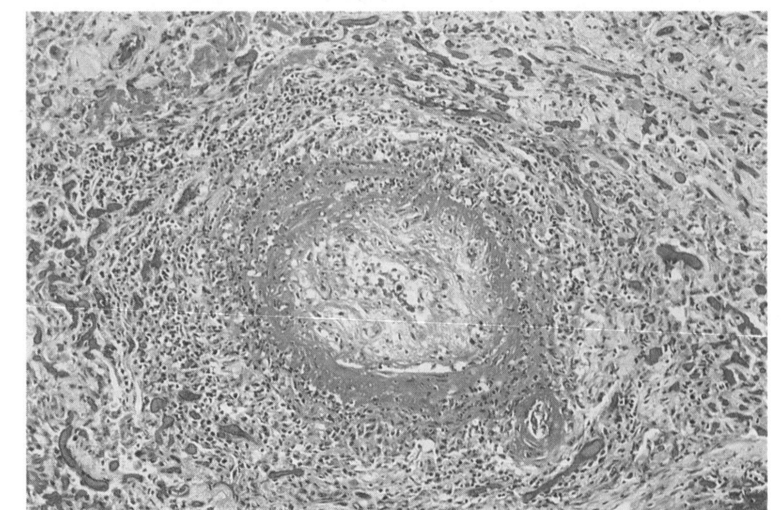

Figure 1–51.

Figures 1–50, 1–51. Pulmonary hypertension in rheumatoid arthritis (RA). Pulmonary hypertension in RA is associated with marked intimal thickening and occlusion in some vessels and with fibrinoid necrosis of other vessel walls (Fig. 1–51).

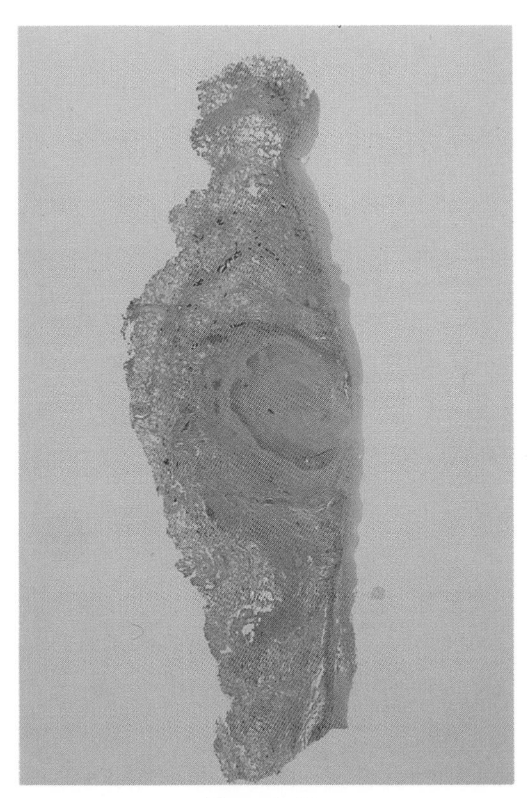

Figure 1 – 52.

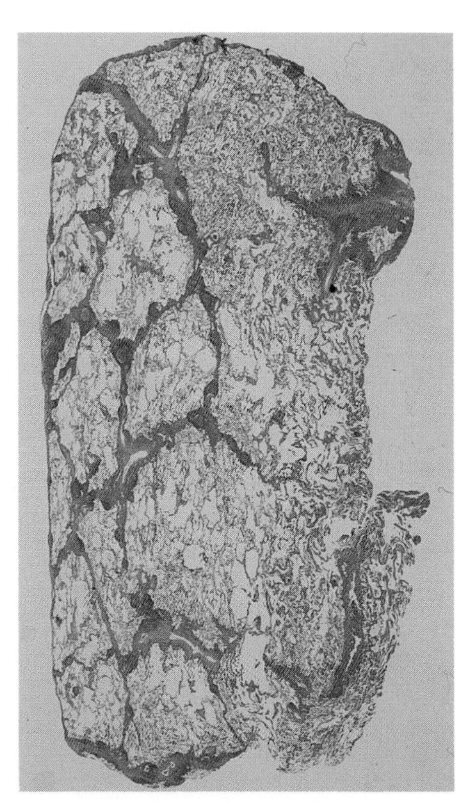

Figure 1 – 54. Lymphoid hyperplasia rheumatoid arthritis (RA). There are germinal centers along lymphatic routes.

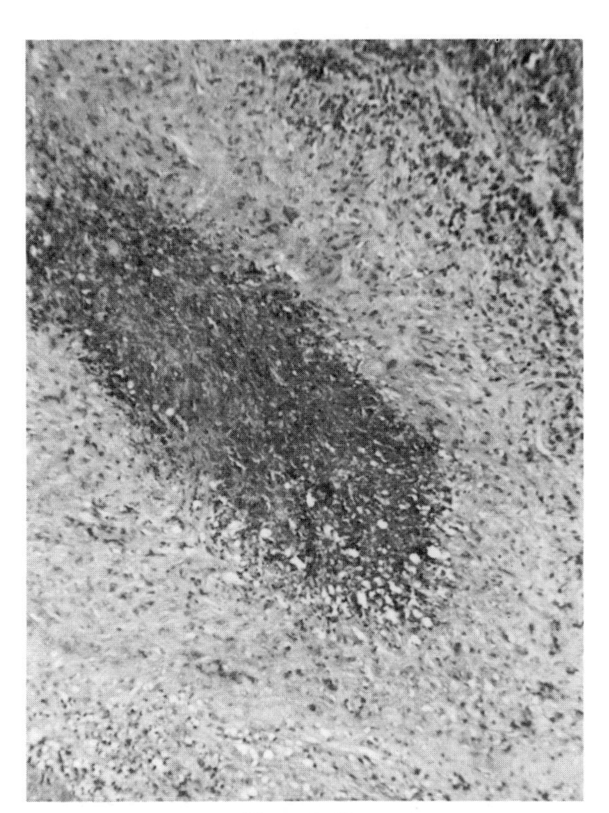

Figure 1 – 53.

Figures 1 – 52, 1 – 53. Rheumatoid nodule. There is a subpleural necrobiotic nodule with central (fibrinoid or basophilic) necrosis surrounded by palisaded histiocytes.

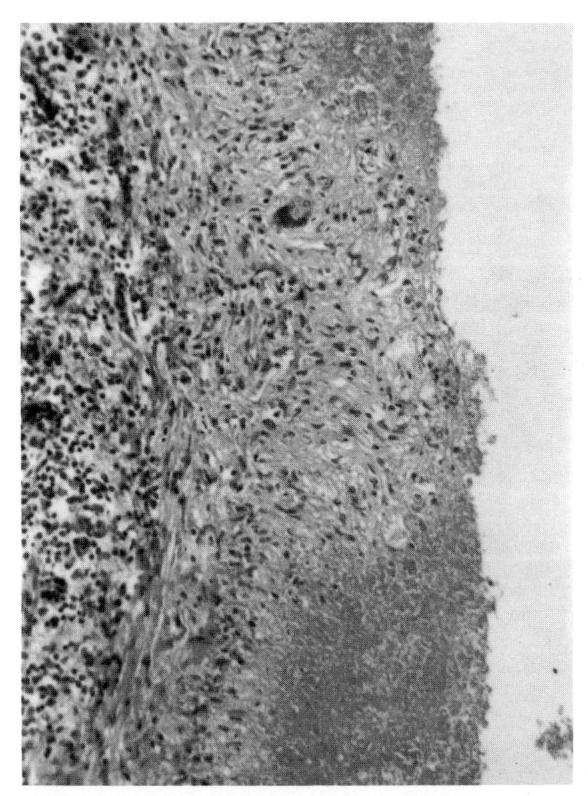

Figure 1 – 55. Rheumatoid pleuritis. There is eosinophilic debris lining the visceral pleural surface with associated palisaded histiocyte and giant cell reaction. The appearances are identical to those of a rheumatoid nodule.

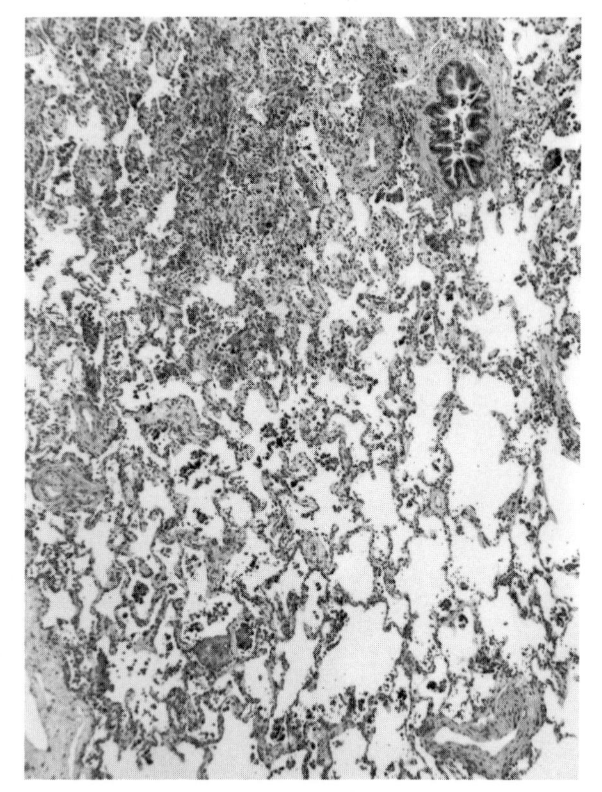

Figure 1-56.

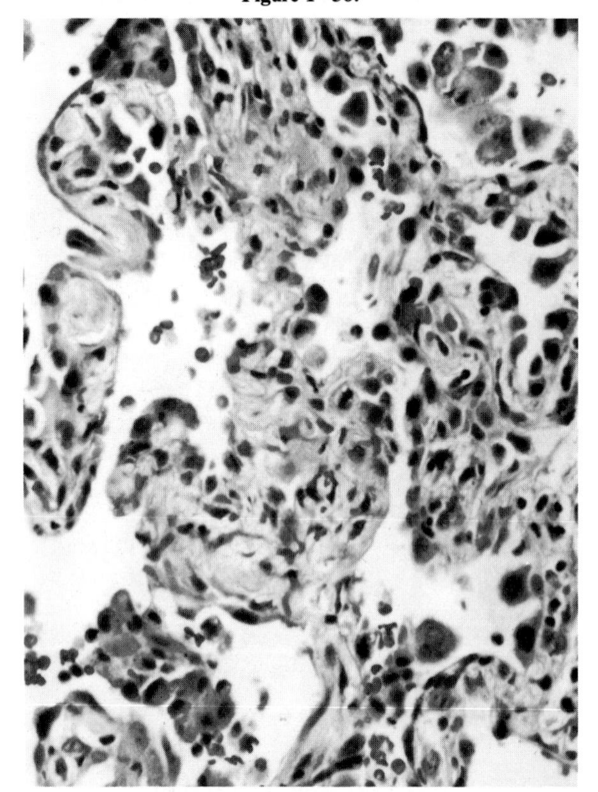

Figure 1-57.

Figures 1-56, 1-57. Diffuse alveolar damage in systemic lupus erythematosus (SLE) ("acute lupus pneumonitis"). There is diffuse interstitial edema with myxoid thickening of alveolar walls, accumulations of macrophages in airspaces (which may contain hemosiderin), and prominent type II cells.

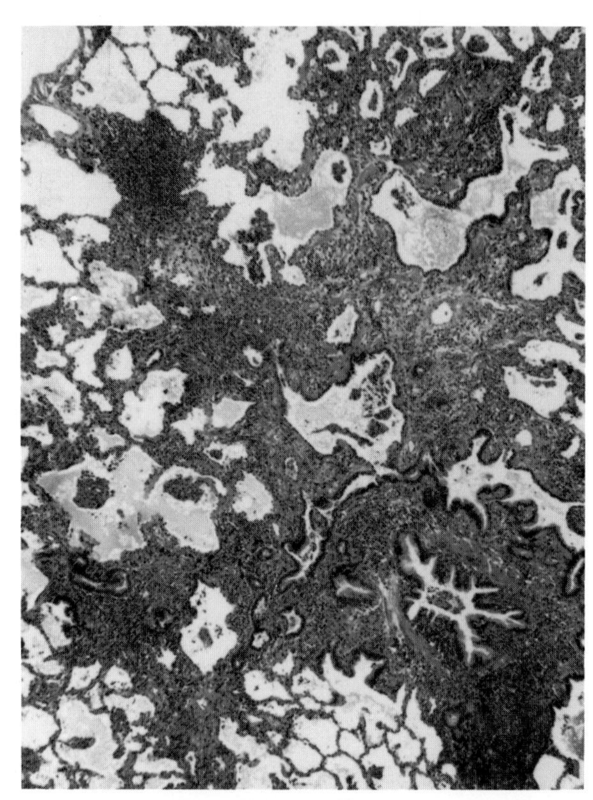

Figure 1-58.

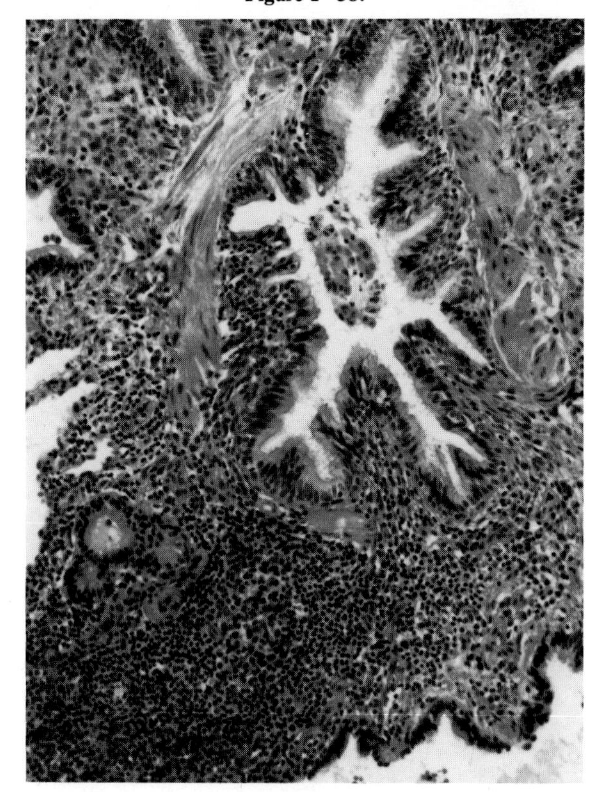

Figure 1-59.

Figures 1-58, 1-59. Lymphocytic interstitial pneumonia in systemic lupus erythematosus (SLE). Interstitial infiltrate, fibrosis, and lymphoid hyperplasia can be seen.

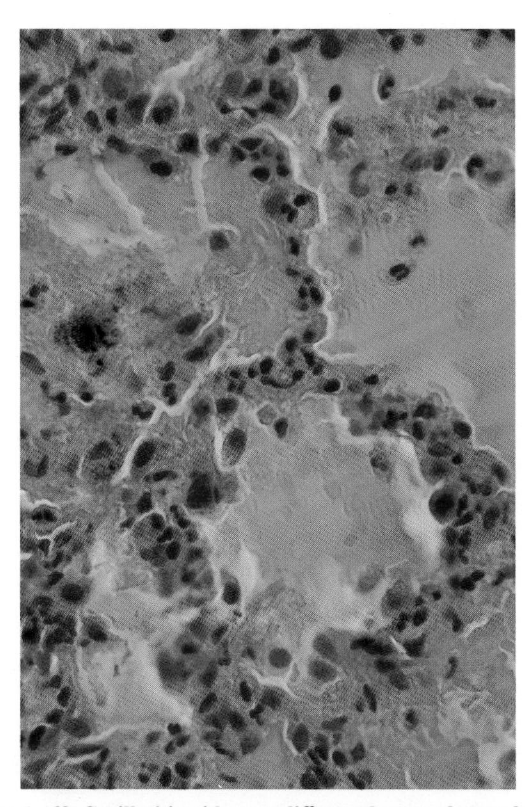

Figure 1–60. Capillaritis with acute diffuse pulmonary hemorrhage in systemic lupus erythematosus (SLE) ("acute lupus pneumonitis"). Large numbers of neutrophils fill the alveolar walls. The alveoli contain edema, red blood cells, and hemosiderin-filled macrophages. Immune complexes were present in the alveolar walls.

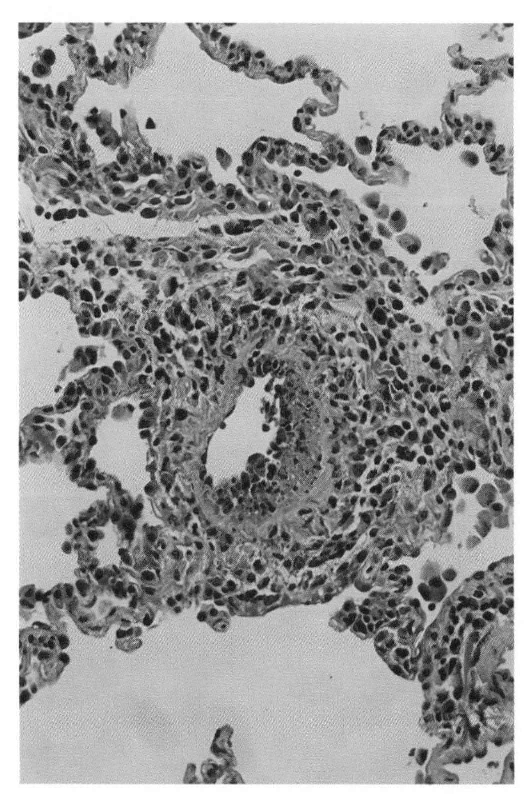

Figure 1–61. Necrotizing venulitis in systemic lupus erythematosus (SLE). This small vein is characterized by acute inflammation and fibrinoid necrosis of a portion of the wall.

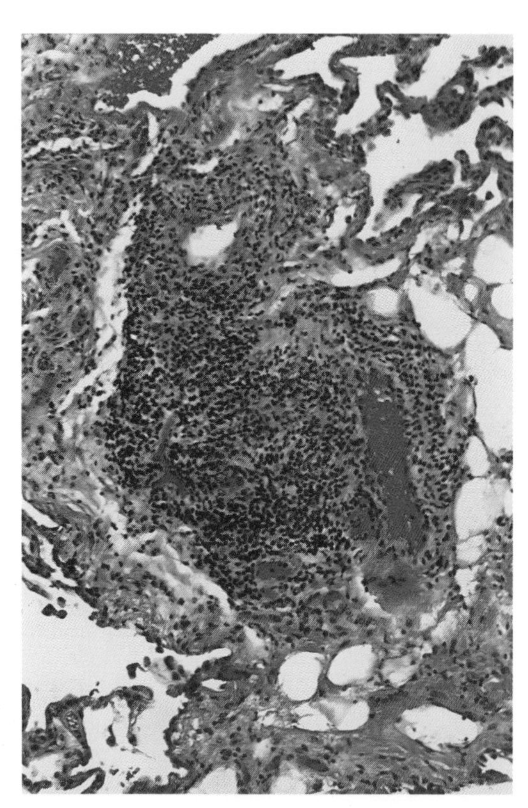

Figure 1–62. Lymphocytic vasculitis in systemic lupus erythematosus (SLE).

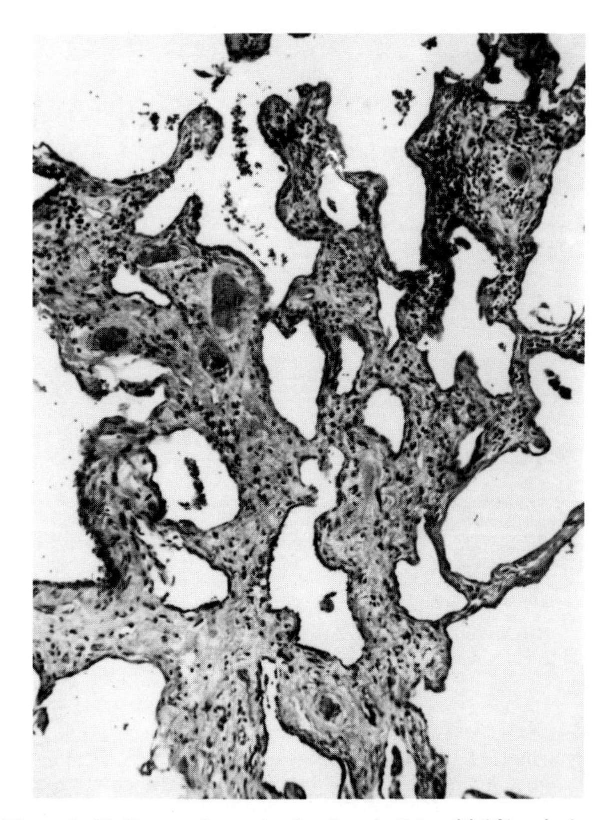

Figure 1–63. Progressive systemic sclerosis. Interstitial fibrosis shows a pattern similar to that of usual interstitial pneumonia.

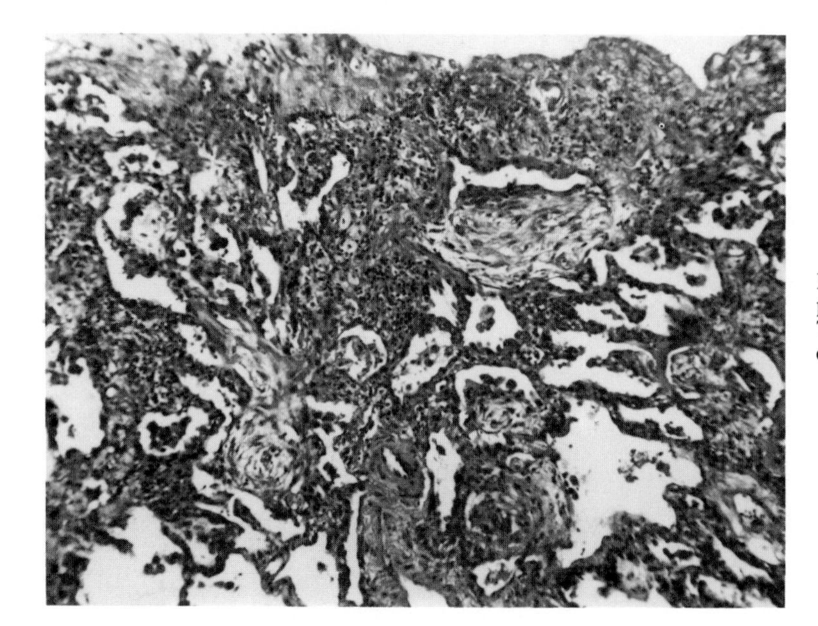

Figure 1-64. Progressive systemic sclerosis. There is a pattern of bronchiolitis obliterans organizing pneumonia. There is inflammation of alveolar walls, and organizing connective tissue is seen as tufts within the airspaces.

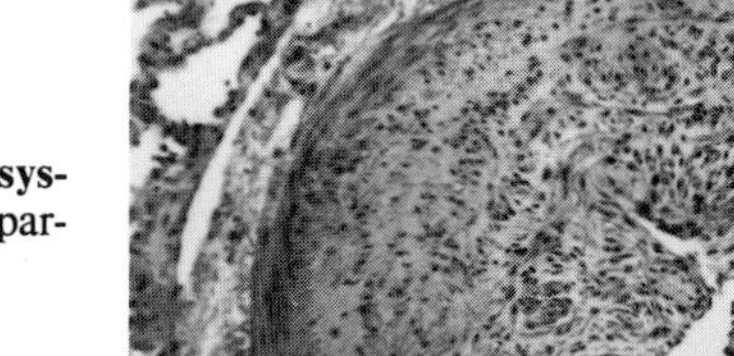

Figure 1-65. Pulmonary hypertension in progressive systemic sclerosis. Marked myointimal thickening is apparent.

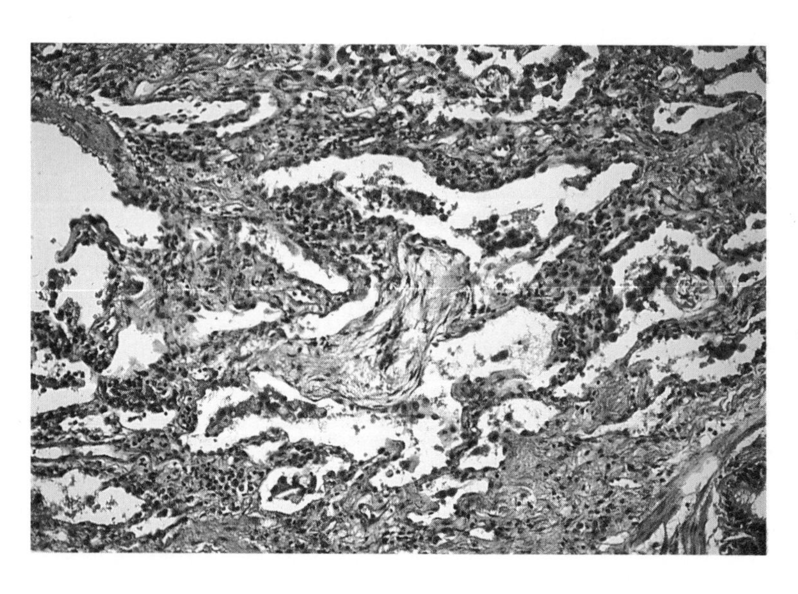

Figure 1-66. Bronchiolitis obliterans organizing pneumonia (BOOP) pattern in polymyositis. An alveolar duct contains a tuft of organizing tissue.

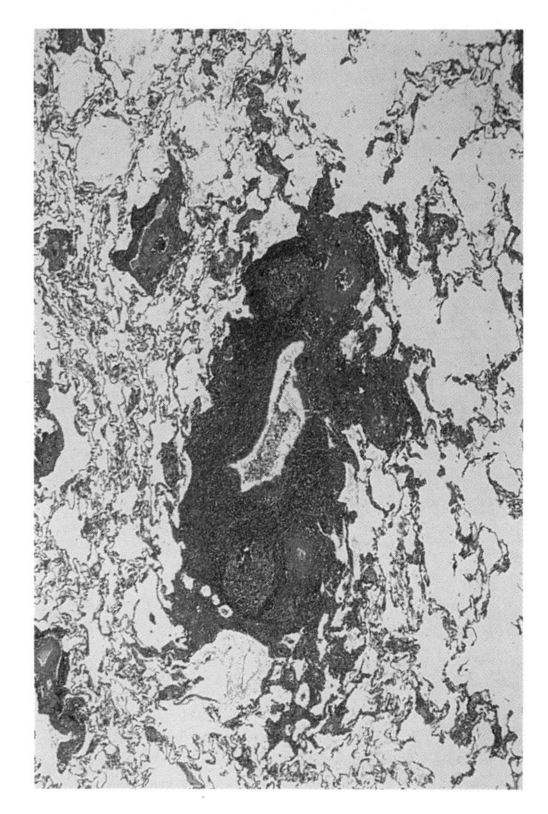

Figure 1-67. Sjögren's syndrome. Lymphoid hyperplasia and acute and chronic cellular bronchiolitis (follicular bronchiolitis) are seen.

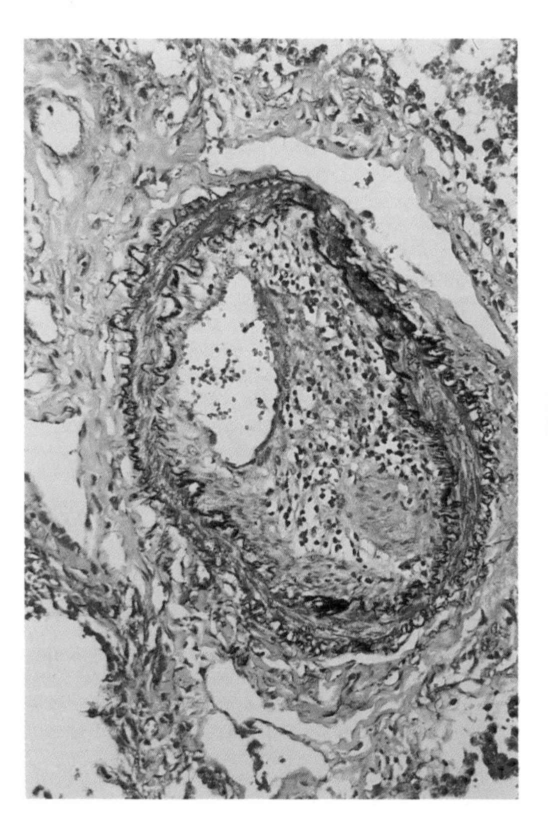

Figure 1-68. Behçet's syndrome. Mild lymphocytic vasculitis associated with a healed thrombus is shown. (Case courtesy of R. Slavin, M.D.)

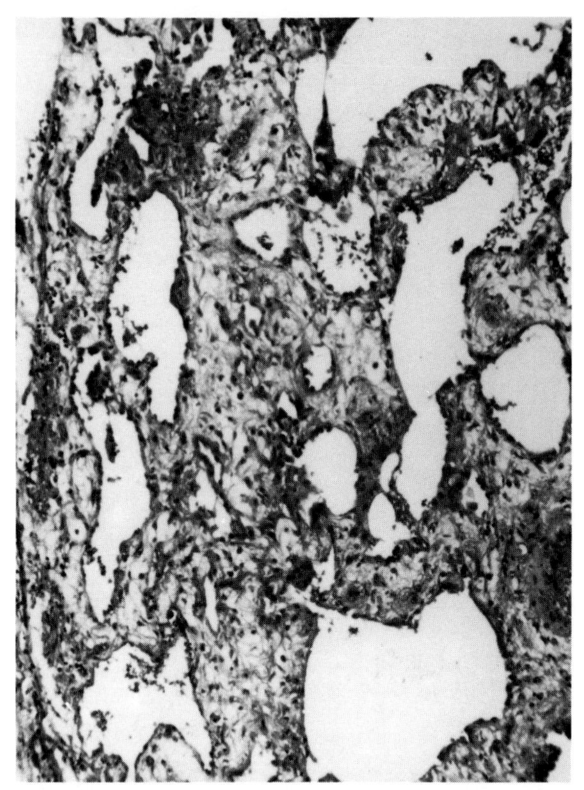

Figure 1-69. Bleomycin-associated alveolar damage. Diffuse alveolar damage is associated with bleomycin. There is marked edema of alveolar walls, a scant inflammatory infiltrate, and prominent type II alveolar lining cells. This histologic pattern is nonspecific and on clinical grounds was ascribed to bleomycin.

■ HISTOLOGIC FINDINGS IN PULMONARY DRUG REACTIONS (Figs. 1-69 to 1-92)

One can recognize three broad groups of drug reactions in the lung:

- Those that are toxic or dose-related
- Those that represent idiosyncratic or allergic reactions in susceptible individuals
- A large group of miscellaneous reactions, a few of which have specific histologic features

Toxic and dose-related reactions usually show the histologic features of diffuse alveolar damage in the early or organizing phases. Occasional cases are seen late in their evolution and have interstitial scarring and honeycombing, which may prove fatal.

Idiosyncratic and allergic reactions show a variety of patterns and are associated with an ever increasing list of drugs; therefore, a history of drug therapy is important in any diagnosis of lung disease, particularly interstitial lung disease. Among diffuse lung diseases, the following patterns may occur:

1. Bronchiolitis obliterans (proliferative or constrictive)
2. Bronchiolitis obliterans organizing pneumonia (BOOP)-like pattern
3. Nonspecific cellular interstitial infiltrates
4. Granulomatous interstitial pneumonia (microgranulomatosis; may resemble extrinsic allergic alveolitis)
5. Eosinophilic pneumonia
6. Usual interstitial pneumonia (UIP)
7. Desquamative interstitial pneumonia (DIP)
8. Lymphocytic interstitial pneumonia (LIP)
9. Vasculitis (predominantly hypersensitivity angiitis of small vessels)
10. Mixtures and combinations of the above

Miscellaneous reactions associated with drugs include the following:

1. Pulmonary edema
2. Alveolar hemorrhage
3. Histiocytic infiltrates and phospholipidosis (amiodarone)
4. Metastatic calcification
5. Asthma
6. Foreign body giant cell reaction (IV [intravenous] talcosis)
7. Pulmonary hypertension
8. Pleuritis (including SLE-like syndromes)
9. Veno-occlusive disease

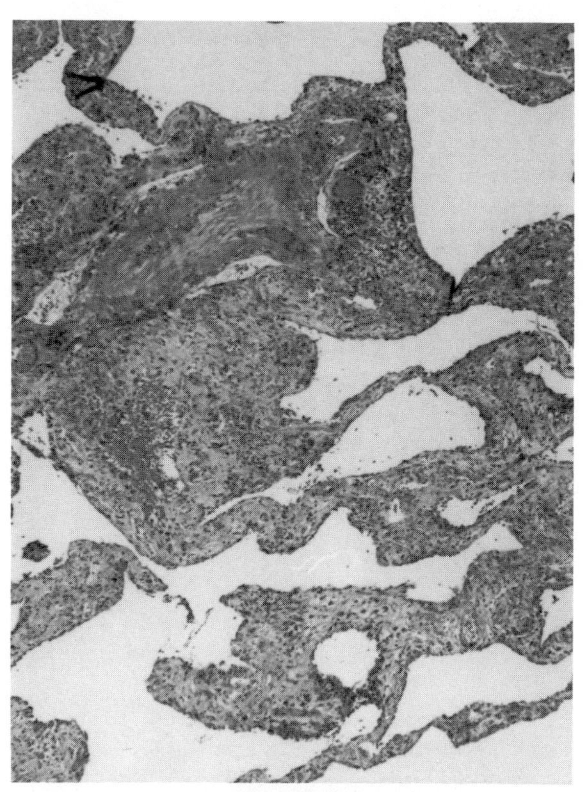

Figure 1-70.

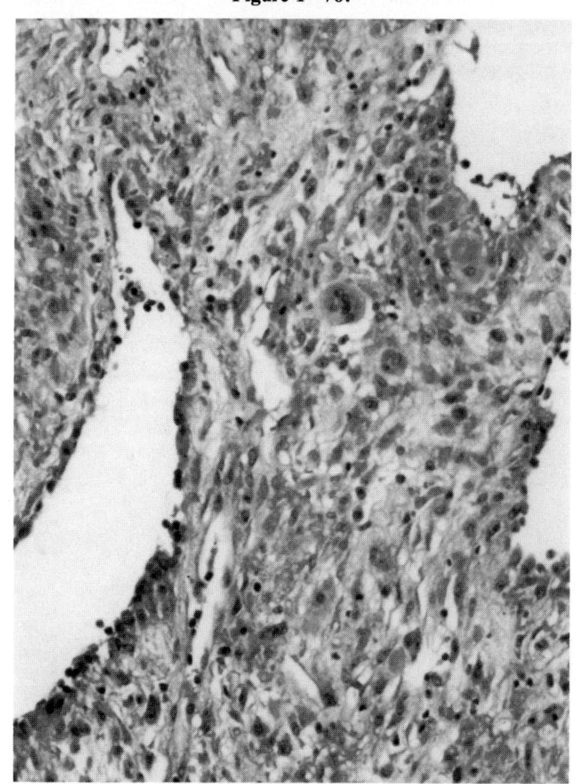

Figure 1-71.

References

Cooper JAD, White DA, Mathay RA. Drug-induced pulmonary disease (Parts 1 and 2). Am Rev Respir Dis 133:321-338; 133:488-502, 1986.

Dail DH, Hammer SP (eds). Pulmonary Pathology. New York, Springer-Verlag, 1988.

Kilburn KH. Pulmonary disease induced by drugs. *In* Fishman AP (ed). Pulmonary Diseases and Disorders. New York, McGraw-Hill, 1980, pp 707-724.

Lombard CL, Churg A, Winokur S. Pulmonary veno-occlusive disease following therapy for malignant neoplasms. Chest 92:871-876, 1987.

Thurlbeck WM (ed). Pathology of the Lung. New York, Thieme, 1988.

Whimster WF, DePoitiers W. The lung. *In* Riddell RH (ed). Pathology of Drug-induced and Toxic Diseases. New York, Churchill Livingstone, 1982, pp 167-200.

Text continued on page 44

Figures 1-70, 1-71. Paraquat pulmonary toxicity. An open lung biopsy specimen shows markedly destructive acute diffuse alveolar damage that could be descriptively termed acute honeycombing. Tissue analysis at autopsy confirmed the presence of paraquat, which was presumed to have been ingested in a suicide attempt. Rapid destruction of lung parenchyma with a hemorrhagic diffuse alveolar damage may be seen in paraquat toxicity. Another well-recognized pattern in paraquat toxicity is edematous fibrosis of alveolar spaces with preservation of alveolar walls.

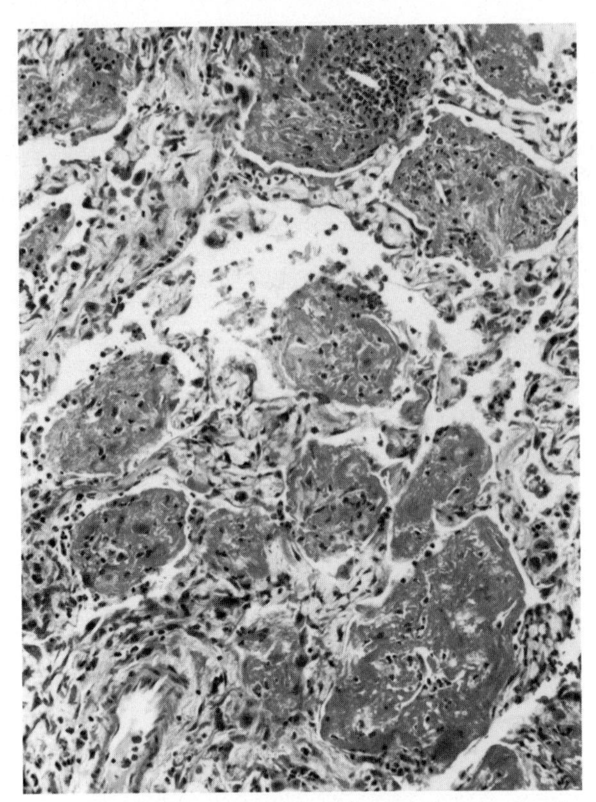

Figure 1–72. Busulfan pneumonitis. This relatively acute case shows acute fibrinous exudate within the airspaces, which are lined by edematous alveolar walls with prominent type II cells.

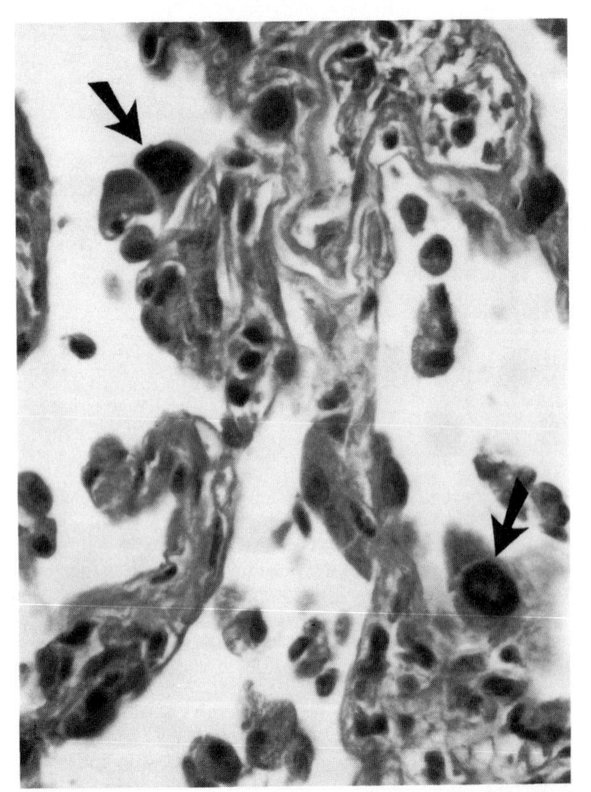

Figure 1–73. Busulfan pneumonitis. A case that evolved somewhat later than the one in Figure 1–72 shows bizarre hyperchromatic type II cells (arrows).

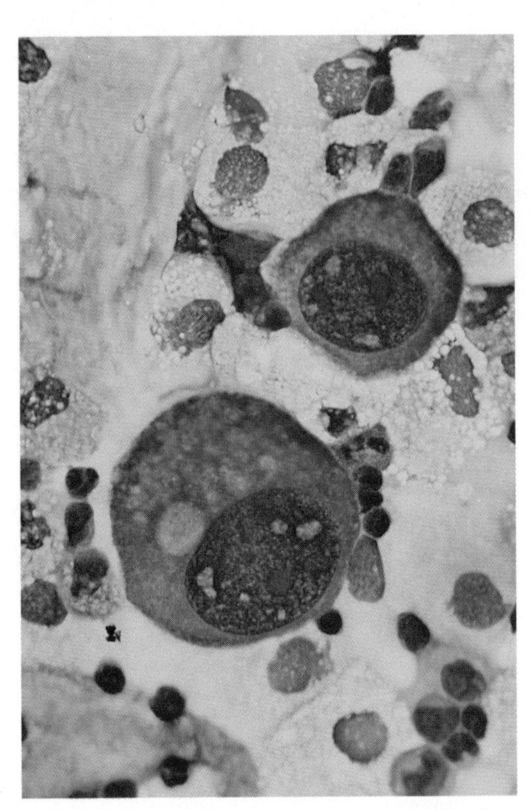

Figure 1–74. Atypical cells from cytotoxic drug reaction. Bronchoalveolar lavage from a patient with a cytotoxic drug reaction is shown. Large bizarre cells (presumed to be type II cells) can be seen in the cytospin preparation of the lavage fluid.

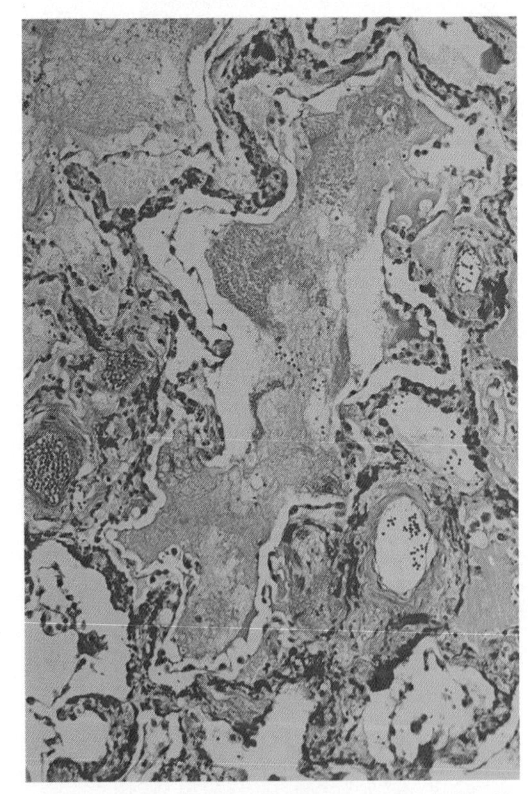

Figure 1–75. Cytosine arabinoside therapy–associated effect. The dense eosinophilic material resembling pulmonary edema in this case was ascribed to cytosine arabinoside therapy.

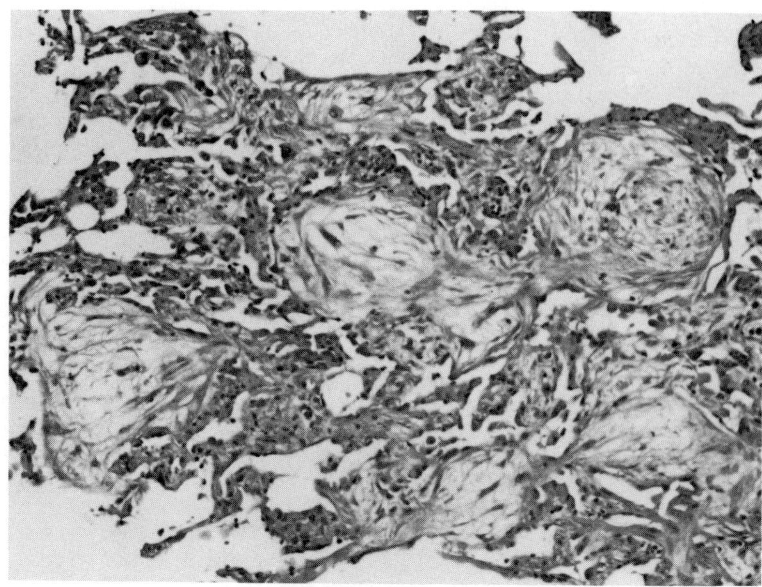

Figures 1–76, 1–77. Methotrexate pneumonitis. There are foci of nonspecific organization (Fig. 1–76) as well as foci of interstitial cellular infiltrate and airspace accumulations of fibrin and histiocytes (Fig. 1–77). The diagnosis of methotrexate pneumonitis was made by clinicopathologic correlation.

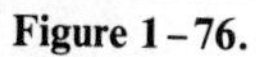

Figure 1–76.

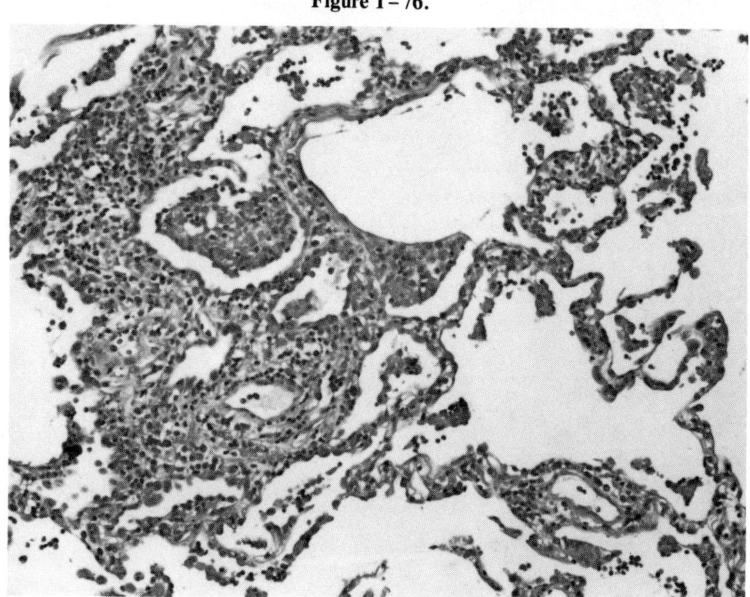

Figure 1–77.

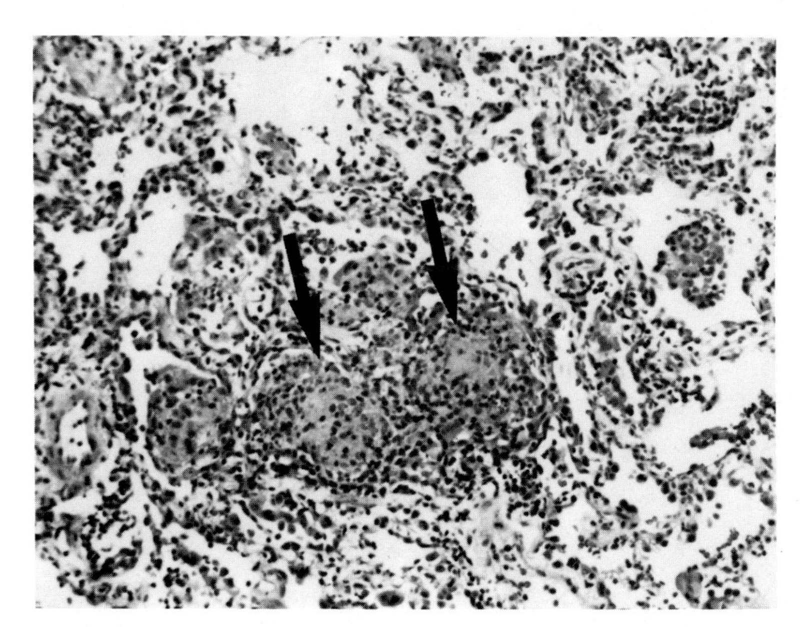

Figure 1–78. Methotrexate pneumonitis. There are patchy interstitial and airspace cellular infiltrates. A few small structures composed of epithelioid histiocytes (arrows) were considered to be small granulomas, which are seen in one third to one half of all cases of methotrexate pneumonitis.

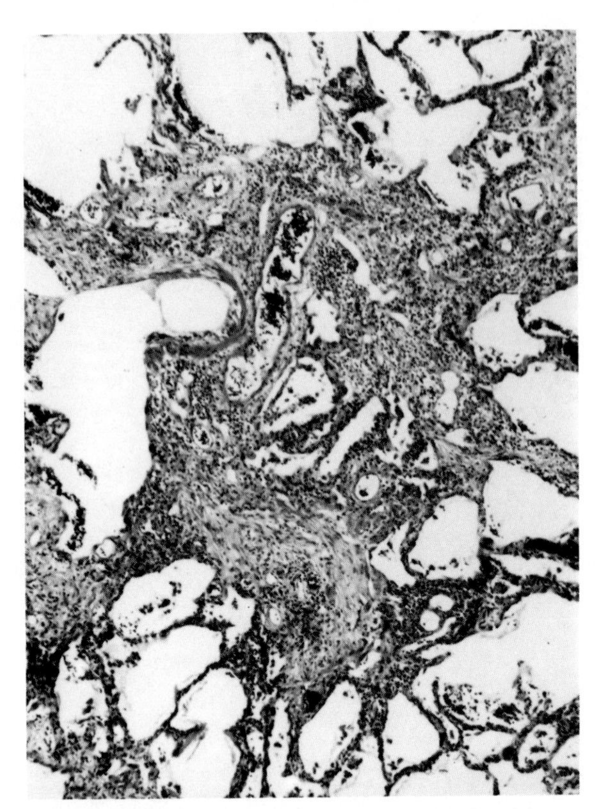

Figure 1-79. Methotrexate pneumonitis. This case is somewhat later in its evolution than those illustrated in Figures 1-76 to 1-78. There has been some incorporation of the organization into the interstitium with interstitial scarring and architectural distortion. The histologic features are nonspecific, and the diagnosis of methotrexate pneumonitis was made by clinicopathologic correlation.

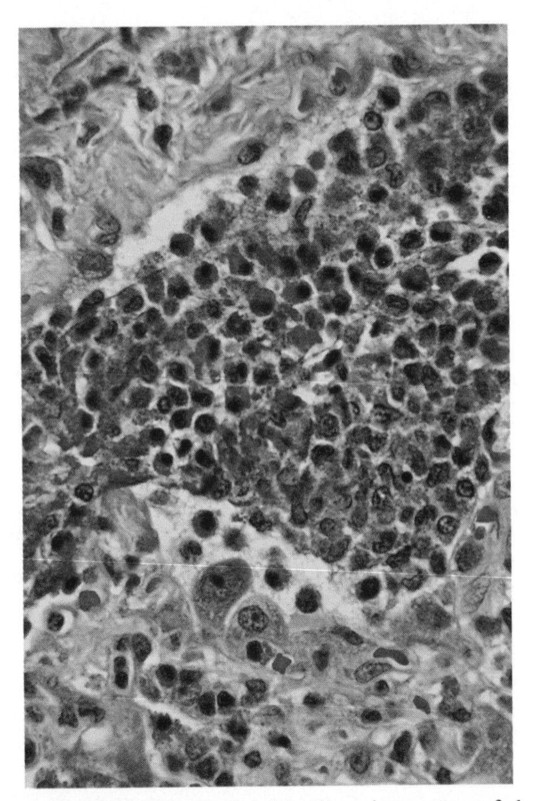

Figure 1-80. Bleomycin pneumonitis. There is a pattern of chronic eosinophilic pneumonia, probably an idiosyncratic reaction to the bleomycin. There are zones of airspace consolidation by histiocytes and clusters of eosinophils.

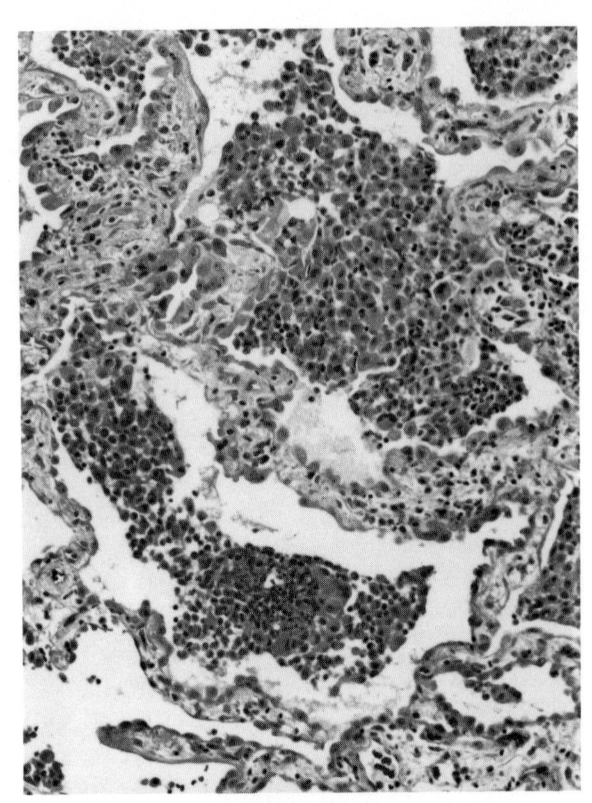

Figure 1-81.

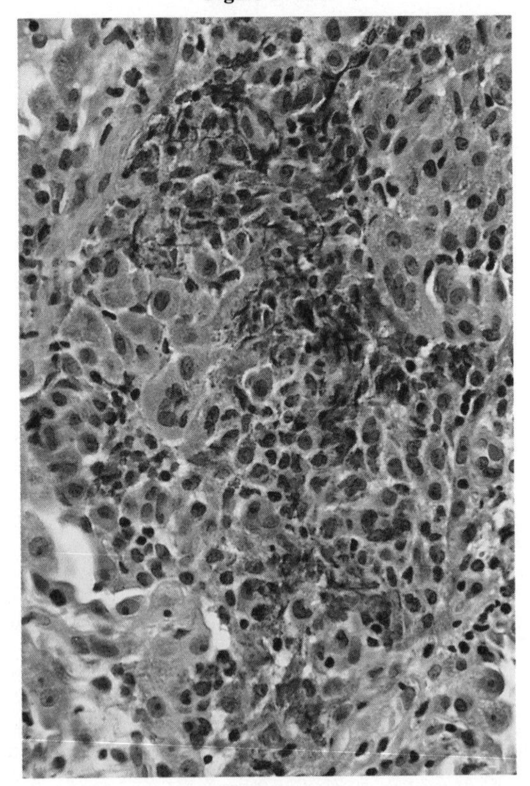

Figure 1-82.

Figures 1-81, 1-82. Procarbazine-associated pneumonitis. Chronic eosinophilic pneumonia ascribed to procarbazine therapy is shown. The open lung biopsy findings showed patchy airspace consolidation by histiocytes with clusters of eosinophils. Metaplasia of the alveolar lining cells is prominent.

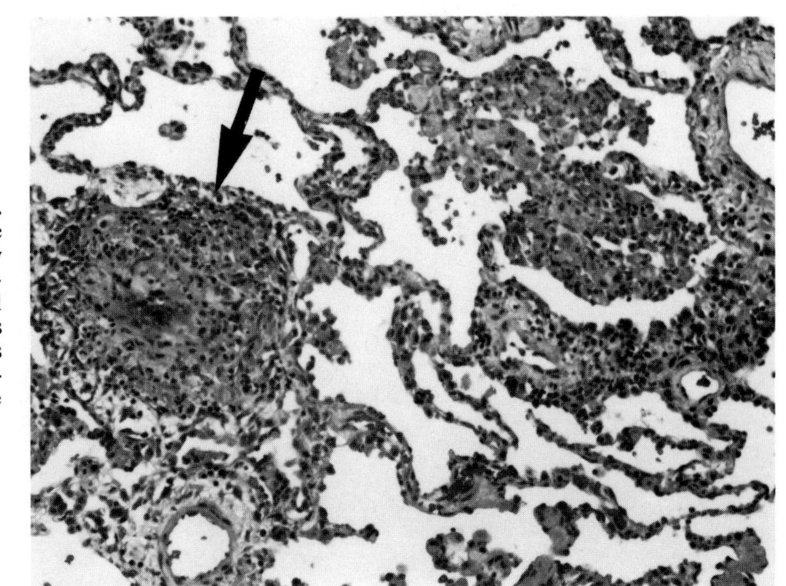

Figure 1-83. Drug-induced granulomatous pneumonitis. Acute diffuse pulmonary infiltrates developed some months after heart transplantation. Open lung biopsy findings show an interstitial pneumonia with chronic inflammatory infiltrates of alveolar walls and occasional small non-necrotizing granulomas (arrow). A rigorous search for an infection was negative. The pneumonitis cleared dramatically with steroid therapy. A drug was implicated by exclusion, although no specific drug could be named.

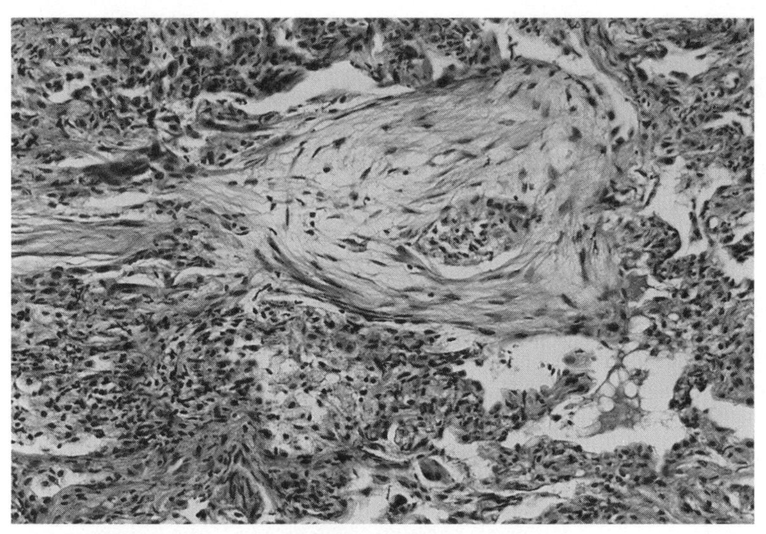

Figure 1-84.

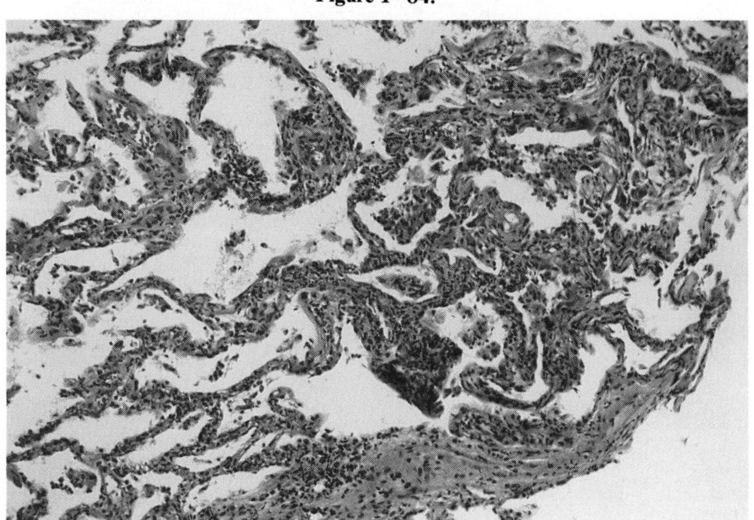

Figure 1-85.

Figures 1-84, 1-85. Nitrofurantoin pneumonitis. Transbronchial biopsy findings show foci of interstitial mononuclear cell infiltrate and airspace organization. The diagnosis of nitrofurantoin toxicity was made on the basis of clinicopathologic correlation. These histologic features are nonspecific.

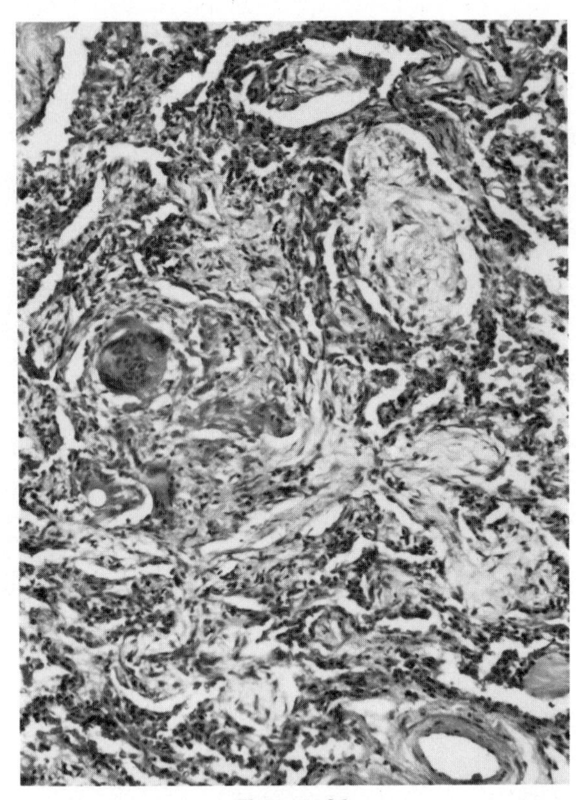

Figure 1-86.

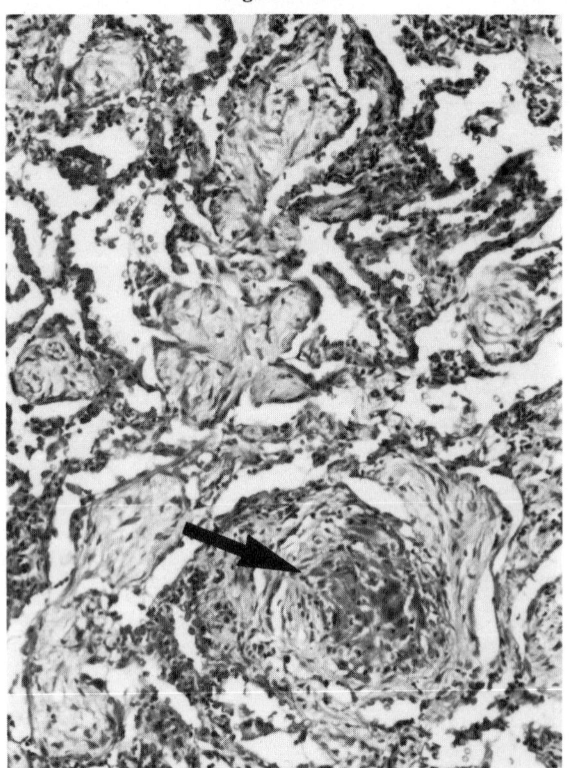

Figure 1-87.

Figures 1-86, 1-87. Chlorambucil pneumonitis. This patient was receiving chlorambucil for rheumatoid arthritis, and acute diffuse pulmonary infiltrates developed. Open lung biopsy findings showed extensive organization with granulomas (arrow) and giant cells within the tufts of organization. The chlorambucil was discontinued, steroid therapy was initiated, and the patient's pulmonary disease cleared entirely. On the basis of clinicopathologic correlation, chlorambucil was implicated.

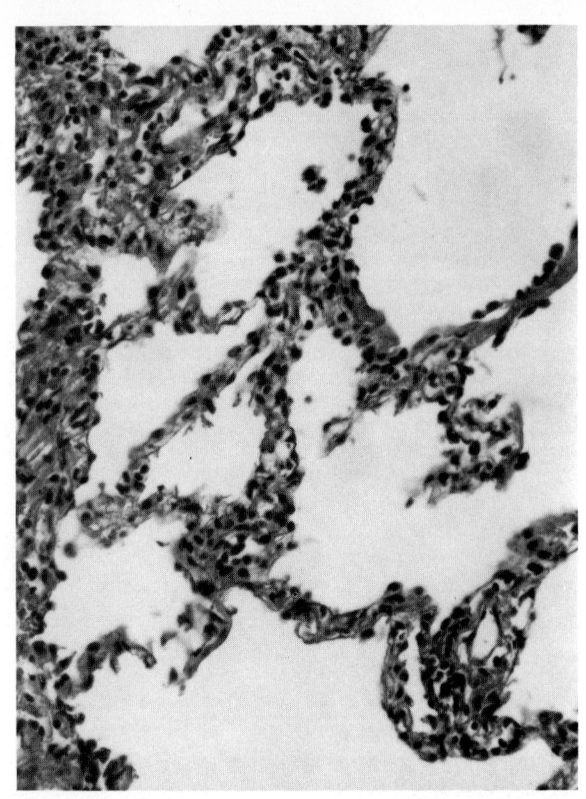

Figure 1-88. Gold pneumonitis. Transbronchial biopsy findings show a nonspecific interstitial infiltrate of chronic inflammatory cells. Gold therapy was implicated on the basis of clinicopathologic correlation.

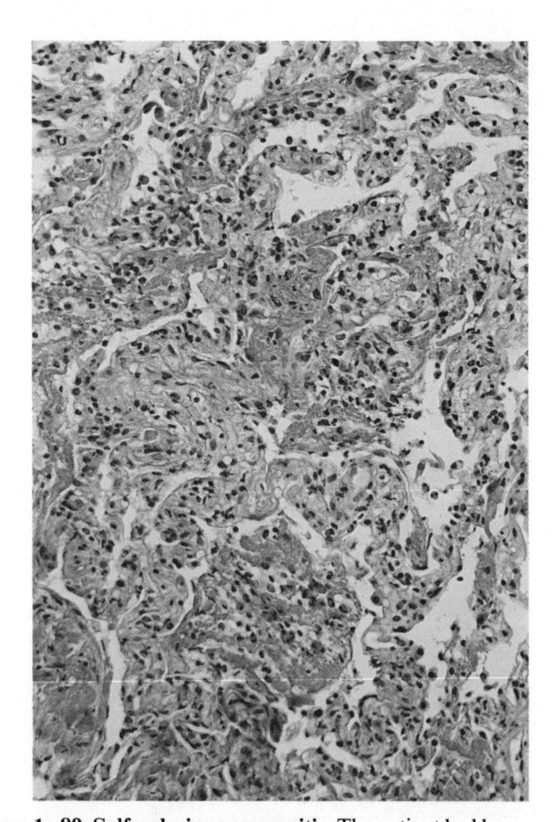

Figure 1-89. Sulfasalazine pneumonitis. The patient had been receiving sulfasalazine for chronic inflammatory bowel disease, and pulmonary infiltrates with peripheral eosinophilia developed. Transbronchial biopsy findings show airspace accumulations of fibrin, histiocytes, and numerous eosinophils. The pattern suggests acute eosinophilic pneumonia, and the drug was implicated by clinicopathologic correlation.

Figures 1–90, 1–91, 1–92. Amiodarone toxicity. There is interstitial inflammation, metaplasia of type II alveolar lining cells, and increased accumulations of histiocytes in the airspaces. The histiocytes in amiodarone toxicity have the appearance of an acquired phospholipidosis with cytoplasmic vacuoles of varying sizes. The pattern is not specific, but any interstitial pneumonia with large numbers of foamy histiocytes in the airspaces that cannot be explained on the basis of obstruction should raise the possibility of amiodarone toxicity.

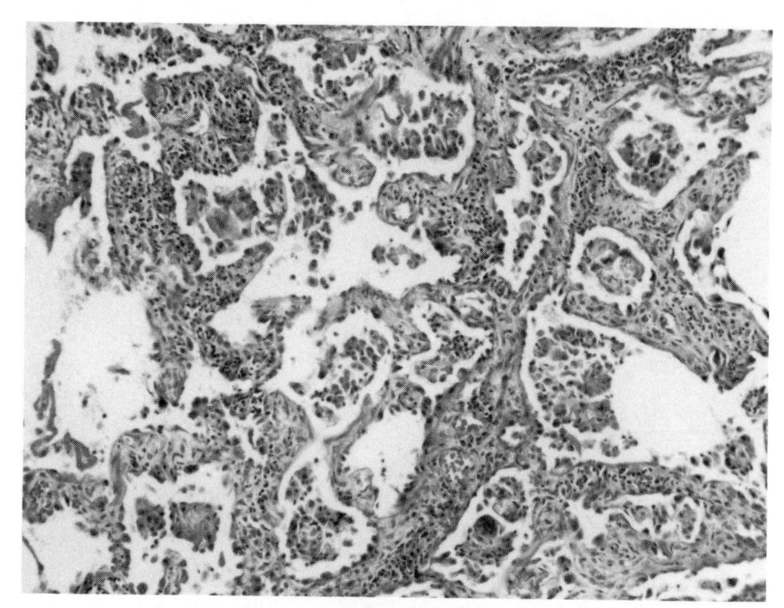

Figure 1–90.

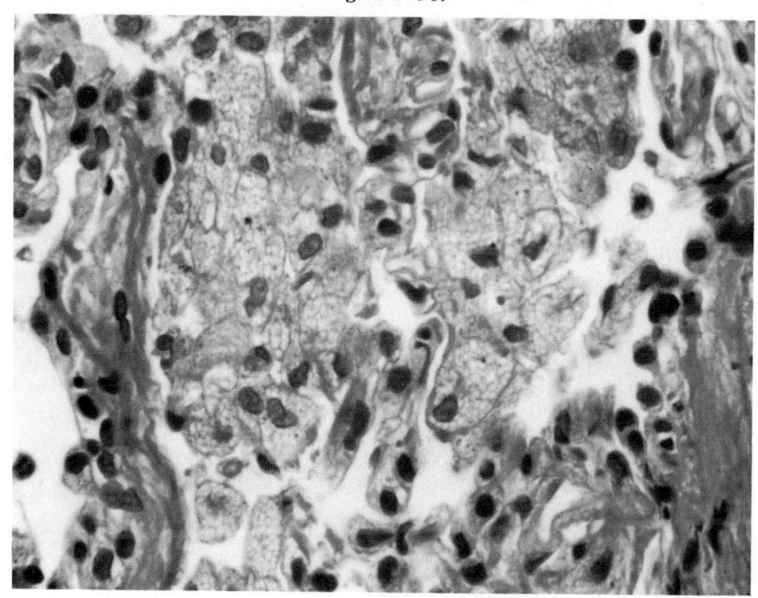

Figure 1–91.

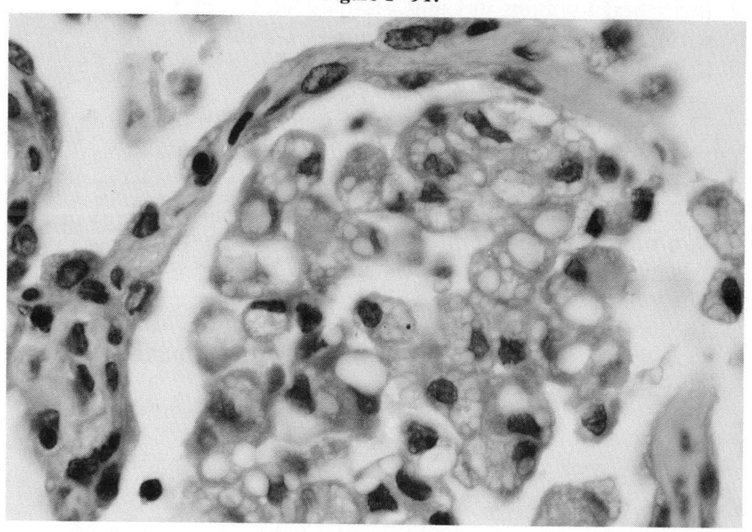

Figure 1–92.

■ HISTOLOGIC FINDINGS IN PATIENTS KNOWN TO HAVE OBSTRUCTIVE LUNG DISEASE

■ Lung Biopsy for the Diagnosis of Obstructive Lung Disease

In obstructive lung disease, one clearly looks for disease in the airways and less often in the alveolar parenchyma. Usually the changes will fall into one of the following groups.

Large Airway Lesions

These lesions include obstructing tumors, tracheobronchial amyloid, chondromalacia, tracheobronchopathia osteoplastica, and so on.

Inflammatory and/or Fibrotic Changes in the Small Airways

Either chronic inflammation or acute and chronic inflammation with or without fibrosis of the airway wall may be seen in airway infections, chronic obstructive pulmonary disease (COPD), bronchiectasis, cystic fibrosis, aspiration, primary and acquired immunodeficiency states, diffuse panbronchiolitis, and idiopathic small airway injury. Sarcoidosis is occasionally associated with airflow obstruction.

Parenchymal Abnormalities

Emphysema, eosinophilic granuloma, and lymphangiomyomatosis may be associated with severe airflow obstruction. The parenchymal changes overshadow the airway changes. In nonsmokers with severe emphysema, $alpha_1$-antitrypsin deficiency should be considered.

■ Incidental Findings in Lung Tissue from Patients with Chronic Obstructive Pulmonary Disease (Chronic Bronchitis and Emphysema)

The changes described below are usually seen in tissue removed for some other problem, often a carcinoma.

1. Pleural blebs, bullae, focal scarring
2. Parenchymal emphysema; anthracosis often prominent; some interstitial scarring, relatively acellular, may be present; increased alveolar macrophages
3. Small airway stenosis, dilation, inflammation, mucostasis, goblet cell metaplasia, basement membrane thickening
4. Large airway inflammation, bronchial submucosal gland hypertrophy, goblet cell metaplasia, basement membrane thickening
5. Pulmonary arteries mildly thickened from chronic hypoxia

■ PULMONARY HISTOLOGIC CHANGES IN PATIENTS WITH INFLAMMATORY BOWEL DISEASE

A number of pulmonary conditions have been described in association with chronic ulcerative colitis. The most common of these has been chronic airway disease, although all are relatively uncommon. The following is a summary of the literature modified from Desai and co-workers and from Prakash.

■ Airway-Associated Diseases

1. Bronchiectasis
2. Bronchitis
3. Sclerosing tracheobronchitis
4. Sclerosing bronchiolitis (presumably constrictive bronchiolitis)
5. Diffuse panbronchiolitis
6. Asthma

■ Pulmonary Vascular Disease

1. Vasculitis
2. Emboli
3. Edema

■ Parenchymal Interstitial Disease

1. Interstitial fibrosis (e.g., UIP, DIP)
2. Apical pulmonary fibrosis
3. Bullous disease

■ Pleural Diseases

Effusion (with or without pericardial effusion) may be apparent.

■ Drug Reaction

May occur, especially with sulfasalazine.

References

Desai SJ, Gephardt GN, Stoller JK. Diffuse panbronchiolitis preceding ulcerative colitis. Chest 45:1342–1344, 1989.
Prakash UBS. Pulmonary manifestations of systemic diseases. *In* Baum GL, Wolinsky E (eds). Textbook of Pulmonary Disease. Boston, Little, Brown & Co, 1989.

■ DIAGNOSTIC CONSIDERATIONS IN PATIENTS WITH PULMONARY RENAL SYNDROMES

1. Goodpasture's disease (antiglomerular basement antibody disease)
2. Wegener's granulomatosis
3. Churg-Strauss syndrome
4. Polyarteritis nodosa
5. Systemic lupus erythematosus
6. Henoch-Schönlein purpura
7. Hemolytic-uremic syndrome
8. Scleroderma
9. Rheumatoid arthritis
10. Mixed connective tissue disease
11. Drug reactions
12. Giant cell arteritis
13. Hypocomplementemic urticarial vasculitis
14. Idiopathic rapidly progressive glomerulonephritis
15. Essential mixed cryoglobulinemia
16. Unclassified (with or without immune complexes)

References

Prakash UBS. Pulmonary manifestations of systemic diseases. *In* Baum GL, Wolinsky E (eds). Textbook of Pulmonary Disease. Boston, Little, Brown & Co, 1989.

CHAPTER 2

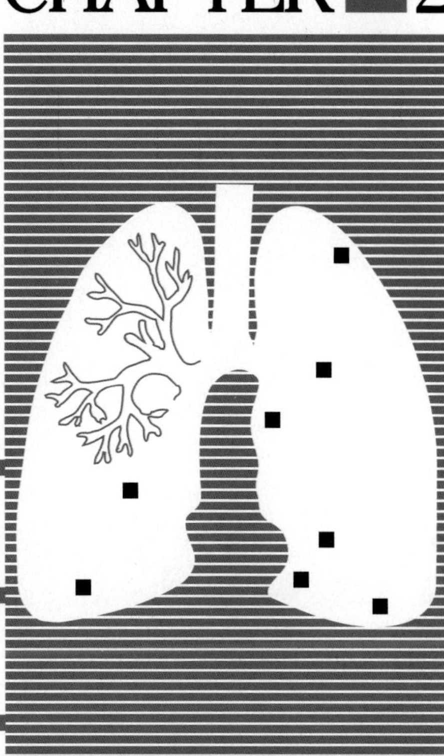

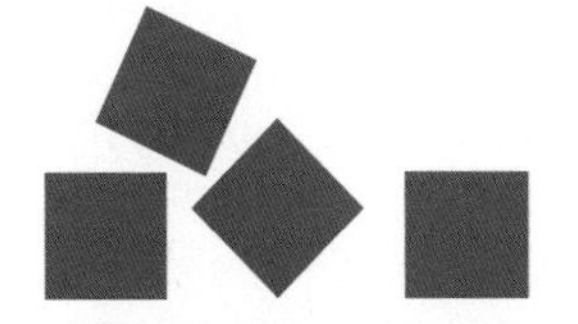

ANOMALIES, CYSTS, PEDIATRIC LESIONS

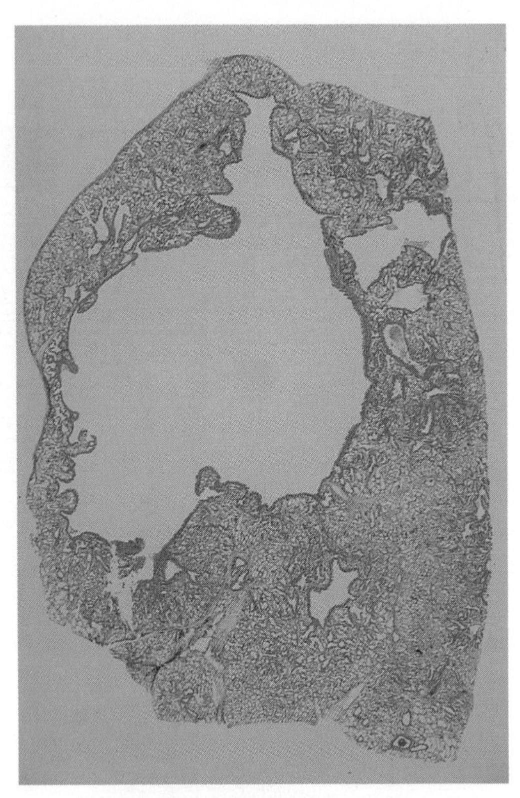

Figure 2–1. Cystic adenomatoid malformation. Irregular cysts and abnormal architecture are apparent.

■ Cystic Adenomatoid Malformation (Figs. 2–1 to 2–4)

A cystic adenomatoid malformation is architecturally abnormal (hamartomatous) immature lung tissue that presents as a mass or a cystic lesion, usually in a neonate (rarely in adults). It often communicates with airways, and the tissue is aerated. Most patients with cystic adenomatoid malformation present with respiratory distress and with a mass or cystic lesion on a chest radiograph. Other congenital anomalies, especially cardiac and genitourinary anomalies, may be present.

Histologic pattern includes malformed lung parenchyma with alveolar-like spaces lined by cuboidal, and occasionally mucinous, cells and scattered bronchiole-like structures, but without normal pulmonary architecture. Large cysts may be present. The lesion may merge imperceptibly with normal lung tissue at its edge. Cartilage and skeletal muscle may be seen. Occasionally, the lesions become superinfected. Stocker and colleagues recognize three subtypes that have clinical and pathologic differences.

Some cystic adenomatoid malformations may be quite subtle histologically. It is useful to know the clinical history and whether a mass or cystic lesion was identified radiographically. Gross visualization may also be helpful in that the cystic or mass character of the lesion can be appreciated. Cystic sarcomas may mimic a cystic adenomatoid malformation.

References

Avitabile AM, et al. Congenital cystic adenomatoid malformation of the lung in adults. Am J Surg Pathol 8:193, 1984.

Buntain WL, Isaacs H, Payne VC, et al. Lobar emphysema, cystic adenomatoid malformation, pulmonary sequestration, and bronchogenic cyst in infancy and childhood, a clinical group. J Pediatr Surg 9:85, 1974.

Carter D, Eggleston JC. Tumors of the Lower Respiratory Tract. AFIP Atlas of Tumor Pathology, Second Series, Fascicle 17. Washington DC, Armed Forces Institute of Pathology, 1980.

Dail DH, Hammer SP (eds). Pulmonary Pathology. New York, Springer-Verlag, 1988.

Katzenstein A-LA, Askin FB. Surgical Pathology of Non-neoplastic Lung Disease, 2nd ed. Philadelphia, WB Saunders Co, 1990.

Landing BH, Dixon LG. Congenital malformations and genetic disorders of the respiratory tract (larynx, trachea, bronchi, and lungs). Am Rev Respir Dis 120:151, 1979.

Miller RK, Sieber WK, Yunis EJ. Congenital adenomatoid malformation of the lung. Part 1. Pathol Annu 15:387, 1980.

Stocker JT, Drake RM, Madewell JE. Cystic and congenital lung disease in the newborn. Perspect Pediatr Pathol 4:93–154, 1978.

Thurlbeck WM (ed). Pathology of the Lung. New York, Thieme, 1988.

Figures 2-2, 2-3. Cystic adenomatoid malformation. Dilated, almost normal-appearing bronchiolar structures are present; an accompanying pulmonary artery is absent. The surrounding airspaces are abnormal but resemble immature alveoli. Papillary epithelial proliferation is apparent in one of the larger cysts. Abnormal airspaces are lined by cuboidal or columnar epithelium with focal mucinous differentiation manifested by pale goblet cells with abundant mucinous cytoplasm.

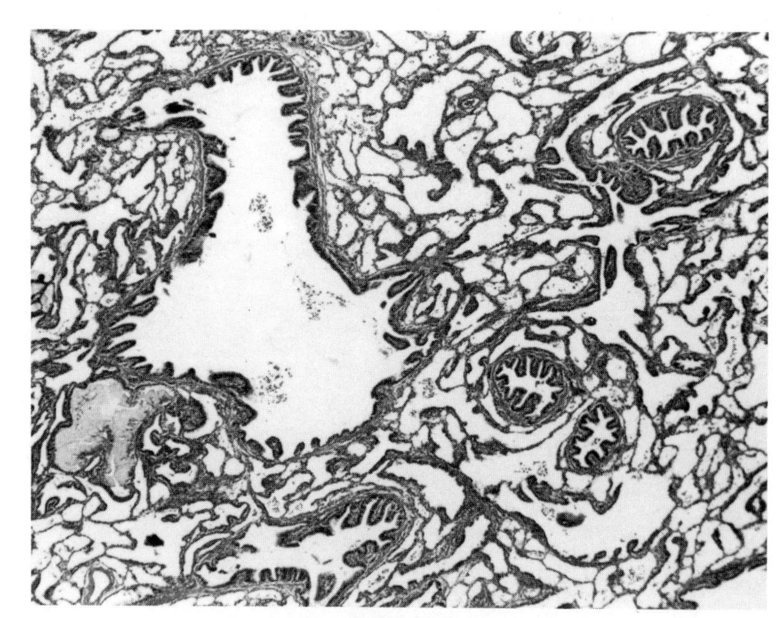

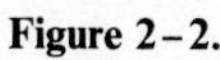

Figure 2-2.

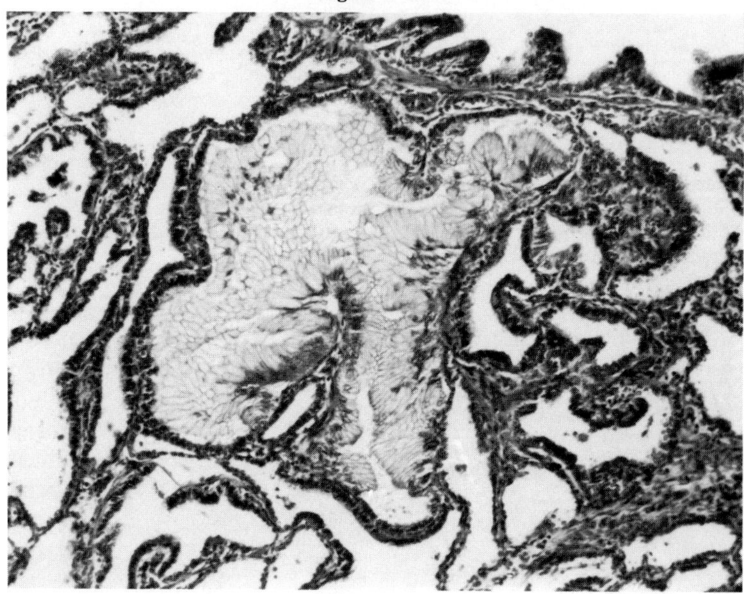

Figure 2-3.

Figure 2-4. Cystic adenomatoid malformation. The lesion is well demarcated from the surrounding compressed lung tissue. The airspaces are irregular in shape and enlarged, with walls that appear thickened compared with those of adjacent normal alveoli.

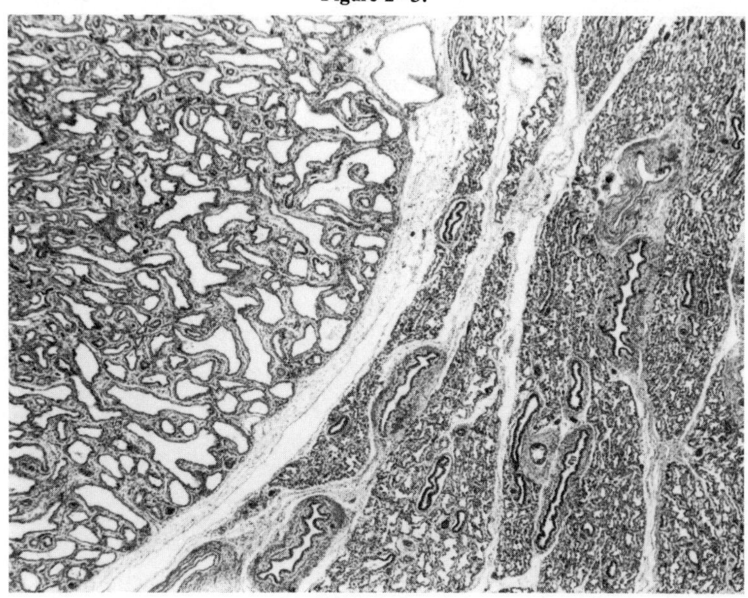

Figure 2-4.

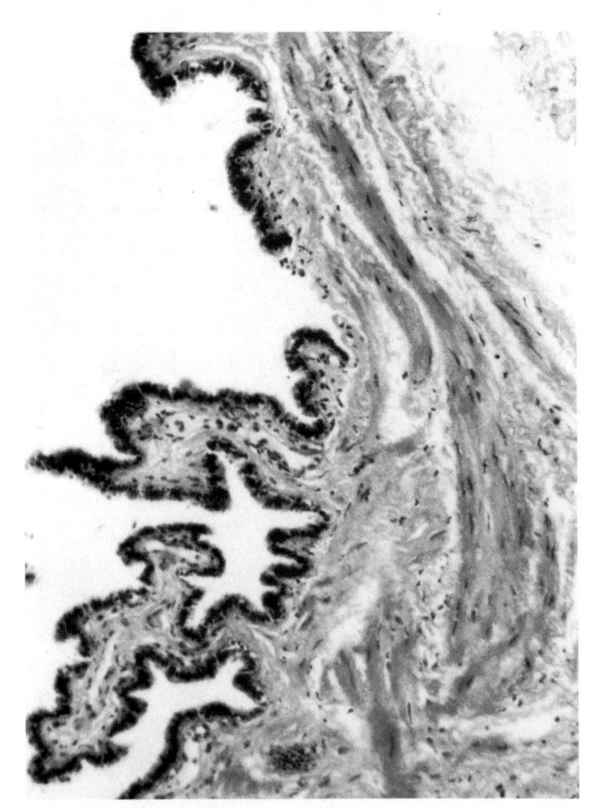

Figure 2-5. Bronchogenic cyst. This cyst is lined by bronchiolar epithelium with a surrounding layer of smooth muscle. Islands of cartilage were absent from the wall in this cyst, which was obtained from a patient with coexisting lymphangioleiomyomatosis.

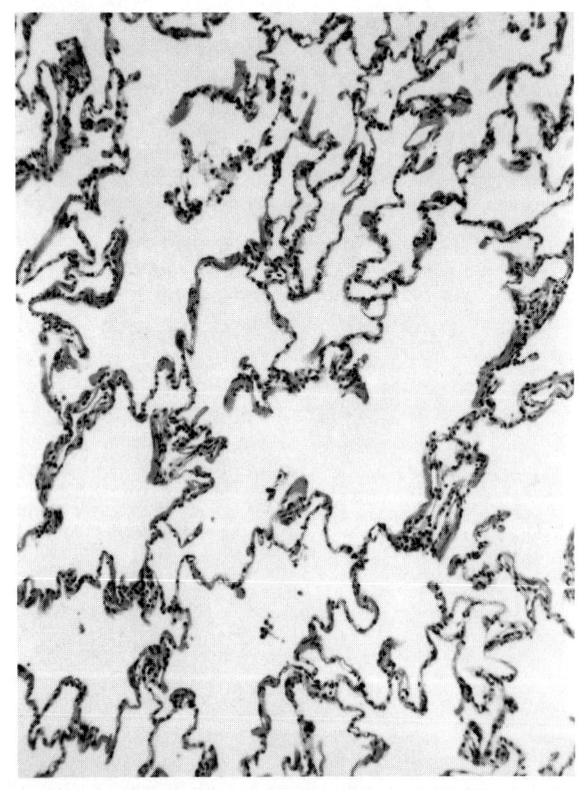

Figure 2-6. Infantile lobar emphysema. The histologic appearance is normal except for the size of the airspaces and their relative hypocellularity compared with the usually small and hypercellular-appearing alveoli seen in infants.

■ Bronchogenic Cyst (Fig. 2-5)

Midline cysts from malformation of the developing tracheobronchial tree are often in a middle or anterior mediastinal or subcarinal location. They may involve the neck and sternal tissues as well.

Histologically, there is a cystic lesion, usually unilocular, lined at least in part by ciliated columnar epithelium, although other metaplastic epithelia may be present. Smooth muscle and islands of cartilage are present in the wall. Multiple sections and careful gross examination may be required to find the islands of cartilage.

Bronchogenic cysts should be distinguished from cystic bronchiectasis, intralobar sequestration, and bronchial atresia. Lack of cartilage and smooth muscle is typical of nonspecific foregut cysts.

References

Dail DH, Hammer SP (eds). Pulmonary Pathology. New York, Springer-Verlag, 1988.

Ramenovsky ML, Leape LL, McCauley RGK. Bronchogenic cyst. J Pediatr Surg 14:219-224, 1979.

Thurlbeck WM (ed). Pathology of the Lung. New York, Thieme, 1988.

■ Infantile Lobar Emphysema (Lobar Hyperinflation) (Fig. 2-6)

Infantile lobar emphysema represents hyperinflation of a segment or a lobe with normal numbers and configuration of alveoli. Distinction from bronchial atresia may be difficult and somewhat arbitrary. This lesion is usually seen in infants.

Bronchial occlusion may or may not be demonstrated, and inflammation is rarely present. A major finding is an increase in alveolar size. Correlation of clinical findings with subtle histologic features is helpful. When bronchial obstruction is present, it may be intrinsic or extrinsic and correlation with the findings at surgery is useful.

References

Berlinger NT, Porto DP, Thompson TR. Infantile lobar emphysema. Am Otol Rhinol Laryngol 96:106-111, 1987.

Dail DH, Hammer SP (eds). Pulmonary Pathology. New York, Springer-Verlag, 1988.

Stocker JT, Drake RM, Madewell JE. Cystic and congenital lung disease in the newborn. Perspect Pediatr Pathol 4:93-154, 1978.

Thurlbeck WM (ed). Pathology of the Lung. New York, Thieme, 1988.

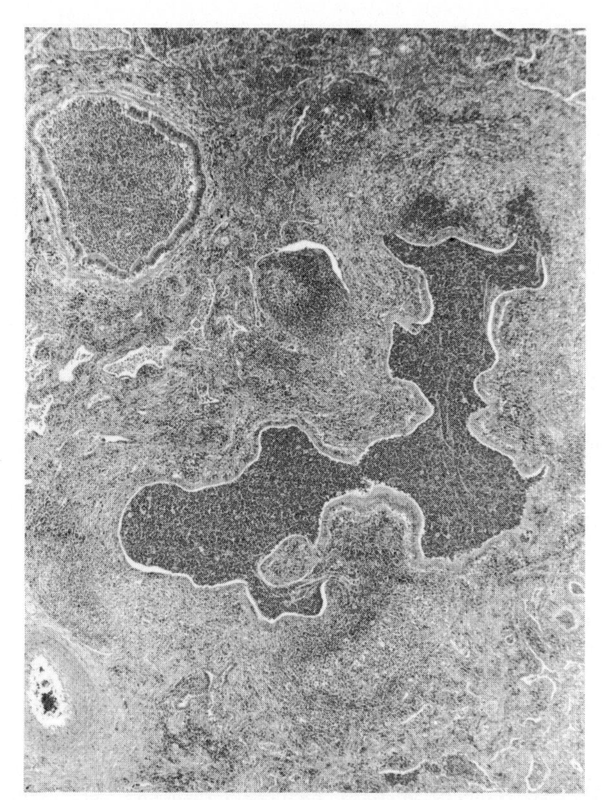

Figure 2–7. Intralobar pulmonary sequestration. The sequestered lung parenchyma is extensively infiltrated by acute and chronic inflammatory cells, and the airways are dilated and contain a mucopurulent exudate.

■ Bronchial Atresia (Segmental Overinflation)

Bronchial atresia is defined as a localized loss of communication of a bronchus with its supplied lung tissue, usually resulting in hyperinflation and hyperlucency. Although possibly related to lobar emphysema of infancy, bronchial atresia is usually segmental and is seen in adults.

Histologically, alveoli are larger than normal. Atresia or stenosis of the segmental bronchus may be difficult to demonstrate. Enlarged alveoli can often be appreciated by comparison with normal alveoli in the specimen, which can be found across a septum from the affected tissue. When this diagnosis is being considered, specimen bronchography, if feasible, may be helpful.

References

Jederlinic PJ, Sicilian LS, Baigelman W, Gaensler EA. Congenital bronchial atresia: A report of four cases and a review of the literature. Medicine 66:73–83, 1987.

■ Polyalveolar Lobe

Polyalveolar lobe occurs as a nonobstructive form of clinical lobar hyperinflation resulting from an abnormally increased number of normal appearing alveoli.

Increased numbers and increased size of alveoli can be demonstrated by morphometric methods. In normal children under 1 year of age, the number of alveoli between the most distal terminal bronchiole and the pleura is five to seven. In polyalveolar lobes, the number is greater than nine.

References

Hislop A, Reid L. New pathologic findings in emphysema of childhood: I. Polyalveolar lobe with emphysema. Thorax 25:682–690, 1970.

■ Pulmonary Sequestration (Fig. 2–7)

Intralobar and extralobar sequestrations are recognized. Extralobar sequestrations are extrapulmonary, rarely extrathoracic, and usually are seen in neonates. They have their own pleural investment, lack connection to the tracheobronchial tree, and may have a blood supply from the systemic or pulmonary arterial system. Intralobar sequestrations are within the visceral pleura, affect the lower lobes, are seen in both children and young adults, lack connections to tracheobronchial tree, and usually have a systemic vascular supply.

In extralobar sequestrations, one sees expanded parenchyma with dilated mucin-filled airways and airspaces. In neonates, the features of neonatal lung are present. A large vascular pedicle is usually seen entering the accessory lobe. Intralobar sequestrations usually have abundant mucostasis, cyst formation, obstructive changes, and acute and chronic inflammation from superinfection that may be severe enough to distort the anatomy. Histologically, they may resemble bronchiectasis or honeycombing, which both are quite nonspecific.

The diagnosis is usually made radiographically, however, a large feeding elastic artery inappropriate for the site in the lung may be a histologic clue and dissection may reveal the lack of bronchial connection. The diagnosis of sequestration is greatly aided by angiographic and operative findings.

References

Dail DH, Hammer SP (eds). Pulmonary Pathology, New York, Springer-Verlag, 1988.
Stocker JT. Sequestration of the lung. Semin Diagn Pathol 3:106–121, 1986.
Thurlbeck WM (ed). Pathology of the Lung. New York, Thieme, 1988.

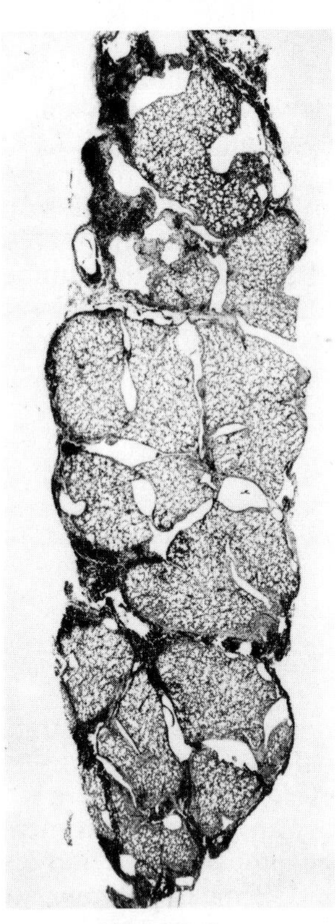

Figure 2–8.

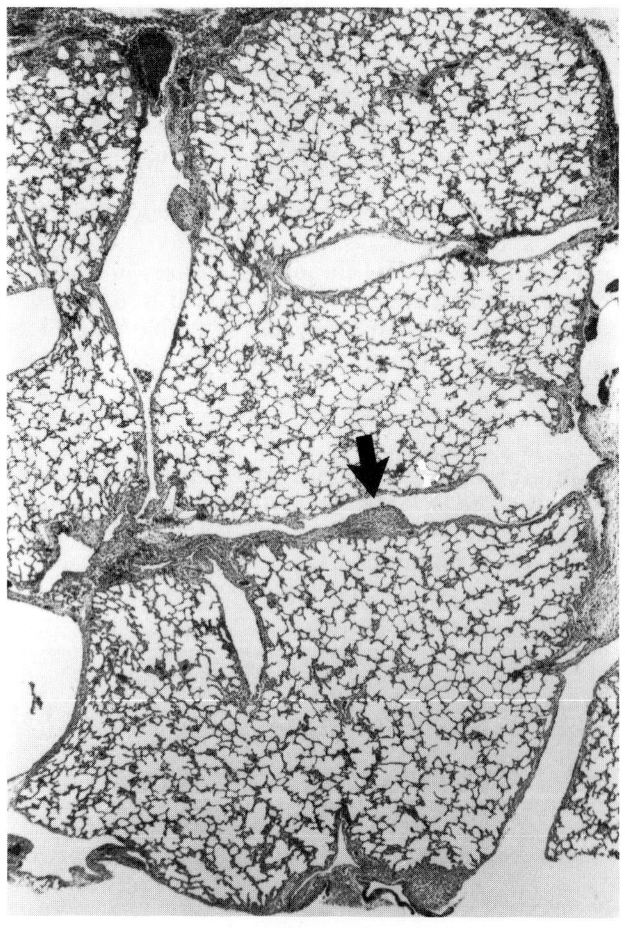

Figure 2–9.

■ Persistent Interstitial Pulmonary Emphysema (PIPE) (Figs. 2–8 to 2–12)

Persistent interstitial pulmonary emphysema is characterized by radiographic hyperlucency and hyperinflation caused by dissection of air into the interstitium. This may be localized to a segment or lobe and is usually associated with a history of assisted ventilation or respiratory distress at birth.

The dissection of air around bronchovascular bundles and into the septa and the pleura leaves ragged spaces that may be missed on cursory examination at scanning power. One may think that the tissue is artifactually torn or that the lymphatics are dilated. In more chronic cases, there is fibrosis and a histiocytic and giant cell reaction that surrounds the abnormal spaces. In severe cases, the air-filled spaces are greatly expanded and the lung tissue is completely atelectatic.

Note: Interstitial air with or without giant cell reaction is an occasional focal and incidental finding in patients with interstitial lung disease, in those with obstructive lung disease accompanied by bullae or blebs, and in those who have been connected to a respirator.

References

Dail DH, Hammer SP (eds). Pulmonary Pathology. New York, Springer-Verlag, 1988.

Stocker JT, Drake RM, Madewell JE. Cystic and congenital lung disease in the newborn. Perspect Pediatr Pathol 4:93–154, 1978.

Thurlbeck WM (ed). Pathology of the Lung. New York, Thieme, 1988.

Figures 2–8, 2–9. Pulmonary interstitial emphysema. Abnormal, dilated, air-containing spaces are seen in the pleura and septa and around the bronchovascular structures. Hemorrhage can be seen in some of these spaces, and valves (which are seen in lymphatic spaces) are absent. A histiocytic reaction to the air is present focally (arrow). This finding, particularly with the presence of giant cells, is typical of chronic pulmonary interstitial emphysema.

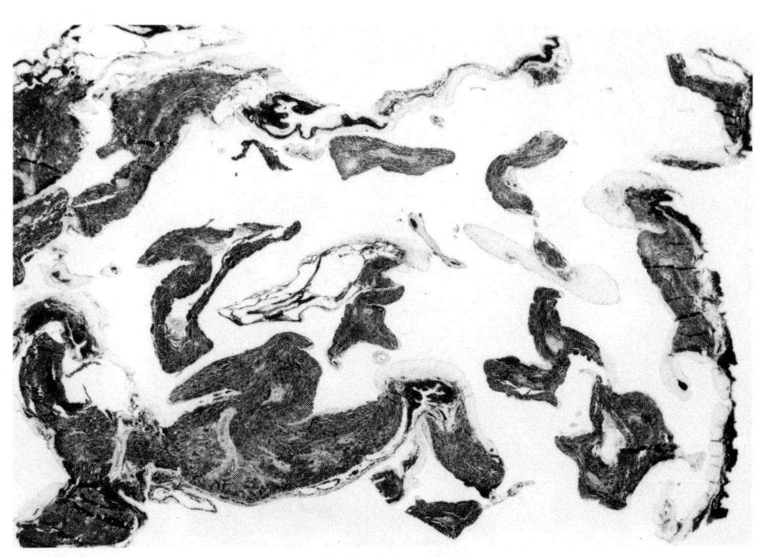

Figure 2–10.

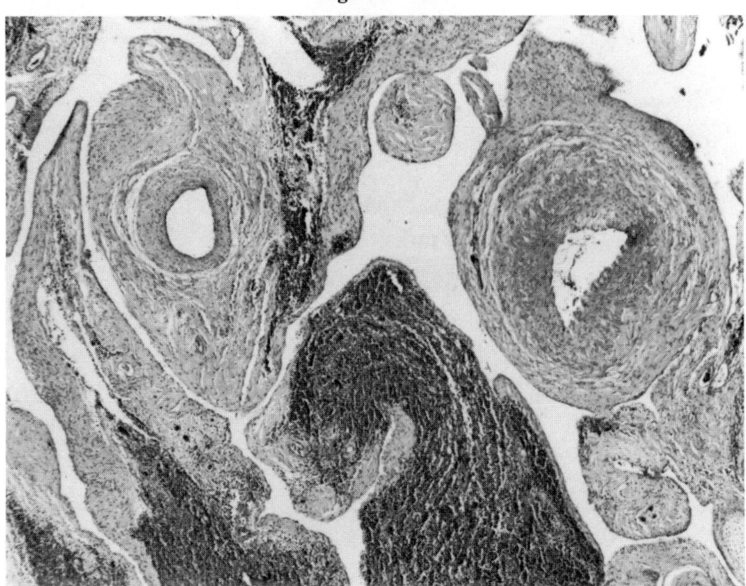

Figure 2–11.

Figures 2–10, 2–11, 2–12. Pulmonary interstitial emphysema. In this case, there is massive expansion of the interstitium by abnormal air pockets with resultant atelectasis of the lung parenchyma, which appears as dark, airless tissue. The architecture is so severely distorted that it is difficult to distinguish anatomic features. The lung parenchyma is anatomically normal but compressed by the interstitial air. A peribronchial region (Fig. 2–12) in this case shows dissection of air into the connective tissue with hemorrhage and a giant cell reaction.

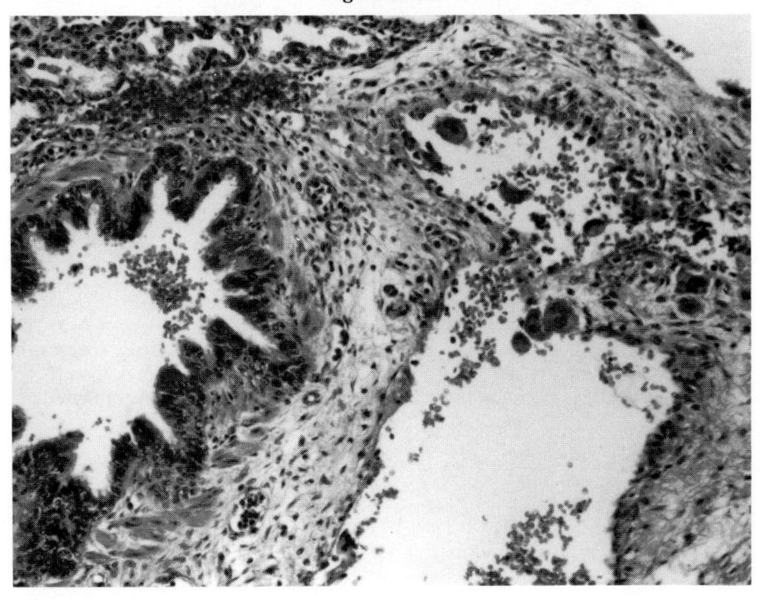

Figure 2–12.

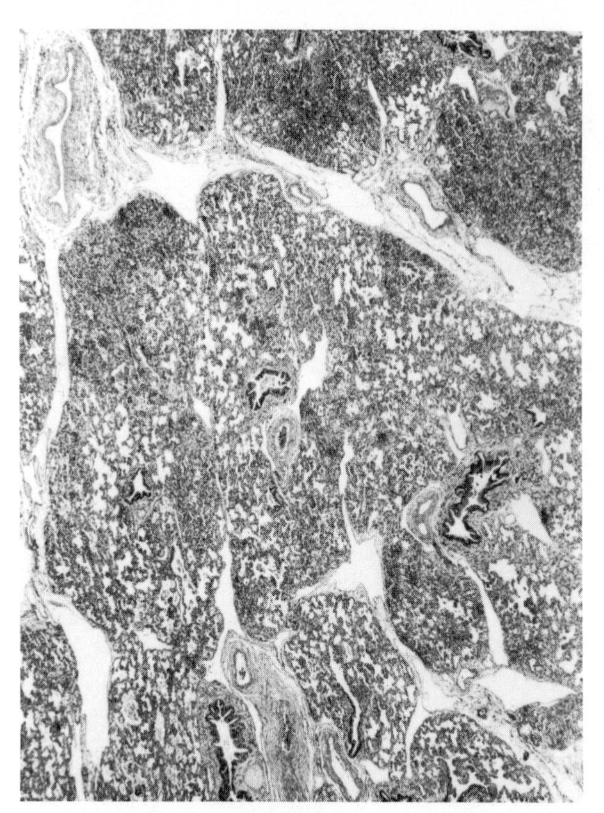

Figure 2-13.

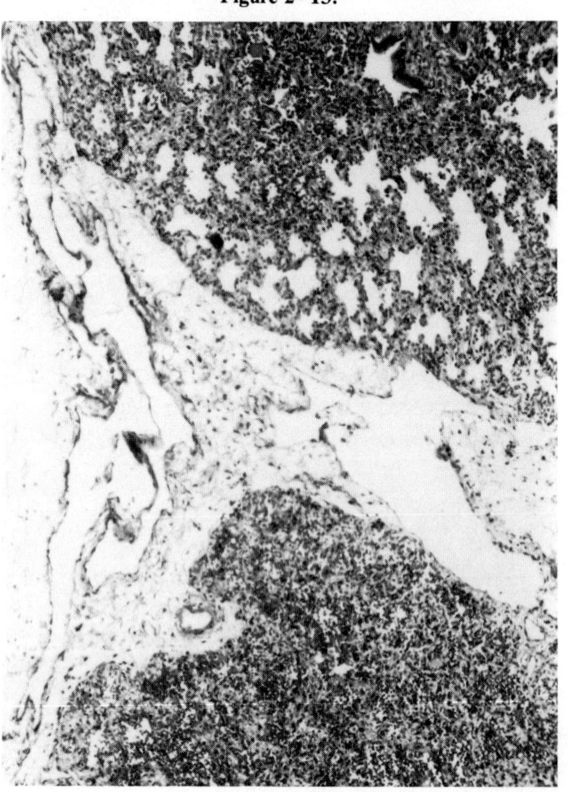

Figure 2-14.

■ Lymphangiectasia (Figs. 2-13, 2-14)

An extremely rare condition that may be restricted to the lungs or that may be part of a systemic abnormality of the lymphatics; secondary lymphangiectasia may occur as a result of cardiovascular anomalies or mediastinal masses that impinge on the thoracic duct. The majority of cases are seen in stillborn infants, as this condition is usually not compatible with life.

There is a diffuse dilatation of the lymphatics in the septa and pleura, and along the bronchovascular structures.

Secondary causes of lymphangiectasia, particularly cardiovascular, should be excluded prior to accepting a diagnosis of primary pulmonary lymphangiectasia, which should also be distinguished from interstitial emphysema.

References

Landing BH, Dixon LG. Congenital malformations and genetic disorders of the respiratory tract (larynx, trachea, bronchi, and lungs). Am Rev Respir Dis 120:151, 1979.

Stocker JT, Drake, RM, Madewell JE. Cystic and congenital lung disease in the newborn. Perspect Pediatr Pathol 4:93-154, 1978.

Figures 2-13, 2-14. Congenital pulmonary lymphangiectasia. Dilated lymphatic spaces are seen in the septa and pleura. In one lymphatic vessel, valves can be discerned (Fig. 2-14), and their presence excludes a diagnosis of interstitial emphysema.

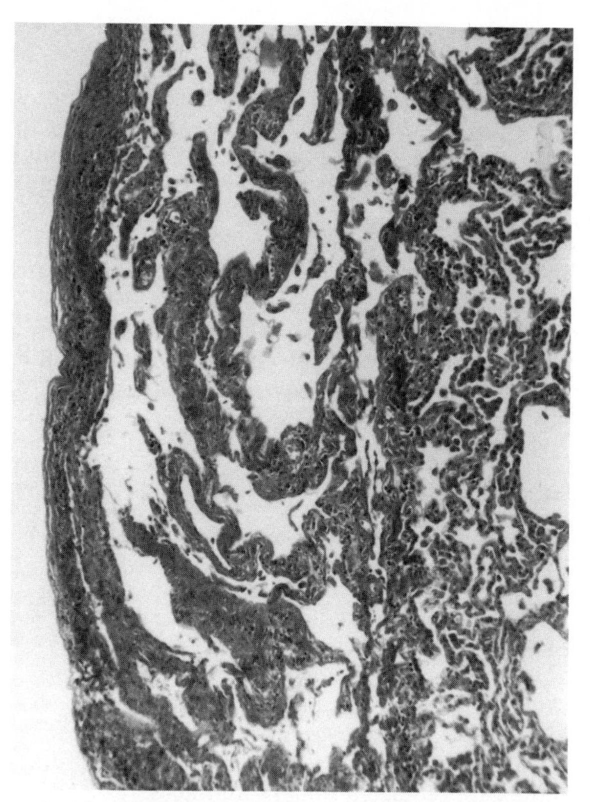

Figure 2-15. Pleural lymphangiomatosis. Dilated, irregular, anastomosing lymphatic channels form a layer between the surface of the visceral pleura and the underlying lung tissue, which can be recognized by the presence of alveolar macrophages. This was a diffuse pleural lesion that was found in a young woman and that clinically mimicked lymphangioleiomyomatosis.

■ Lymphangioma and Lymphangiomatosis (Fig. 2-15)

Lymphangioma and lymphangiomatosis are hamartomatous or benign neoplastic proliferations of lymphatics. Although usually seen in the soft tissues of the head and neck, they may extend into the mediastinum, lung, and pleura. They may recur if incompletely excised. Some cases have been interpreted as localized lymphangiectasia. A few cases are associated with Turner's syndrome.

Anastomosing, usually dilated, lymphatic spaces are apparent. The spaces may be associated with nodular aggregates of lymphocytes; and they may contain eosinophilic chylous material.

References

Wagenaar SJSC, Swierenga J, Wagenvoort CA. Late presentation of primary pulmonary lymphangiectasis. Thorax 33:791-795, 1978.

■ Other Rare Anomalies

A number of unusual anomalies may also affect the lung, including displaced lung tissue, supernumerary lobes and segments, airway stenosis, congenital bronchiectasis, and tracheoesophageal fistulas. Tracheoesophageal fistulas may be dominated by the features of aspiration.

References

Landing BH, Dixon LG. Congenital malformations and genetic disorders of the respiratory tract (larynx, trachea, bronchi, and lungs). Am Rev Respir Dis 120-151, 1979.

Stocker JT, Drake RM, Madewell JE. Cystic and congenital lung disease in the newborn. Perspect Pediatr Pathol 4:93-154, 1978.

■ Pneumatoceles

Pneumatoceles are postinflammatory cystic spaces in the lung that are connected to an airway, usually seen in infants and children. The diagnosis may be suggested radiographically; rarely is a biopsy performed.

Histologically, the cavity is usually lined by bronchiolar or cuboidal metaplastic epithelium that may have some fibrosis and inflammation in the walls. Secondary infection or even a fungus ball may be present.

References

Landing BH, Dixon LG. Congenital malformations and genetic disorders of the respiratory tract (larynx, trachea, bronchi, and lungs). Am Rev Respir Dis 120:151, 1979.

Thurlbeck WM (ed). Pathology of the Lung. New York, Thieme, 1988.

■ Arteriovenous Malformation

Arteriovenous malformation is a vascular anomaly with an abnormal communication between the arteries and veins often associated with abnormal elastica and muscularis components. The diagnosis is commonly made radiographically, and the pathologist confirms the diagnosis following resection. When multifocal, Osler-Weber-Rendu syndrome should be considered. Extrathoracic vascular malformations and Berry aneurysms may accompany findings.

In such cases, one need only identify abnormal vasculature. The majority of arteriovenous malformations are supplied by pulmonary arteries and drain via the pulmonary veins. The vessels often show intimal thickening. Hemorrhage may be seen in the surrounding lung tissue.

References

Anabtawi IN, Ellison RG, Ellison LT. Pulmonary arteriovenous aneurysms and fistulas. Anatomical variations, embryology, and classification. Ann Thorac Surg 1:277-285, 1965.

Carter D, Eggleston JC. Tumors of the Lower Respiratory Tract. AFIP Atlas of Tumor Pathology, Second Series, Fascicle 17. Washington DC, Armed Forces Institute of Pathology, 1980.

Dail DH, Hammer SP (eds). Pulmonary Pathology. New York, Springer-Verlag, 1988.

Mark EJ. Lung Biopsy Interpretation. Baltimore, Williams & Wilkins, 1984.

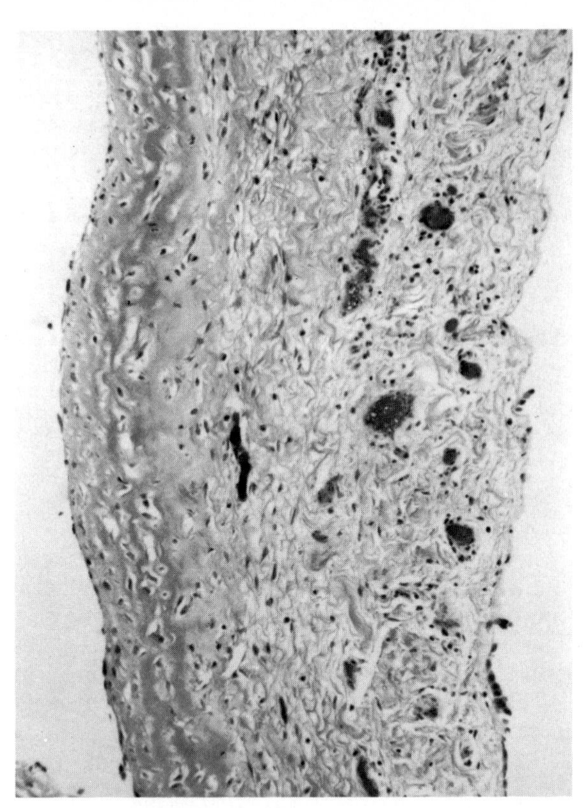

Figure 2–16. Bulla. The wall of a bulla is composed of thick fibrovascular tissue, often with dense, somewhat hyaline fibrosis, and is lined on one side by hyperplastic mesothelial cells and on the other side by metaplastic type II cells. A histiocytic reaction, sometimes with giant cells, is not uncommon in the walls of bullae.

■ **Bulla** (Fig. 2–16)

Bullae are air-filled spaces usually seen in emphysematous lungs and are arbitrarily defined as larger than 1 cm in diameter. Large expansive bullae may compromise function of surrounding lung tissue. Bullectomy may be performed if the nonbullous tissue is normal or has only mild emphysema.

Bullae are seen histologically as irregular collapsed cavities, with a relatively thin fibrous wall that shows some chronic inflammation and metaplastic epithelial lining. If air has dissected into the adjacent interstitium, gaping clefts lined by histiocytes and giant cells may be seen.

References

Thurlbeck WM. Chronic Airflow Obstruction in Lung Disease. Philadelphia, WB Saunders Co, 1976.

■ Bleb

Blebs are intrapleural collections of air usually smaller than 1 cm in diameter and are often associated with subpleural scarring. They may be the only finding in patients with recurrent pneumothoraces.

References

Thurlbeck WM. Chronic airflow obstruction in lung disease. Philadelphia, WB Saunders Co, 1976.
Thurlbeck WM (ed). Pathology of the Lung. New York, Thieme, 1988.

■ Apical Fibrobullous Change

Apical fibrobullous change is a term used for *radiographically apparent* changes usually seen in a number of conditions, especially ankylosing spondylitis in which the pulmonary apices show increased stranding and bullous change. The diagnosis is made radiographically, and biopsies are not necessary.

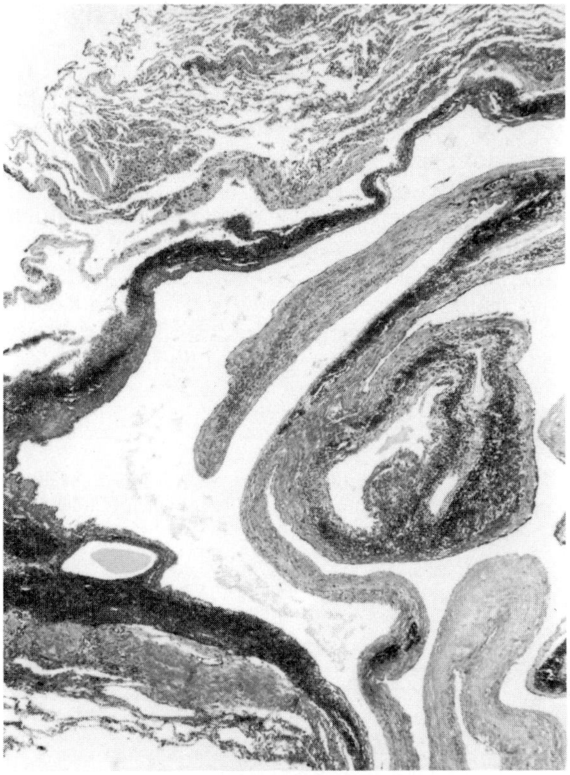

■ Mesenchymal Cystic Hamartoma (Figs. 2-17, 2-18)

Mesenchymal cystic hamartoma usually presents as multifocal cystic nodules or round masses occurring in adults who may have a variety of pulmonary symptoms.

Multiloculated cysts are lined by low cuboidal epithelium with papillae and septa formed by immature mesenchymal cells that may resemble a cambium layer or may suggest smooth muscle differentiation. If mitoses and atypia are prominent, a sarcoma should be excluded. Hemorrhage into the cysts may occur.

The differential diagnosis includes benign metastasizing leiomyoma; multiple fibromyomatous hamartomas; lymphangioleiomyomatosis in women in the childbearing years; cystic primary and metastatic sarcomas, especially stromal sarcoma of the uterus; and multiple cystic fibrohistiocytic tumors.

References

Mark EJ. Mesenchymal cystic hamartoma of the lung. N Engl J Med 315:1255-1259, 1986.

Figure 2-17.

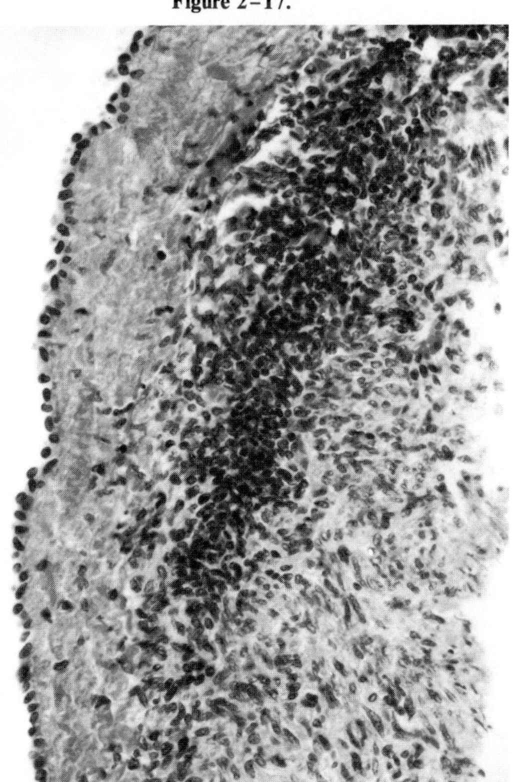

Figure 2-18.

Figures 2-17, 2-18. Mesenchymal cystic hamartoma. A multicystic structure is lined by thin walls in which there are compact, cytologically benign cells that show some tendency toward spindling. The cyst itself is lined by benign metaplastic cuboidal epithelium (Case courtesy of E. J. Mark, M. D., Boston).

■ Multiple Cystic Fibrohistiocytic Tumors of the Lung (Figs. 2–19 to 2–21)

This rare condition presents as bilateral nodular and/or cystic lesions that progress slowly over many years. Cysts of gigantic size may be attained with only minimal symptomatology.

Histologically, there is a benign-appearing cellular proliferation resembling a dermatofibroma (fibrous histiocytoma) in the skin. The proliferation is interstitial and is associated with secondary cystic change with hemorrhage and cholesterol clefts in the cysts. Large cysts are air-filled with a metaplastic epithelial lining.

References

Joseph MG, Colby TV, Swenson S, Gaensler EA, Mikus P. Multiple bilateral fibrohistiocytic tumors of the lung. Mayo Clinic Proc 65:192–197, 1990.

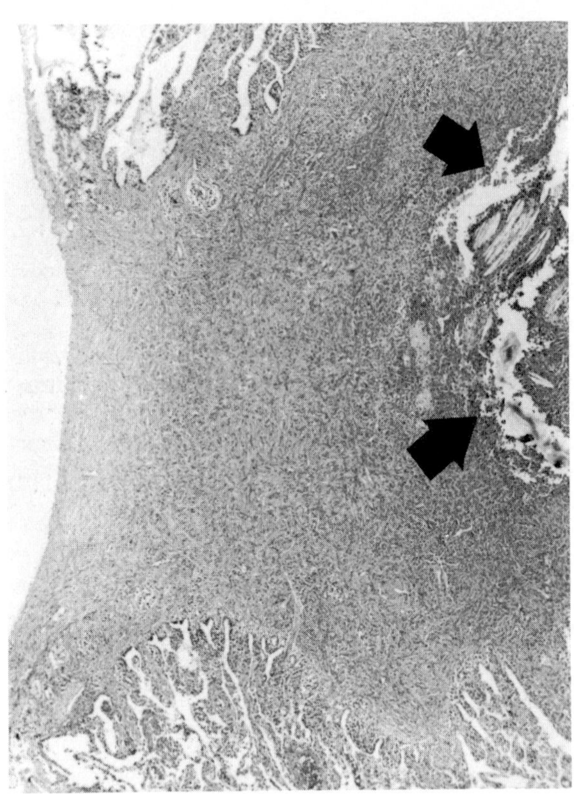

Figure 2–19.

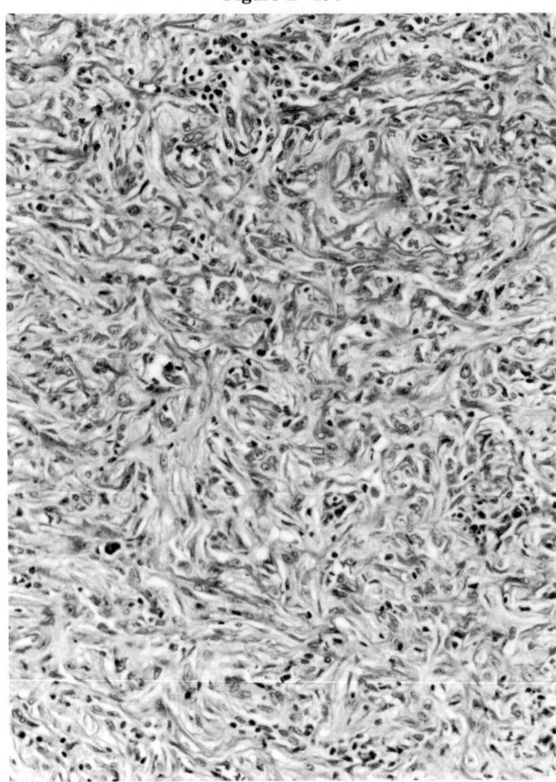

Figure 2–20.

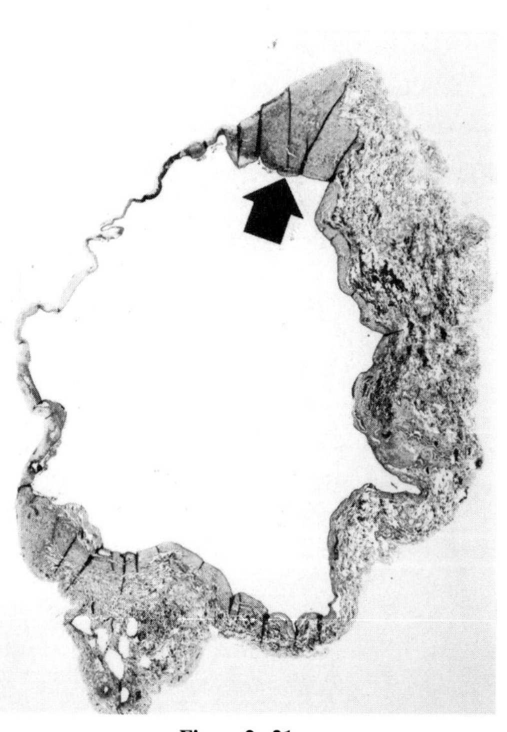

Figure 2–21.

Figures 2–19, 2–20, 2–21. Cystic fibrohistiocytic tumor of the lung. There is an interstitial, subpleural proliferation of cells that is identical to a dermatofibroma. In the central regions (arrows), there is hemorrhage and cholesterol cleft formation. In another case (Fig. 2–21), there is formation of large, thin-walled cysts. The fibrohistiocytic proliferation was identified focally in the cyst wall (arrow). Reproduced with permission from Joseph MG, Colby TV, Swenson S, et al. Multiple bilateral fibrohistiocytic tumors of the lung. Mayo Clinic Proc. 65:192–197, 1990.

CHAPTER 3

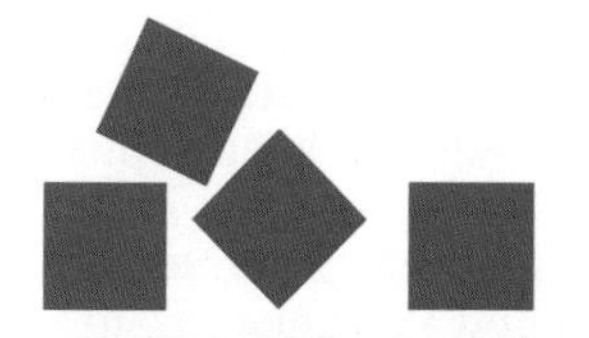

TUMORS, MASSES, LOCALIZED INFILTRATES

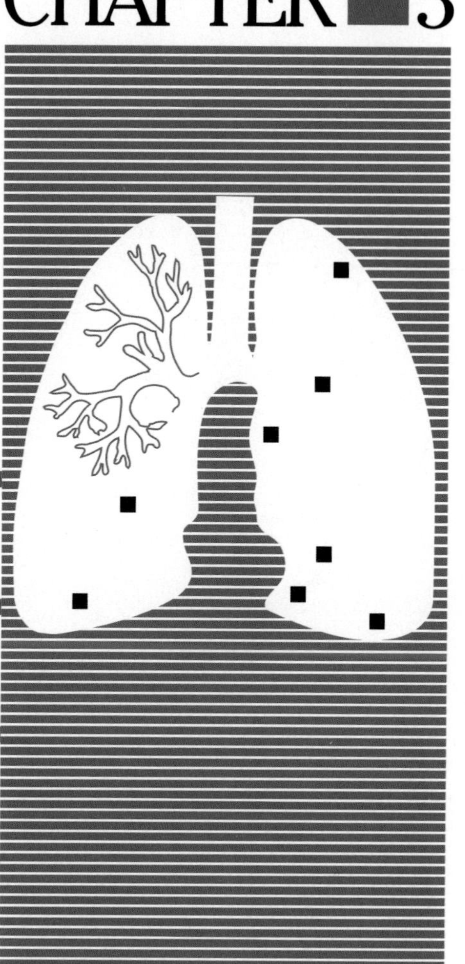

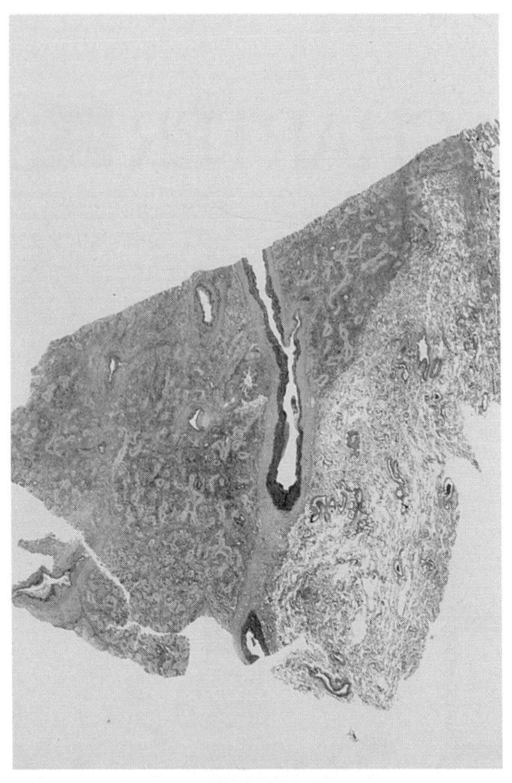

Figure 3–1.

■ Focal Organizing Pneumonia (Figs. 3–1 to 3–3)

Focal organizing pneumonia is a nonspecific, *localized,* inflammatory lesion that is known by a number of names, including chronic pneumonitis and inflammatory pseudotumor. It presents as a coin lesion or localized infiltrate that is usually resected and to exclude neoplasm.

A prior bronchopneumonia or inflammatory event is rarely documented, but many cases may be the result of a healing residue of a prior infection. Serologic evaluations for specific agents may be indicated.

Histologically, lung parenchyma shows organizing pneumonia with tufts of granulation tissue within bronchioles, alveolar ducts, and distal airspaces associated with chronic inflammation in alveolar septa. There is usually some evidence of obstructive pneumonia as well as a component of chronic bronchitis or bronchiolitis. Some cases show foci of acute fibrinous exudate in the airspaces, and occasional granulomas may be present. If any necrosis is present, infection and Wegener's granulomatosis should be considered.

Note: Lesions should be well sampled, since an organizing pneumonia may be a nonspecific reaction around some other lesions, such as a tumor, abscess, or a noninfectious inflammatory process (i.e., Wegener's granulomatosis).

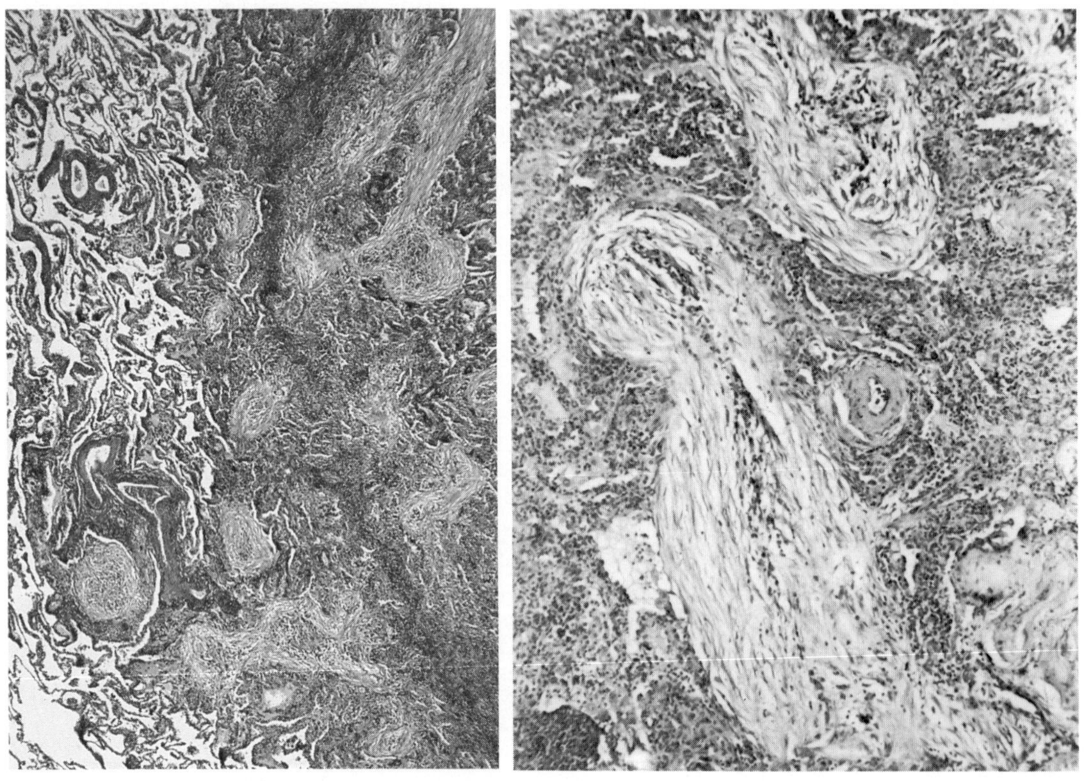

Figure 3–2. Figure 3–3.

Figures 3–1, 3–2, 3–3. Focal organizing pneumonia. This well-demarcated nodule shows evenly spaced, pale masses of organizing connective tissue with pockets of chronic inflammatory cells in the center. Compressed alveolar walls can be barely discerned between these connective tissue polyps, which are predominantly within alveolar ducts. The color pictures are of elastic tissue-stained sections with connective tissue staining red; the airspace proliferative tissue is faintly red in comparison with the dark red color of the mature collagen. In Figure 3–2, proliferative bronchiolitis obliterans is seen at the edge of the main lesion.

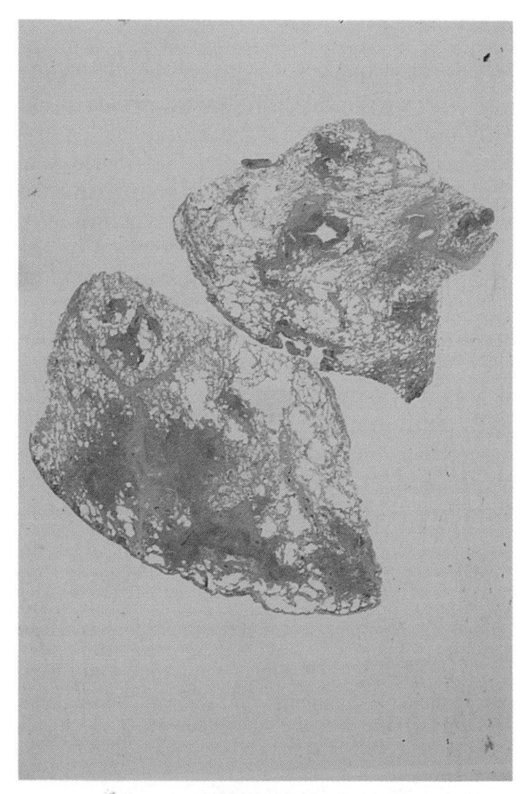

Figure 3–4.

Because of the histologic similarity, focal organizing pneumonia has also been called focal bronchiolitis obliterans organizing pneumonia (BOOP), but the clinical and radiographic findings of BOOP, as described below, are entirely different.

See references for Plasma Cell Granuloma section.

■ Right Middle Lobe Syndrome (Figs. 3–4 to 3–6)

The right middle lobe, and sometimes the lingula, appear prone to recurrent bouts of pneumonia, possibly owing to the anatomy and/or to partial obstruction by enlarged hilar nodes. Lobectomy is sometimes necessary.

Histologically, there is acute and chronic inflammation of the airways, patchy organizing pneumonia, and a variable degree of scarring. Lymphoid hyperplasia may be marked.

References

Katzenstein A-LA, Askin FB. Surgical Pathology of Non-Neoplastic Lung Disease, 2nd ed. Philadelphia, WB Saunders Co, 1990.
Thurlbeck WM (ed). Pathology of the Lung. New York, Thieme, 1988.

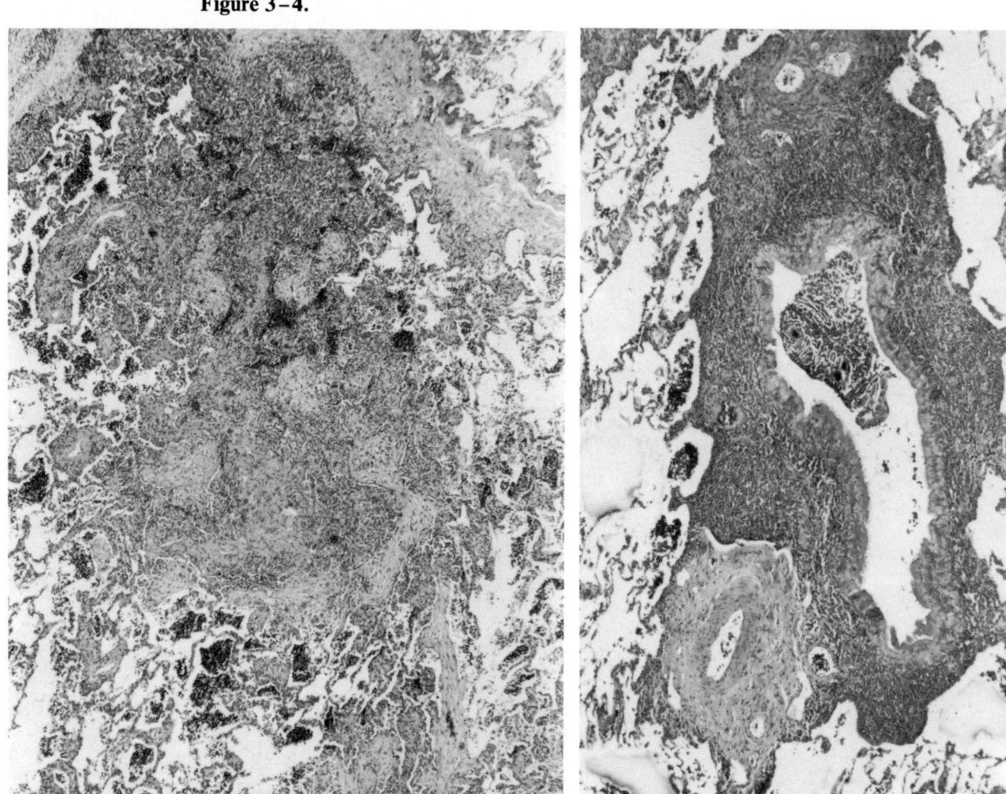

Figure 3–5. Figure 3–6.

Figures 3–4, 3–5, 3–6. Right middle lobe syndrome. Chronic inflammation centers on airways, and there are adjacent zones of consolidation (Fig. 3–5) representing foci of organizing pneumonia. The airway inflammation (Fig. 3–6) is an acute and chronic cellular bronchiolitis, and the zones of organization are typical of nonspecific organizing pneumonia.

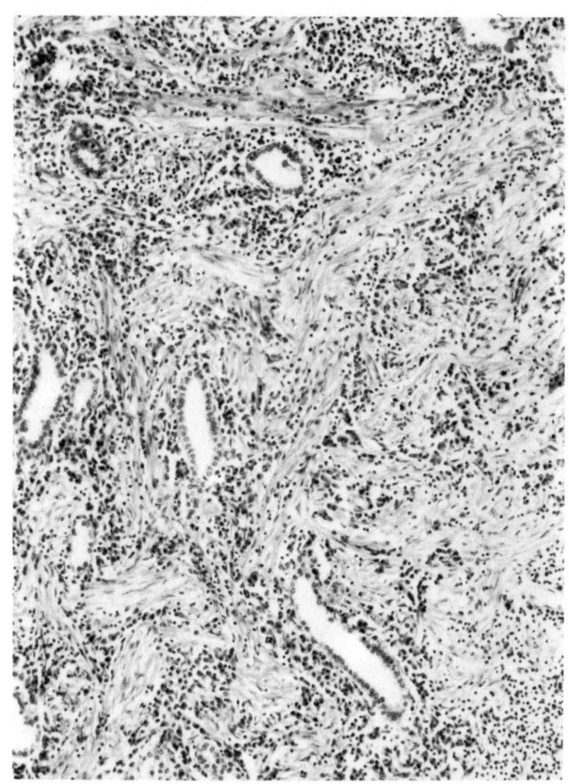

Figure 3-7.

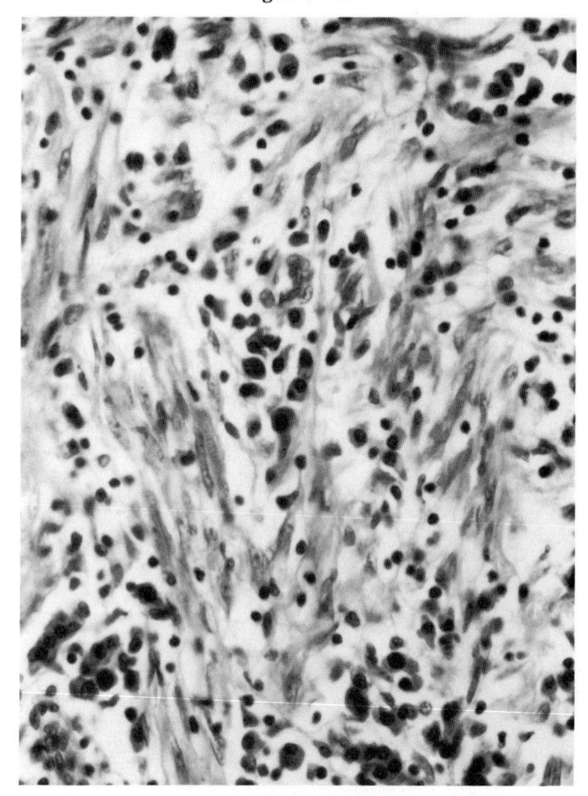

Figure 3-8.

Figures 3-7, 3-8. Plasma cell granuloma. There is an interstitial expansion by proliferating spindle cells and plasma cells that surround alveolar spaces lined by metaplastic epithelium. The spindle cells resemble fibroblasts and myofibroblasts.

■ Plasma Cell Granuloma (Inflammatory Pseudotumor, Inflammatory Myofibroblastic Tumor) (Figs. 3-7 to 3-10)

Plasma cell granuloma is a localized, histologically benign tumor with a cellular fibroblastic proliferation that frequently contains abundant plasma cells, spinal cells, histiocytes, and xanthoma cells. Storiform foci may be present. Dense fibrosis or myxoid change may be seen in some cases. When lymphoid tissue is prominent, lymphoma and pseudolymphoma are included in the differential diagnosis and immunophenotyping may be helpful.

This lesion has also been called inflammatory pseudotumor and benign fibrous histiocytoma. It may evolve from a focal organizing pneumonia.

Plasma cell granuloma, seen in children and adults, sometimes appears as an endobronchial lesion; in children, recurrence and/or "invasion" may be seen, but metastases do not develop. In adults the course is benign.

References

Bahadori H, Liebow AA. Plasma cell granulomas of the lung. Cancer 31:191-208, 1973.

Carter D, Eggleston JC. Tumors of the Lower Respiratory Tract. AFIP Atlas of Tumor Pathology, Second Series, Fascicle 17. Washington, DC, Armed Forces Institute of Pathology, 1980.

Dail DH, Hammer SP (eds). Pulmonary Pathology. New York, Springer-Verlag, 1988.

Matsubara O, Tau-Liu NS, Kenney RM, Mark EJ. Inflammatory pseudotumors of the lung. Hum Pathol 19:807-814, 1988.

Pettinato G, Manivel JC, Dehner LP. Inflammatory myofibroblastic tumor of the lung (abstr). Lab Invest 57:73A, 1989.

Sajjad SM, Begin LR, Dail DH, Lukeman JM. Fibrous histiocytoma of lung: A clinicopathologic study of two cases. Histopathology 5:325-334, 1981.

Spencer H. The pulmonary plasma cell/histiocytoma complex. Histopathology 8:903-916, 1984.

Thurlbeck WM (ed). Pathology of the Lung. New York, Thieme, 1988.

■ Benign Fibrous Histiocytoma (Figs. 3-11, 3-12)

This histologically benign lesion is composed of a fusiform or storiform arrangement of spindled or stellate fibroblasts, foamy histiocytes, and variable mixtures of lymphocytes and plasma cells. The features overlap with those of plasma cell granuloma.

References

Carter D, Eggleston JC. Tumors of the Lower Respiratory Tract. AFIP Atlas of Tumor Pathology, Second Series, Fascicle 17. Washington DC, Armed Forces Institute of Pathology, 1980.

Dail DH, Hammer SP (eds). Pulmonary Pathology. New York, Springer-Verlag, 1988.

Spencer H. The pulmonary plasma cell/histiocytoma complex. Histopathology 8:903-916, 1984.

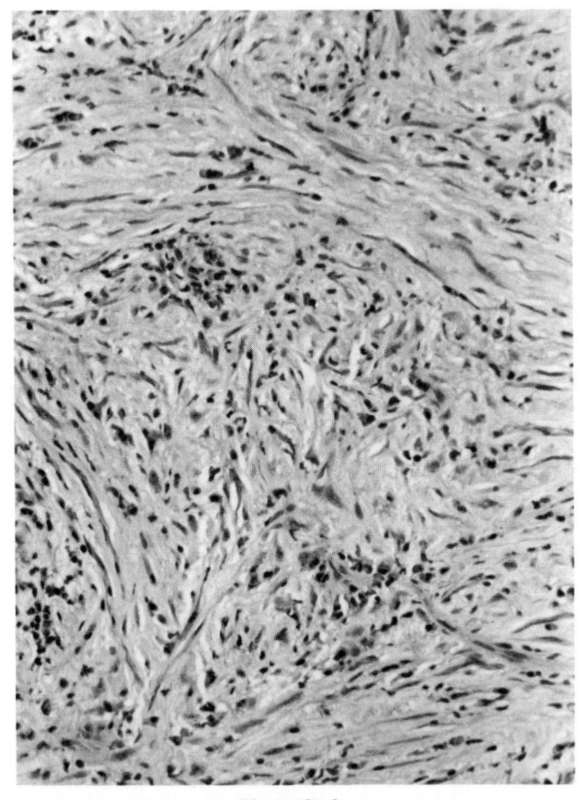

Figure 3-9.

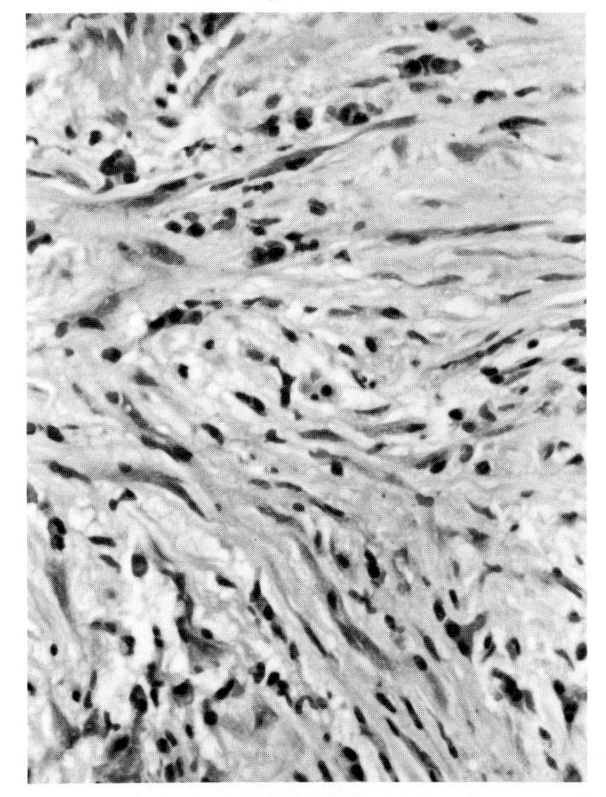

Figure 3-10.

Figures 3-9, 3-10. Plasma cell granuloma. A spindle cell proliferation in a somewhat fascicular arrangement is associated with scattered lymphocytes and plasma cells. The cytoplasm of many of the spindle cells is eosinophilic, which is typical of myofibroblastic differentiation.

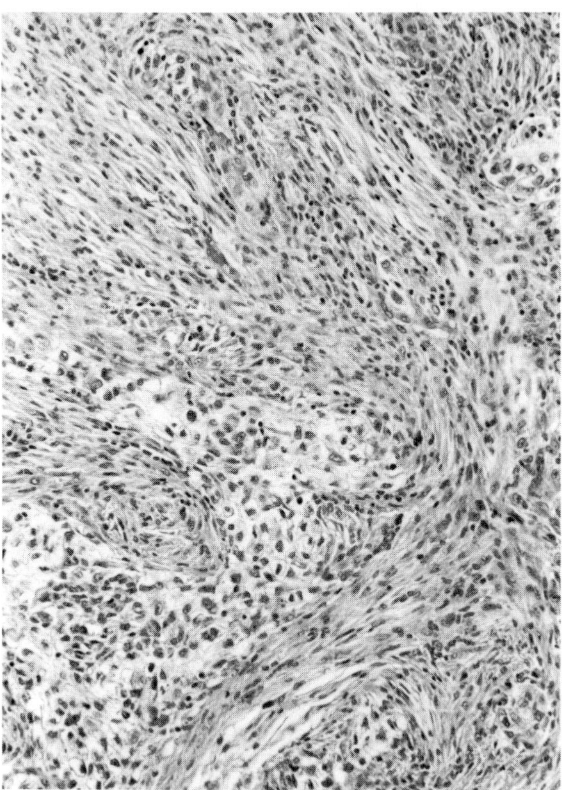

Figure 3-11.

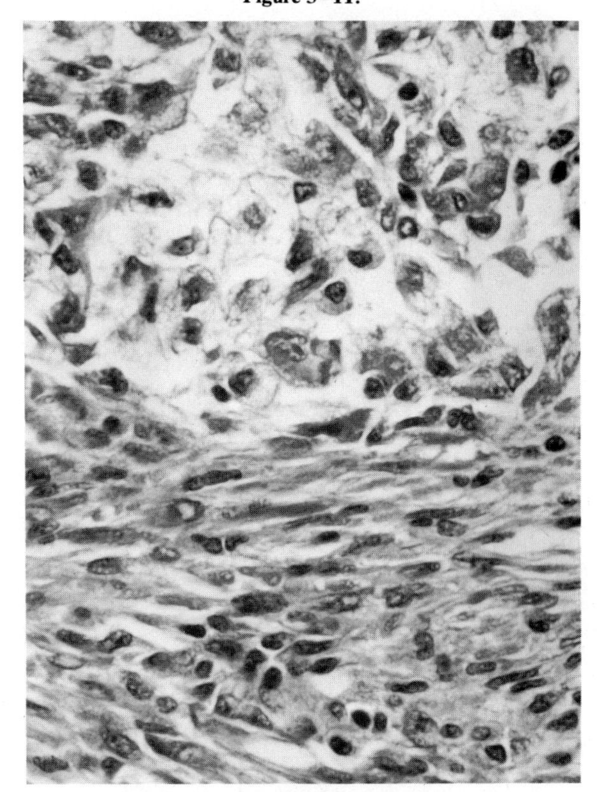

Figure 3-12.

Figures 3-11, 3-12. Fibrous histiocytoma. There is a proliferation of plump spindle cells with mild cytologic atypia that is associated with pockets of histiocytes, some of which are foamy.

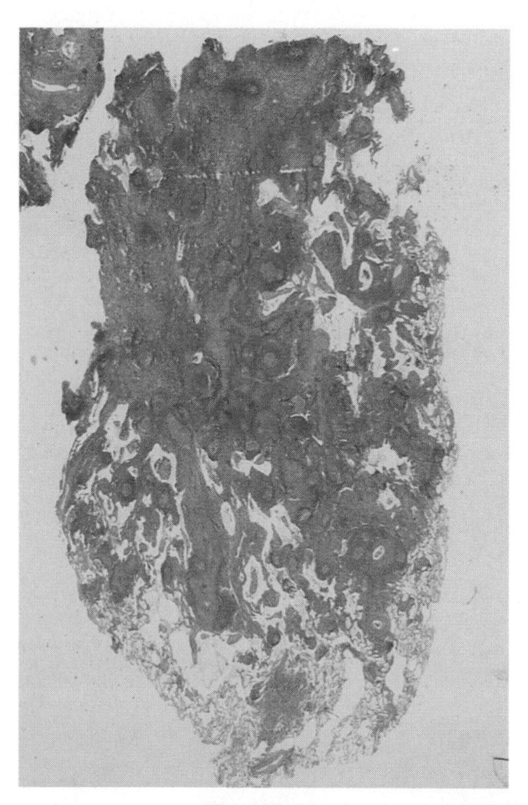

Figure 3-13.

■ Pseudolymphoma (Figs. 3-13 to 3-15)

Pseudolymphoma is a circumscribed localized mass or infiltrate with prominent lymphoid hyperplasia simulating a lymphoma. Large numbers of lymphocytes and plasma cells are associated with fibrosis with hyalinization and germinal centers. Some cases have been called inflammatory pseudotumors. These lesions may occasionally recur.

Note: Differential diagnosis with lymphoma is important, especially when sheets of small lymphocytes are present; immunologic marker studies are also useful in such cases.

References

Dail DH, Hammer SP (eds). Pulmonary Pathology. New York, Springer-Verlag, 1988.

Koss MN, Hochholzer L, Nichols PW, et al. Primary non-Hodgkin's lymphoma and pseudolymphoma of the lung: a study of 161 patients. Hum Pathol 14:1024-1038, 1983.

Focal organizing pneumonia, plasma cell granuloma, benign fibrous histiocytoma, and pseudolymphoma may all show some overlapping of histologic features, and this has led to some overlapping in labeling. There is no universally accepted terminology. Pulmonary hyalinizing granuloma should be considered in cases with marked hyalinization.

Common features in all of these lesions include lymphocytes and plasma cells, germinal centers, epithelial metaplasia in entrapped airspaces, fibroblasts in whorls and fascicles, obstructive changes with foamy macrophages, and cholesterol clefts and giant cells.

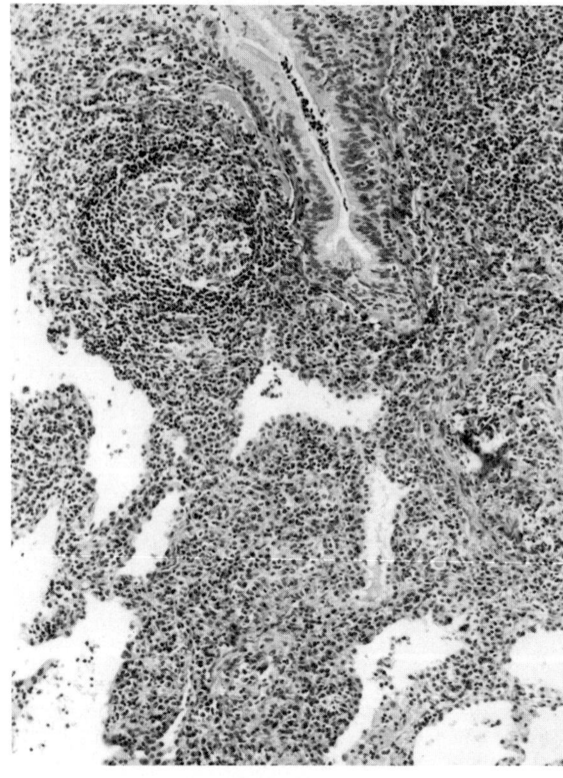

Figure 3-14.

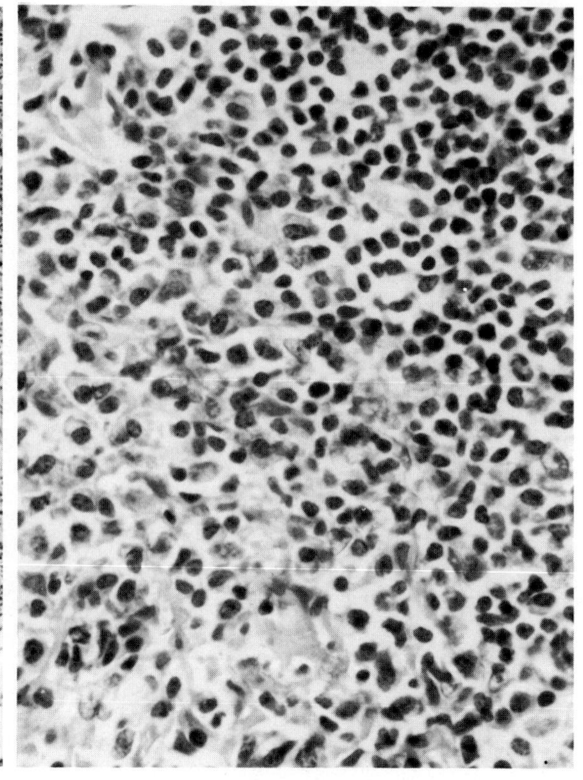

Figure 3-15.

Figures 3-13, 3-14, 3-15. Pseudolymphoma. There is a localized, well-circumscribed mass, composed of lymphoid tissue and traversed by fibrous bands with scattered germinal centers. Cytologically, the lesion is quite polymorphous with lymphocytes, plasma cells, and histiocytes.

■ Apical Cap (Figs. 3–16, 3–17)

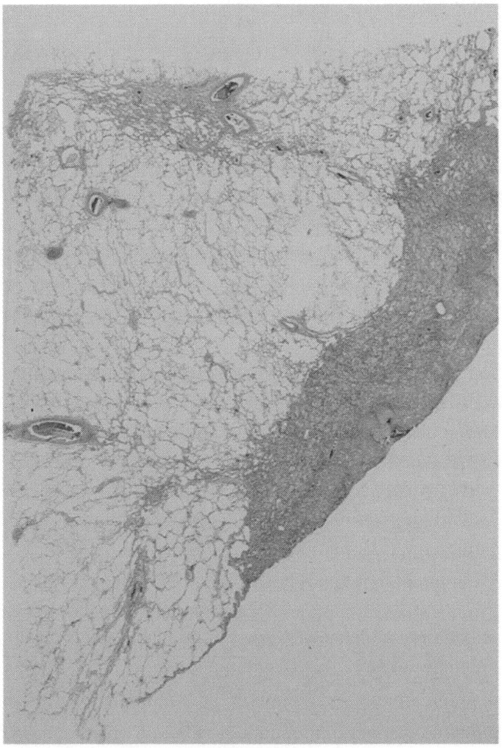

An apical cap is a localized apical thickening that is sometimes visible on chest radiographs and that may be biopsied to exclude the possibility of a tumor. It usually occurs as a bilateral convex thickening of the visceral pleura and subpleural lung in the apical regions. At one time, this was thought to represent healed tuberculosis; however, it is now believed to be a result of chronic ischemia.

Histologically a convex zone of elastotic fibrous tissue is apparent in the apices with patchy mild inflammation and prominent vascular sclerosis and thrombosis; alveolar structure with collapse may still be appreciated.

A similar histologic character may occasionally be seen elsewhere in the lung in ancient scars or infarcts.

References

Renner RR, Markarian B, Pernice NJ, Heitzman ER. The apical cap. Radiology 110:569–582, 1974.

Figure 3–16.

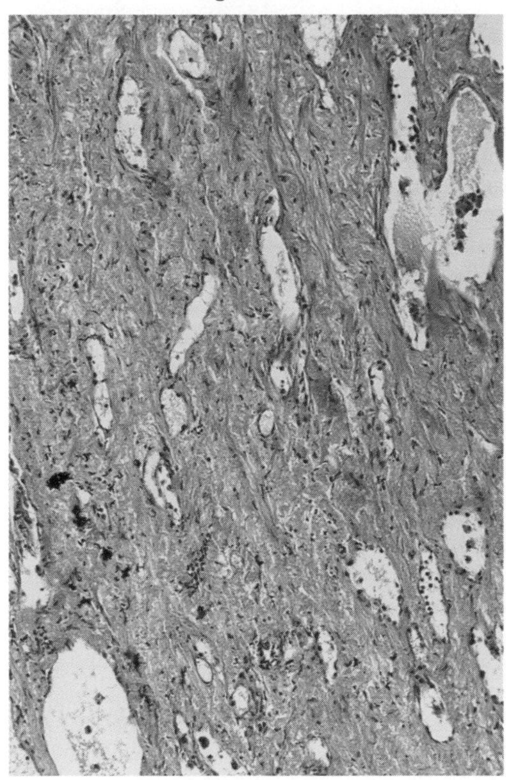

Figure 3–17.

Figures 3–16, 3–17. Apical cap. This tissue from the apex of the lung shows a localized, biconvex fibrous lesion in the visceral pleura. The lesion is composed of relatively hypocellular fibrous tissue that is rich in elastic tissue fibers. Sometimes the ghost outlines of alveoli can be discerned.

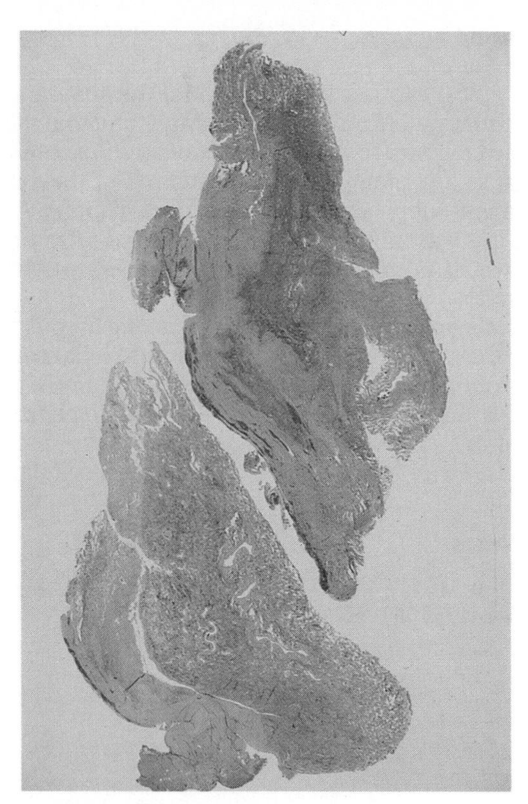

Figure 3–18. Rounded atelectasis. Low power shows marked pleural thickening with extension of fibrosis along septa that surround and compress lung tissue.

■ Rounded Atelectasis (Fig. 3–18)

Rounded atelectasis consists of pleural and subpleural fibrosis associated with septal contraction and trapping of parenchyma, producing a coin lesion on chest radiograph that is resected to exclude the possibility of a tumor. The "comet-tail" is almost radiographically pathognomonic, reflecting traction on the bronchovascular structures.

Rounded atelectasis is not uncommonly seen in patients who were previously exposed to asbestos and is thought to be the result of asbestos-induced pleural fibrosis.

Pleural and septal fibrosis is apparent with secondary parenchymal atelectasis, inflammation, and scarring.

Note: In these cases, the surgeon often suspects that a tumor is present but the pathologists' findings show only dense septal and pleural fibrosis and atelectatic lung tissue.

References

Cases of the Massachusetts General Hospital. Case 24:1983. N Engl J Med 308:1466–1472, 1983.

Hanke R, Kretzschmar R. Round atelectasis. Semin Roentgenol 15:174–182, 1980.

Thurlbeck WM (ed). Pathology of the Lung. New York, Thieme, 1988.

■ Nonspecific Fibrous and Inflammatory Nodules

Nonspecific fibrous and inflammatory nodules may be the residue of old infarcts, granulomas, healed abscesses, and so forth. These lesions are rarely of clinical significance and are encountered as incidental findings.

■ Benign Clear Cell Tumor (Sugar Tumor) (Figs. 3-19 to 3-21)

This rare, benign, localized lung tumor usually presents as a coin lesion.

This is a well-circumscribed tumor with clear or faintly eosinophilic cells with central nuclei and a delicate vascular pattern around the nests. Atypia and mitotic figures are inconspicuous. Giant cells are not uncommon. Neuroendocrine differentiation may be demonstrated immunohistochemically but the histogenesis remains uncertain.

It is extremely difficult to exclude metastatic renal cell carcinoma histologically, and before a diagnosis of benign clear cell tumor is rendered, a radiographic examination of the kidneys is warranted. The differential diagnosis also includes other primary and metastatic clear cell tumors. Clear cell carcinoma of the lung and sclerosing hemangioma, epithelioid hemangioendothelioma, and carcinoid tumors all may have some clear cell features.

References

Dail DH, Hammer SP (eds). Pulmonary Pathology. New York, Springer-Verlag, 1988.

Gaffey MJ, Mills SE, Ross MD, Askin FB, Yousem SA, Colby TV. Benign clear cell tumor of the lung. Am J Surg Pathol 14:248-259, 1990.

Mark EJ. Lung Biopsy Interpretation. Baltimore, Williams & Wilkins, 1984.

Thurlbeck WM (ed). Pathology of the Lung. New York, Thieme, 1988.

Figure 3-19.

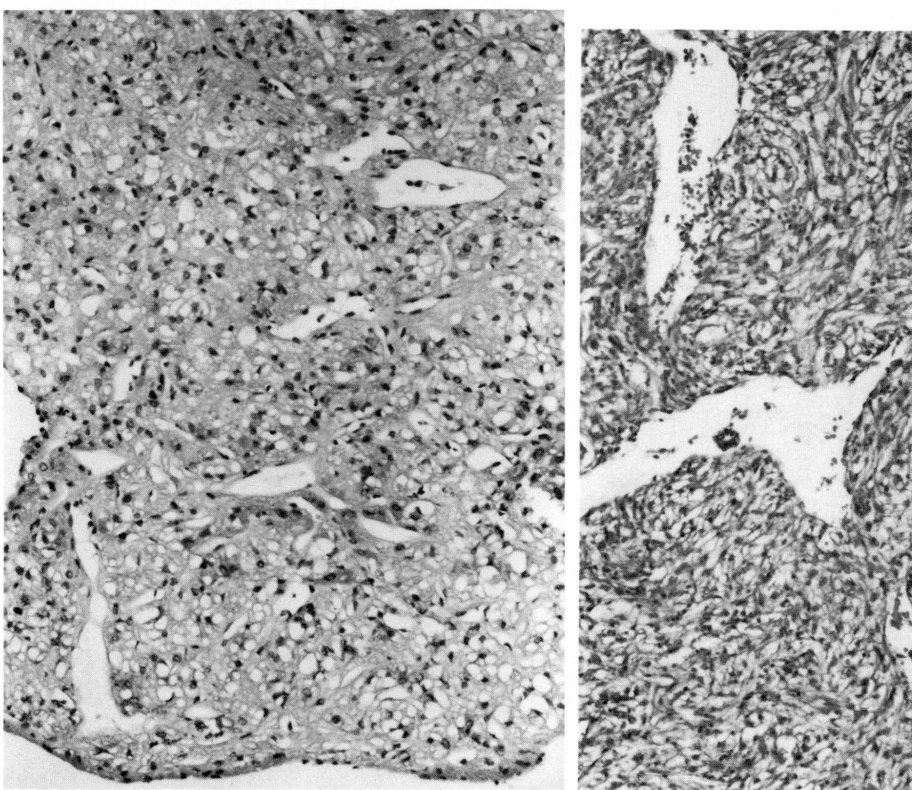

Figure 3-20.

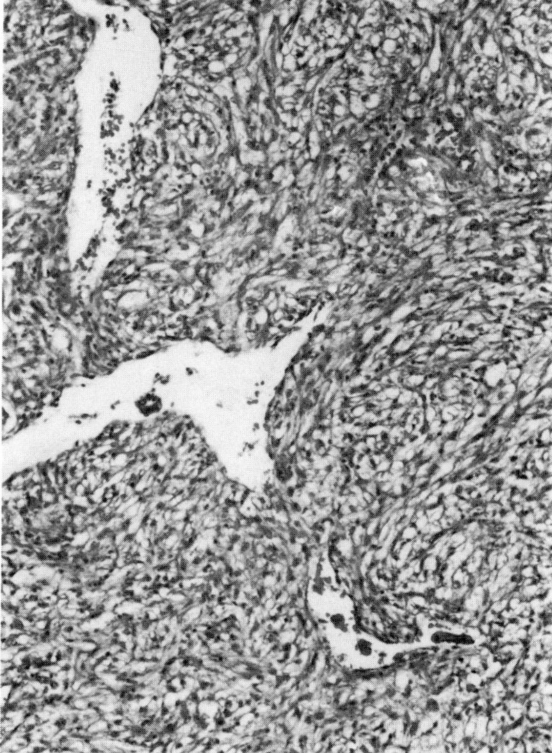

Figure 3-21.

Figures 3-19, 3-20, 3-21. Benign clear cell tumor. In these three cases there are dilated vascular spaces and relatively acellular collagenous or vascularized trabeculae separating clusters of clear or vacuolated cells with small nuclei. In some instances the cells have faintly eosinophilic cytoplasm; in others, the cells may show a tendency toward spindling.

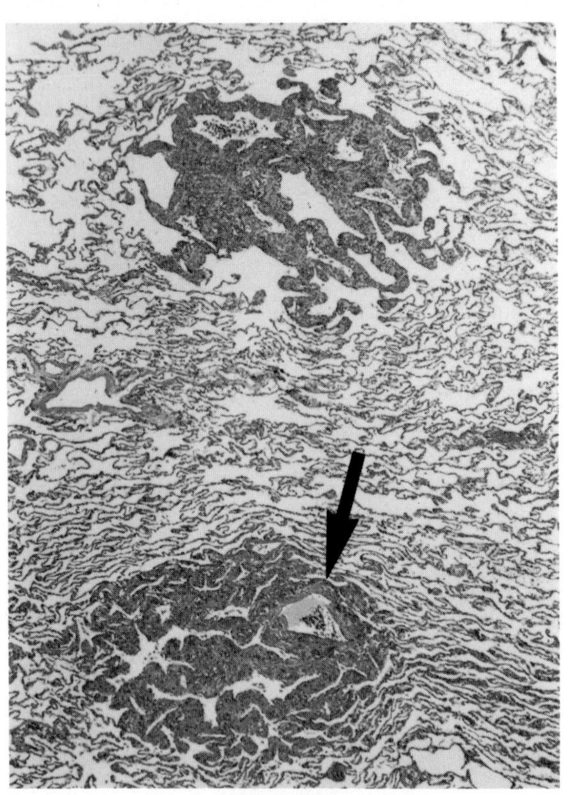

Figure 3-22.

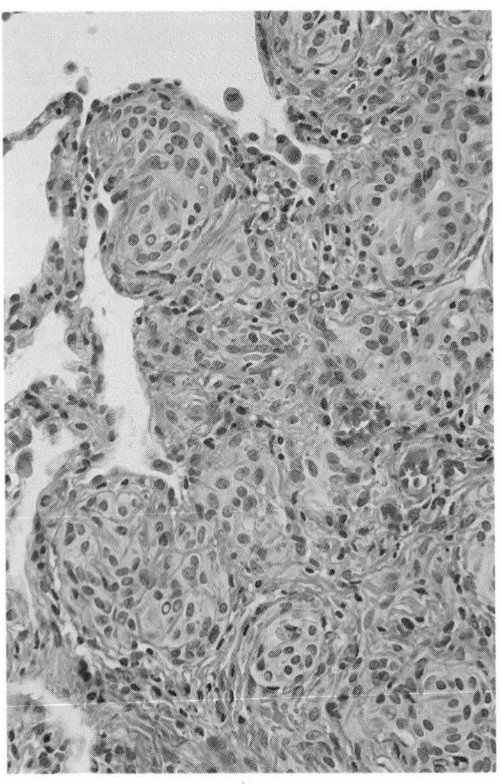

Figure 3-23.

■ Minute Pulmonary Chemodectoma (Minute Pulmonary Meningothelial-Like Nodules)
(Figs. 3-22, 3-23)

Minute pulmonary chemodectoma occurs as a perivenular nodule composed of cells resembling meningothelial cells. These tiny nodules are usually identified as an incidental microscopic finding in tissue removed for some other reason. Originally, the cells were thought to be related to paraganglia, and the term "minute pulmonary chemodectoma" was suggested. These lesions are extremely common.

Nested balls of interstitial cells surrounded by a delicate fibrous stroma occur in a perivenular distribution. The cytologic appearance, ultrastructural, and immunohistochemical findings of these cells are indistinguishable from those of meningothelial cells.

Minute pulmonary chemodectomas and carcinoid tumorlets (see the following discussion) are often confused, but they are readily separable when strict criteria are applied.

References

Carter D, Eggleston JC. Tumors of the Lower Respiratory Tract. AFIP Atlas of Tumor Pathology, Second Series, Fascicle 17, Washington, DC, Armed Forces Institute of Pathology, 1980.

Churg A, Warnock ML. So-called "minute pulmonary chemodectoma": a tumor not related to paragangliomas. Cancer 37:1759-1769, 1976.

Dail DH, Hammer SP (eds). Pulmonary Pathology. New York, Springer-Verlag, 1988.

Gaffey MJ, Mills SE, Askin FB. Minute pulmonary meningothelial-like nodules. Am J Surg Pathol 12:167-175, 1988.

Korn D, Bensch K, Liebow AA, Castleman B. Multiple minute pulmonary tumors resembling chemodectomas. Am J Pathol 37:641-672, 1960.

Thurlbeck WM (ed). Pathology of the Lung. New York, Thieme, 1988.

Figures 3-22, 3-23. Minute pulmonary chemodectoma. Two-minute pulmonary chemodectomas are seen amidst surrounding normal lung tissue. These lesions sometimes center on small pulmonary veins (arrow) and are composed of whorled band cells that are similar to arachnoidal cells of the meninges.

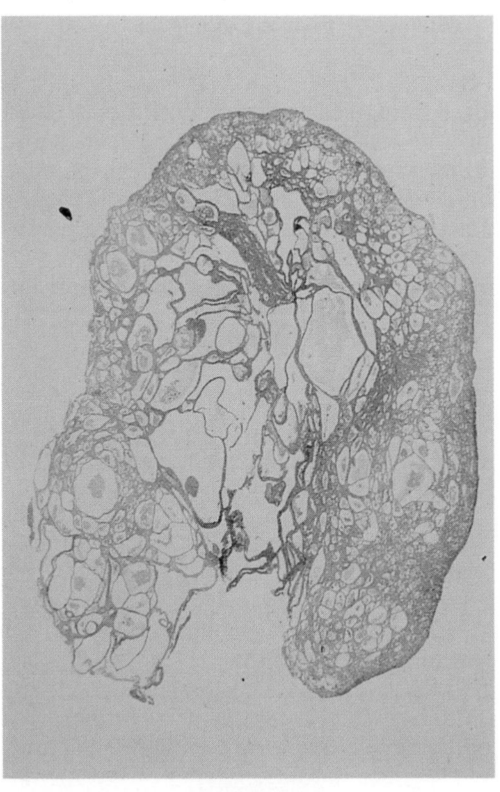

Figure 3 – 24.

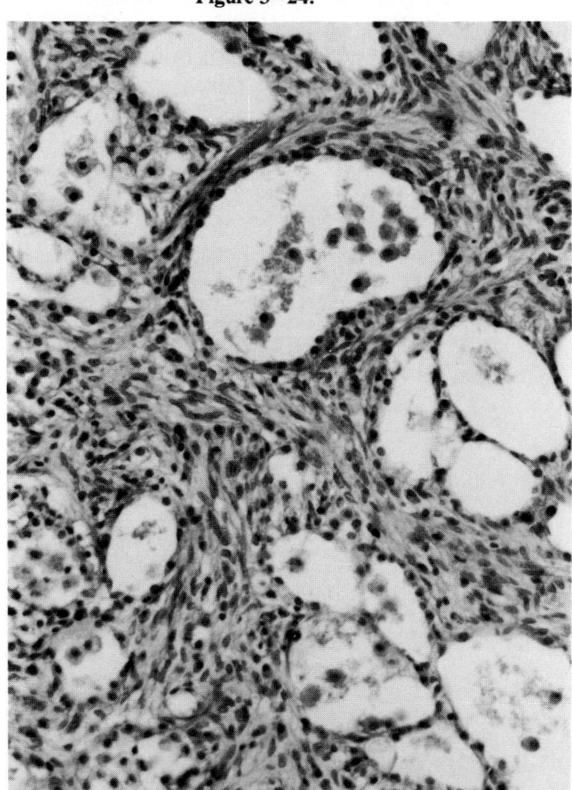

Figure 3 – 25.

■ Alveolar Adenoma (Figs. 3 – 24, 3 – 25)

An alveolar adenoma is a benign tumor composed of dilated alveolar spaces with intervening septa that contain spindle cells, capillaries, and a few inflammatory cells.

Histologically, there is a discrete nodule composed of varying-sized cystic spaces lined by type II cells and separated by septa containing benign spindle cells. The lesion is sharply circumscribed from the surrounding lung tissue and has a pushing margin.

Differential diagnosis includes lymphangioma, bronchioloalveolar carcinoma, papillary adenoma of type II cells, sclerosing hemangioma, and noncartilaginous hamartomas.

References

Yousem SA, Hocholzer L. Alveolar adenoma. Hum Pathol 17:1066 – 1071, 1986.

Figures 3 – 24, 3 – 25. Alveolar adenoma. There is a circumscribed, cytologically benign lesion with cystic spaces of varying sizes lined by type II cells. A benign interstitial spindle cell proliferation is present between the cysts.

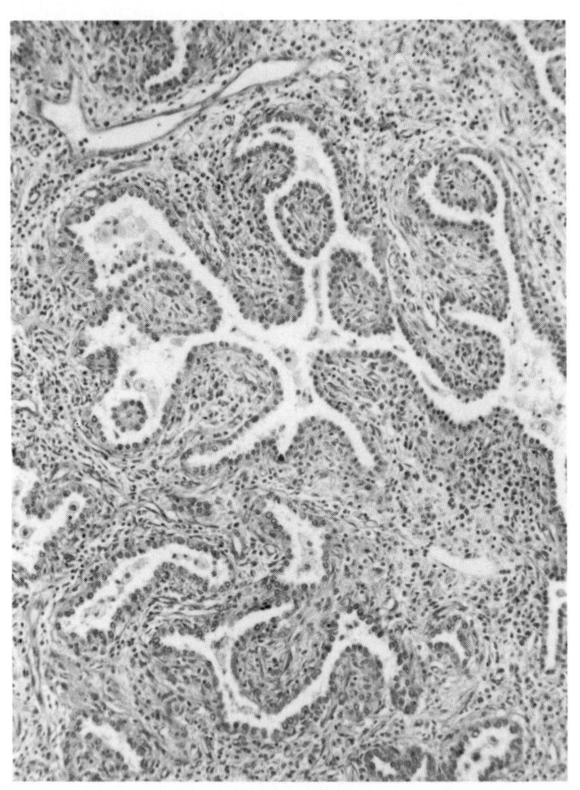

Figure 3–26.

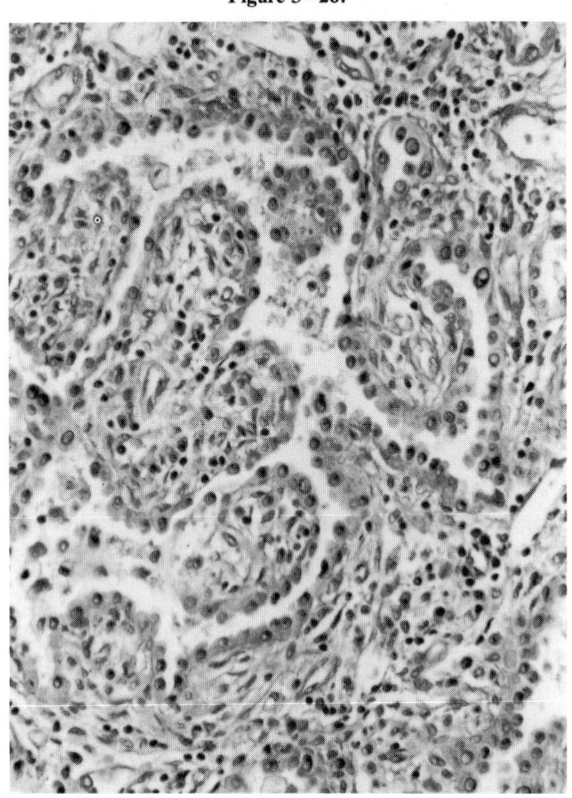

Figure 3–27.

Figures 3–26, 3–27. **Papillary adenoma of type II cells.** This well-circumscribed lesion is composed of papillae lined by type II cells, many of which contain nuclear vacuoles. Significant atypia and mitotic figures are absent.

■ Papillary Adenoma of Type 2 Cells (Figs. 3–26, 3–27)

This localized benign tumor usually presents as an asymptomatic coin lesion. It is a non-encapsulated and well-circumscribed tumor composed of delicate papillae lined by prominent type II cells. Cells with intranuclear inclusions may be present. These tumors may be parenchymal or endobronchial in location.

The differential diagnosis includes: Sclerosing hemangioma, bronchioloalveolar carcinoma, and alveolar adenoma.

References

Noguchi M, Kodama T, Shimosato Y, et al. Papillary adenoma of type II pneumocytes. Am J Surg Pathol 10:134–139, 1986.

■ Mucous Gland Adenoma (Figs. 3–28 to 3–31)

Mucous gland adenoma is a benign tumor derived from bronchial submucosal glands.

Mucous gland adenoma is a histologically well-circumscribed endobronchial tumor that is composed of goblet and columnar cells that form glands, papillae, and cystic spaces. They lack cytologic atypia or mitotic figures. Some cases feature a myxomatous stroma.

The differential diagnosis includes low-grade mucoepidermoid carcinoma with abundant mucinous differentiation and noncartilaginous hamartomas with a prominent myxoid stroma.

References

Carter D, Eggleston JC. Tumors of the Lower Respiratory Tract. AFIP Atlas of Tumor Pathology, Second Series, Fascicle 17. Washington, DC, Armed Forces Institute of Pathology, 1980.

Dail DH, Hammer SP (eds). Pulmonary Pathology. New York, Springer-Verlag, 1988.

Thurlbeck WM (ed). Pathology of the Lung. New York, Thieme, 1988.

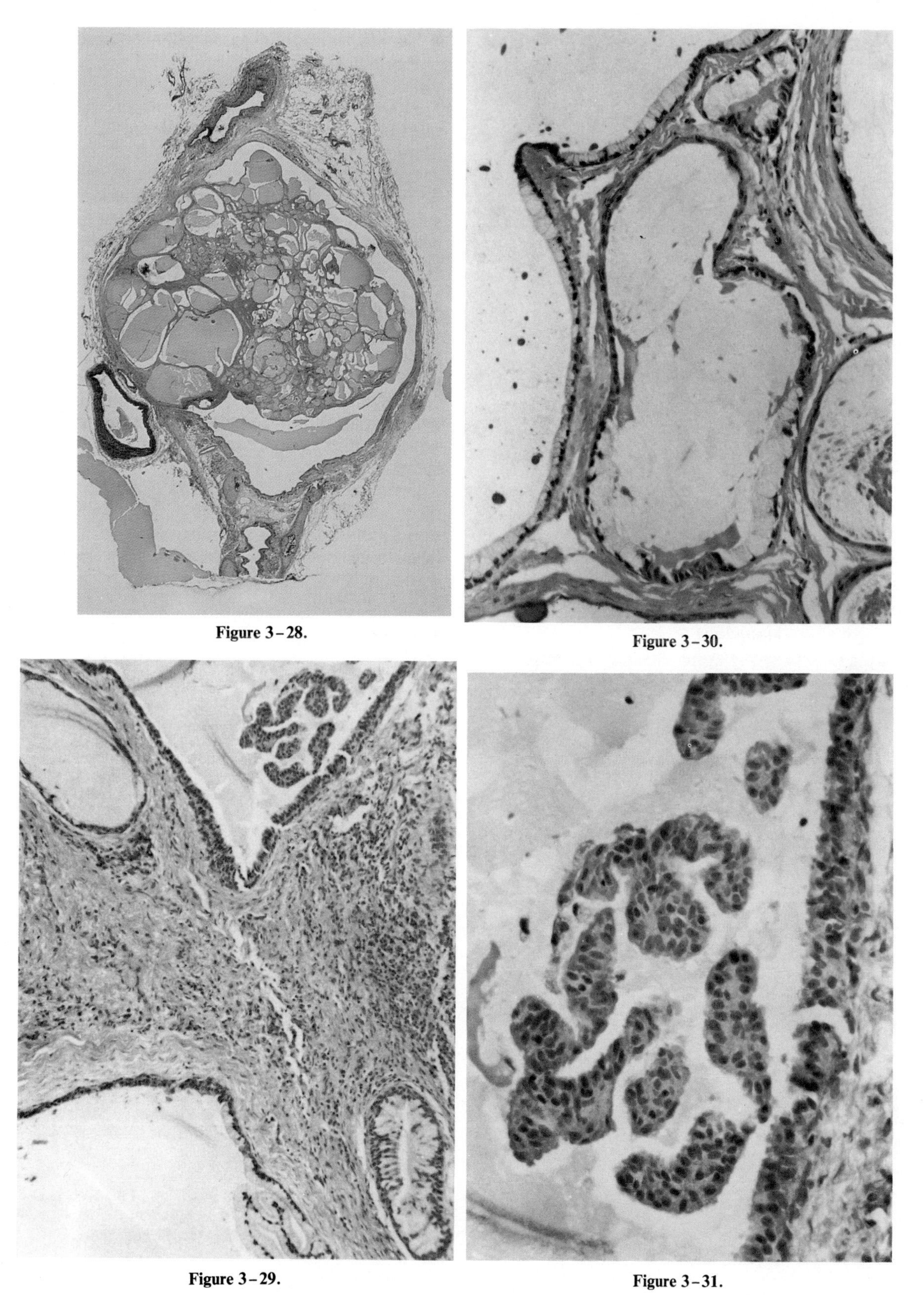

Figure 3–28.

Figure 3–30.

Figure 3–29.

Figure 3–31.

Figures 3–28, 3–29, 3–30, 3–31. Bronchial gland cystadenoma. Foci of mucous gland adenoma and foci of papillary adenoma are seen. The lesion is composed of cysts of varying sizes, lined in part by benign mucinous cells and in part by bland papillae resembling those of a papillary adenoma. The cysts are filled with Alcian green positive mucus. The differential diagnosis in this case includes an extremely well-differentiated mucoepidermoid tumor.

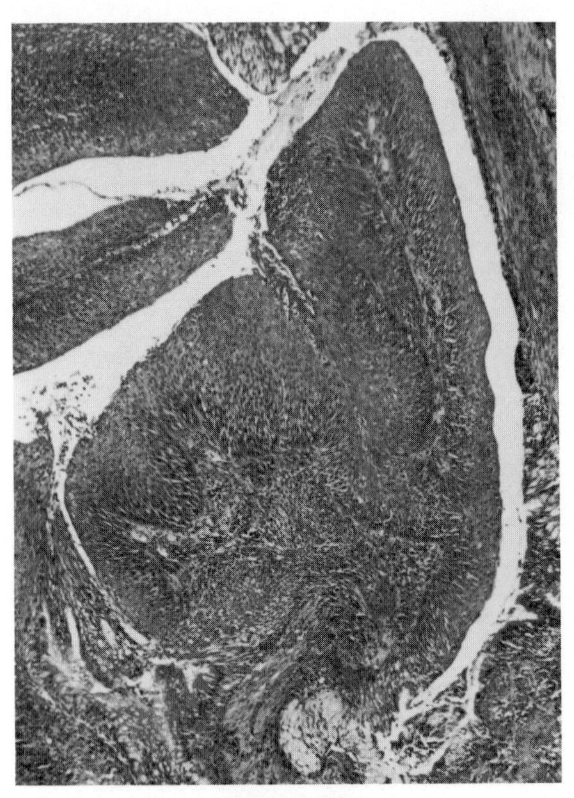

Figure 3-32.

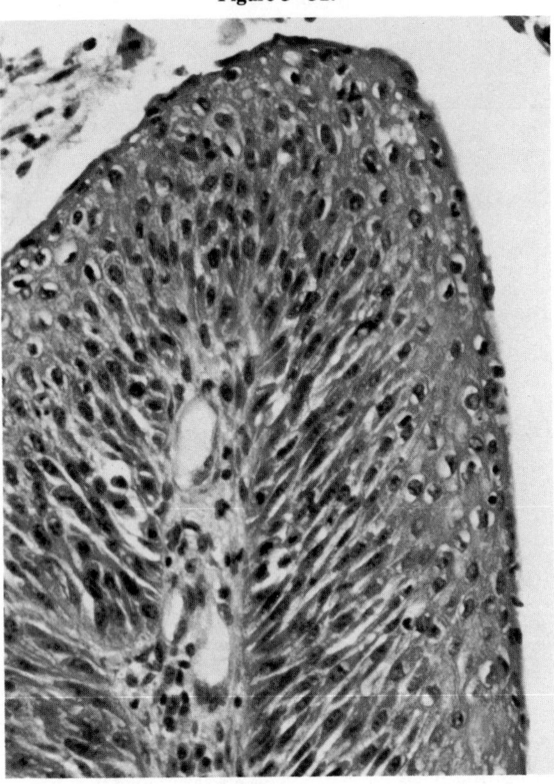

Figure 3-33.

■ Squamous Papillomas, Papillomatosis, and Other Papillomas (Figs. 3-32 to 3-35)

This group includes benign endobronchial papillary tumors that may be single (papilloma) or multiple (papillomatosis), and the latter may be associated with laryngeal papillomatosis. These lesions vary from incidental findings to major clinical problems associated with severe obstruction. Solitary lesions can often be cured with resection. In children with papillomatosis, cysts may be apparent on chest radiographs.

Cytologically benign, endobronchial papillary growths are present without underlying stromal invasion. The majority of papillomas are covered by bland squamous epithelium with or without keratinization; however, other cell types, including cuboidal, columnar, ciliated, and mucinous, may also partially or completely line the papillae. In the bronchial counterpart of laryngeal papillomatosis, condylomatous features may be present.

Differential diagnosis includes mucoepidermoid tumors, well-differentiated papillary squamous carcinoma, and papillary adenocarcinomas. Careful attention should be paid to cytologic details and evidence of invasion.

References

Carter D, Eggleston JC. Tumors of the Lower Respiratory Tract. AFIP Atlas of Tumor Pathology, Second Series, Fascicle 17. Washington, DC, Armed Forces Institute of Pathology, 1980.

Dail DH, Hammer SP (eds). Pulmonary Pathology. New York, Springer-Verlag, 1988.

Figures 3-32, 3-33. Solitary squamous papilloma of the bronchus. There is a complex benign papillary proliferation of squamous epithelium, which at higher power, suggests the possibility of koilocytotic atypia.

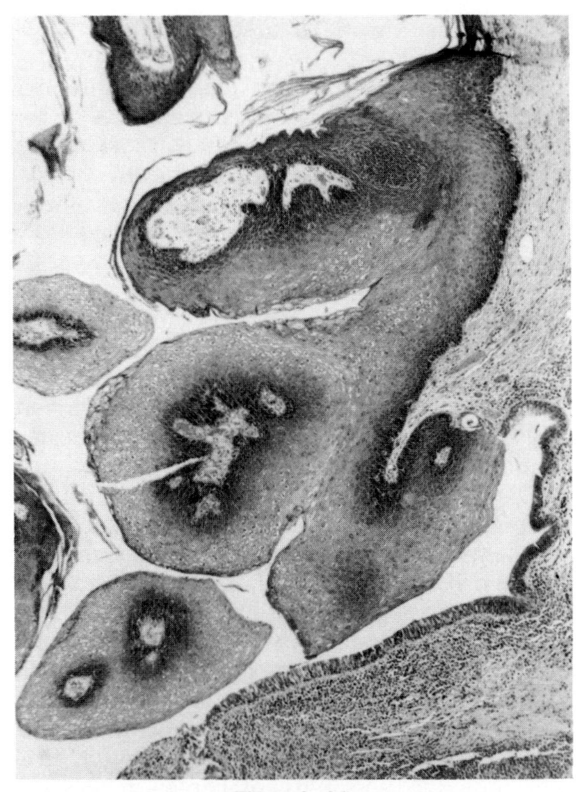

Figure 3-34.

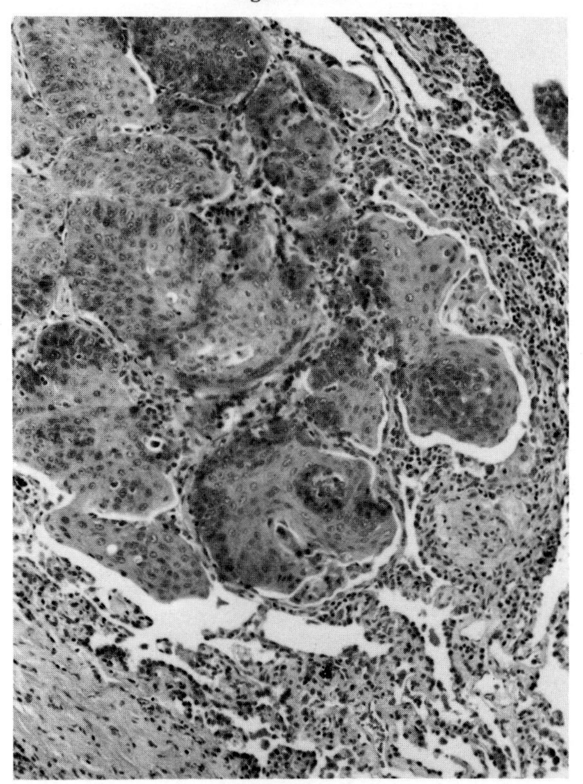

Figure 3-35.

Figures 3-34, 3-35. Papillomatosis. There was a several-decade history of laryngeal papillomatosis, which eventually spread down the airways into the lung parenchyma (Fig. 3-35). There was also a history of recurrent obstructive pneumonias and multiple surgical procedures.

■ Oncocytoma (Fig. 3-36)

Oncocytoma is a rare endobronchial or parenchymal tumor presenting as a coin lesion, analogous to salivary gland oncocytomas. Pure oncocytomas lack neuroendocrine differentiation. Mixtures of oncocytic cells with cells more typical of carcinoid tumors also occur (oncocytic carcinoid).

References

Thurlbeck WM (ed). Pathology of the Lung. New York, Thieme, 1988.

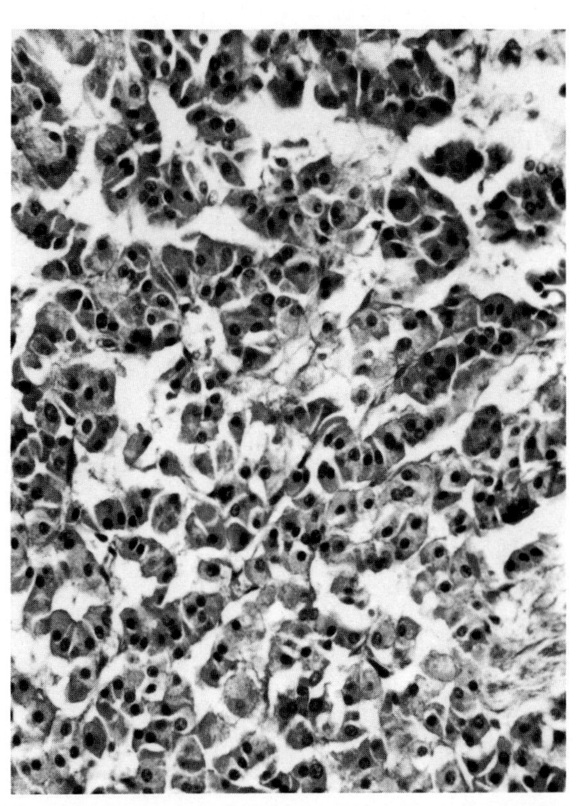

Figure 3-36. Pulmonary oncocytoma. This small, tan, well-circumscribed nodule was an incidental finding at autopsy. The lesion is composed of large, polygonal eosinophilic cells with small, round nuclei. Ultrastructurally, large numbers of mitochondria were demonstrated.

Figures 3-37, 3-38, 3-39. Hamartoma. These figures show the typical lobulated appearance with epithelium-lined clefts around the lobules. In one case (Figures 3-37, 3-38), the lobules are both cartilaginous and fatty; in the other (Figure 3-39), they are composed only of smooth muscle and fat.

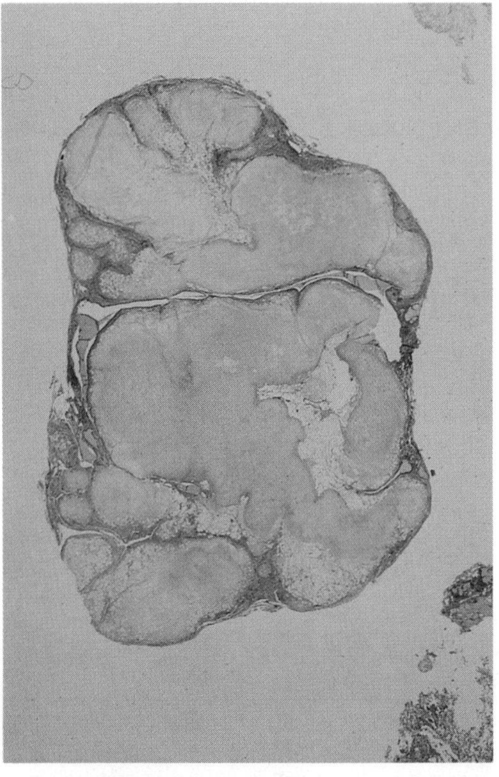

Figure 3-37.

■ Hamartomas (Figs. 3-37 to 3-43)

A hamartoma is a parenchymal or endobronchial nodule that presents with airway obstruction if the lesion is endobronchial. It may also present as an asymptomatic, sometimes calcified (radiographically "popcorn-like") coin lesion or as an incidental finding at surgery or autopsy. Classically, these lesions are "shelled out" by the surgeon. They are rarely multiple.

The classic hamartoma is a lobulated, mature, cartilaginous nodule with epithelial-lined clefts surrounding the lobules. Other mesenchymal tissues that may be seen include fat, smooth muscle, and undifferentiated myxoid mesenchymal tissue. In some cases, cartilage is completely lacking. The most characteristic features are the lobulation and the epithelial-lined clefts.

The differential diagnosis includes epithelioid hemangioendothelioma (IVBAT), chondromas, chondrosarcomas, teratomas (both primary and metastatic), other mesenchymal tumors (when hamartomas show other than cartilaginous differentiation) and mixed tumor of salivary origin. A chondroma in a young woman should raise the possibility of Carney's triad: multiple pulmonary chondromas, epithelioid smooth muscle tumors of the stomach, and extra-adrenal paragangliomas. Multiple nodules with prominent smooth muscle stroma should raise the possibility of benign metastasizing leiomyoma.

References

Carter D, Eggleston JC. Tumors of the Lower Respiratory Tract. AFIP Atlas of Tumor Pathology, Second Series, Fascicle 17. Washington, DC, Armed Forces Institute of Pathology, 1980.

Dail DH, Hammer SP (eds). Pulmonary Pathology, New York, Springer-Verlag, 1988.

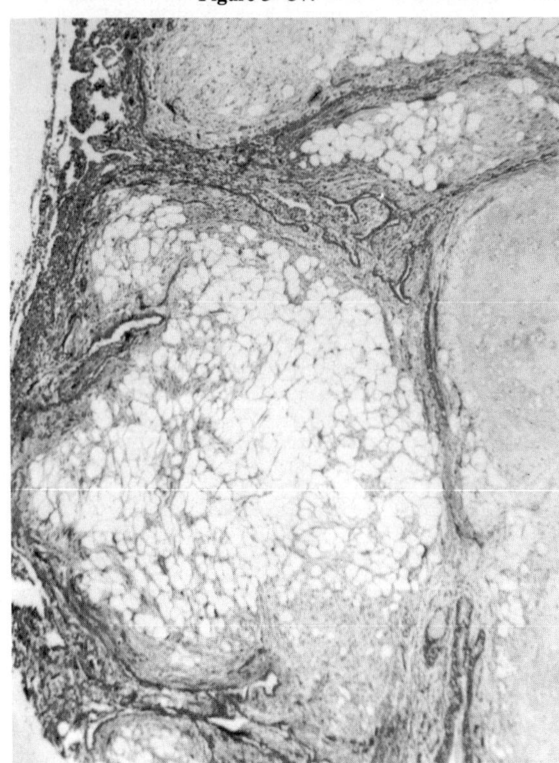

Figure 3-38.

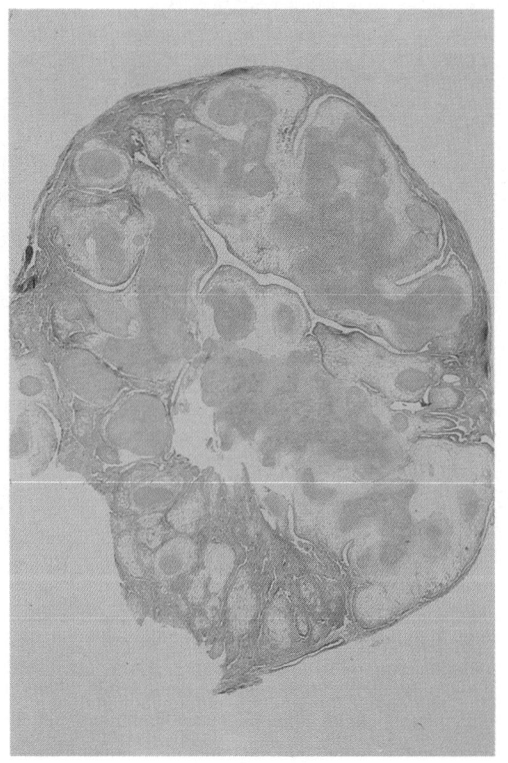

Figure 3-39.

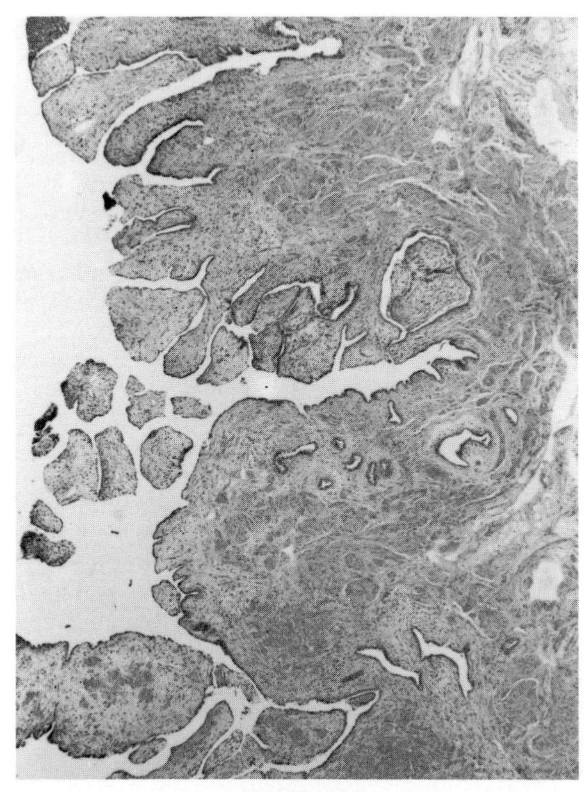

Figure 3-40.

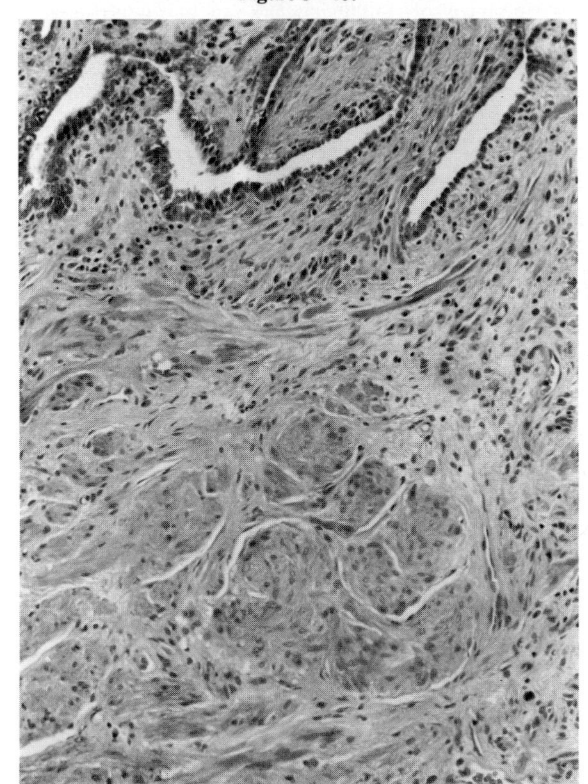

Figure 3-41.

Figures 3-40, 3-41. Hamartoma. This shelled-out hamartoma shows a lobulated appearance with extensive smooth muscle proliferation and absence of cartilage.

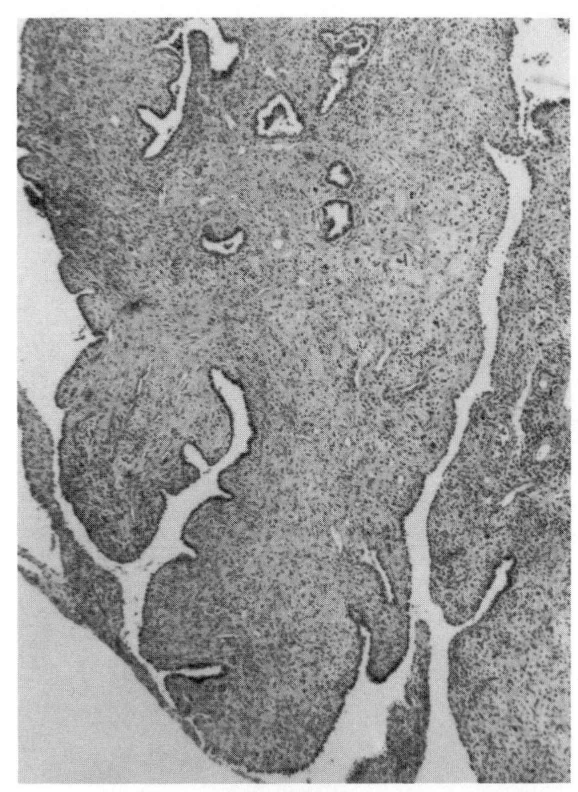

Figure 3-42.

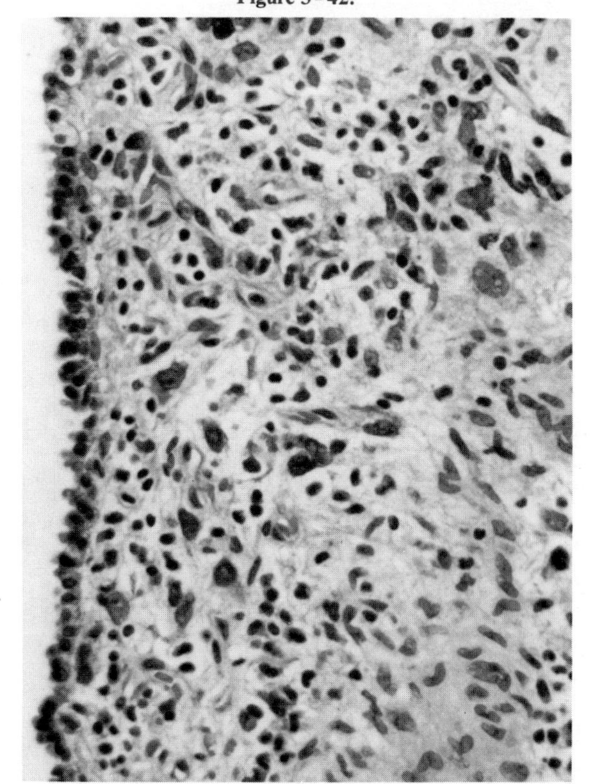

Figure 3-43.

Figures 3-42, 3-43. Hamartoma. The lobules are composed of non-descript mesenchymal cells with prominent lymphoid cells. At the periphery of the lobules, mild cytologic atypia is apparent.

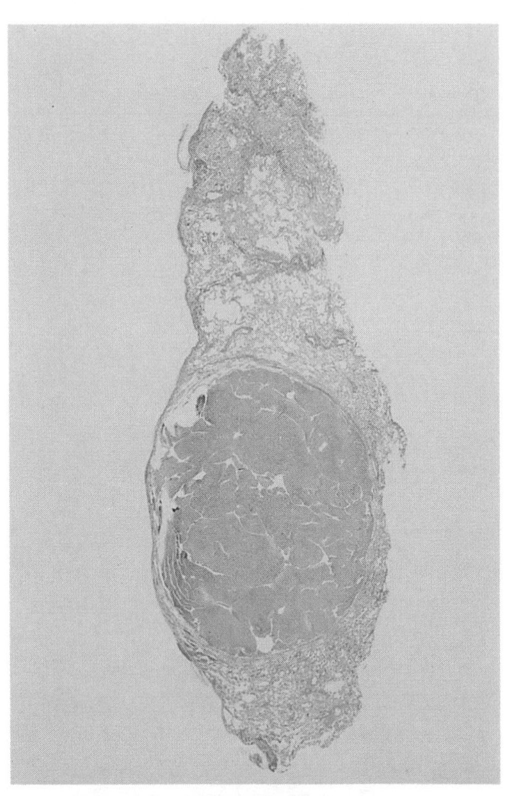

Figure 3–44.

■ Intrapulmonary Fibrous Mesothelioma (Intrapulmonary Localized Fibrous Tumor, Subpleural Fibroma) (Figs. 3–44 to 3–49)

Intrapulmonary fibrous mesothelioma is a nodule, often septal or subpleural in location, that shows histologic features identical to those of localized fibrous mesothelioma of the pleura. A connection to the pleura may or may not be present.

Histologically, this tumor is composed of haphazardly arranged, stubby, spindled, bipolar fibroblastic cells with interspersed, thick, hyalinized collagenous bands with variation in cellularity from one portion of the tumor to the next. The majority of cases are histologically benign; however, some may show foci of marked cellularity with mitotic figures, and these lesions may recur and even show aggressive behavior if incompletely excised. A typical feature of fibrous mesotheliomas is interstitial growth at the edge and inclusion of airspaces lined by metaplastic cells, thereby mimicking a biphasic tumor.

Differential diagnosis includes plasma cell granulomas and other spindle cell tumors. Resection is the treatment of choice and nearly always can be performed.

References

England DM, Hochholzer L, McCarthy MJ. Localized benign and malignant fibrous tumors of the pleura. Am J Surg Pathol 13:640–658, 1989.

Yousem SA, Flynn SD. Intrapulmonary localized fibrous tumor. Am J Clin Pathol 89:365–369, 1988.

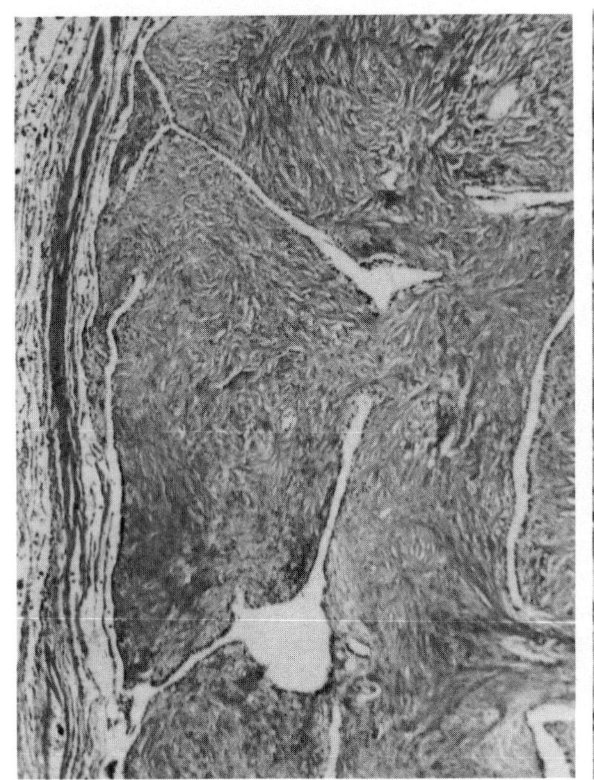

Figure 3–45.

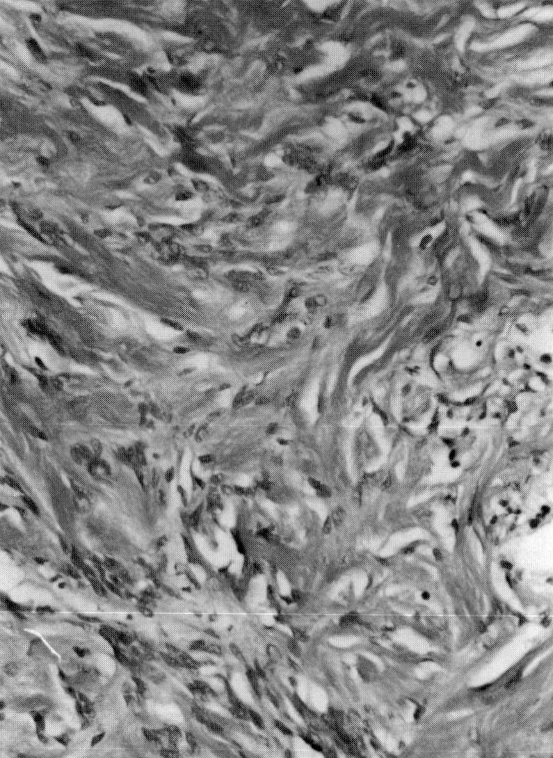

Figure 3–46.

Figures 3–44, 3–45, 3–46. Intrapulmonary fibrous mesothelioma. A highly sclerotic, pauci-cellular, intraparenchymal lesion is well demarcated from the surrounding tissue, although some epithelium-lined clefts are present at the periphery. Benign spindle cells are seen among thick, hyalinized bundles of collagen.

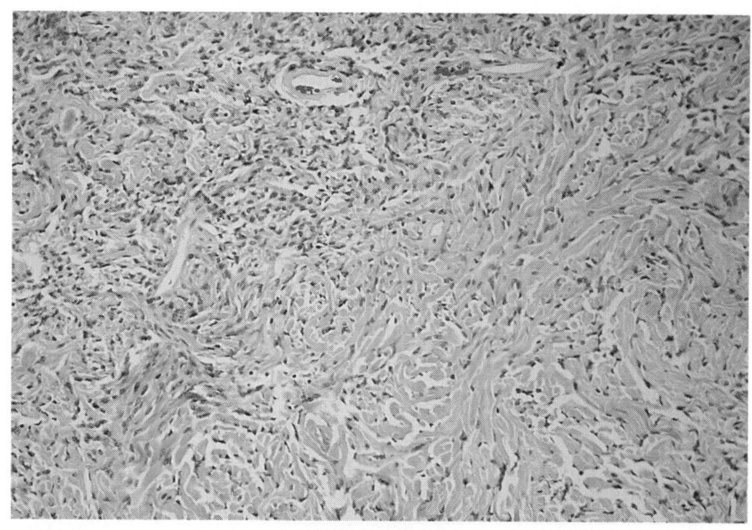

Figure 3–47.

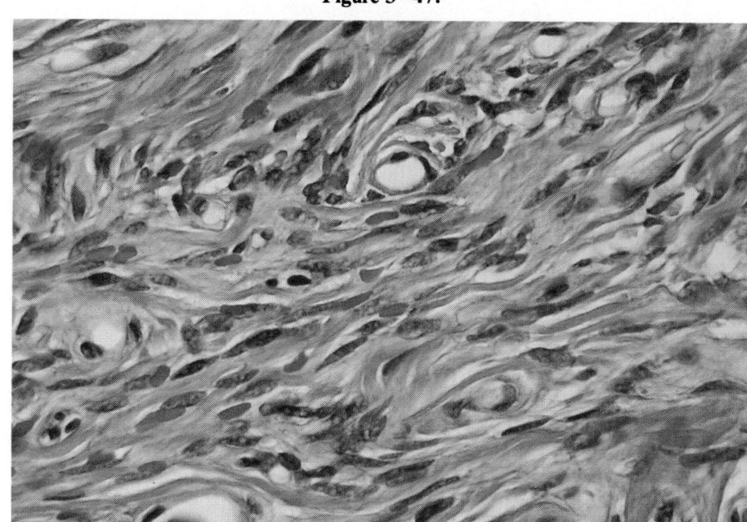

Figure 3–48.

Figures 3–47, 3–48, 3–49. Intrapulmonary fibrous mesothelioma. These three examples illustrate typical features. Cytologic atypia and mitotic figures are absent. The waviness of the nuclei in some cases is reminiscent of a neural tumor. The variation in cellularity from field to field and dense hyalinized collagenous bands are characteristic.

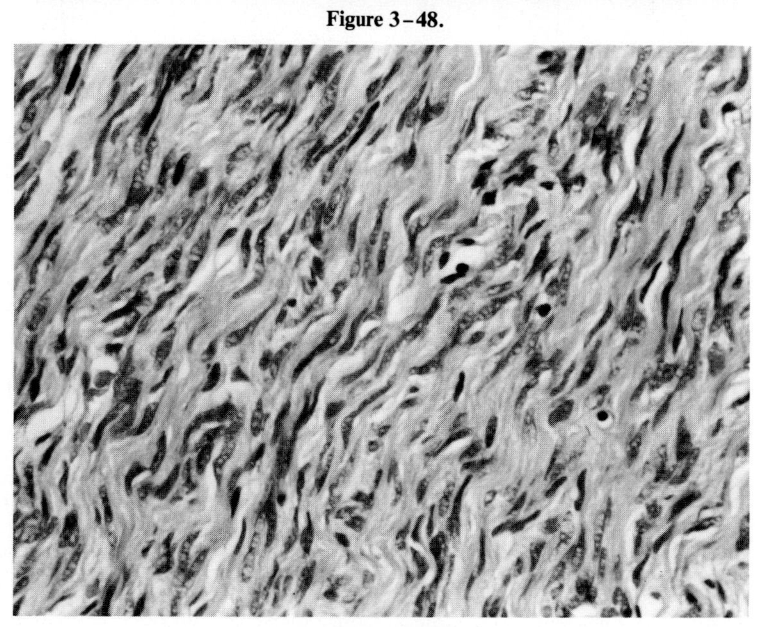

Figure 3–49.

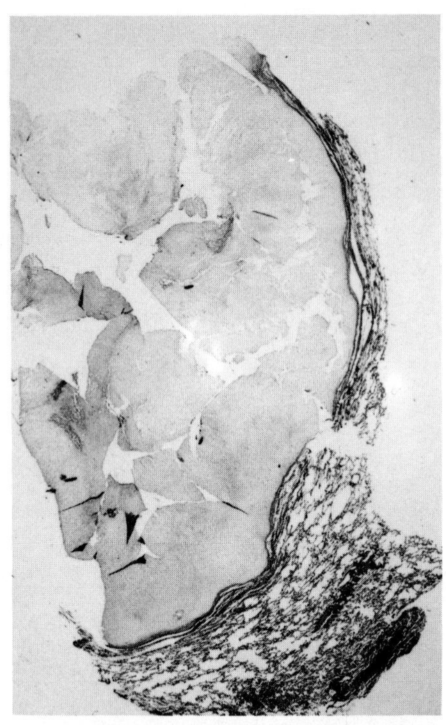

Figure 3–50. Chondroma. Chondroma in Carney's triad. This cartilaginous lung tumor from a young woman with Carney's triad is composed of histologically benign cartilage. It is well circumscribed from the surrounding lung parenchyma and lacks the lobulation of a cartilaginous hamartoma. (Courtesy of J. A. Carney, M.D.).

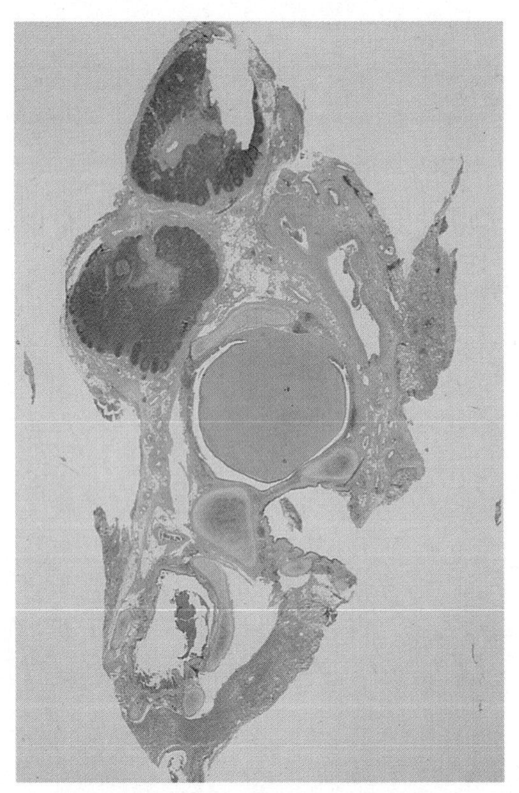

Figure 3–51. Endobronchial leiomyoma. A small segmental bronchus is occluded by a polypoid tumor composed of benign, mature smooth muscle cells. The lesion had caused recurrent bouts of obstructive pneumonia.

■ Chondroma (Fig. 3–50)

A chondroma is a benign cartilaginous tumor that may be either endobronchial or parenchymal in location.

Bland hyaline cartilage without malignant features is present, and generally there is less cellularity than seen in hamartomas.

Differential diagnosis includes other lesions that appear cartilaginous, including hamartomas, epithelioid hemangioendothelioma, chondrosarcoma (both primary and metastatic), teratomas with cartilage, the chondroma of Carney's triad (smooth muscle tumors of the stomach, extra-adrenal paragangliomas, and pulmonary parenchymal chondromas), and mixed tumors of salivary origin.

References

Thurlbeck WM (ed). Pathology of the Lung. New York, Thieme, 1988.

■ Sclerosing Hemangioma (Figs. 3–52 to 3–59)

Sclerosing hemangioma is a tumor of disputed histogenesis (probably derived from developing bronchopulmonary epithelium) presenting as a coin lesion, usually in asymptomatic middle-aged women. The tumors are well circumscribed, frequently hemorrhagic, and may be "shelled out."

Sclerosing hemangioma has a variegated histologic appearance with papillae lined by prominent type II cells; recent and old hemorrhage; sclerotic zones, which may contain small "hemangiomatous-like" vessels; and polygonal interstitial cells, which occur singly or in sheets and which may appear to merge with type II cells. These polygonal cells are thought to be the proliferating cells, with all the other changes being secondary. Foam cells and hemorrhage may be prominent.

Recent evidence suggests that the sclerosing hemangioma is a tumor of primitive bronchopulmonary cells akin to type II cells. Despite the disputed histogenesis, this is a well-recognized and well-defined clinicopathologic lesion that is benign and curable with resection. Because of the papillary foci lined by prominent type II cells, bronchoalveolar carcinoma, alveolar adenoma, hamartoma, and papillary adenoma of type II cells enter the differential diagnosis.

References

Carter D, Eggleston JC. Tumors of the Lower Respiratory Tract. AFIP Atlas of Tumor Pathology, Second Series, Fascicle 17. Washington, DC, Armed Forces Institute of Pathology, 1980.

Dail DH, Hammer SP (eds). Pulmonary Pathology. New York, Springer-Verlag, 1988.

Katzenstein AL, Gmelich JT, Carrington CB. Sclerosing hemangioma of the lung: a clinicopathologic study of 51 cases. Am J Surg Pathol 4:343–356, 1980.

Yousem SA, Wick M, et al. Sclerosing hemangioma: an immunohistochemical and clinicopathologic study. Am J Surg Pathol 12:582–590, 1988.

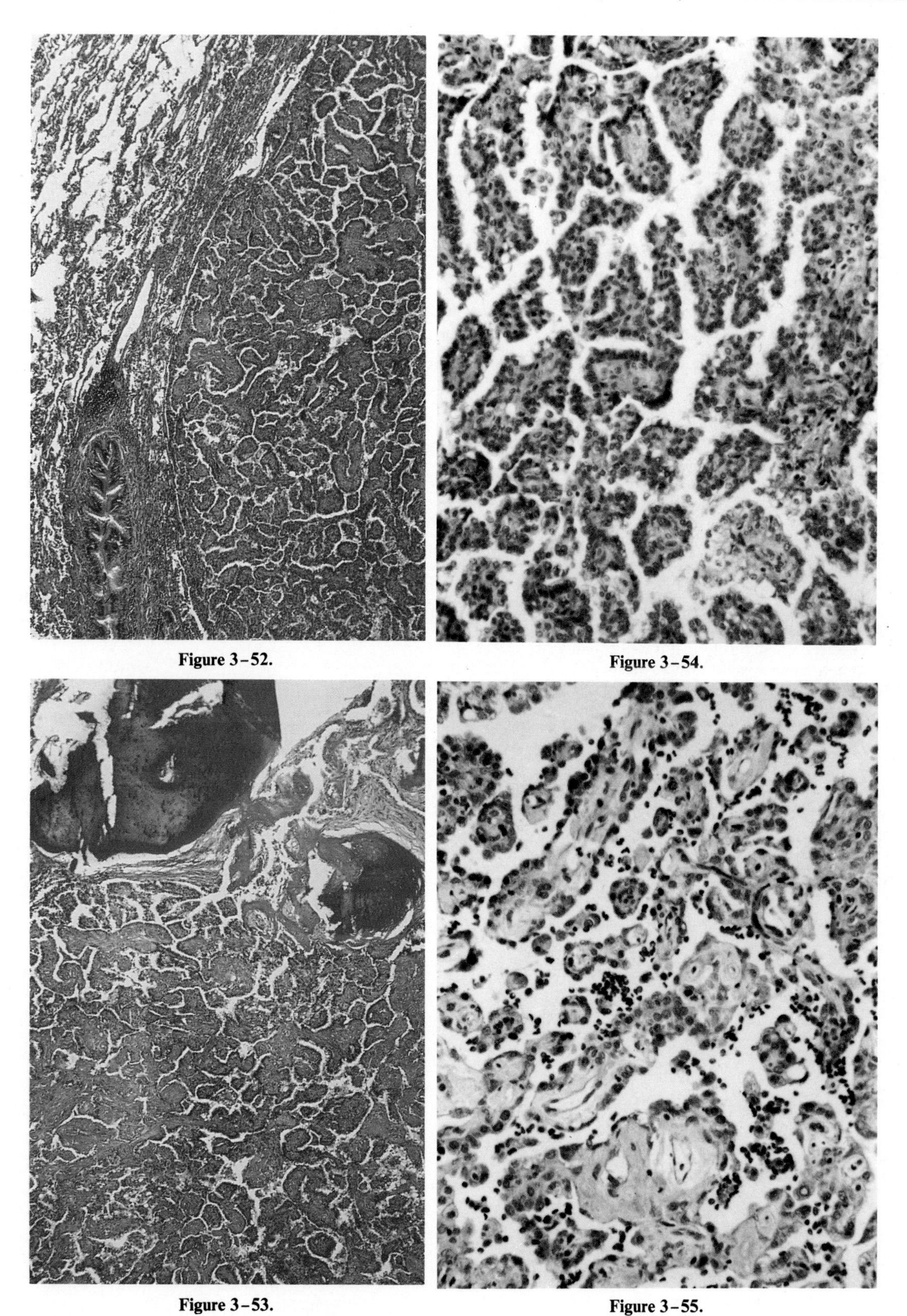

Figure 3-52.

Figure 3-54.

Figure 3-53.

Figure 3-55.

Figures 3-52, 3-53, 3-54, 3-55. Sclerosing hemangioma. Central sclerosis, calcification, or ossification may be seen. The lesions are well circumscribed with papillary structures in the periphery. Some sclerosing hemangiomas are composed almost entirely of papillae. The papillae are lined by monotonous polygonal cells resembling type II cells with connective tissue cores with variable amounts of sclerosis.

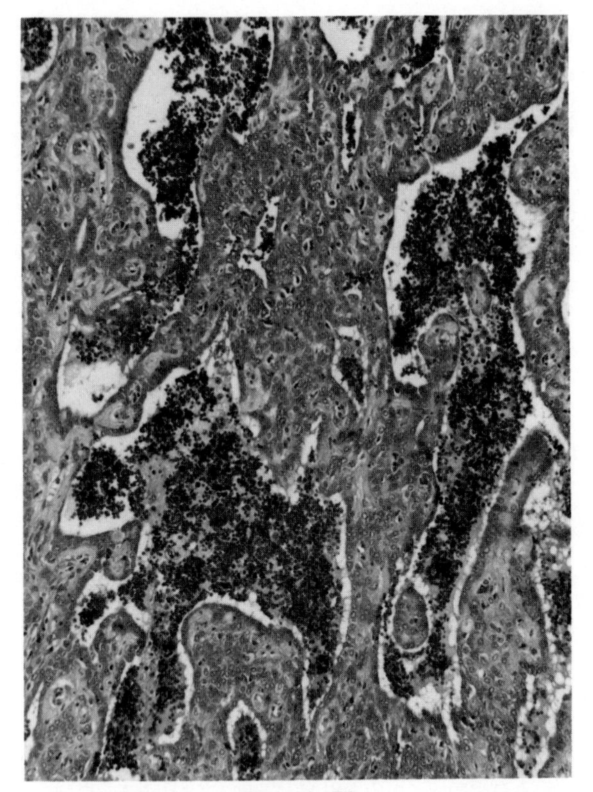

Figure 3–56.

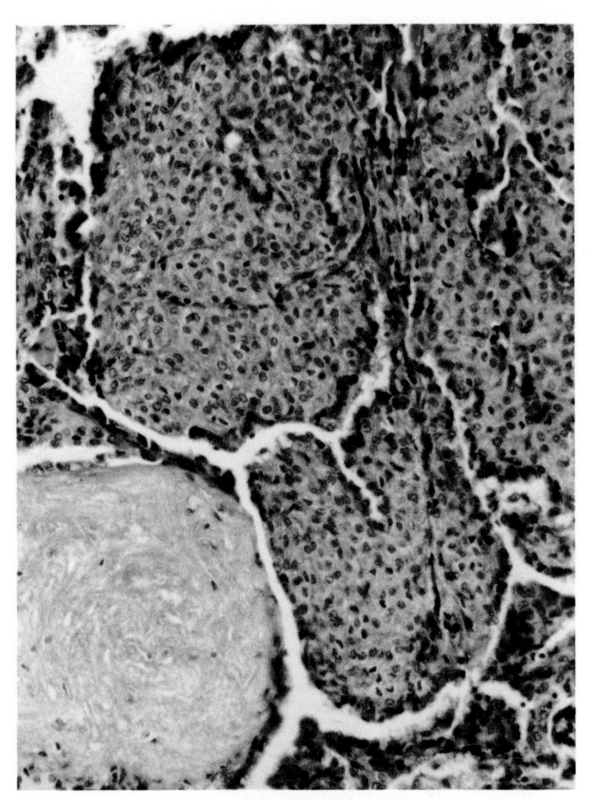

Figure 3–58.

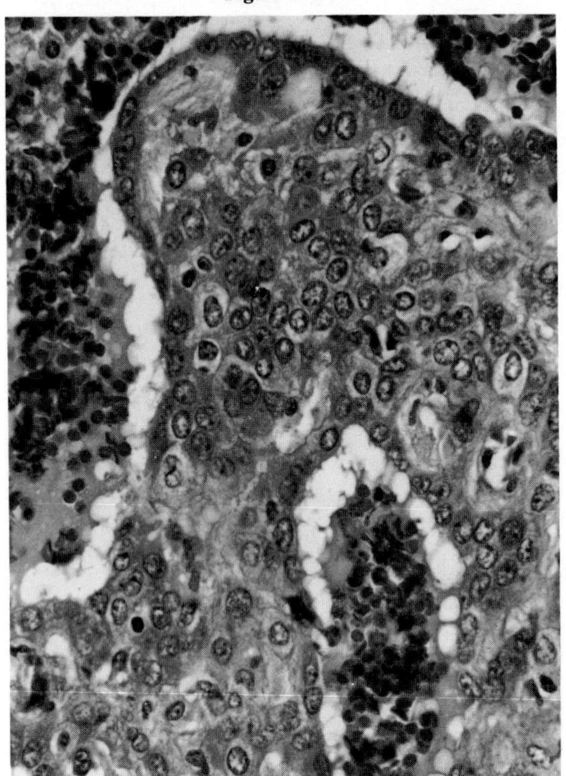

Figure 3–57.

Figures 3–56, 3–57. Sclerosing hemangioma. Irregular spaces filled with blood are separated by cellular trabeculae that are both lined by and composed in part of benign polygonal cells with epithelial features.

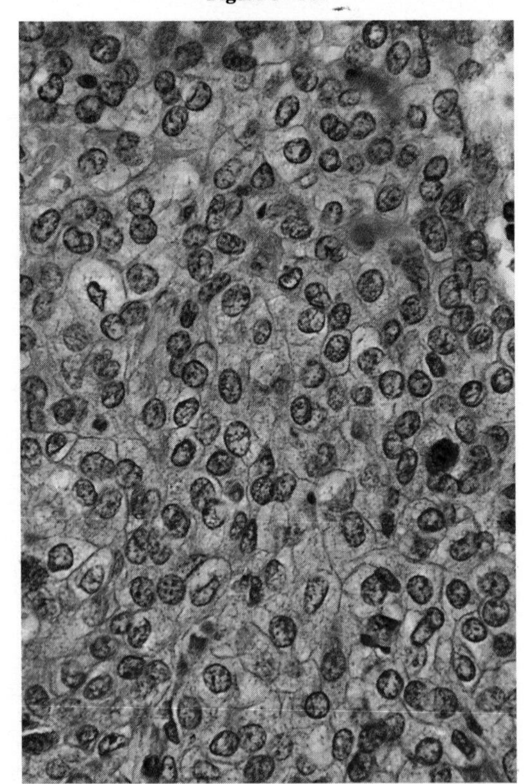

Figure 3–59.

Figures 3–58, 3–59. Sclerosing hemangioma. The bland, proliferating polygonal cells produce small nodules within papillae and interstitial infiltrates. Recent studies suggest that these are primitive bronchopulmonary cells with differentiation toward type II cells.

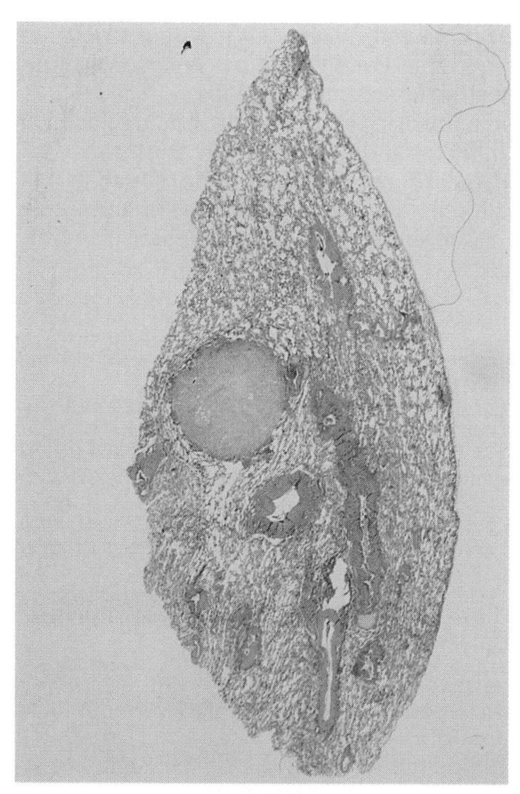

Figure 3-60.

■ Epithelioid Hemangioendothelioma (Intravascular Bronchioloalveolar Tumor or IVBAT) (Figs. 3-60 to 3-70)

Epithelioid hemangioendothelioma is a low-grade angiosarcoma that may involve multiple sites in the body but often presents in the lung as multiple bilateral nodules, sometimes in an asymptomatic patient. The lesion was originally called intravascular bronchioloalveolar tumor (IVBAT) because it sometimes shows a marked propensity toward intravascular growth, and in one of the early cases, there was a concomitant bronchioloalveolar carcinoma. Some patients have an indolent course despite bilateral disease; in others, a rapidly fatal course is experienced. There is no known therapy.

Nodules are appreciated grossly and microscopically; they contain a relatively acellular center and polygonal cells with vesicular nuclei irregularly dispersed within a myxohyaline or chondroid matrix. The nodules are lobulated with growth into alveolar spaces, bronchioles, lymphatics, and blood vessels. There is greater cellularity in the periphery of the nodules where small clusters, cords, and individual cells are seen, some of which contain cytoplasmic vacuoles thought to be indicative of endothelial lumen differentiation. Coagulative necrosis may occur in the center of large nodules. The degree of atypia is usually mild, but some cases do show moderate nuclear hyperchromasia. Spindling may occur with

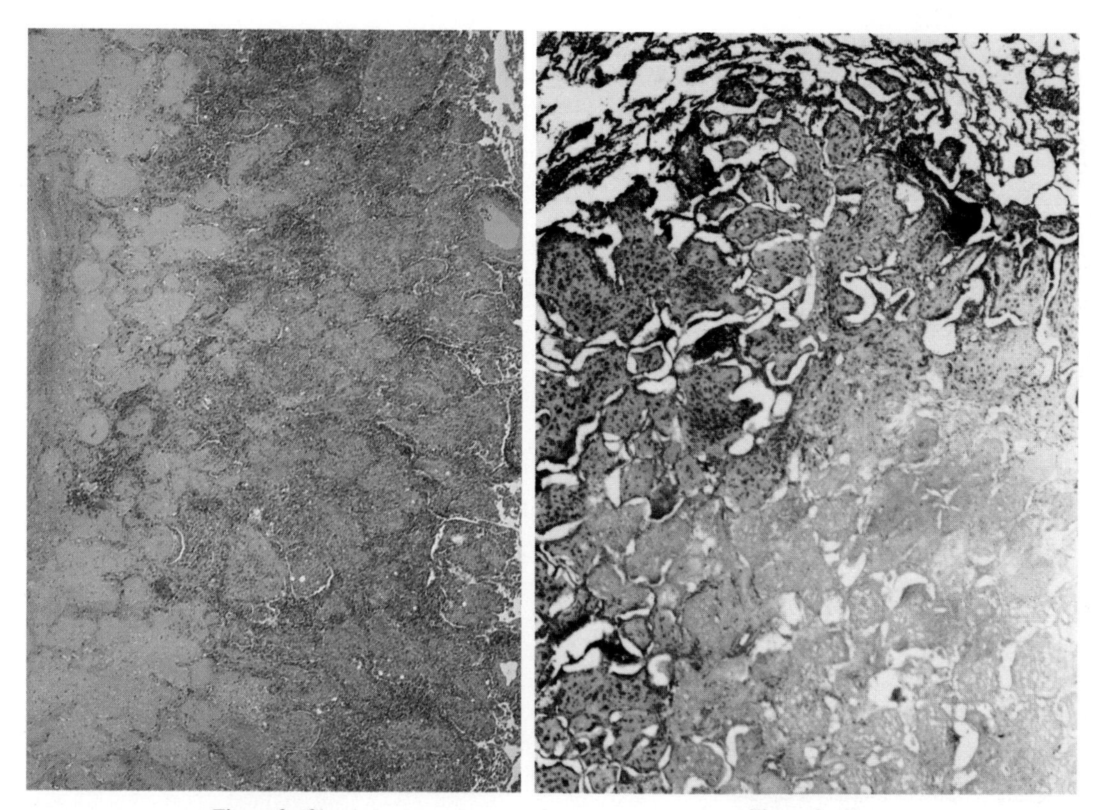

Figure 3-61. Figure 3-62.

Figures 3-60, 3-61, 3-62. Epithelioid hemangioendothelioma. A well-circumscribed nodule with necrotic, acellular myxochondroid center is surrounded by intra-alveolar nodules of myxochondroid cells.

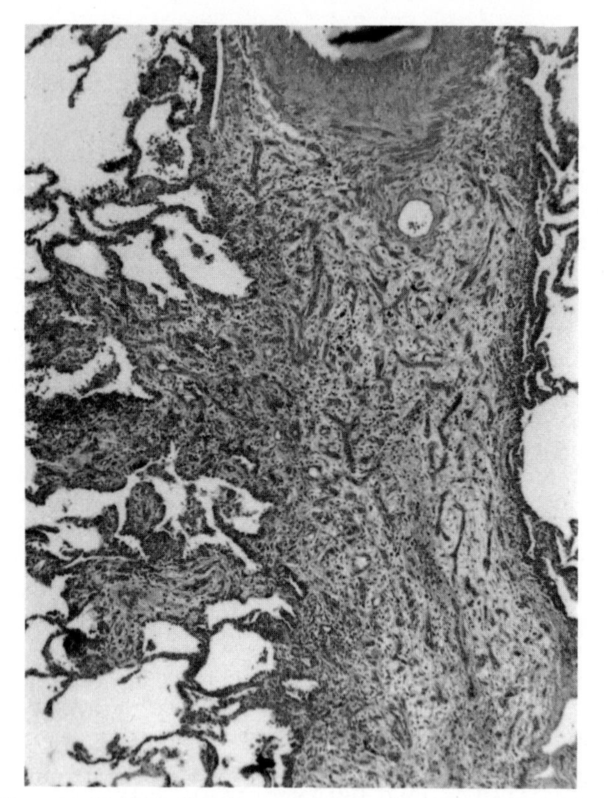

Figure 3-63. Epithelioid hemangioendothelioma. There is septal expansion by a vascular neoplasm, producing elongated, epithelioid vascular channels.

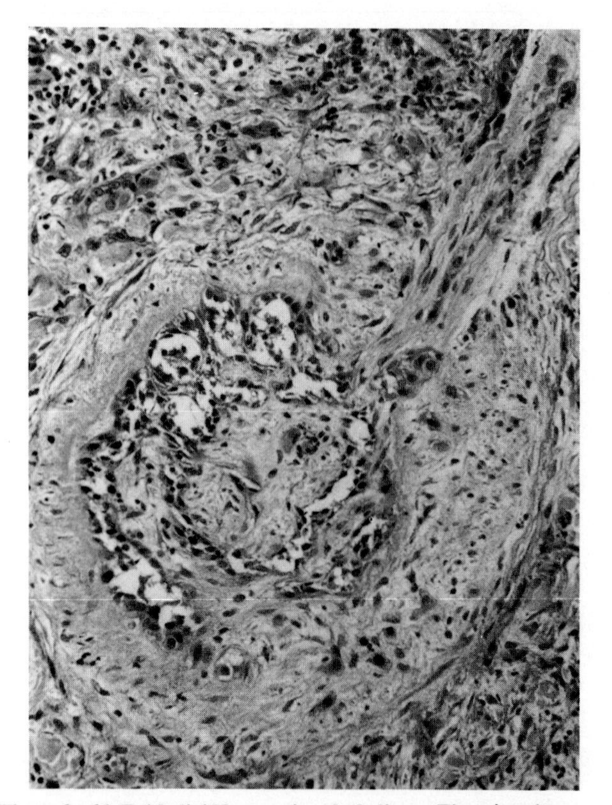

Figure 3-64. Epithelioid hemangioendothelioma. There is pulmonary arterial invasion. Neoplastic vascular spaces are lined by epithelioid cells.

growth in the septa and/or pleura. Growth restricted to the pleura can mimic a mesothelioma. Widespread lymphatic permeation sometimes develops.

Epithelioid hemangioendothelioma should be considered in the differential diagnosis of any tumor that appears chondroid or myxohyaline. The possibility of metastatic epithelioid hemangioendothelioma from the liver or soft tissue should also be considered.

References

Dail DH, Hammer SP (eds). Pulmonary Pathology. New York, Springer-Verlag, 1988.

Dail DH, Liebow AA, Gmelich JT, et al. Intravascular, bronchiolar and alveolar tumor of the lung. Cancer 51:452-463, 1983.

Eggleston JC. The intravascular bronchioalveolar tumor and sclerosing hemangiomas of the lung. Semin Diagn Pathol 2:270-279, 1985.

Thurlbeck WM (ed). Pathology of the Lung. New York, Thieme, 1988.

Weiss SW, Enzinger FM. Epithelioid hemangioendothelioma. Cancer 50:970-981, 1982.

Yousem SA, Hochholzer LH. Unusual thoracic manifestations of epithelioid hemangioendothelioma. Arch Pathol Lab Med 111:459-463, 1987.

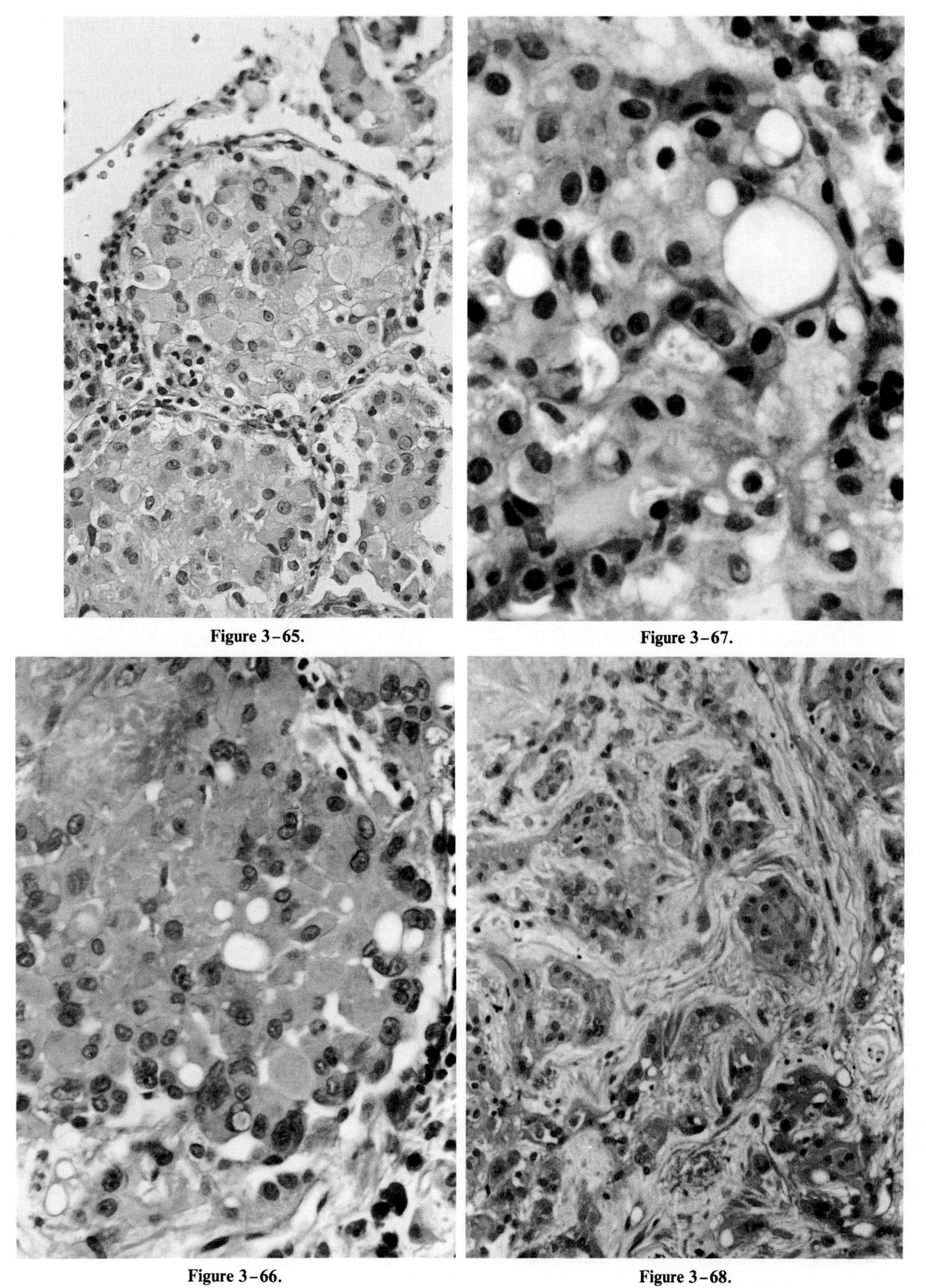

Figure 3-65.

Figure 3-67.

Figure 3-66.

Figure 3-68.

Figures 3-65, 3-66, 3-67, 3-68. Epithelioid hemangioendothelioma. Cytologic detail shows eosinophilic epithelioid cells with somewhat opaque and glassy cytoplasm. Clear, sharply demarcated cytoplasmic vacuoles can be seen.

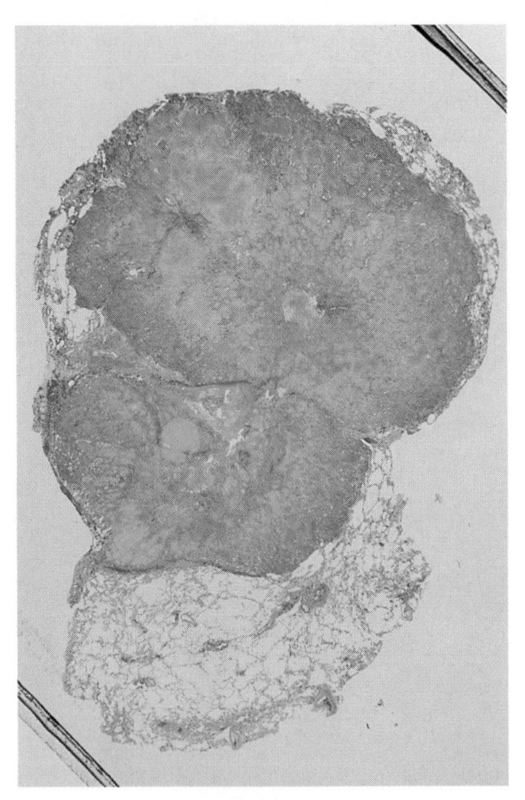

Figure 3-69.

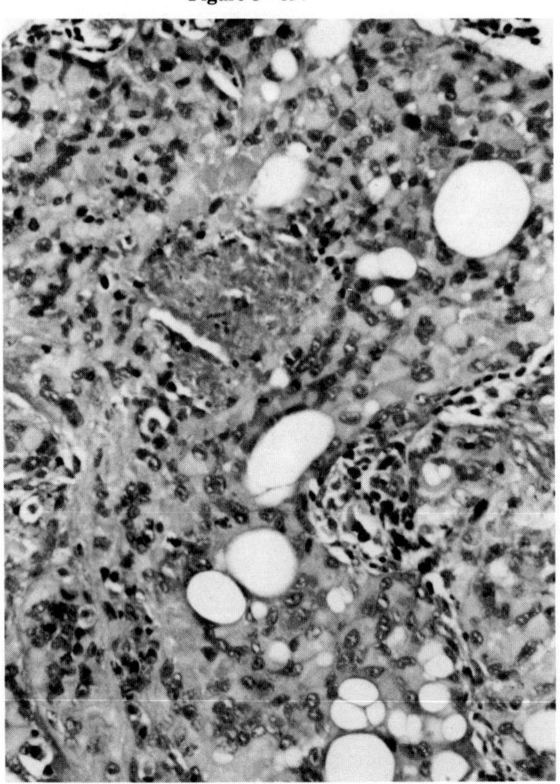

Figure 3-70.

■ Carcinoid Tumorlets (Carcinoid Atypical Proliferation) (Figs. 3-71, 3-72)

Carcinoid tumorlets consist of peribronchiolar proliferations of neuroendocrine cells forming small nodules that are usually identified microscopically. These tumorlets are more common in zones of airway scarring and bronchiectasis.

Tumorlets are characterized by nested polygonal to spindled cells showing granular chromatin typical of neuroendocrine differentiation without necrosis, atypia, or frequent mitotic figures. They typically occur in a fibrotic region around a small airway. An intraepithelial component in the airway may be present.

The differential diagnosis of a large tumorlet is a small carcinoid, and the exact point of separation may be somewhat arbitrary, particularly since tumorlets may occur in lung tissue containing a carcinoid tumor. In fact, some believe tumorlets are just tiny carcinoid tumors. Crush artifact in tumorlets may simulate small cell undifferentiated carcinoma.

References

Churg A, Warnock ML. Pulmonary tumorlet. A form of peripheral carcinoid. Cancer 37:1469-1477, 1976.

D'Agati VD, Perzin KH. Carcinoid tumorlets of the lung with metastasis to peribronchial lymph node. Cancer 55:2472-2476, 1985.

Ranchod M. The histogenesis and development of pulmonary tumorlets. Cancer 39:1135-1145, 1977.

Figures 3-69, 3-70. Epithelioid hemangioendothelioma. In this case, there is increased cellularity with cytologic atypia and foci of necrosis. Nevertheless, characteristic cells with the glassy eosinophilic cytoplasm, which contains sharp vacuoles, are apparent.

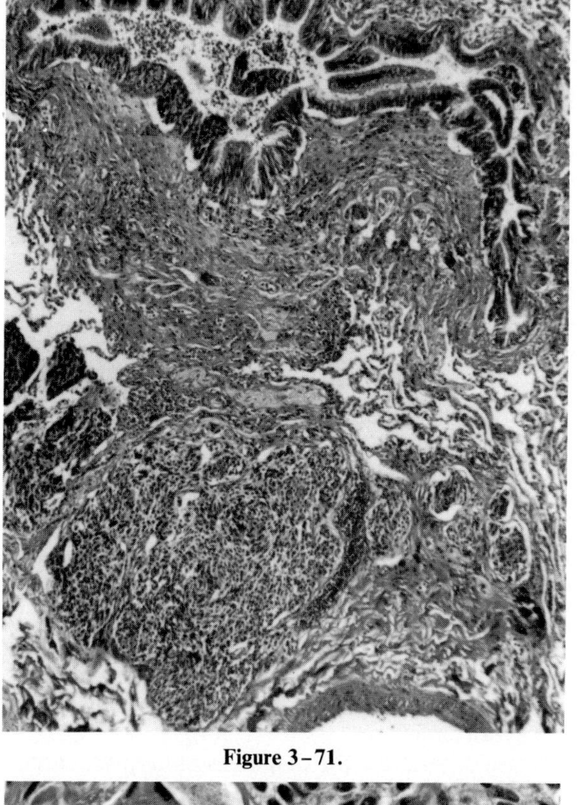

Figure 3–71.

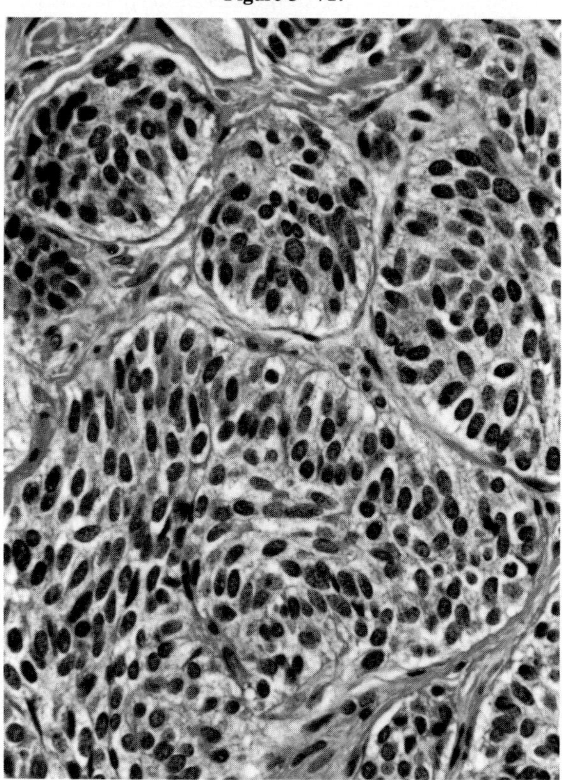

Figure 3–72.

Figures 3–71, 3–72. Carcinoid tumorlet. There is a microscopic nodular proliferation of nested spindle and polygonal cells adjacent to a small airway. The vascular septa are typical of neuroendocrine proliferations.

■ Carcinoid Tumors and Atypical Carcinoid Tumors (Figs. 3–73 to 3–83)

These neuroendocrine neoplasms vary in clinical aggressiveness from low grade (typical carcinoid) to higher grade (atypical carcinoid). These tumors may be central or peripheral. Although central carcinoids classically are characterized by trabecular or insular patterns and peripheral tumors tend to show more spindling, there is considerable overlap. Carcinoid tumors may be discovered incidentally; they may also present either as recurrent pneumonias due to obstruction or, rarely, with syndromes due to hormone secretion (e.g., adrenocorticotropic hormone [ACTH]).

Carcinoid tumors are often totally or partially endobronchial, although some invasion of the bronchial submucosa is nearly always present. The tumors usually resemble carcinoids at other sites with organoid cell clusters, rich arborizing vascularity, and insular or trabecular patterns. Nuclei show a salt-and-pepper chromatin pattern. Peripheral carcinoids tend to show spindling, and a reticulin stain may help outline the nesting of cells. Other patterns include papillary and oncocytic types. Dystrophic calcification, ossification, and amyloid may be concomitant findings. Tumorlets may be identified in surrounding lung tissue and, presumably, represent separate de novo growths, rather than metastases. Typical carcinoids lack necrosis and show uniform architectural organization and an organoid pattern. Appreciable mitotic figures and cellular atypia are absent.

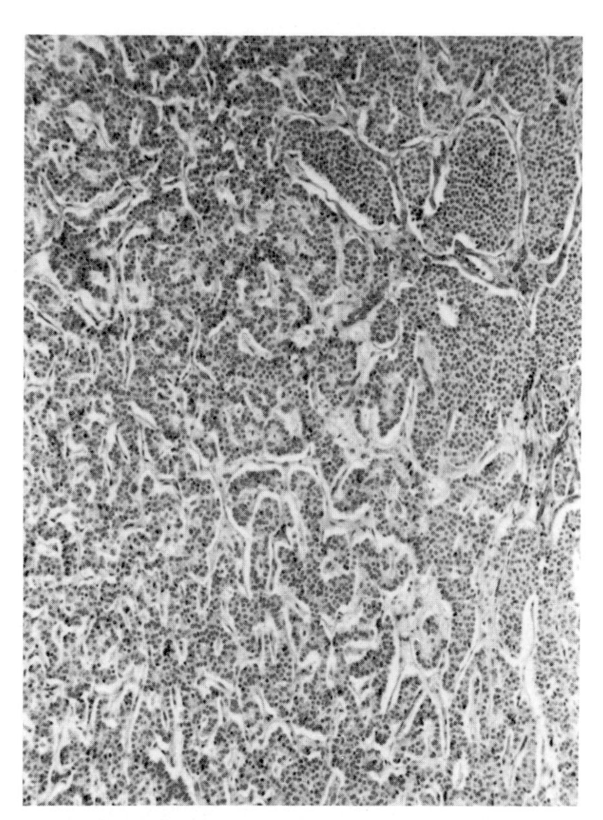

Figure 3–73. Carcinoid tumor. This typical carcinoid tumor shows insular and trabecular patterns.

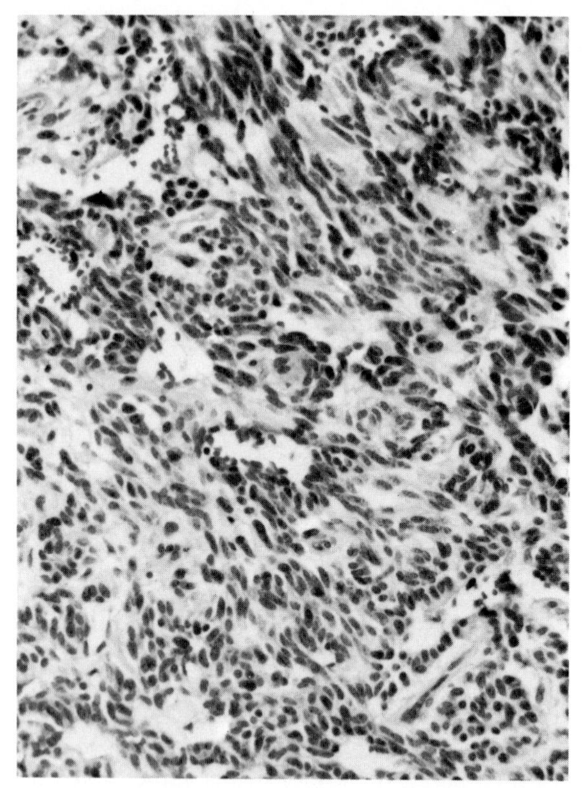

Figure 3–74. Carcinoid tumor. Typical carcinoid tumor with spindling. The vascular pattern is not easy to discern, although the stippled chromatin is characteristic. The vascular pattern in such cases can be enhanced by special stains.

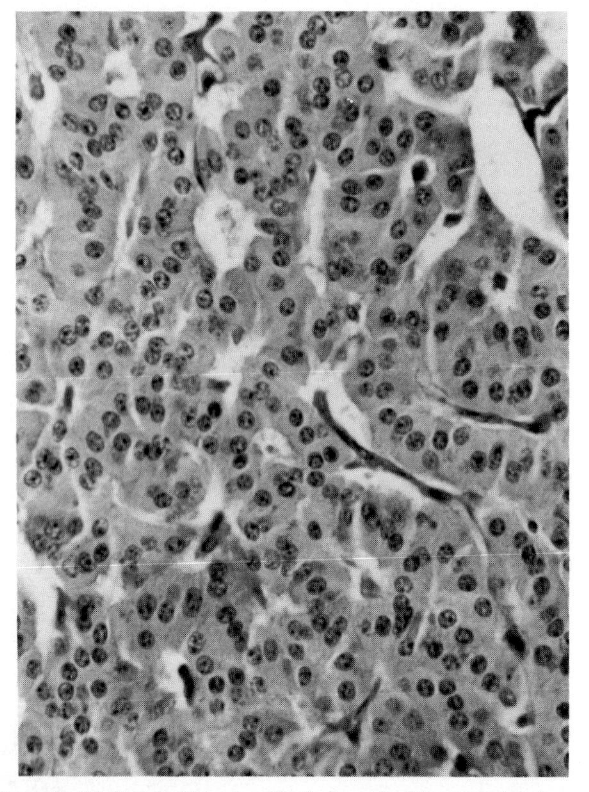

Figure 3–75. Carcinoid tumor. Typical carcinoid tumor showing eosinophilic and oncocytic cytoplasmic features.

Argyrophil stains are commonly positive, as are immunostains for a number of peptides, especially serotonin, bombesin, synaptophysin, and chromogranin.

Atypical carcinoids show necrosis, increased mitotic figures, nuclear atypia, and some loss of the organoid architectural pattern. At the extreme end of the spectrum, some atypical carcinoids merge with high-grade malignancies, either small cell undifferentiated carcinoma or large cell carcinoma with neuroendocrine features.

All carcinoid tumors should be considered low-grade malignancies because they may recur and/or metastasize. Lymph node metastases do not appear to adversely affect survival in typical carcinoids. Complete surgical resection, most often necessitating lobectomy, is recommended.

Papillary carcinoids should be distinguished from sclerosing hemangiomas and papillary adenomas of type II cells. Spindle cell carcinoids should be distinguished from sarcomas (particularly hemangiopericytoma). In small biopsy specimens with crush artifact, carcinoid tumors may be extremely difficult to distinguish from small cell undifferentiated carcinoma or other bronchogenic carcinomas. An endobronchial biopsy specimen showing metastatic breast, prostate, or renal carcinoma may be mistaken for a carcinoid tumor. If sufficient tissue is available, it is worthwhile to freeze a portion for special studies, particularly if there are associated endocrine syndromes.

Precise criteria for the diagnosis of atypical carcinoid are difficult to lay out and have varied in the literature: large size, vascular invasion, necrosis, appreciable mitotic figures, and loss of organoid architecture favor atypical carcinoid over typical carcinoid. Sheet-like growth of pleomorphic cells with relatively little resemblance to carcinoid, marked atypia that is frankly malignant, extensive necrosis, and numerous mitotic figures favor either large cell carcinoma with neuroendocrine features or small cell undifferentiated carcinoma. The treatment for typical and atypical carcinoid tumors is surgical resection of the lobe and associated lymph nodes. Occasionally, a pneumonectomy is necessary.

References

Arrigoni MG, Woolner LB, Bernatz PE. Atypical carcinoid tumors of the lung. J Thorac Cardiovasc Surg 64:413–421, 1972.

Carter D, Eggleston JC. Tumors of the Lower Respiratory Tract. AFIP Atlas of Tumor Pathology, Second Series, Fascicle 17. Washington, DC, Armed Forces Institute of Pathology, 1980.

Dail DH, Hammer SP (eds). Pulmonary Pathology. New York, Springer-Verlag, 1988.

Gould VE, Linnoila RI, Memoli VA, Warren WH. Neuroendocrine cells and neuroendocrine neoplasms of the lung. Pathol Annu 18:287–330, 1983.

Mark EJ, Ramirez JF. Peripheral small cell carcinoma of the lung resembling carcinoid tumor. Arch Pathol Lab Med 109:263–269, 1985.

McCaughan BC, Martini N, Bains MS. Bronchial carcinoids: review of 124 cases. J Thorac Cardiovasc Surg 89:8–17, 1985.

Mills SE, Cooper PH, Walker AN, Kron IL. Atypical carcinoid tumors of the lung. Am J Surg Pathol 6:643–654, 1982.

Okike N, Bernatz PE, Woolner LB. Carcinoid tumors of the lung. Ann Thorac Surg 22:270–275, 1976.

Thurlbeck WM (ed). Pathology of the Lung. New York, Thieme, 1988.

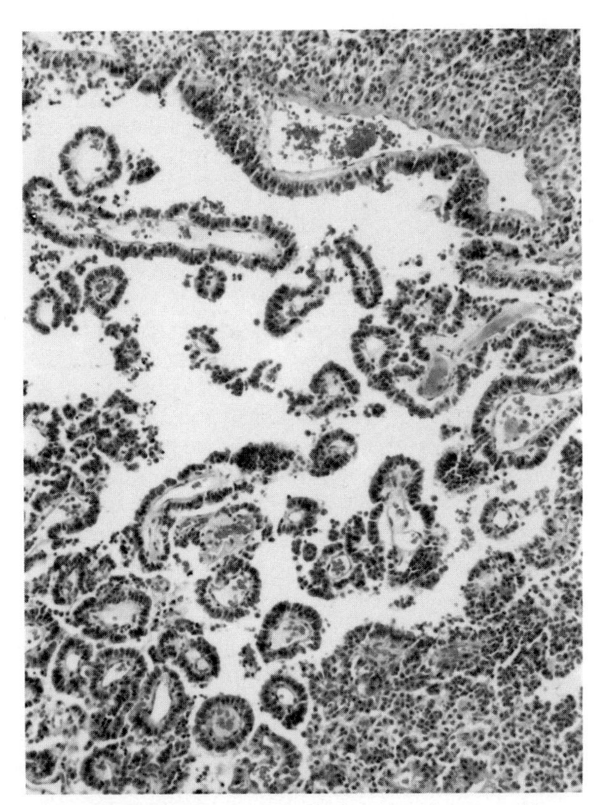

Figure 3–76. Carcinoid tumor. Typical carcinoid tumor with central dyscohesion imparting a papillary appearance.

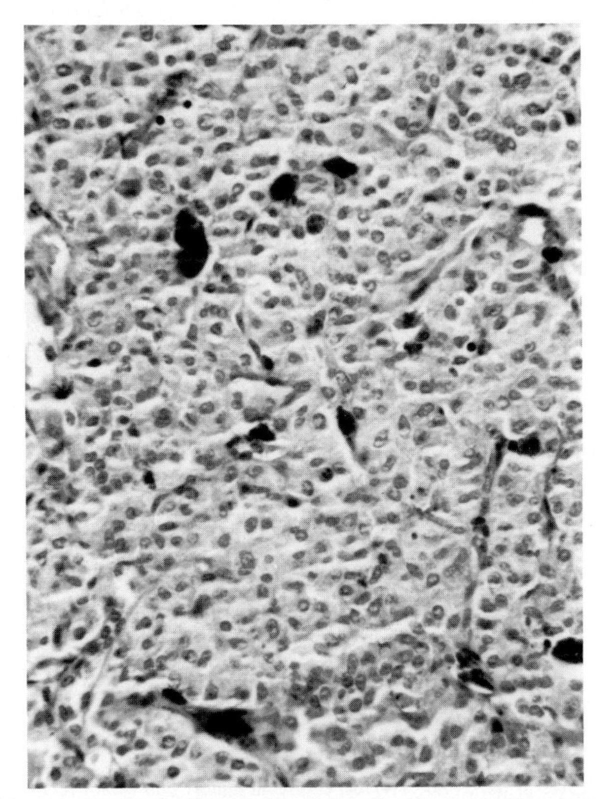

Figure 3–77. Carcinoid tumor. Typical carcinoid tumor with melanin-like pigmentation (dark material). This predominantly solid carcinoid tumor has an inconspicuous vascular pattern, although some cellular packeting is apparent. This tumor produced adrenocorticotropic hormone (ACTH) and Cushing's syndrome.

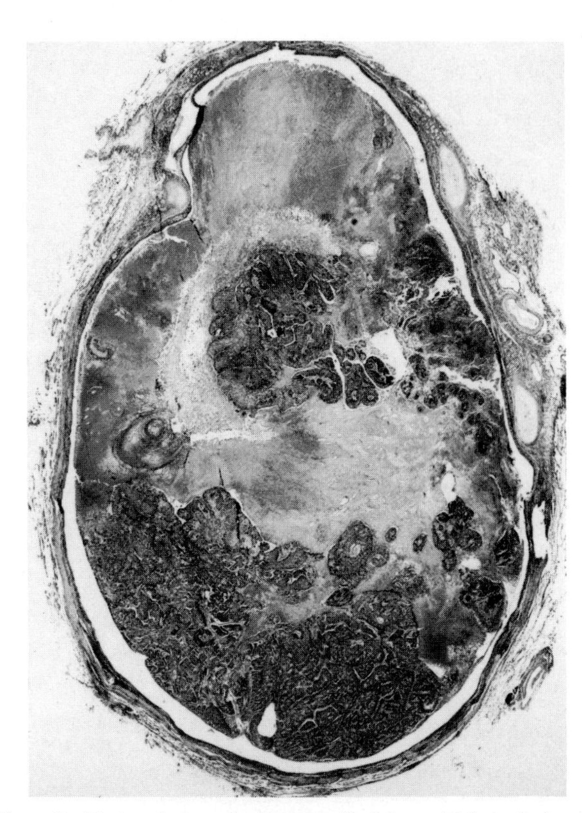

Figure 3–78. Atypical carcinoid tumor. Endobronchial atypical carcinoid tumor with extensive necrosis.

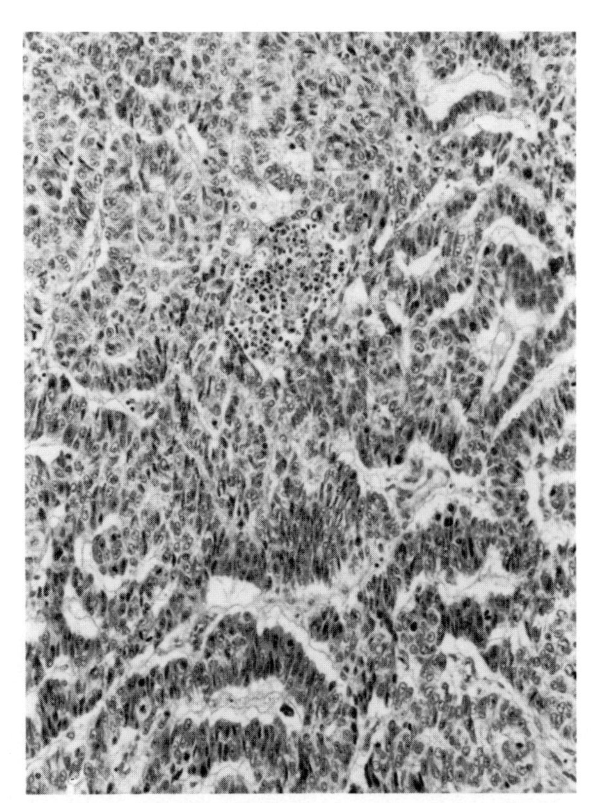

Figure 3–79. Atypical carcinoid tumor. A trabecular pattern is evident. Even at medium power, variation in nuclei and mitotic figures can be seen.

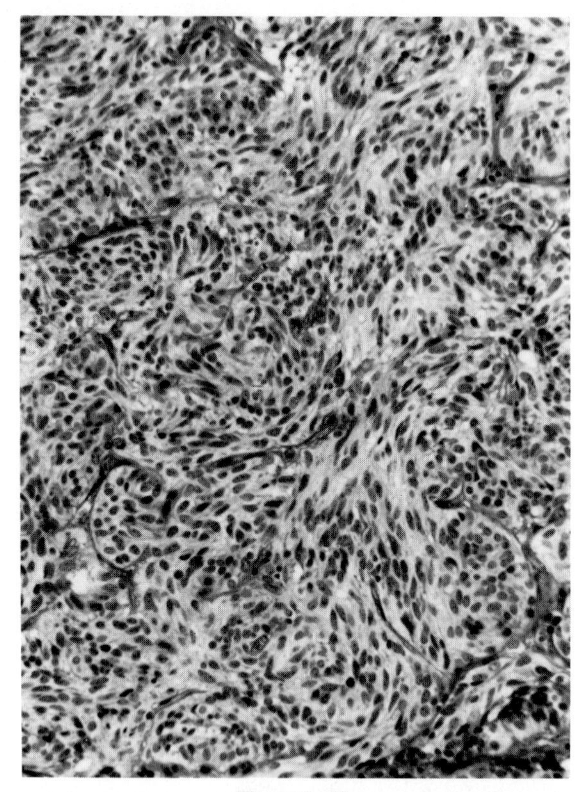

Figure 3–80.

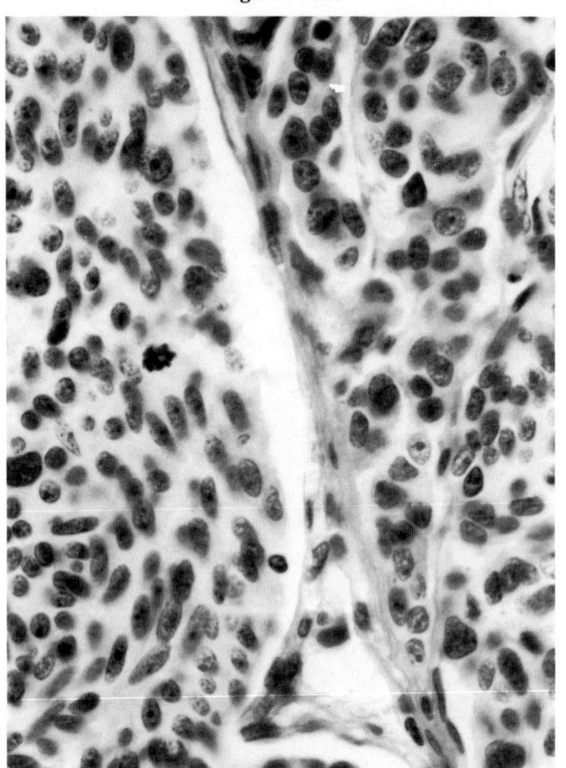

Figure 3–81.

Figures 3–80, 3–81. Spindle cell atypical carcinoid tumor. Vascular pattern and organoid pattern are apparent; detail shows significant nuclear variation, prominent nucleoli, and mitotic figures.

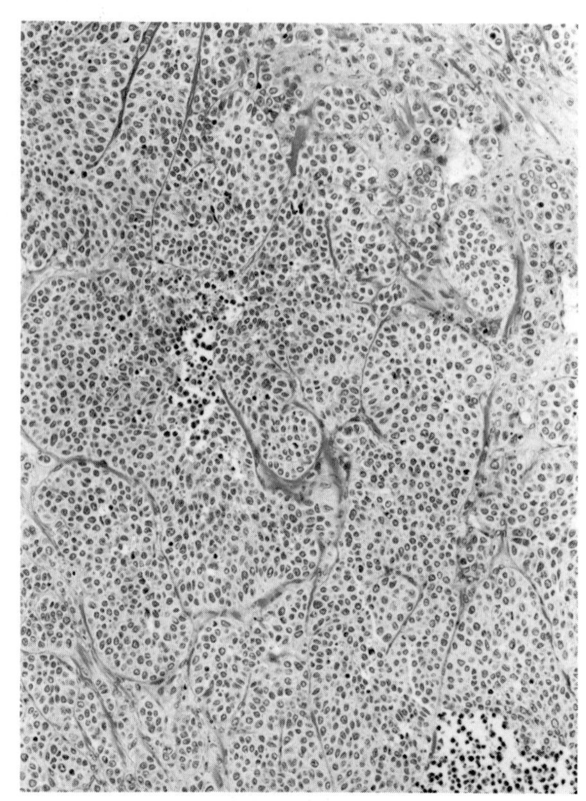

Figure 3–82.

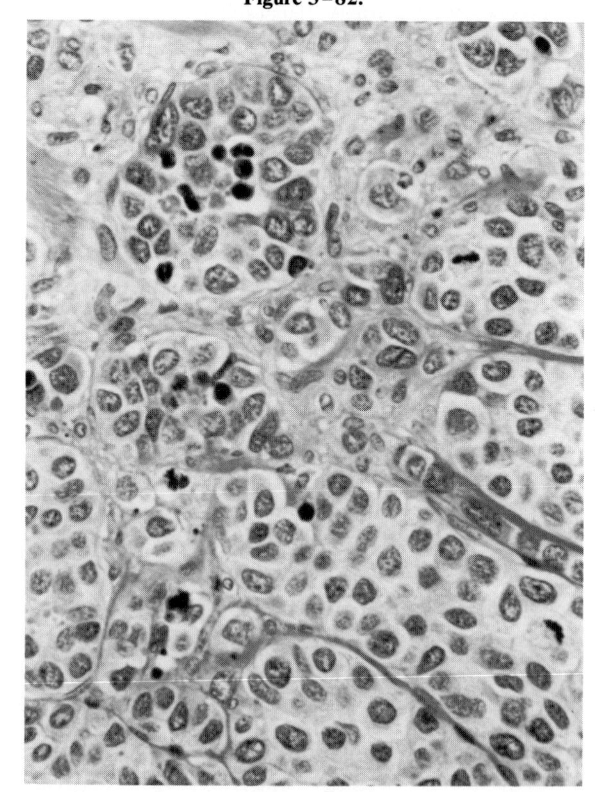

Figure 3–83.

Figures 3–82, 3–83. Atypical carcinoid tumor. This tumor retains its insular pattern with prominent vascularity, although nuclear atypia and mitotic figures are prominent. This lesion is at the threshhold for large cell carcinoma with neuroendocrine features.

■ Mucoepidermoid Tumor (Figs. 3-84 to 3-91)

Pulmonary mucoepidermoid tumors are similar to mucoepidermoid tumors of the major salivary glands, showing mucinous and epidermoid cell differentiation.

The majority of these tumors are low grade and show variable histologic features, including cysts lined by mucinous cells filled with mucin and sheets of squamoid (intermediate) cells in which foamy goblet cells may be interspersed and highlighted with mucin stains. Keratinization and keratin pearl formation should be absent. Cytologic features are generally bland with few mitotic figures. In high-grade tumors, transitional foci from a low-grade histology should be apparent; otherwise, adenosquamous carcinoma should be considered.

The treatment of mucoepidermoid tumor is resection of the involved lobe.

References

Yousem SA, Hochholzer L. Mucoepidermoid tumors of the lung. Cancer 60:1346-1352, 1987.

Figure 3-84.

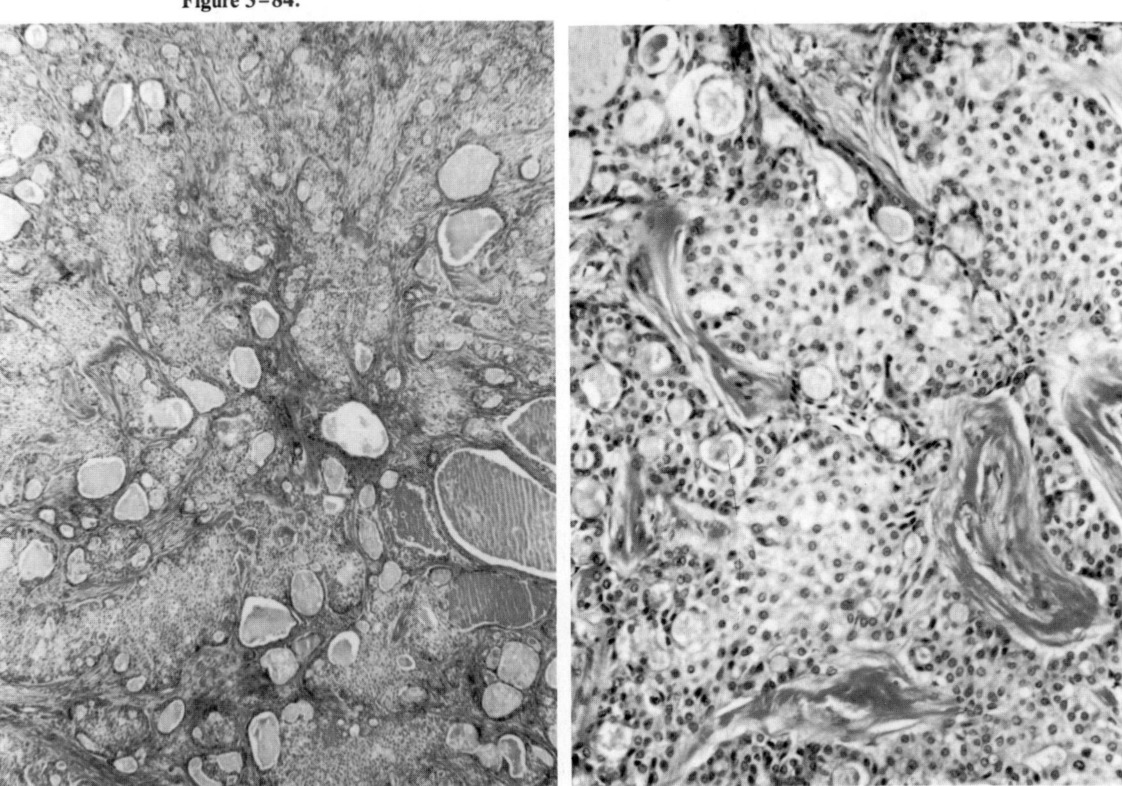

Figure 3-85. **Figure 3-86.**

Figures 3-84 through 3-89. Mucoepidermoid tumor. There is a polypoid endobronchial tumor composed of cystic and solid foci. Solid zones and microcysts containing proteinaceous material are evident. Epidermoid cells in sheet-like arrays have interspersed microscopic cysts and periodic acid-Schiff (PAS)-positive goblet cells (Fig. 3-89), some of which form glands. Acellular collagenous bands may be prominent.

Illustrations continued on following page

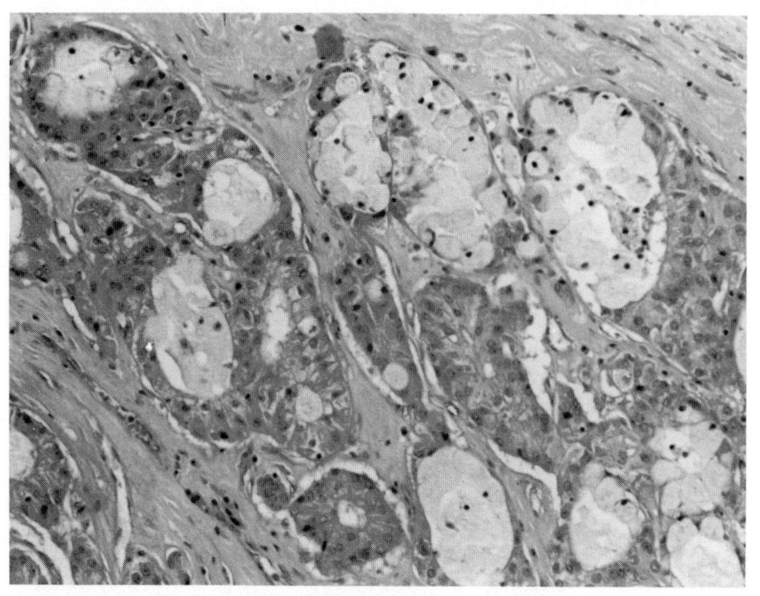

Figure 3-87.

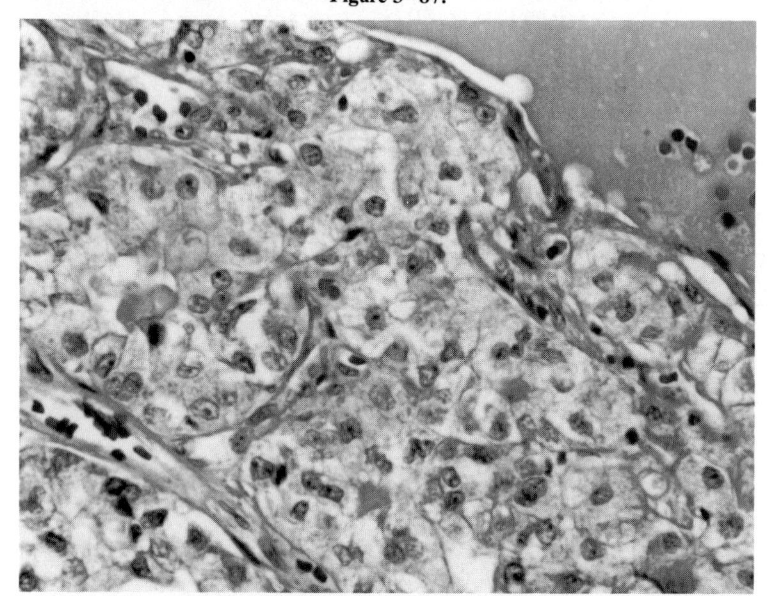

Figure 3-88.

Illustrations continued from page 89. See legend on preceding p

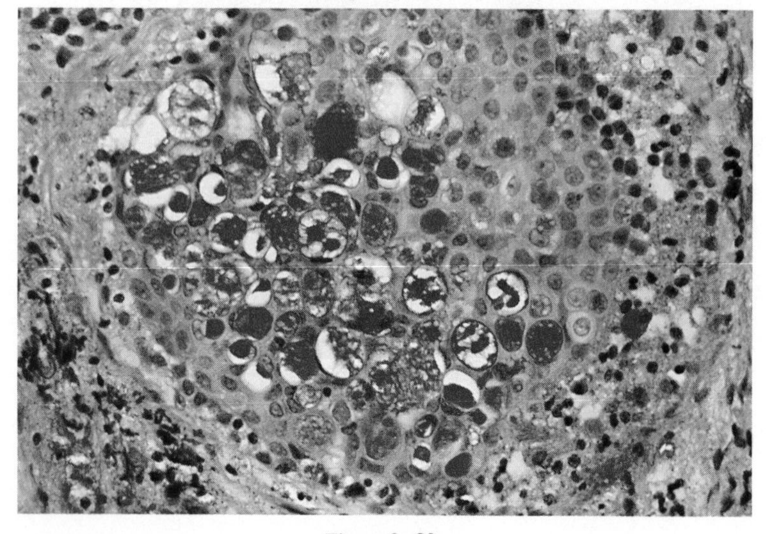

Figure 3-89.

Figures 3–90, 3–91. Atypical mucoepidermoid tumor. This high-grade polypoid endobronchial tumor is composed of a mixed cellular population showing glandular and squamous differentiation separated by delicate connective tissue septa. The cells show moderate cytologic atypia, best appreciated in the squamous component. Mitotic figures were easy to find.

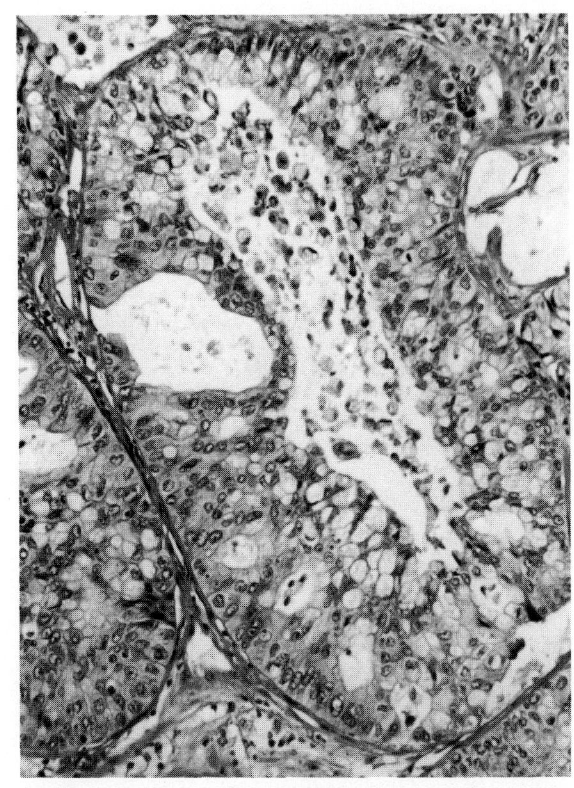

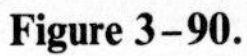

Figure 3–90.

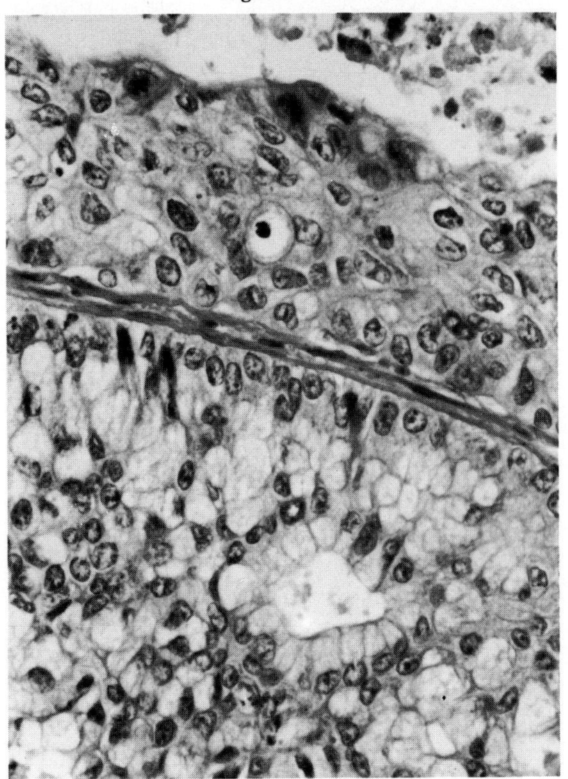

Figure 3–91.

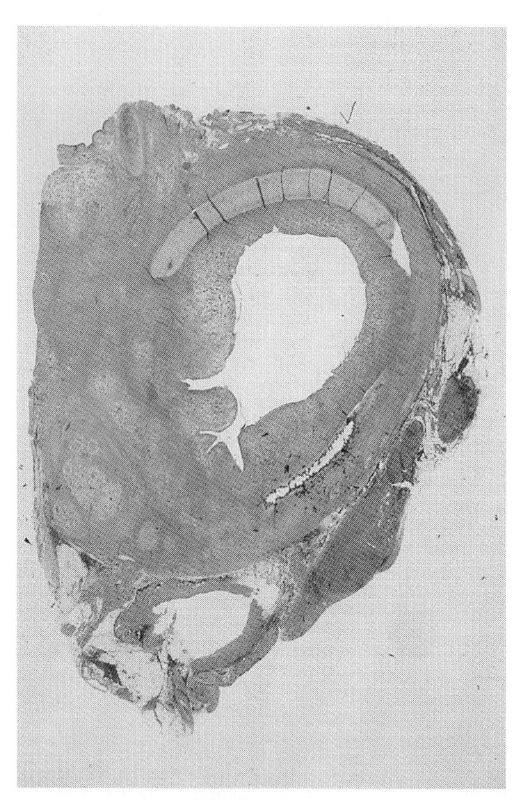

Figure 3–92.

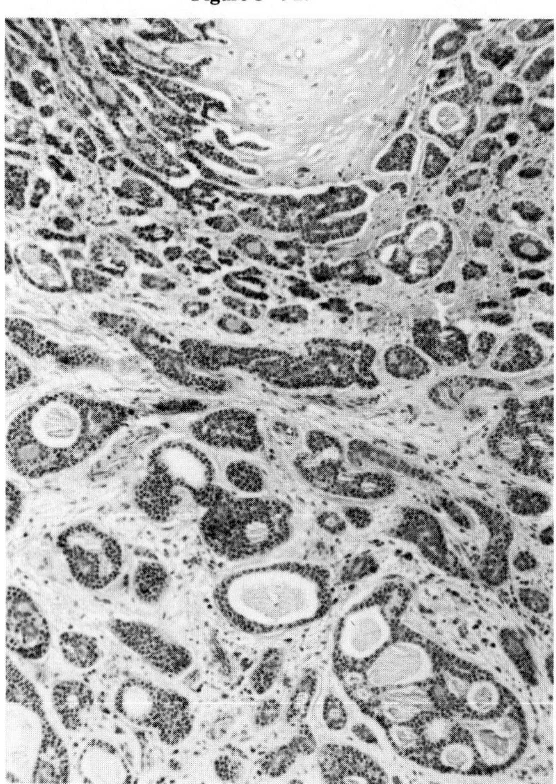

Figure 3–93.

■ Adenoid Cystic Carcinoma (Figs. 3–92, 3–93)

Adenoid cystic carcinoma in the lung is similar to adenoid cystic carcinoma of the major salivary glands. The majority involve large airways.

Adenoid cystic carcinomas may be amenable to cure with resection, but late recurrences occur. Some tumors have a slow but relentless course with multiple local recurrences related to perineural and perivascular invasion.

References

Carter D, Eggleston JC. Tumors of the Lower Respiratory Tract. AFIP Atlas of Tumor Pathology, Second Series, Fascicle 17. Washington, DC, Armed Forces Institute of Pathology, 1980.

Dail DH, Hammer SP (eds). Pulmonary Pathology. New York, Springer-Verlag, 1988.

Thurlbeck WM (ed). Pathology of the Lung. New York, Thieme, 1988.

Figures 3–92, 3–93. Adenoid cystic carcinoma. There is fusiform thickening of a large bronchus by an infiltrate that extends from the submucosa around cartilaginous plates into the adventitia. The histologic features are typical of adenoid cystic carcinomas at other sites.

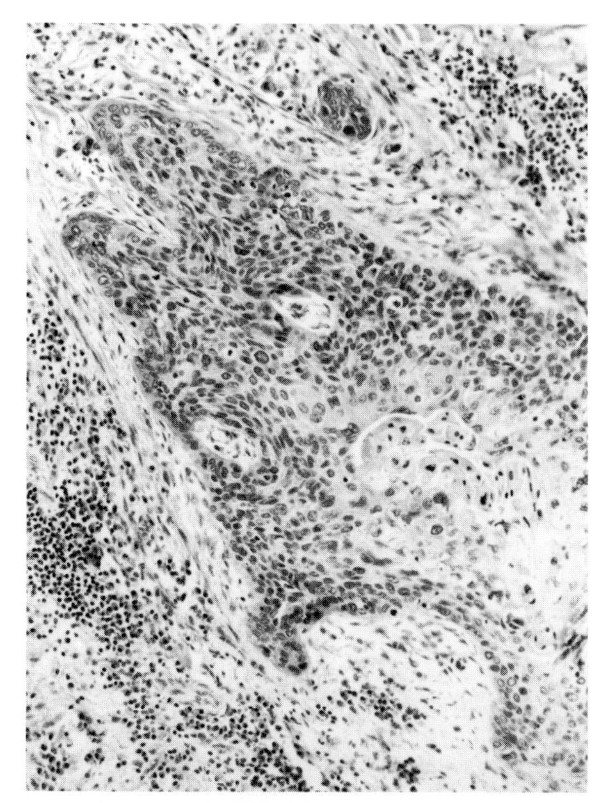

Figure 3-94. Moderately differentiated keratinizing squamous carcinoma. This case is associated with a moderate lymphoid infiltrate.

■ Squamous Cell (Epidermoid) Carcinoma (Figs. 3-94 to 3-96)

This bronchogenic carcinoma shows squamous differentiation. This tumor is more often central than peripheral and has a tendency to cavitate. It may be associated with dysplasia and carcinoma in situ in adjacent bronchial epithelium.

Squamous cell carcinomas vary in their differentiation from the papillary exophytic well-differentiated keratinizing carcinomas to very poorly differentiated tumors with bizarre cytology that are only arbitrarily distinguished from large cell undifferentiated carcinoma. Defining features of squamous cell carcinoma include keratin production, keratin pearl formation, and intercellular bridges. Mucin stains are negative. A squamoid appearance of the cells is not sufficient for the diagnosis because this may be seen in large cell undifferentiated carcinomas and in adenocarcinomas. Clear cell variants of squamous carcinoma occur.

References

Carter D, Eggleston JC. Tumors of the Lower Respiratory Tract. AFIP Atlas of Tumor Pathology, Second Series, Fascicle 17. Washington, DC, Armed Forces Institute of Pathology, 1980.

Dail DH, Hammer SP (eds). Pulmonary Pathology. New York, Springer-Verlag, 1988.

Thurlbeck WM (ed). Pathology of the Lung. New York, Thieme, 1988.

World Health Organization Monograph: Histologic Typing of Lung Tumors, 2nd ed. Geneva, WHO, 1981.

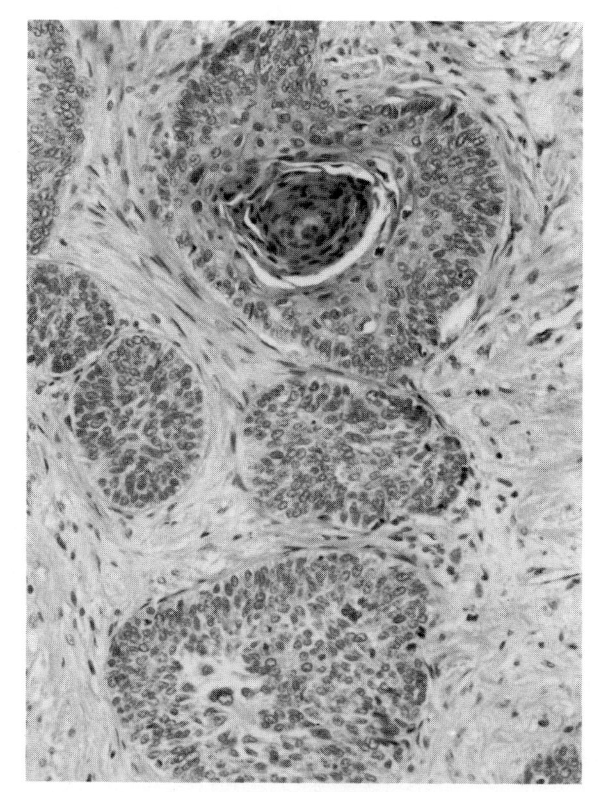

Figure 3-95. Basaloid squamous carcinoma. This pulmonary tumor bears a distinct resemblance to a basal cell carcinoma. A small biopsy specimen could be misinterpreted as small cell undifferentiated carcinoma.

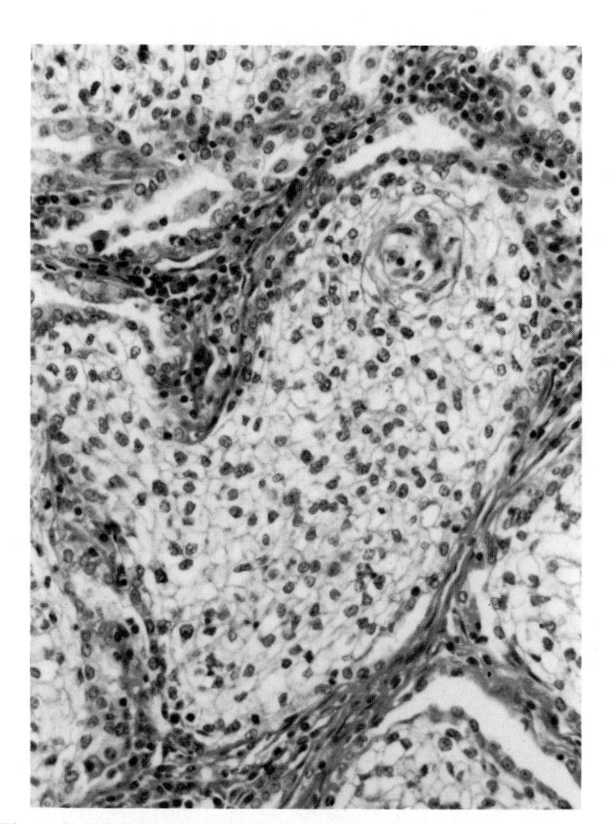

Figure 3-96. Squamous carcinoma with clear cells. Within the nests of clear cells, a small keratin pearl can be seen.

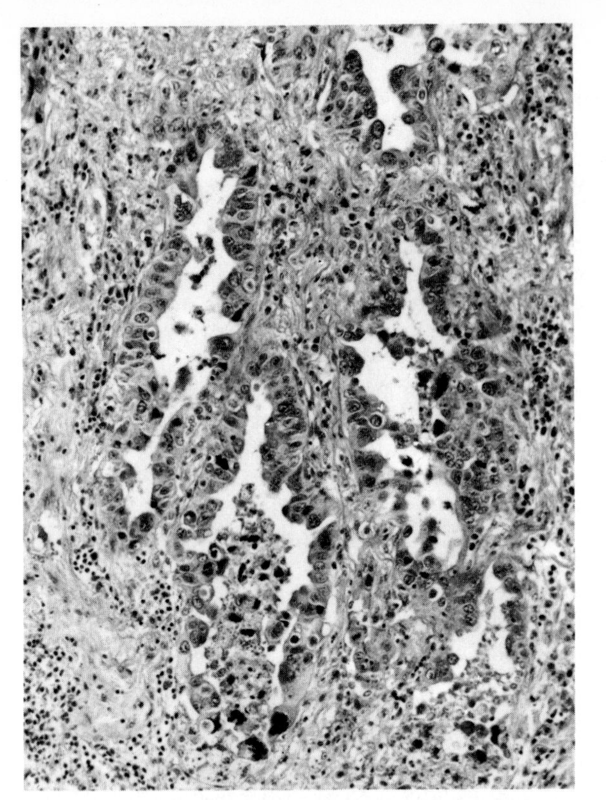

Figure 3-97. Adenocarcinoma. There is glandular differentiation by cytologically malignant cells and a fibrous stroma.

■ Adenocarcinoma (Figs. 3-97 to 3-101)

Bronchogenic adenocarcinoma shows glandular differentiation and/or mucus production by the tumor cells. This tumor tends to be more often peripheral than central, with the classic lesion being a subpleural nodule that puckers the overlying pleura.

Glandular differentiation is manifested by papillary, glandular, and tubular growth patterns; these may be interspersed with a sheetlike growth pattern or a bronchioloalveolar growth pattern. Variable differentiation in different zones of the same tumor is common. Adenocarcinomas are frequently associated with a scar, and although in some cases the scar may have predated the tumor (by radiographic studies), in many other cases the tumors appear to induce collagen production. Thus, the concept of "scar carcinoma" is in a state of flux. The degree of differentiation in adenocarcinoma varies enormously; in some cases, only rare foci of mucin production by tumor cells or gland formation may be seen.

References

Cagle PT, Cohle SD, Greenberg SD. Natural history of pulmonary scar cancers: clinical and pathologic implications. Cancer 56:2031-2035, 1985.

Carter D, Eggleston JC. Tumors of the Lower Respiratory Tract. AFIP Atlas of Tumor Pathology, Second Series, Fascicle 17. Washington DC, Armed Forces Institute of Pathology, 1980.

Dail DH, Hammer SP (eds). Pulmonary Pathology, New York, Springer-Verlag, 1988.

Kung ITM, Lui IOL, Loke SL, et al. Pulmonary scar cancer: a pathologic reappraisal. Am J Surg Pathol 9:391-400, 1985.

Madri JA, Carter D. Scar cancers of the lung: origin and significance. Hum Pathol 15:625-631, 1984.

Thurlbeck WM (ed). Pathology of the Lung. New York, Thieme, 1988.

World Health Organization Monograph: Histologic Typing of Lung Tumors, 2nd ed. Geneva, WHO, 1981.

Figures 3-98, 3-99. Adenocarcinoma. This poorly differentiated adenocarcinoma shows little glandular differentiation; however, numerous intracytoplasmic periodic acid-Schiff (PAS) with diatase-positive, mucin-containing vacuoles are present.

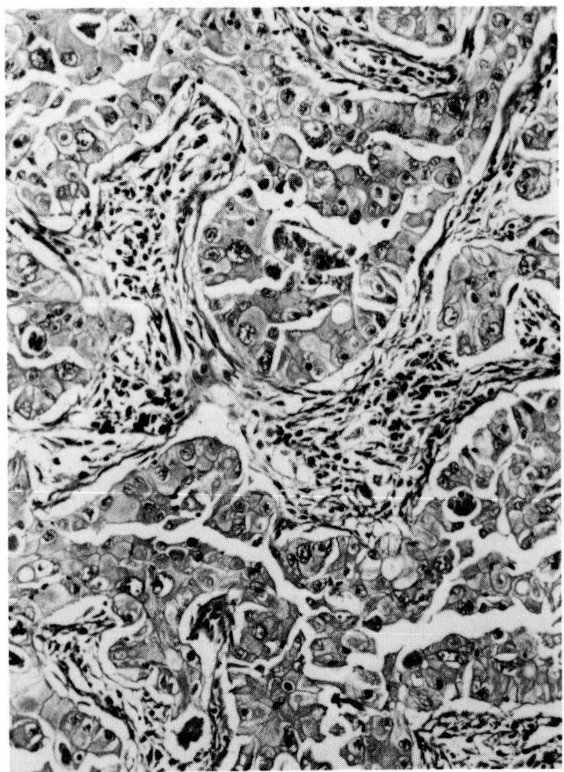

Figure 3-98.

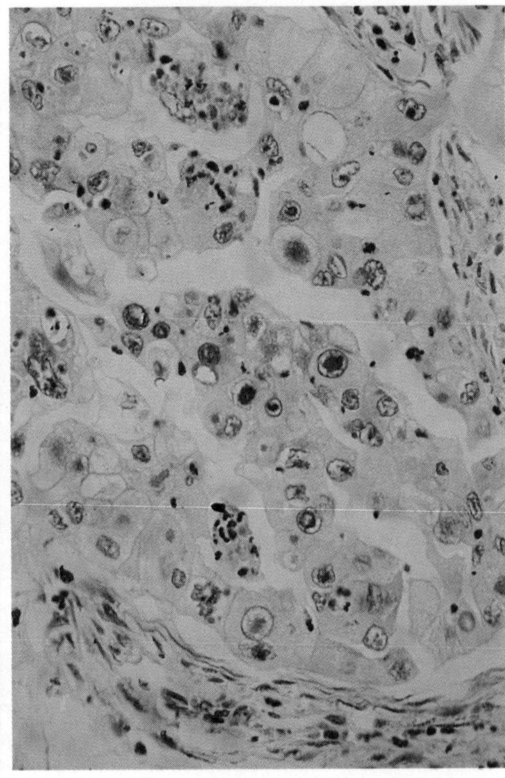

Figure 3-99.

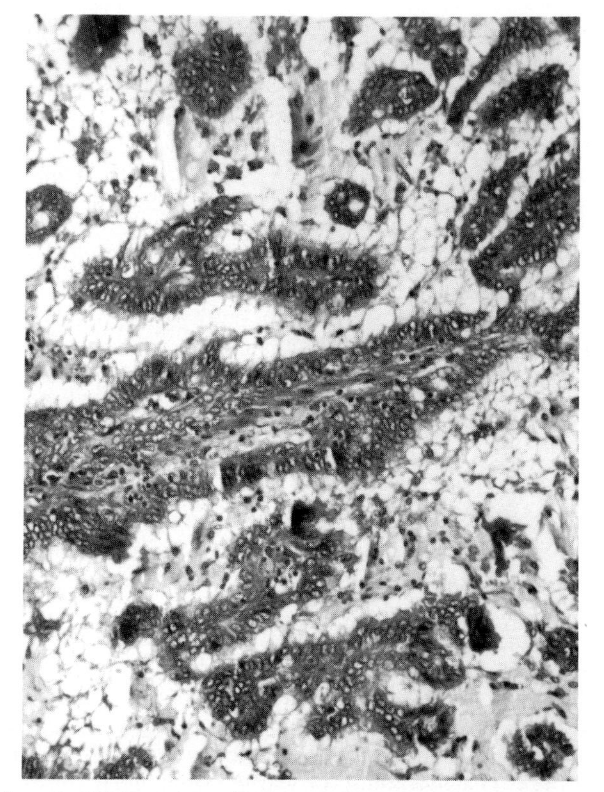

Figure 3-100. Bronchogenic adenocarcinoma with papillae and cytologic features reminiscent of papillary carcinoma of the thyroid. A primary lesion in the thyroid was carefully excluded in this case.

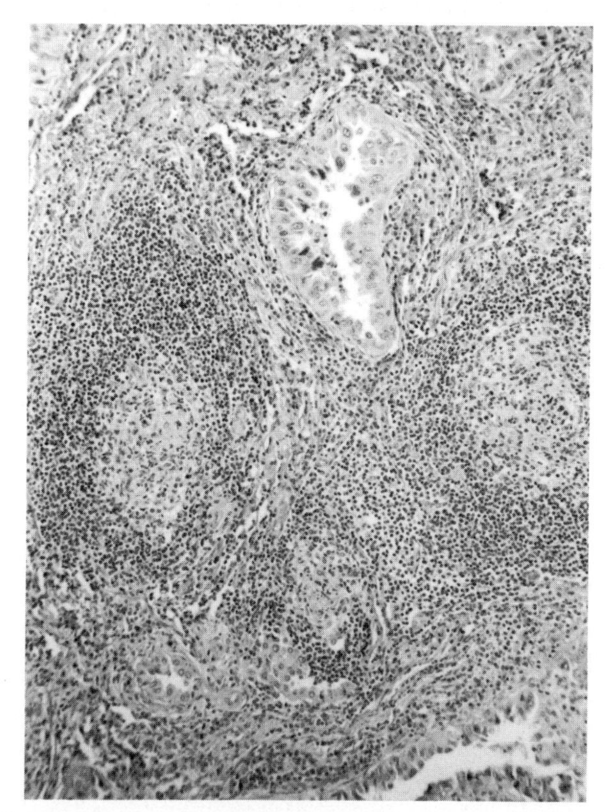

Figure 3-101. Bronchogenic adenocarcinoma associated with marked lymphoid stroma, including the germinal centers. The neoplastic gland is surrounded by two germinal centers.

■ Bronchogenic Carcinoma—A Practical Approach

1. Arrive at a *confirmed* diagnosis of malignancy by whatever technique is available, e.g., exfoliative cytologic study, fine needle aspiration, bronchoscopic biopsy, biopsy of metastasis.
2. Consider (and exclude) the possibility of metastatic carcinoma to the lung.
3. Small cell undifferentiated carcinoma versus non-small cell carcinoma represents the *major decision point.* Neither electron microscopy nor sophisticated immunostaining is usually necessary for routine patient management, even though these techniques may be more sensitive than routine light microscopy to identify differentiation.
4. Subclassification of non-small cell carcinoma is not critical in patient management but is helpful to remember in diagnosis.
5. The diagnosis may change in subsequent specimens. A significant percentage of patients (20 percent or more) treated for small cell undifferentiated carcinoma may later show other histologic differentiation. It is not known whether this represents sampling error, effects of therapy, or inherent change in the tumor itself.
6. The diagnosis of a mixed carcinoma may be an appropriate diagnosis in some cases that are hard to classify.
7. Give the patient the benefit of the doubt. If the tumor is surgically resectable, that is the treatment of choice, even if histologic findings suggest a small cell undifferentiated carcinoma.
8. A few cases of bronchogenic carcinomas defy classification (particularly small cell versus non-small cell), and hope for a consensus among colleagues is wishful thinking.

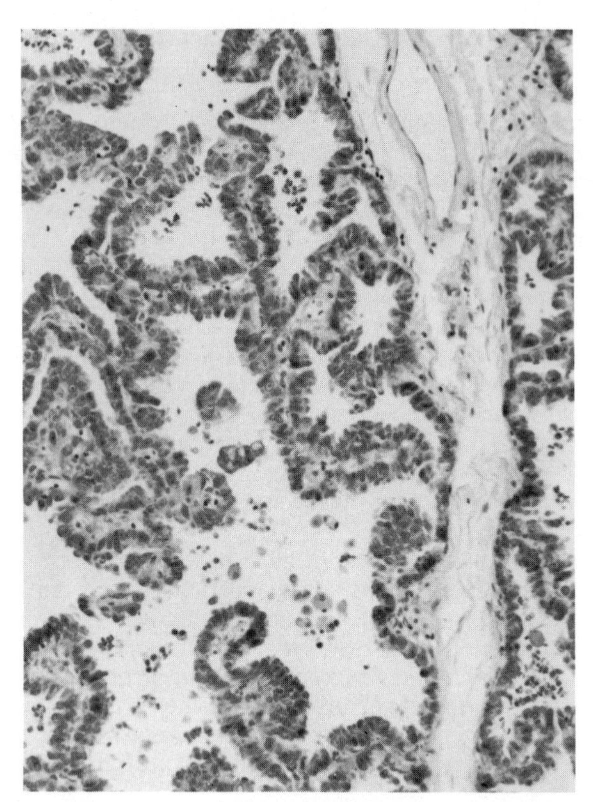

Figure 3-102.

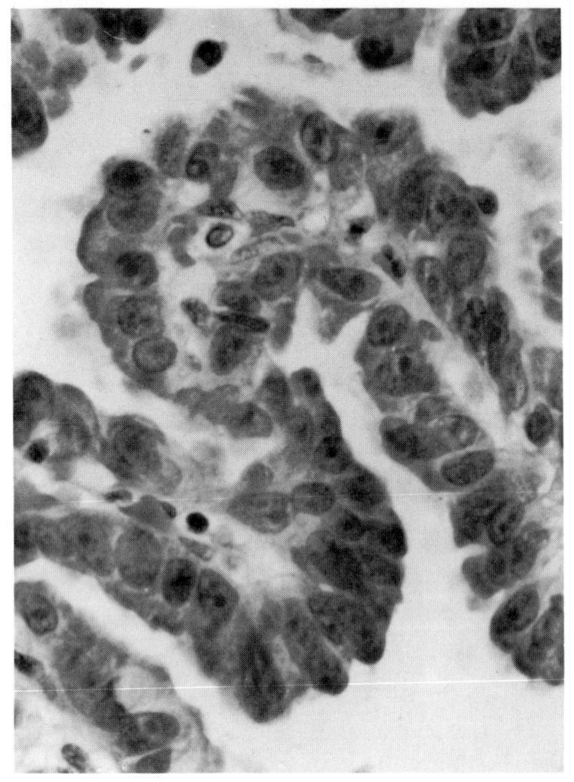

Figure 3-103.

Figures 3-102, 3-103. Bronchioloalveolar carcinoma. In this nonmucinous type of carcinoma, intact alveolar walls are lined by cuboidal cells with atypical nuclei and prominent nucleoli.

■ Bronchioloalveolar Carcinoma (Figs. 3-102 to 3-116)

Bronchioloalveolar carcinoma (BAC) is a subset of adenocarcinoma in which a growth pattern is apparent along pre-existing alveolar walls without frank invasive or destructive growth. Such a growth has been described as "lepidic" (derived from the genus *Lepidoptera,* which includes butterflies) to describe how the tumor cells alight on alveolar walls. The entire lesion (at least as sampled) must show this pattern before the diagnosis of BAC is appropriate, since in any adenocarcinoma some foci resembling BAC may be apparent. If high-grade and invasive foci with stromal reaction are seen, the diagnosis of BAC is not appropriate. BAC may involve scarred lung tissue, and this should be distinguished from true stromal invasion. BAC often has a characteristic gross consolidated appearance without necrosis. Favorable prognostic features include localization and small size. BAC may present as a solitary nodule, bilateral infiltrates, or a localized "pneumonic" focus on chest radiographs. Intrapulmonary spread may take place via aerogenous spread or lymphatic means.

The tumor cells are generally columnar or cuboidal in shape and grow along pre-existing alveolar walls; the cells may show mucinous, Clara, or type II cell features as individual cells or papillary tufts. Cytologic features of malignancy are usually apparent, although the mucinous (goblet cell) variant may be extremely well differentiated and cytologically bland. The diagnosis rests on the fact that tufts of well-differentiated mucinous cells are found on normal alveolar walls away from airways, thus excluding the possibility of metaplasia in an area of scarring. Some tumors show papillary growth in alveolar spaces. Clara cells have a hobnail appearance, and the differentiation may be appreciated ultrastructurally or by the apical periodic acid-Schiff (PAS)-positive granules. Cells with pale eosinophilic intranuclear vacuoles are characteristic of BAC with type II cell differentiation.

The differential diagnosis includes a sclerosing hemangioma, papillary adenoma of type II cells, alveolar adenoma, and metastatic adenocarcinoma growing in a bronchioloalveolar pattern. Distinction from markedly reactive type II pneumocytes is based primarily on cellular monotony, lepidic growth, and abrupt transition to normal alveolar walls at the tumor edge in BAC.

References

Carter D, Eggleston JC. Tumors of the Lower Respiratory Tract. AFIP Atlas of Tumor Pathology, Second Series, Fascicle 17. Washington DC, Armed Forces Institute of Pathology, 1980.

Clayton F. The spectrum and significance of bronchioloalveolar carcinomas. Part 2. Pathol Annu 23:361-394, 1988.

Dail DH, Hammer SP (eds). Pulmonary Pathology, New York, Springer-Verlag, 1988.

Thurlbeck WM (ed). Pathology of the Lung. New York, Thieme, 1988.

World Health Organization Monograph: Histologic Typing of Lung Tumors, 2nd ed. Geneva, WHO, 1981.

Text continued on page 101

Figures 3-104, 3-105. Bronchioloalveolar carcinoma, nonmucinous type. At the lesion's edge, growth along intact alveolar walls is seen and there is an abrupt transition from the tumor to normal alveolar walls. A modest amount of interstitial thickening and inflammation is present. The tumor cells are somewhat oncocytic in appearance.

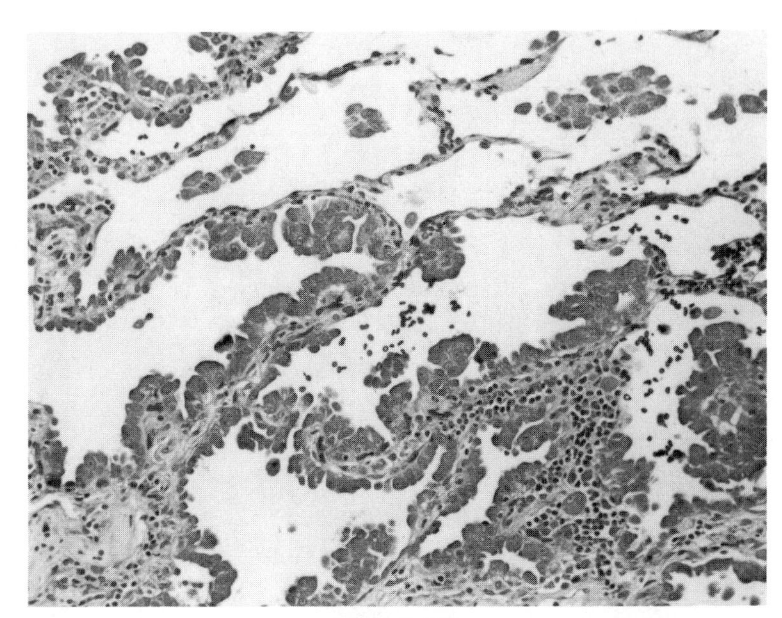

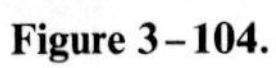

Figure 3-104.

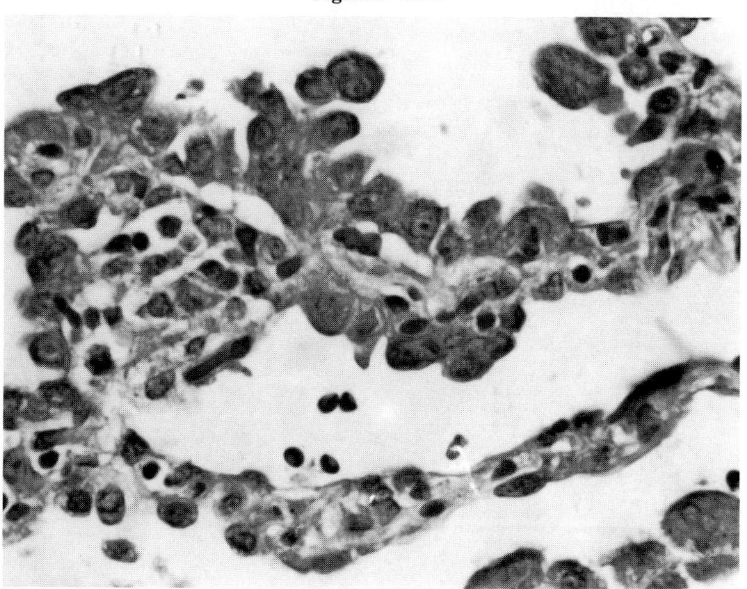

Figure 3-105.

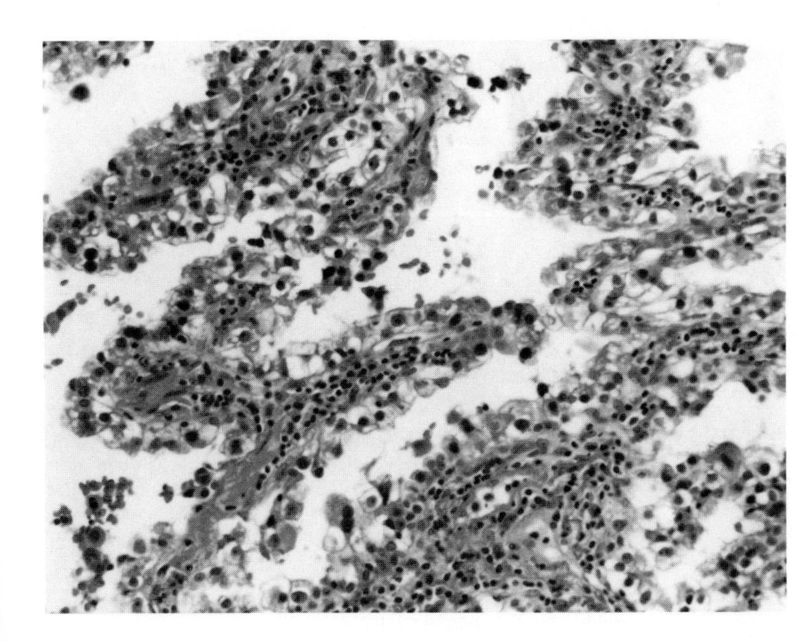

Figure 3-106. Bronchioloalveolar carcinoma. Clear cell change and moderate stromal inflammatory infiltrate are evident.

Figure 3-107.

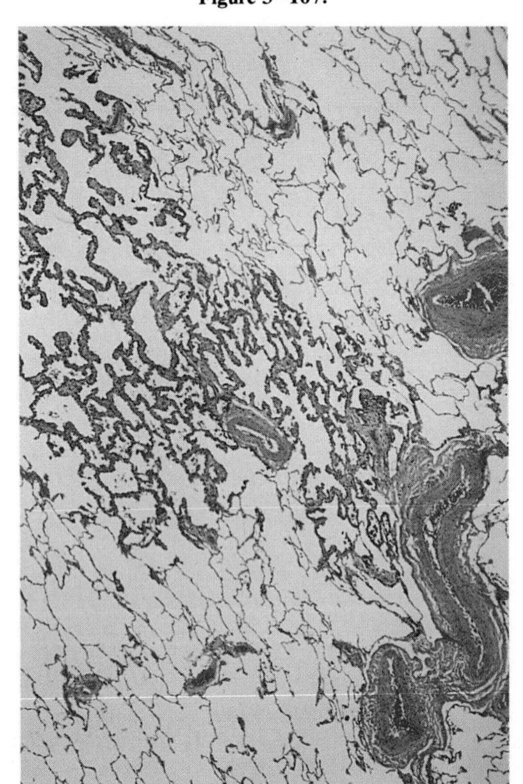

Figure 3-108.

Figures 3-107, 3-108. Bronchioloalveolar carcinoma. A lesion had been present on chest radiographs for several decades and had shown recent enlargement. Biopsy and subsequent resection showed a nonmucinous bronchioloalveolar carcinoma arising adjacent to the scar. The tumor shows extensive involvement of intact alveolar walls.

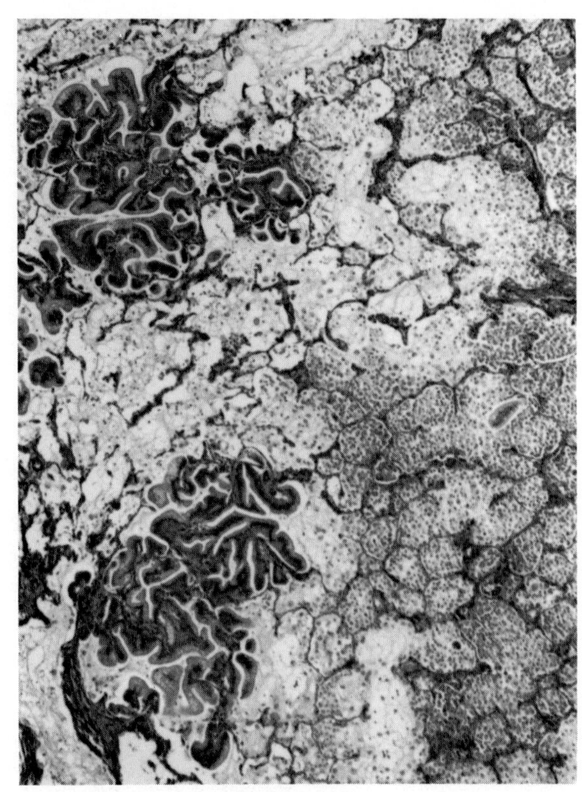

Figure 3-109.

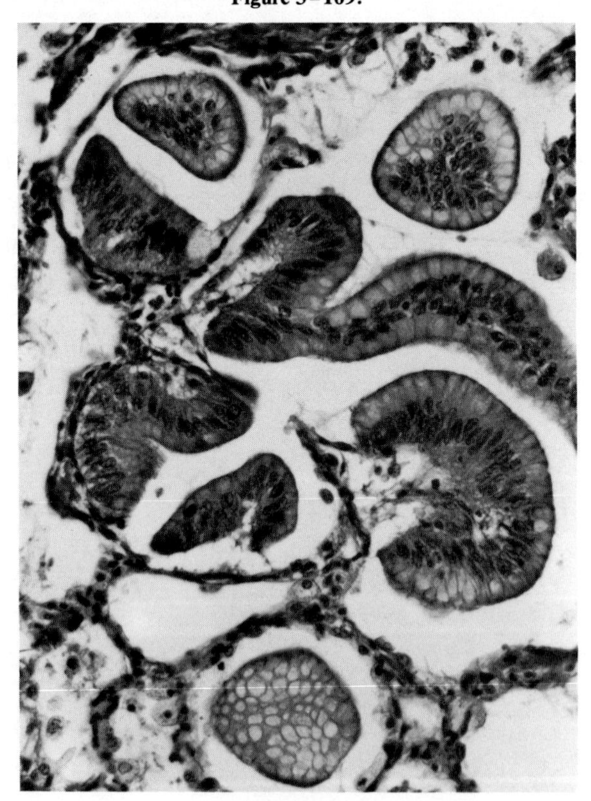

Figure 3-110.

Figures 3-109, 3-110. Bronchioloalveolar carcinoma, mucinous type. Numerous nests of well-differentiated goblet cells grow along alveolar walls. Uninvolved alveoli contain abundant mucus and macrophages. In some foci, nests of tumor float free in the alveoli.

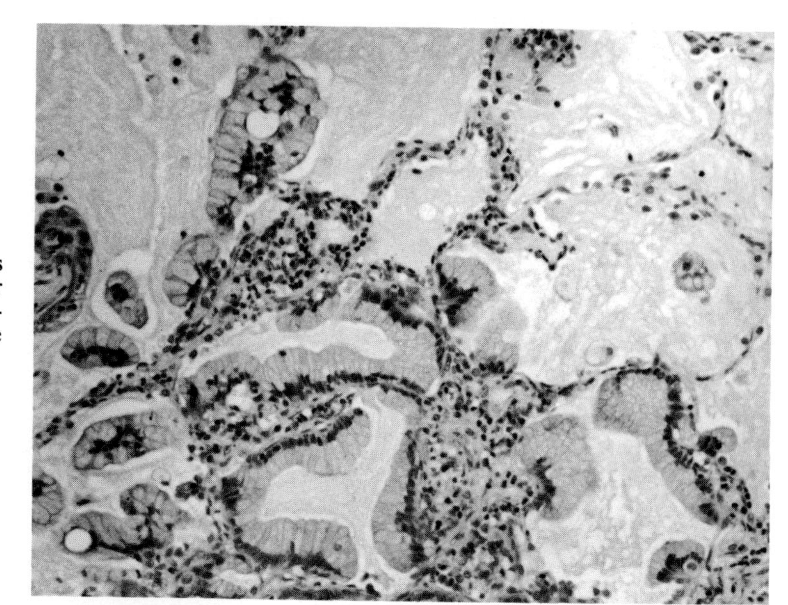

Figure 3–111. Bronchioloalveolar carcinoma, mucinous type. Columnar mucinous cells grow along intact alveolar walls that show prominent interstitial thickening and inflammation. Note abrupt transition at the edge of the tumor cells.

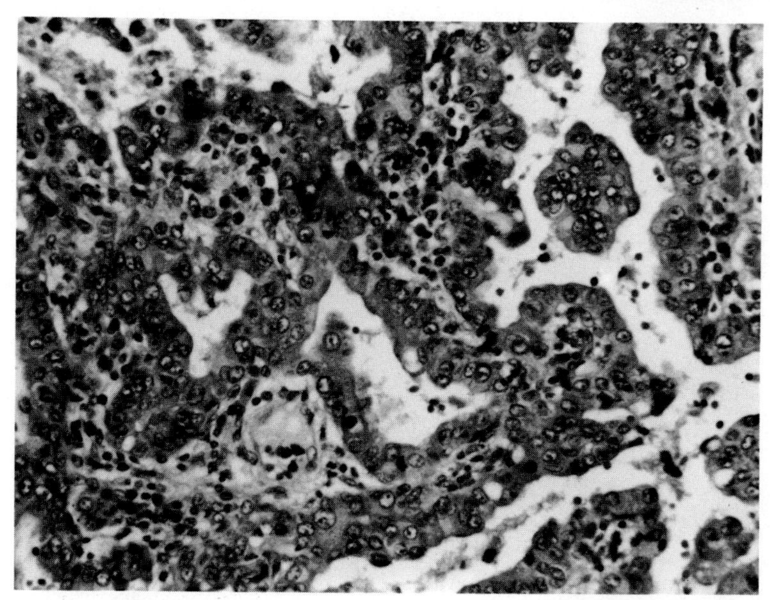

Figure 3–112. Bronchioloalveolar carcinoma with moderate nuclear atypia and numerous mitotic figures.

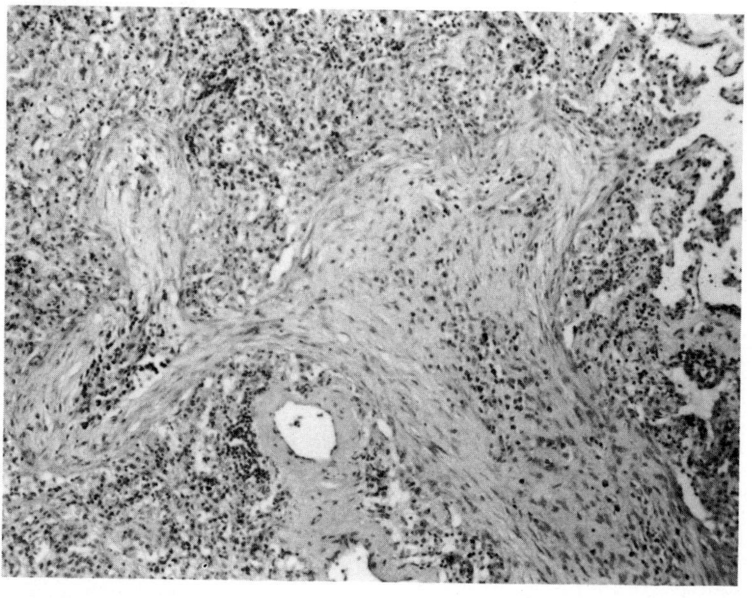

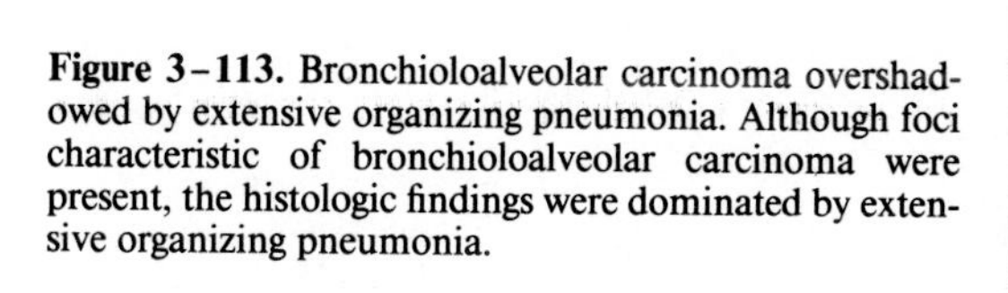

Figure 3–113. Bronchioloalveolar carcinoma overshadowed by extensive organizing pneumonia. Although foci characteristic of bronchioloalveolar carcinoma were present, the histologic findings were dominated by extensive organizing pneumonia.

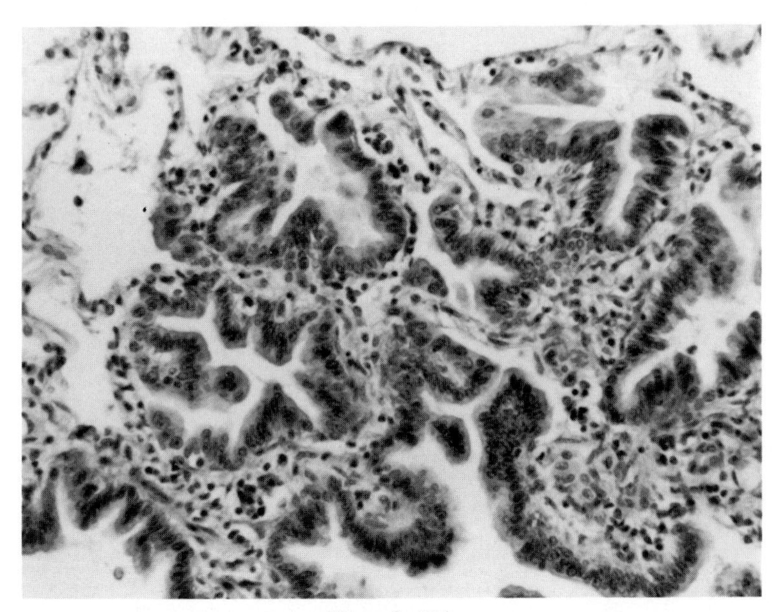

Figure 3-114.

Figures 3-114, 3-115. Bronchioloalveolar carcinoma. The tumor is associated with extensive zones resembling pulmonary alveolar proteinosis.

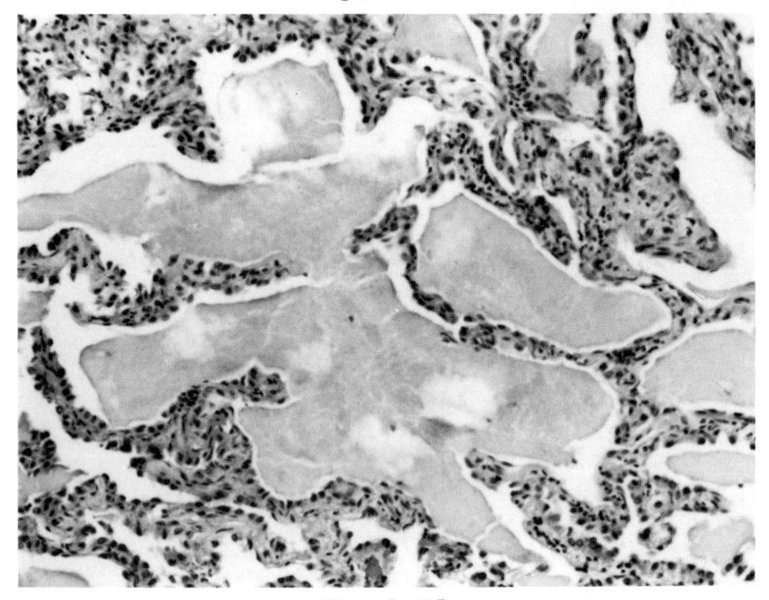

Figure 3-115.

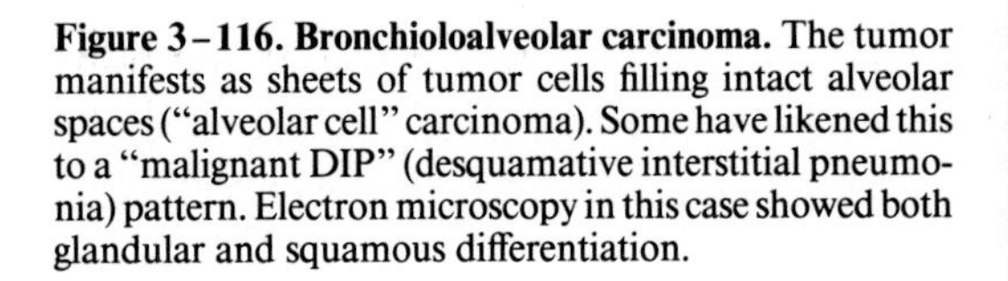

Figure 3-116. Bronchioloalveolar carcinoma. The tumor manifests as sheets of tumor cells filling intact alveolar spaces ("alveolar cell" carcinoma). Some have likened this to a "malignant DIP" (desquamative interstitial pneumonia) pattern. Electron microscopy in this case showed both glandular and squamous differentiation.

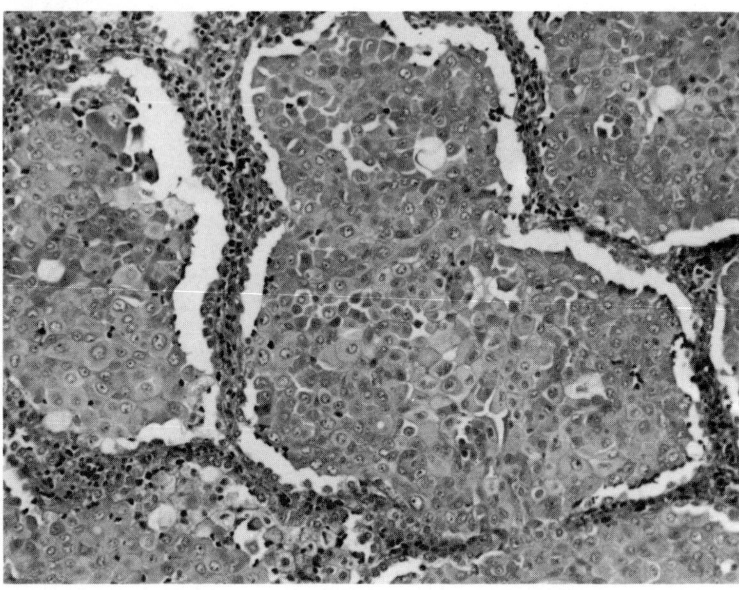

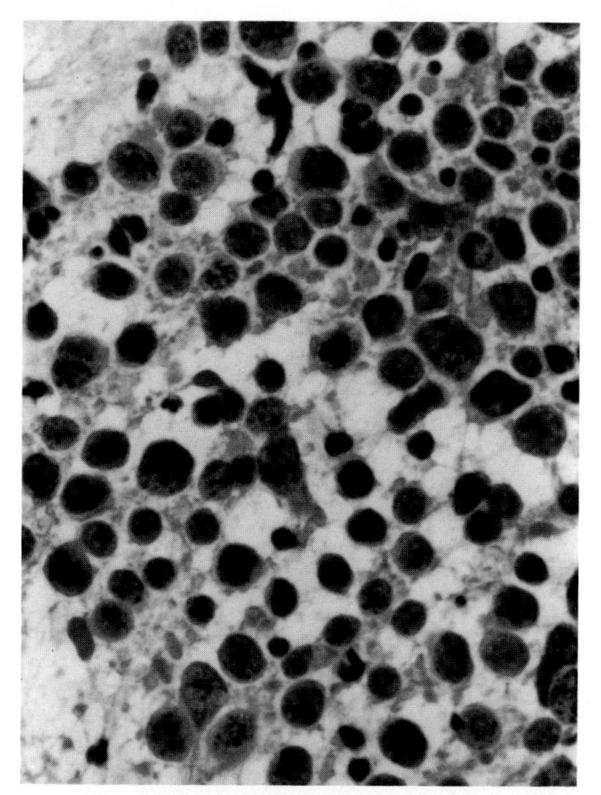

Figure 3-117. Small cell undifferentiated carcinoma. An alcohol-fixed, hematoxylin and eosin (H&E) touch preparation shows a degree of nuclear variation. Dark blobs in the background represent necrotic nuclear debris. Mitotic figures are numerous. The chromatin is coarse, and the nucleoli are inconspicuous. Dyscohesion is marked.

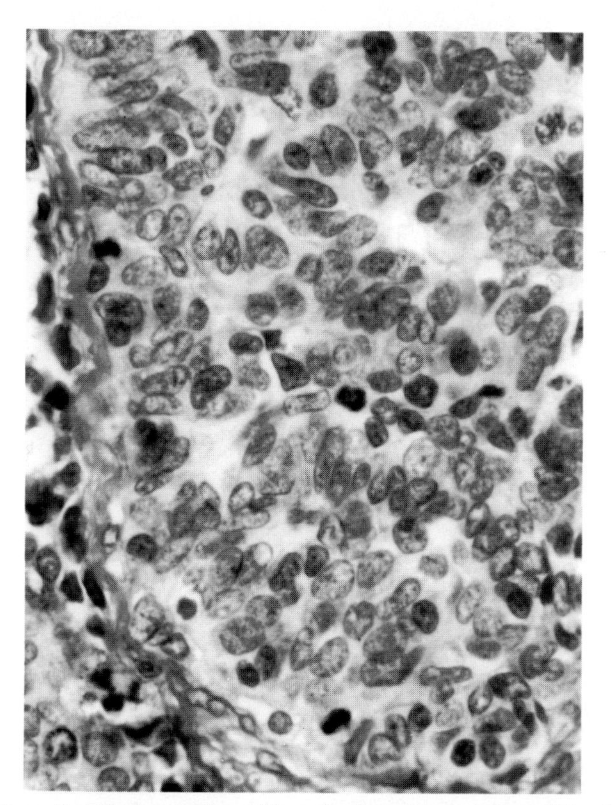

Figure 3-118. Small cell undifferentiated carcinoma. This well-fixed lymph node metastasis shows the typical chromatin features of small cell undifferentiated carcinoma, numerous mitotic figures, and a trabecular growth pattern.

■ Small Cell Undifferentiated (Oat Cell) Carcinoma (Figs. 3-117 to 3-122)

This is a bronchogenic carcinoma composed of a distinctive population of small cells with a high nuclear to cytoplasmic ratio and dispersed granular chromatin without prominent nucleoli. The polygonal variant shows somewhat more cytoplasm and slightly more prominent nucleoli; in general, however, the cells that compose oat cell carcinoma are much smaller than those composing other bronchogenic carcinomas. Some spindling or trabecular growth is common. Extensive necrosis and karyorrhexis, numerous mitotic figures, bronchial submucosal growth, DNA impregnation of vessels in foci of necrosis ("Azzopardi phenomenon"), and nuclear molding are all characteristic. Pagetoid spread along basement membranes also is seen.

By current recommendations (see Hirsch et al., 1988, and Bepler et al, 1989), small cell carcinoma need not be subclassified. Thus, the small cell carcinoma diagnosis encompasses classic oat cell carcinoma, the polygonal variant with larger cells with more prominent cytoplasm and small or indistinct nucleoli, and the small cell/large cell carcinoma, which usually resembles the polygonal variant with intermixed larger cells with relatively prominent nucleoli and considerable cytoplasm. This last group is distinct from mixed small cell and non-small cell carcinomas, which have discrete and separable carcinomatous components. An occasional cell with a prominent nucleolus or an occasional large bizarre cell should not exclude the diagnosis of small cell carcinoma.

Since many lesions (especially lymphomas and carcinoid tumors) may simulate small cell carcinoma in small biopsy specimens with crush artifact, mitotic figures and/or the classic nuclear features of small cell carcinoma should be *clearly* seen before a diagnosis is rendered.

Prognosis and therapy are based on clinical staging, and histologic subtyping of small cell undifferentiated carcinoma does not appear to be useful.

A morphologic diagnosis of small cell undifferentiated carcinoma should not preclude surgery *if the tumor is resectable.* Occasional examples of small cell undifferentiated carcinoma are cured by resection, and some cases carrying the diagnosis as a result of small biopsy or cytologic findings are found to represent other lesions that have been misinterpreted, particularly carcinoid and atypical carcinoid tumors and lymphomas with crush artifact.

References

Azzopardi JG. Oat cell carcinoma of the bronchus. J Path Bact 78:513-519, 1959.

Bepler G, Neumann K, Holle R, Havemann K, Kalbfleisch H. Clinical relevance of histologic subtyping in small cell lung cancer. Cancer 64:74-79, 1989.

Carter D. Small cell carcinoma of the lung. Am J Surg Pathol 7:787-795, 1983.

Carter D, Eggleston JC. Tumors of the Lower Respiratory Tract. AFIP Atlas of Tumor Pathology, Second Series, Fascicle 17. Washington, DC, Armed Forces Institute of Pathology, 1980.

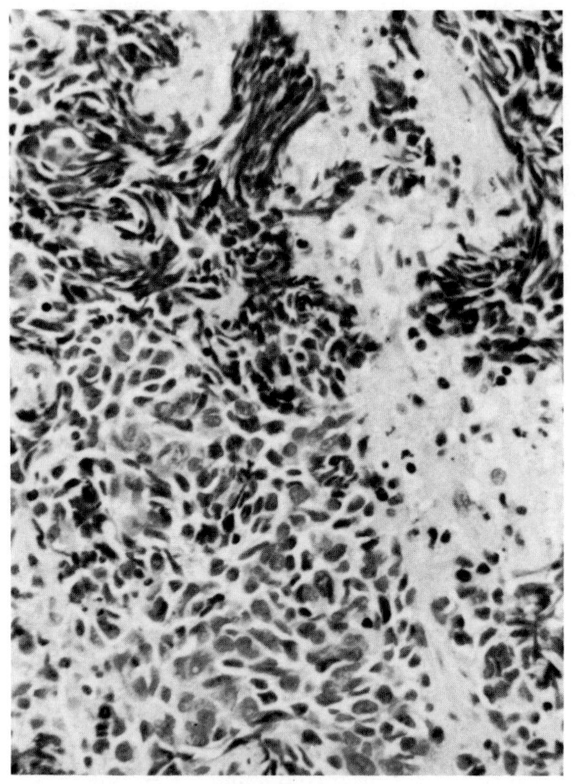

Figure 3-119.

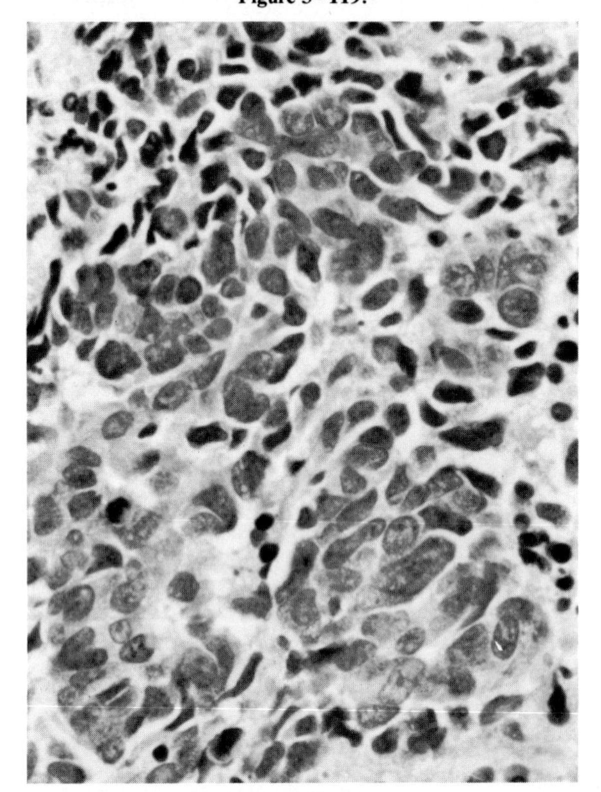

Figure 3-120.

Figures 3-119, 3-120. Small cell undifferentiated carcinoma. This lymph node metastasis shows smearing artifact characteristic of small cell undifferentiated carcinoma. There is some variation in nuclear size, but the coarse chromatin pattern with inconspicuous nucleoli and prominent nuclear molding is apparent.

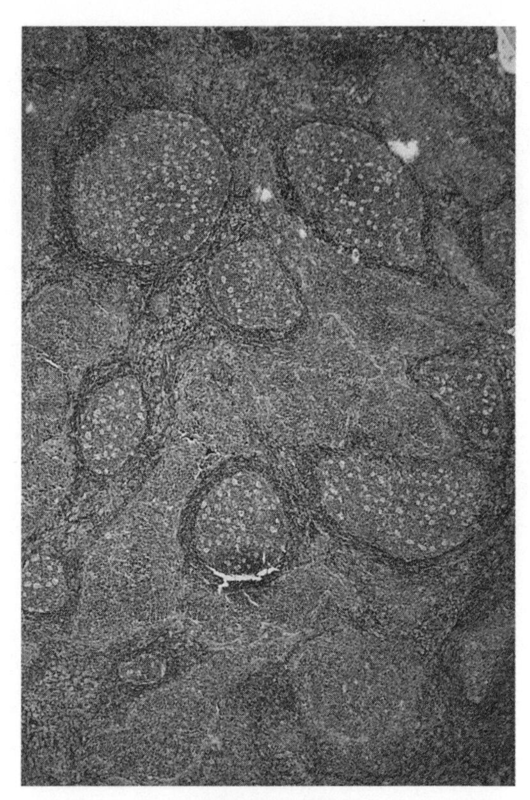

Figure 3-121.

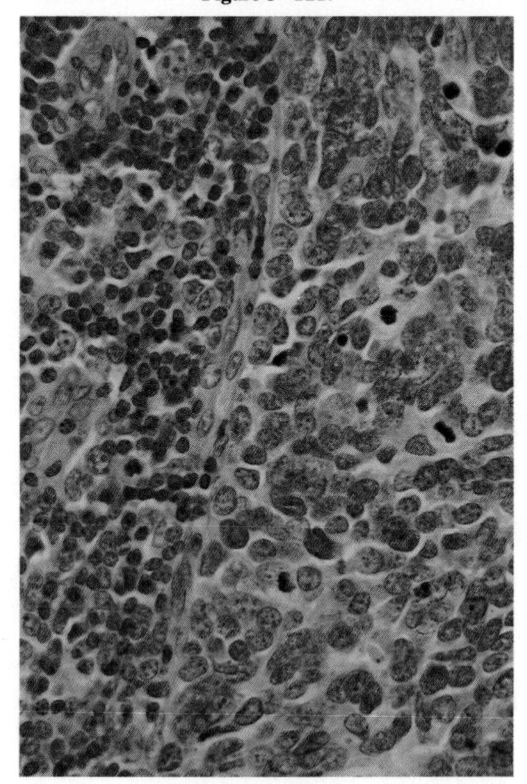

Figure 3-122.

Figures 3-121, 3-122. Small cell undifferentiated carcinoma. This mediastinal lymph node, which is harboring a sinusoidal infiltrate of small cell undifferentiated carcinoma, is characterized by a marked reactive follicular lymphoid hyperplasia.

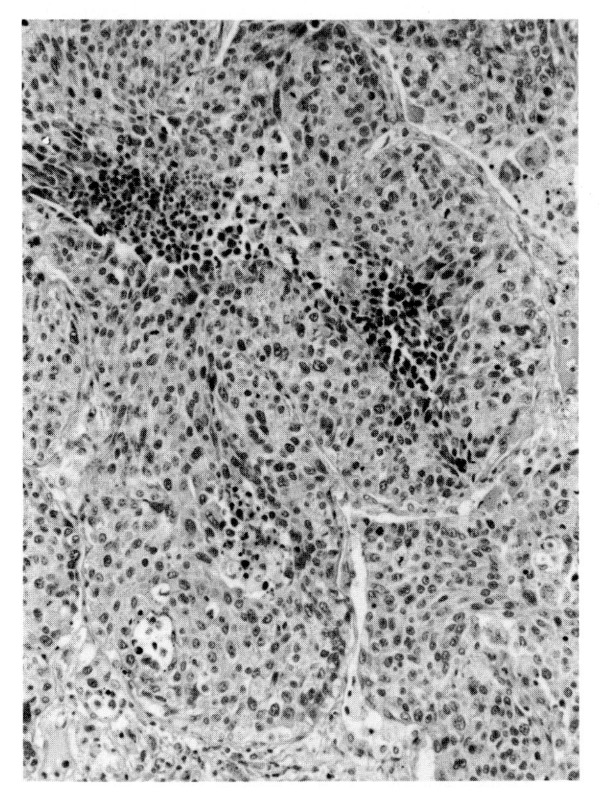

Figure 3-123. Large cell undifferentiated carcinoma. Sheets of large carcinoma cells with abundant cytoplasm and nuclei with prominent nucleoli show no discernible squamous or glandular differentiation.

Dail DH, Hammer SP (eds). Pulmonary Pathology, New York, Springer-Verlag, 1988.
Hirsch FR, Mathews MJ, Aisner S, et al. Histopathologic classification of small cell lung cancer: changing concepts and terminology. Cancer 62:973-977, 1988.
Thurlbeck WM (ed). Pathology of the Lung. New York, Thieme, 1988.
Yesner R. Small cell tumors of the lung. Am J Surg Pathol 7:775-785, 1983.

■ Large Cell Undifferentiated Carcinoma (Figs. 3-123 to 3-128)

This bronchogenic carcinoma lacks histologic features of adenocarcinoma, squamous cell carcinoma, and small cell undifferentiated carcinoma. In other words, it is a poorly differentiated non-small cell carcinoma.

Large cell undifferentiated carcinoma usually manifests as sheets of carcinoma without differentiating features; the cells may often appear squamoid, although defining features for squamous carcinoma are lacking. Clear cell, spindling, and giant cell forms occur (see also below).

The diagnosis of large cell undifferentiated carcinoma is considered by some to be a "wastebasket" diagnosis and thus is dependent on one's criteria and methods of evaluation. Sophisticated techniques (such as ultrastructural examination and immunostaining) show that a number of large cell undifferentiated carcinomas actually are characterized by glandular or squamous differentiation. The distinction from small cell carcinoma is discussed above.

References

Carter D, Eggleston JC. Tumors of the Lower Respiratory Tract. AFIP Atlas of Tumor Pathology, Second Series, Fascicle 17. Washington, DC, Armed Forces Institute of Pathology, 1980.
Churg A. The fine structure of large cell undifferentiated carcinoma of the lung. Evidence for its relation to squamous cell carcinomas and adenocarcinomas. Hum Pathol 9:143-156, 1978.
Dail DH, Hammer SP (eds). Pulmonary Pathology, New York, Springer-Verlag, 1988.
Delmonte VC, Alberti O, Saldiva PHN. Large cell carcinoma of the lung. Chest 90:524-527, 1986.
Thurlbeck WM (ed). Pathology of the Lung. New York, Thieme, 1988.
World Health Organization Monograph: Histologic Typing of Lung Tumors, 2nd ed. Geneva, WHO, 1981.
Yesner R. Large cell carcinoma of the lung. Semin Diagn Pathol 2:255-269, 1985.

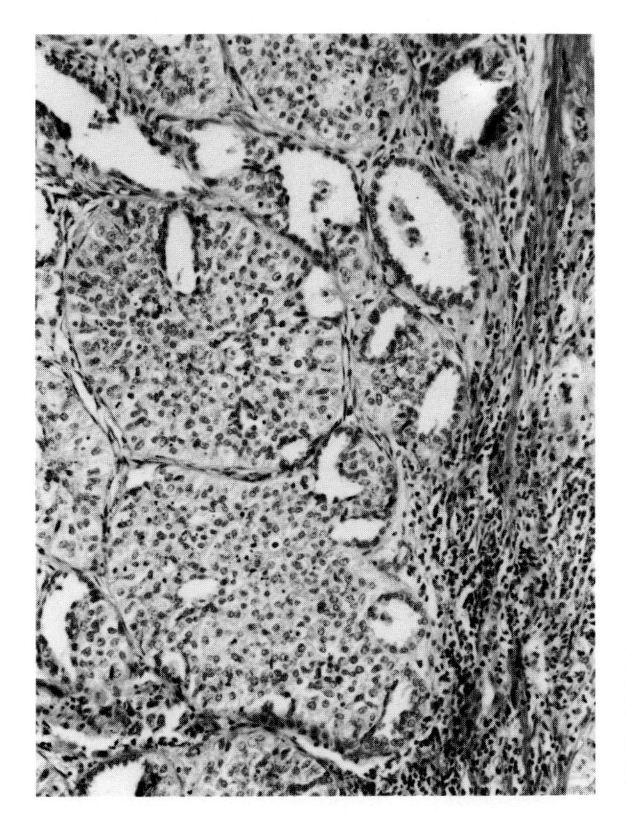

Figure 3-124. Large cell undifferentiated carcinoma. The sheets of carcinoma cells in this case showed intra-alveolar growth. The tumor cells have lifted the normal alveolar lining off the alveolar septum and crowded them toward the center, and they resemble small glandular spaces. The small glandlike spaces depicted represent the original alveolar spaces lined by reactive type II cells, which, in turn, are surrounded by the sheets of large cell undifferentiated carcinoma.

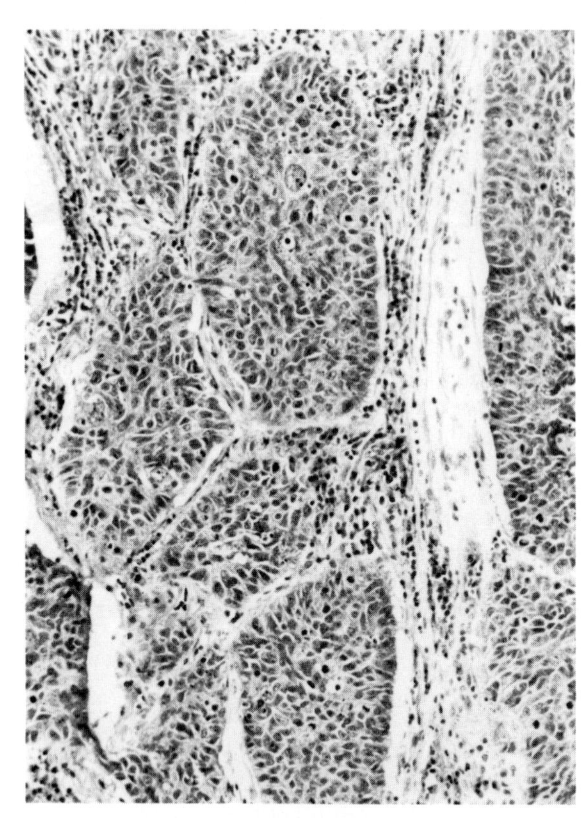

Figure 3-125.

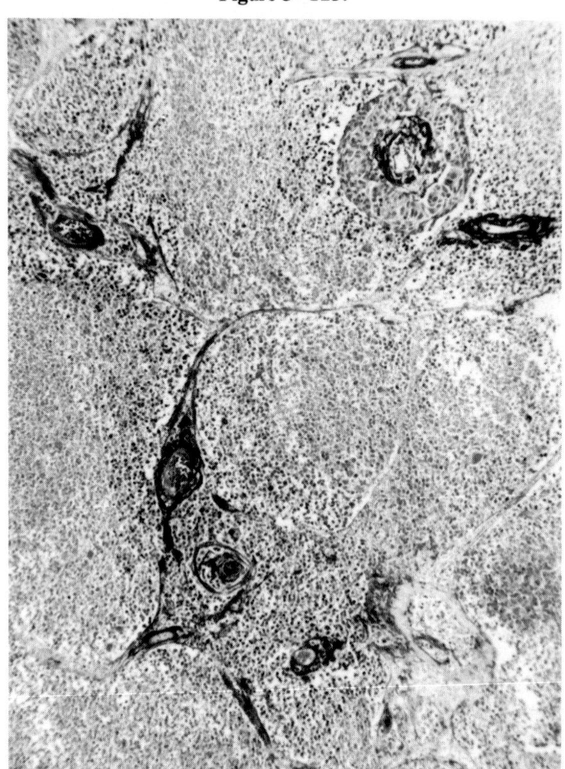

Figure 3-126.

Figures 3-125, 3-126. Large cell undifferentiated carcinoma. Vascular impregnation by nuclear material ("Azzopardi phenomenon") is shown. This carcinoma is characterized by a vaguely insular growth pattern, and one would not be surprised if neuroendocrine differentiation were found on either ultrastructural or immunohistochemical studies. The cells are too large and have too much cytoplasm for small cell undifferentiated carcinoma, although in areas of necrosis, this case illustrated a phenomenon that is usually seen in small cell undifferentiated carcinoma, namely impregnation of the interstitium and vascular walls by nuclear material.

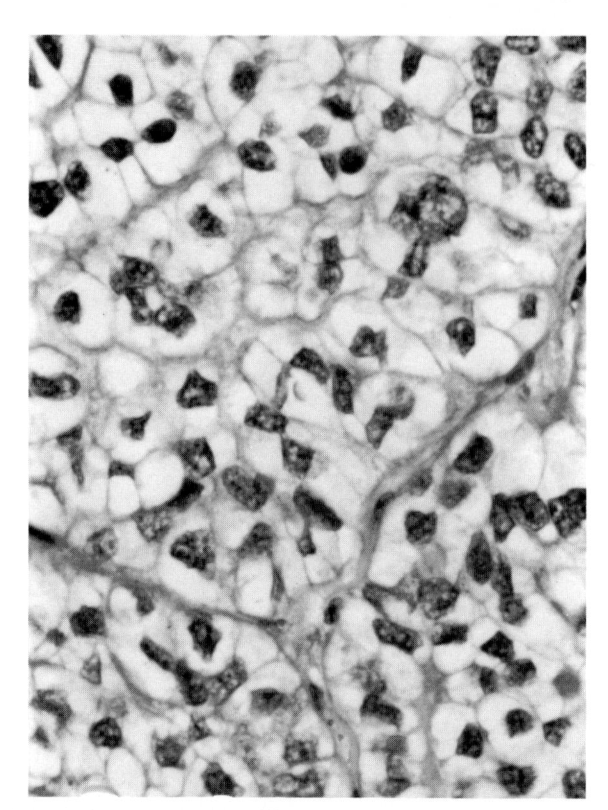

Figure 3-127. Large cell undifferentiated carcinoma with cytoplasmic clearing (clear cell carcinoma). Cytoplasmic clearing can be seen in adenocarcinomas, squamous carcinomas, and large cell undifferentiated carcinoma. The possibility of metastatic renal cell carcinoma should be considered prior to acceptance of such a case as a primary carcinoma of the lung.

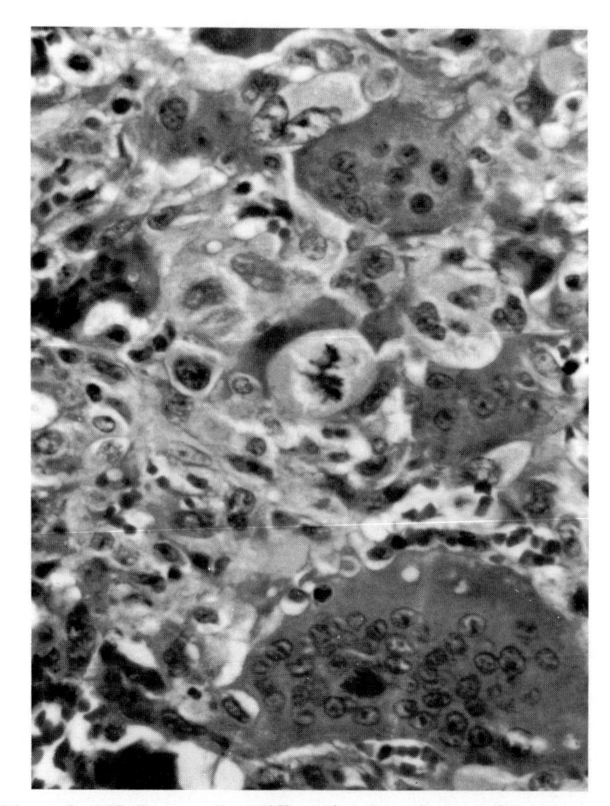

Figure 3-128. Large cell undifferentiated carcinoma with numerous multinucleated giant cells. This carcinoma lacked squamous or glandular differentiation.

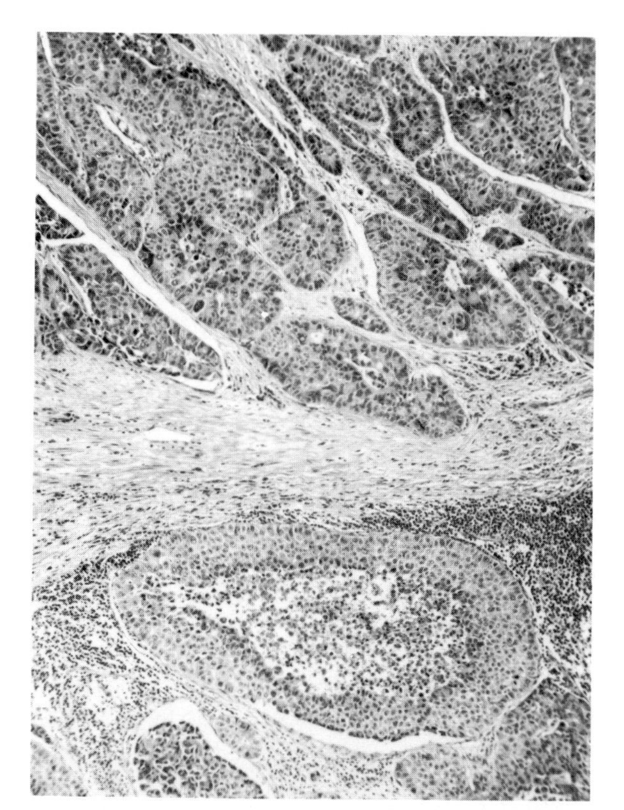

Figure 3-129. Large cell carcinoma with neuroendocrine differentiation. This tumor has a neuroendocrine appearance with rounded clusters of cells with central necrosis and trabecular and glandular patterns. Neuroendocrine differentiation was confirmed by immunohistochemical means.

■ Large Cell Carcinomas with Neuroendocrine Features (Atypical Endocrine Carcinomas) (Fig. 3-129)

High-grade bronchogenic carcinomas not uncommonly have a neuroendocrine appearance on routine light microscopy. There may be trabecular or insular patterns and stippled chromatin with prominent vascularity and/or neuroendocrine differentiation confirmed with electron microscopy or immunostaining. Although these tumors could arbitrarily be called atypical carcinoids, they have routine histologic and cytologic features of a frank carcinoma and we prefer to exclude them from the atypical carcinoid category. It is currently controversial whether they should be treated as small cell undifferentiated carcinomas simply on the basis of their neuroendocrine differentiation, but such an approach is supported in some reports.

References

Delmonte VC, Alberti O, Saldiva PHN. Large cell carcinoma of the lung. Chest 90:524-527, 1986.
Gould VE, Linnoila RI, Memoli VA, Warrne WH. Neuroendocrine cells and neuroendocrine neoplasms of the lung. Pathol Annu 18:287-330, 1983.
Hammond ME, Sause WT. Large cell neuroendocrine tumors of the lung. Cancer 56:1624-1629, 1985.
Linnoila RI, Mulshine JL, Steinberg SM, et al. Neuroendocrine differentiation in endocrine and nonendocrine lung carcinomas. Am J Clin Pathol 90:641-652, 1988.
McDowell EM, Wilson TS, Trump BF. Atypical endocrine tumors of the lung. Arch Pathol Lab Med 105:20-28, 1981.

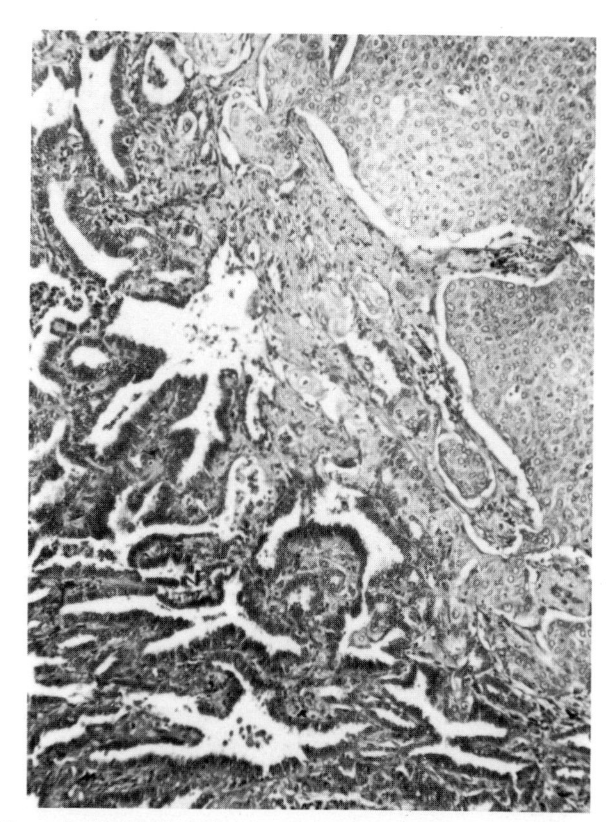

Figure 3-130. Mixed adenocarcinoma and squamous carcinoma. Islands of moderately differentiated squamous carcinoma can be seen adjacent to an adenocarcinoma with a bronchioloalveolar growth pattern.

■ Mixed Bronchogenic Carcinomas (Fig. 3-130)

Histologic heterogeneity in lung cancer is common. Examples include tumors with discrete and separable components of small cell undifferentiated carcinoma, squamous, and/or adenocarcinoma, and the number of cases that show such heterogeneity increases with the sophistication of one's techniques in detecting tumor differentiation (e.g., electron microscopy and batteries of immunostains).

When confronted with a mixed carcinoma, pathologists are often pressed into answering therapeutic questions, particularly if there is a component of small cell undifferentiated carcinoma. These are difficult questions to answer, and they should often be left to the oncologists and treating physicians, who can individualize each case.

References

Adelstein DJ, Tomashefski JF, Snow NJ, et al. Mixed small cell and non-small cell lung cancer. Chest 89:699-704, 1986.
Churg A, Johnston WH, Stulbarg M. Small cell squamous and mixed small cell squamous—small cell anaplastic carcinomas of the lung. Am J Pathol 4:255-263, 1980.
McDowell EM, Trump BF. Pulmonary small cell carcinoma showing tripartite differentiation in individual cells. Hum Pathol 12:286-294, 1981.
Roggli VL, Vollmer RT, Greenberg SE, et al. Lung Cancer heterogeneity. Hum Pathol 16:569-579, 1985.
Yesner R. Classification of lung cancer. N Engl J Med 312:652-653, 1985.

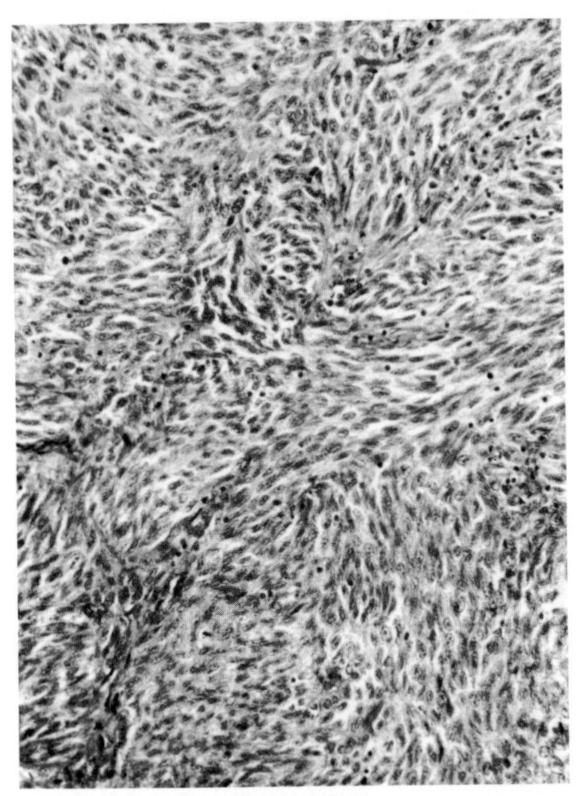

Figure 3-131.

■ Unusual Bronchogenic Carcinomas

There are a number of unusual patterns of bronchogenic carcinoma that bear separate discussion, although some are often included among the traditional categories of bronchogenic carcinoma. Generically, many of the lesions discussed in the next sections might be classified as large cell undifferentiated carcinoma, but the patterns are distinctive.

Spindle Cell Carcinomas (Figs. 3-131 to 3-136)

There is sufficient spindling to mimic a sarcoma. Sometimes squamous differentiation is seen. The differential diagnosis includes sarcomas, carcinosarcoma, metastatic sarcoma, and metastatic spindle cell carcinoma, especially renal cell carcinoma. Reticulin staining, PAS staining for glycogen, immunostaining and other studies for epithelial markers may prove helpful in the diagnosis.

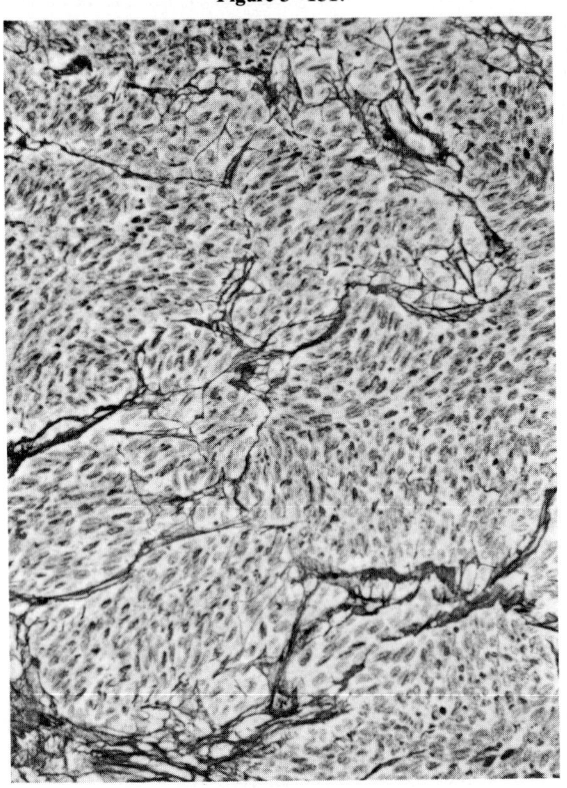

Figure 3-132.

Figures 3-131, 3-132. Spindle cell carcinoma. Epithelial nests are highlighted by reticulin stain. The spindled foci blended with areas of large cell undifferentiated carcinoma.

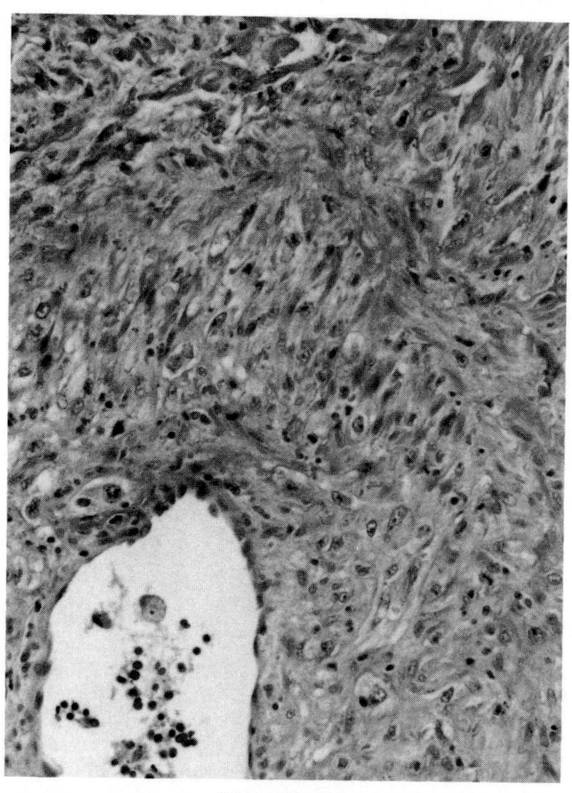

Figure 3–133.

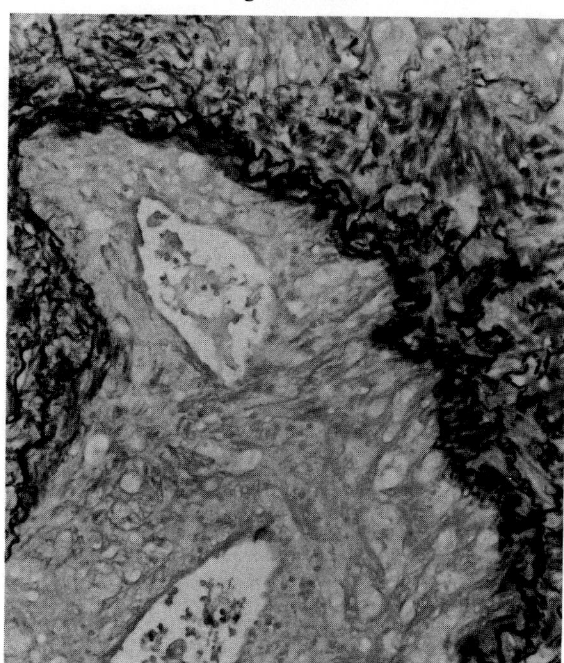

Figure 3–134.

Figures 3–133, 3–134. Spindle cell squamous carcinoma with prominent vascular invasion. Individual tumor cells infiltrate the wall of a medium-sized pulmonary vein that is highlighted by an elastic tissue stain. In other foci, squamous differentiation was prominent.

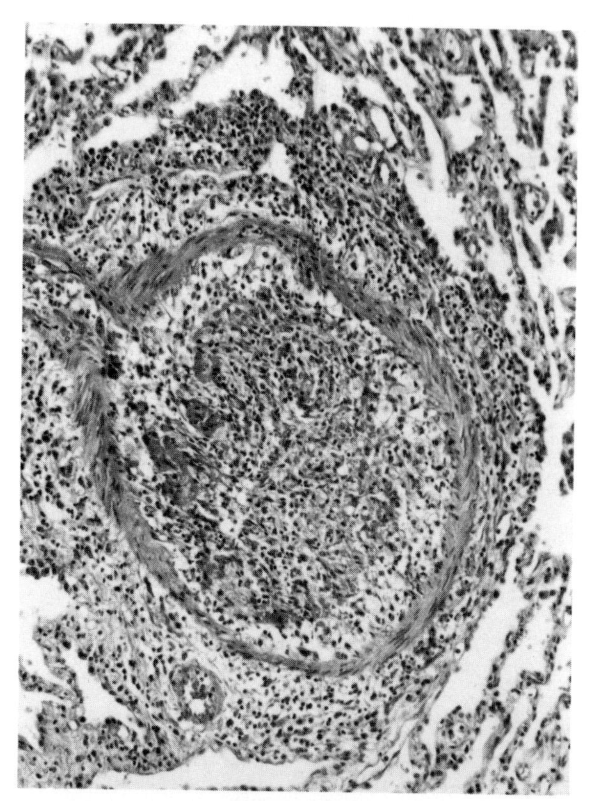

Figure 3–135.

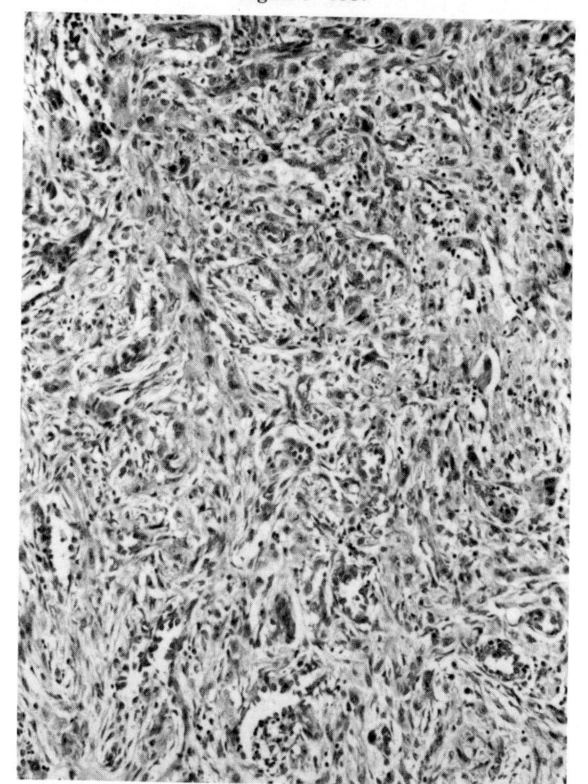

Figure 3–136.

Figures 3–135, 3–136. Spindle cell carcinoma. Marked vascular invasion and foci resembling malignant fibrous histiocytoma are shown. Extensive immunohistochemical studies in this case showed only carcinomatous differentiation.

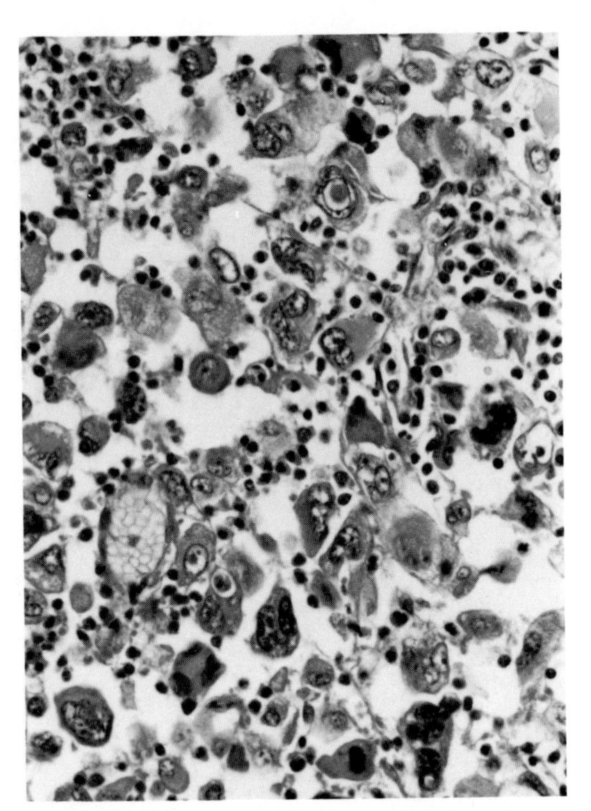

Figure 3–137. Giant cell carcinoma. Loosely cohesive cells are infiltrated by large numbers of neutrophils, some of which are in tumor cell cytoplasm.

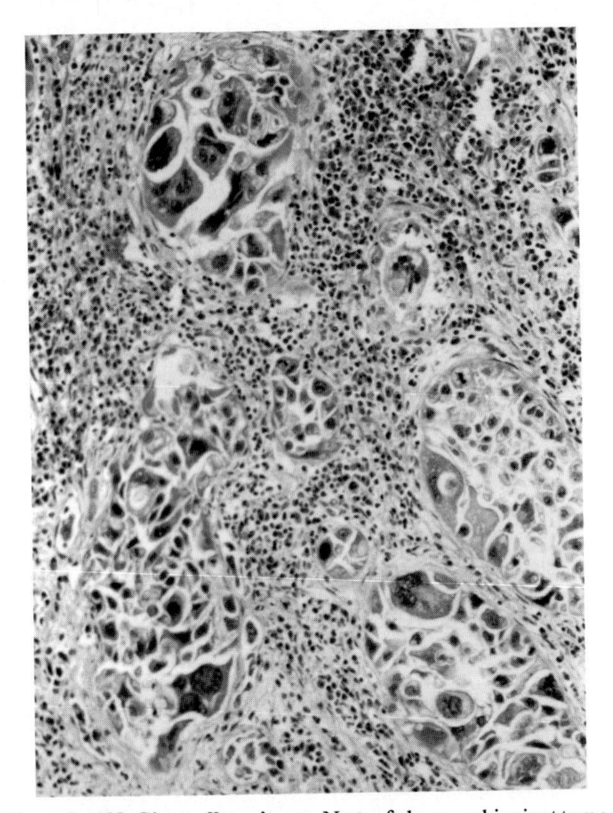

Figure 3–138. Giant cell carcinoma. Nests of pleomorphic giant tumor cells are surrounded by a lymphocyte-rich stroma.

Giant Cell Carcinoma (Figs. 3–137, 3–138)

Giant cell carcinoma consists of tumor cells that are pleomorphic and bizarre and that may sometimes be combined with spindling features. Some cases show sheets of tumor cells infiltrated by neutrophils, both extracellularly and intracellularly ("neutrophil phagocytosis"). Glandular differentiation may occur. Some cases are associated with fever, elevated sedimentation rate, and leukocytosis. In such cases, the differential diagnosis includes Hodgkin's disease, the inflammatory variant of malignant fibrous histiocytoma, and rarely malakoplakia. Radiated carcinomas often have a similar appearance (Figs. 3–139 and 3–140).

References

Addis BJ, Dewar A, Thurlow NP. Giant cell carcinoma of the lung—immunohistochemical and ultrastructural evidence of dedifferentiation. J Pathol 155:231–240, 1988.

Carter D, Eggleston JC. Tumors of the Lower Respiratory Tract. AFIP Atlas of Tumor Pathology, Second Series, Fascicle 17. Washington, DC, Armed Forces Institute of Pathology, 1980.

Dail DH, Hammer SP (eds). Pulmonary Pathology, New York, Springer-Verlag, 1988.

Herman DL, Bullock WK, Waken JK. Giant cell adenocarcinoma of the lung. Cancer 19:1337–1346, 1966.

Nash G, Stout AP. Giant cell carcinoma of the lung: report of 5 cases. Cancer 11:369–376, 1958.

Thurlbeck WM (ed). Pathology of the Lung. New York, Thieme, 1988.

Clear Cell Carcinoma (see Figs. 3–96, 3–106, 3–127)

Clear cell zones may be seen in squamous cell carcinoma, adenocarcinoma, and large cell undifferentiated carcinoma. Some lung tumors are composed entirely of clear cells, which may be glycogen-rich, and the distinction from metastatic renal cell carcinoma is obviously important. Clinical evaluation of the kidneys is indicated in these cases. Distinction from benign clear (sugar) tumor is based on malignant cytology, mitotic activity, necrosis, and large size.

References

Edward C, Carlisle A. Clear cell carcinoma of the lung. J Clin Pathol 38:880–885, 1985.

Katzenstein A-LA, Prioleau PG, Askin FB. The histologic spectrum and significance of clear cell change in lung carcinoma. Cancer 45:943–947, 1980.

Morgan A, Mackenzie D. Clear-cell carcinoma of the lung. J Pathol Bacteriol 87:25–29, 1964.

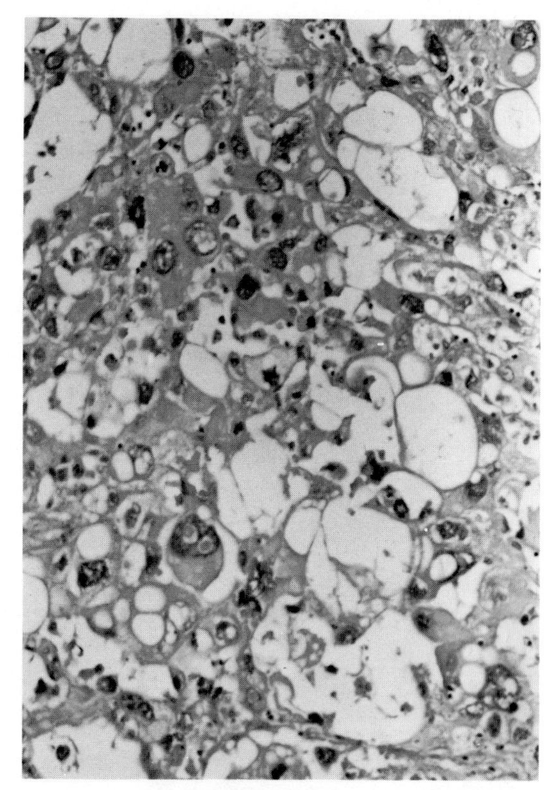

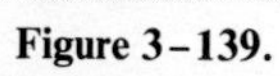

Figure 3–139.

Figures 3–139, 3–140. Large cell undifferentiated carcinoma following radiation therapy. Two different cases show marked tumor cell pleomorphism and nuclear and cytoplasmic vacuolization. The appearance is reminiscent of giant cell carcinoma.

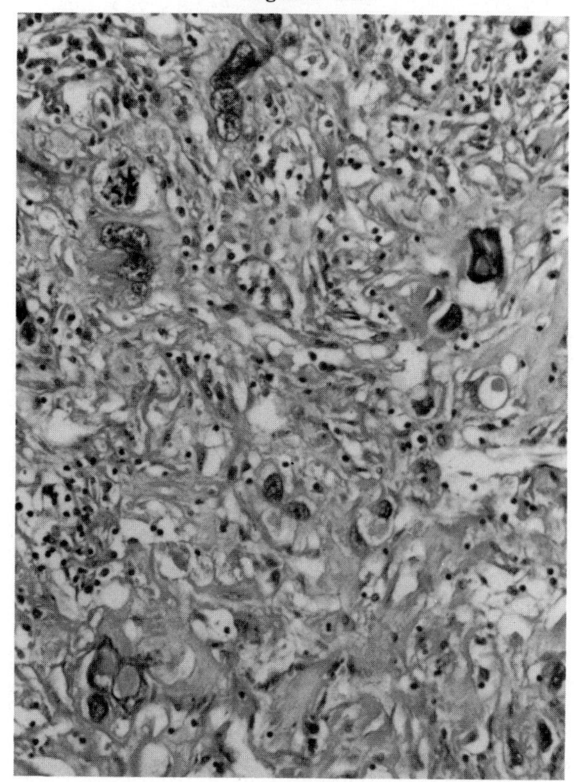

Figure 3–140.

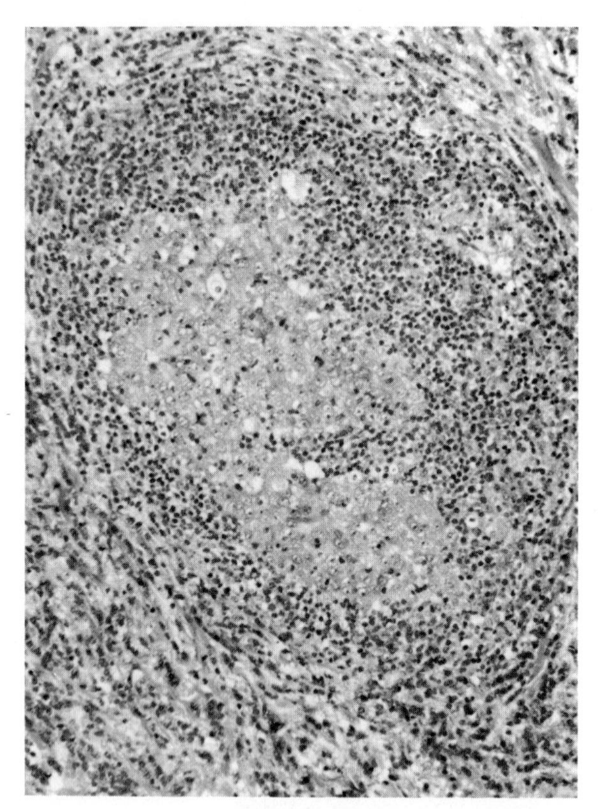

Figure 3-141.

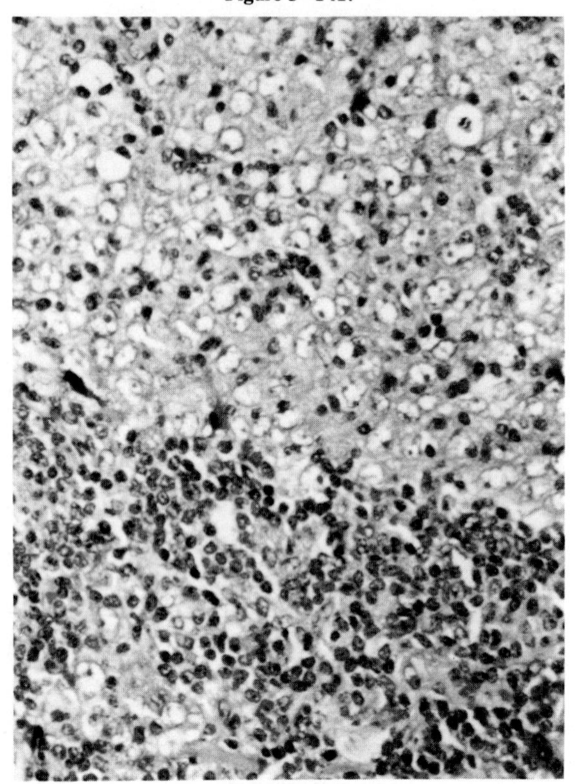

Figure 3-142.

Lymphoepithelioma-like Carcinoma (Figs. 3-141, 3-142)

This tumor is identical to lymphoepithelioma in the nasopharynx but is primary in the lung. The appearance is also similar to metastatic nasopharyngeal lymphoepithelioma to the lung (Figs. 3-143, 3-144).

References

Butler A, Colby TV, Weiss LM, Lombard C. Lymphoepithelioma-like carcinoma of the lung. Am J Surg Pathol 13:632-639, 1989.

Figures 3-141, 3-142. Lymphoepithelioma-like carcinoma. Nests of tumor cells are surrounded by a lymphocyte-rich stroma. The lymphocytes percolate through the tumor cells, which have prominent vesicular nuclei with nucleoli.

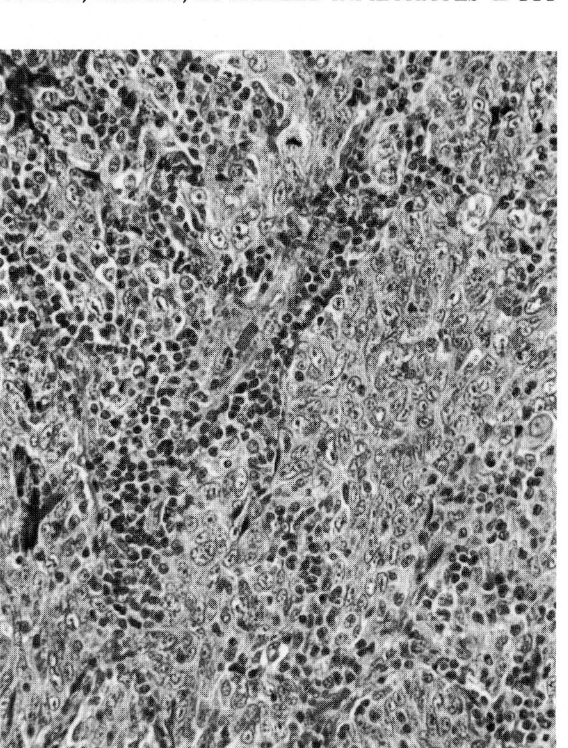

Figure 3–143.

Figures 3–143, 3–144. Nasopharyngeal carcinoma metastatic to the lung. Two cases show carcinoma cells forming small sheets surrounded by lymphocyte-rich stroma and individual tumor cells amidst a dense lymphoid infiltrate.

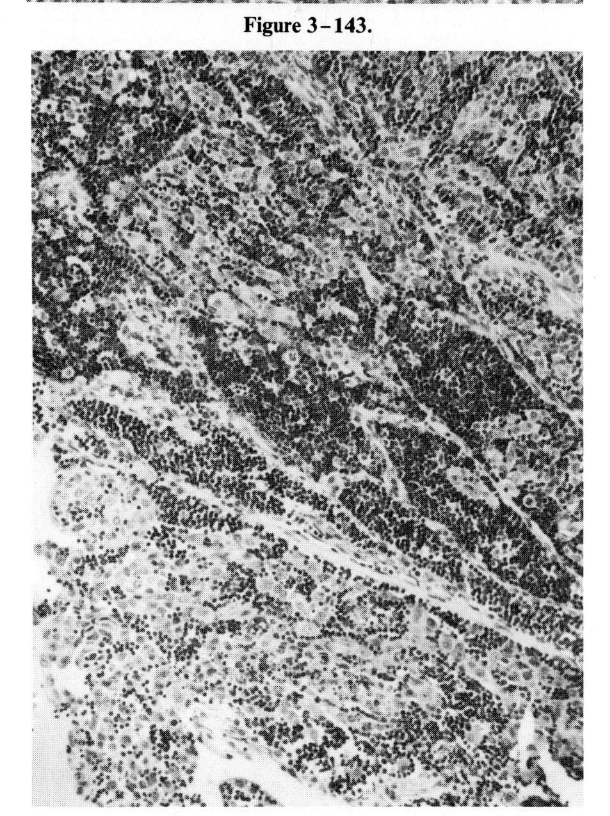

Figure 3–144.

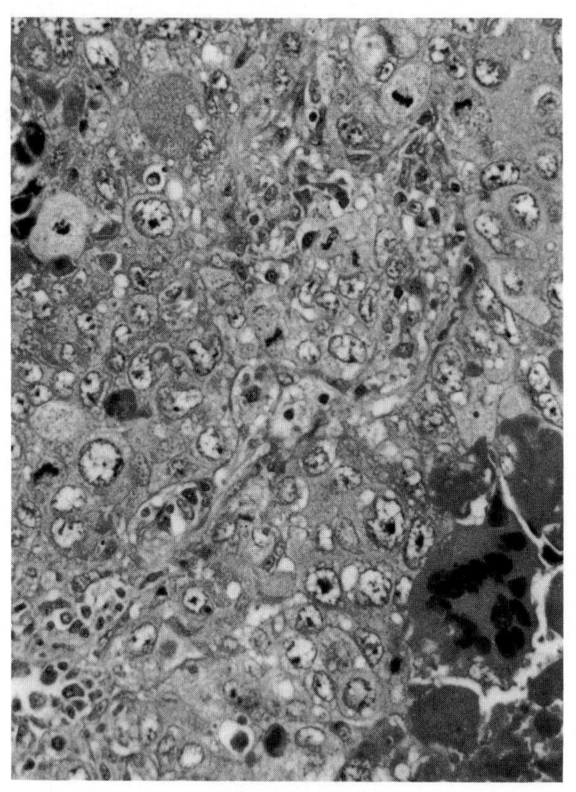

Figure 3-145.

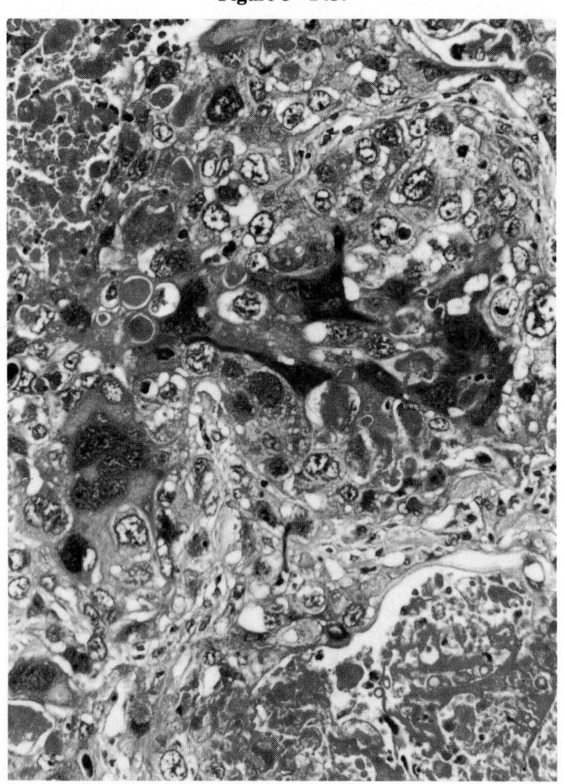

Figure 3-146.

■ Primary Choriocarcinoma of the Lung (Figs. 3-145, 3-146)

Carcinomas with histologic features of choriocarcinoma, but unassociated with gestation, have been described as primary in the lung. Some prefer to regard these tumors as giant cell carcinomas with ectopic human chorionic gonadotropin (HCG) production. Others feel that these represent epithelial neoplasms with divergent differentiation along purely choriocarcinomatous lines.

References

Pushchak MJ, Farhi DC. Primary choriocarcinoma of the lung. Arch Pathol Lab Med 115(5):477-479, 1987.

■ Adenocarcinoma Resembling Fetal Lung

See blastoma (page 123).

Figures 3-145, 3-146. Primary choriocarcinoma of the lung. Poorly differentiated carcinoma with cells resembling cytotrophoblast and multinucleated cells resembling syncytial trophoblast is shown. This tumor was found in a patient with elevated serum human chorionic gonadotropin (hCG) levels, and tumor cells stained positively for hCG.

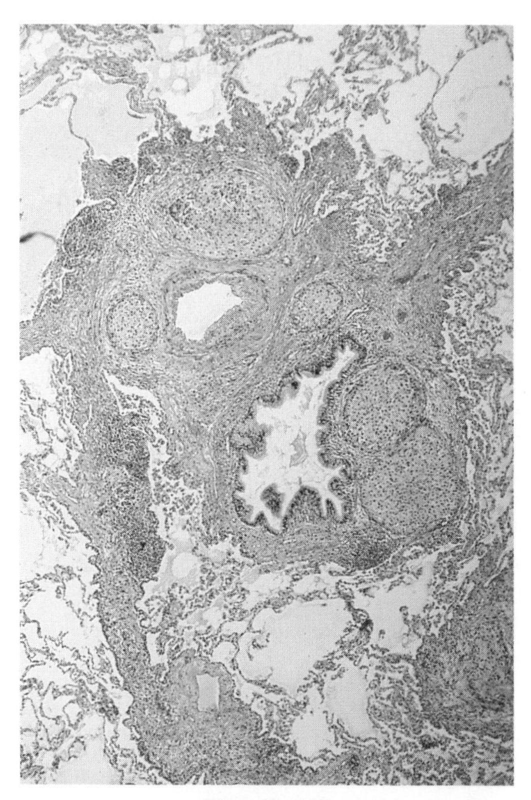

Figure 3–147.

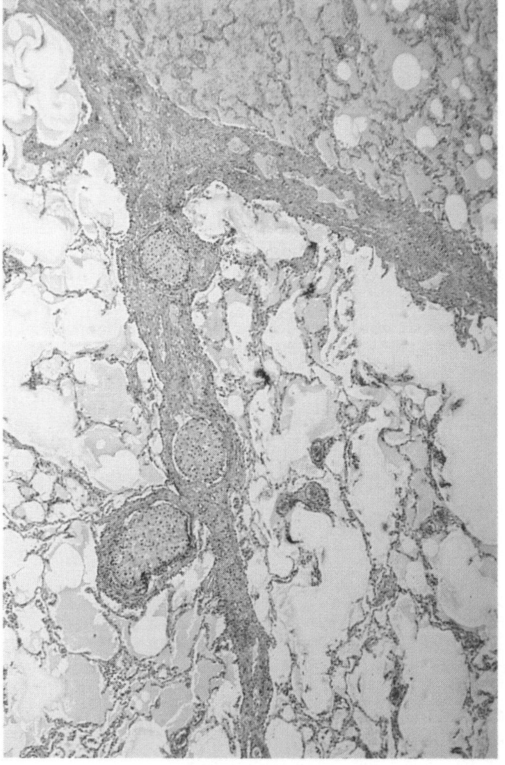

Figure 3–148.

■ **Metastatic Carcinomas to the Lung** (Figs. 3–147 to 3–165)

The lung is an extremely common site for metastatic carcinomas. Metastases may present as single or multiple endobronchial or parenchymal masses, or localized or diffuse infiltrations.

Before a diagnosis of primary bronchogenic carcinoma is made in a patient with a previous carcinoma, the two tumors should be compared and the clinical circumstances evaluated. Special studies including electron microscopy and immunohistochemistry may prove useful. In a patient with prior breast carcinoma, estrogen and progesterone receptor studies are appropriate.

Text continued on page 119

Figures 3–147, 3–148. Metastatic breast carcinoma. Diffuse intralymphatic tumor nodules that are peribronchiolar and septal in location have developed.

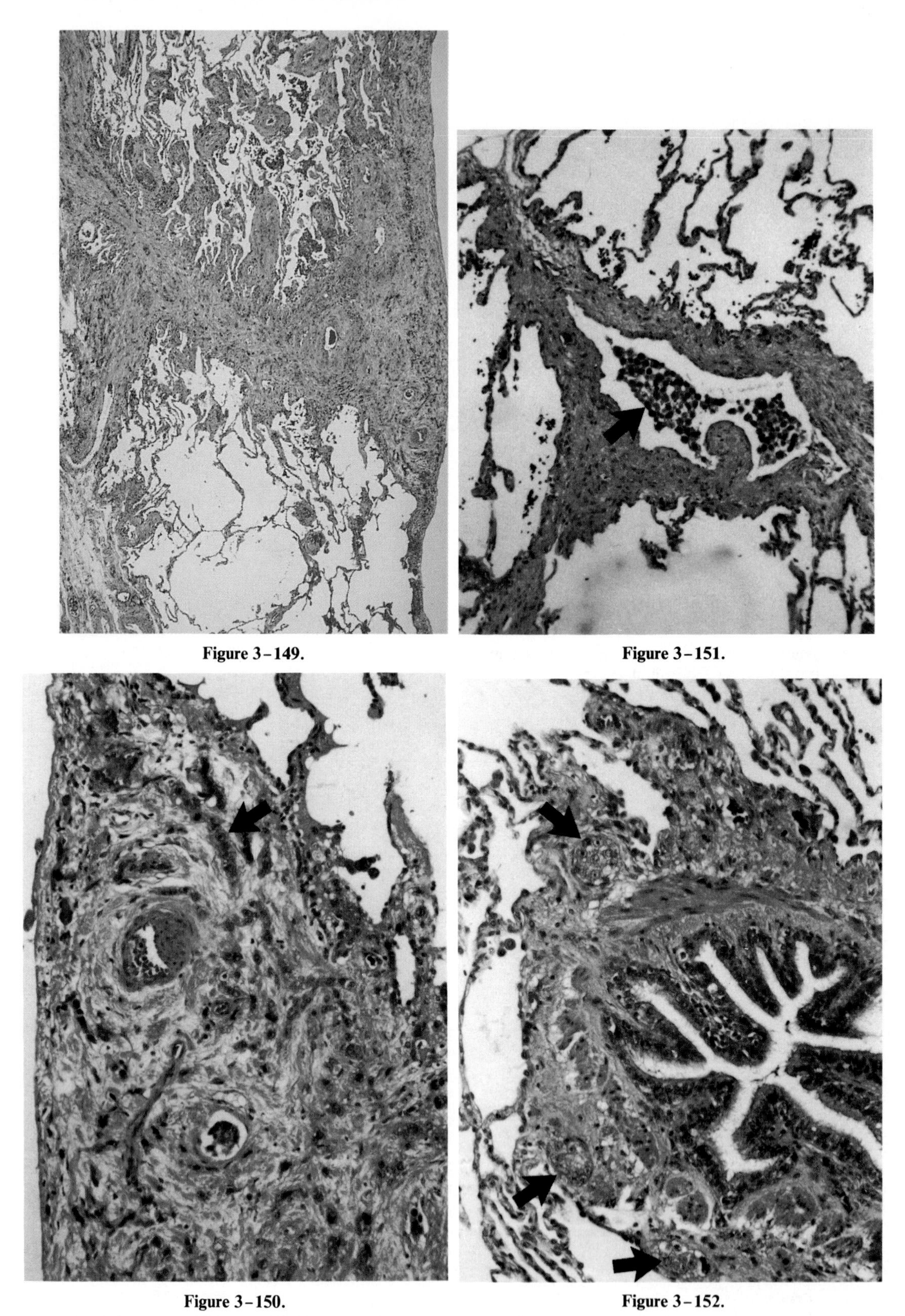

Figure 3–149.

Figure 3–151.

Figure 3–150.

Figure 3–152.

Figures 3–149, 3–150, 3–151, 3–152. Metastatic breast carcinoma. Carcinoma is indicated by the arrows. Pleural and septal infiltration and expansion are shown in Figures 3–149 and 3–150, and involvement of septal and peribronchiolar lymphatics in Figures 3–151 and 3–152.

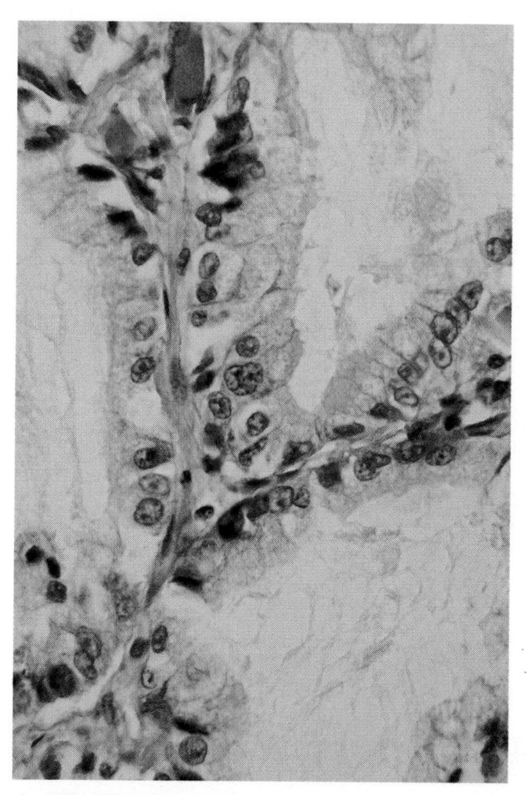

Figure 3-153. Metastatic pancreatic adenocarcinoma. This tumor mimics a mucinous bronchoalveolar carcinoma.

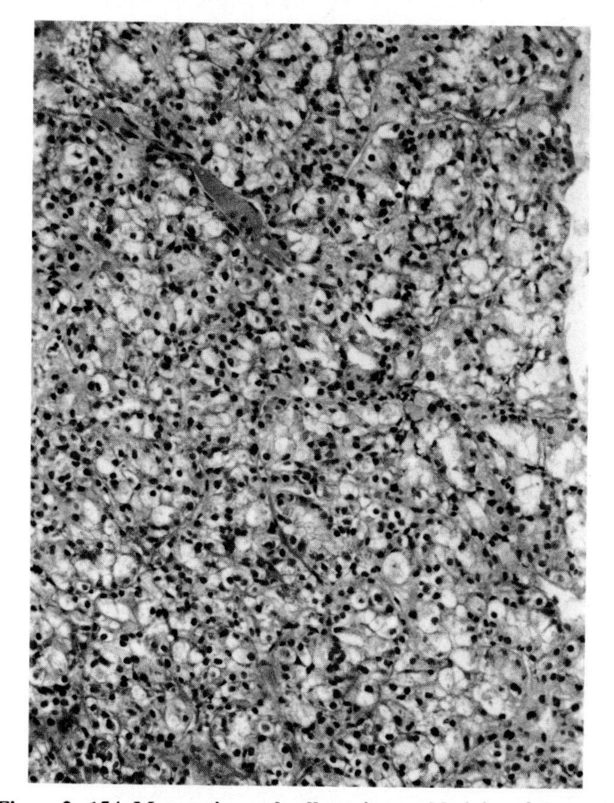

Figure 3-154. Metastatic renal cell carcinoma. Nodules of clear cell carcinoma have developed.

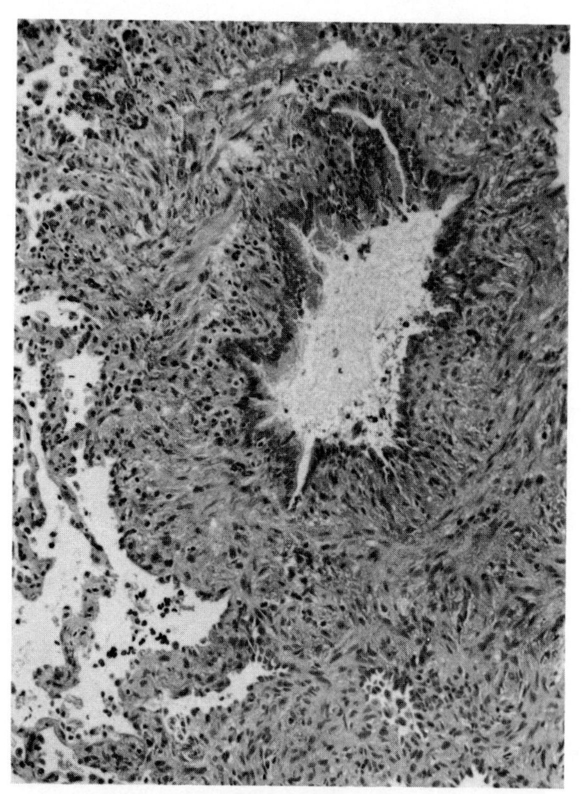

Figure 3-155.

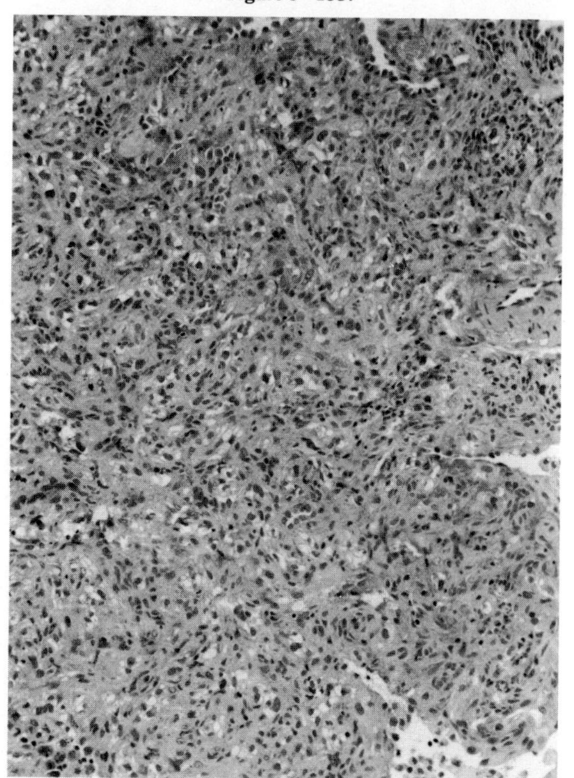

Figure 3-156.

Figure 3-155, 3-156. Metastatic renal cell carcinoma. There are peribronchiolar and interstitial spindle cell infiltrates with minimal clear cell change.

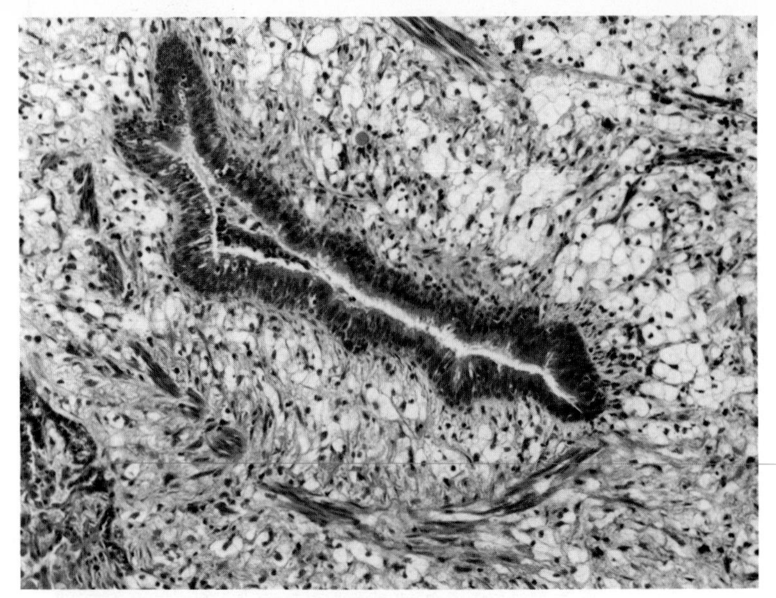

Figure 3-157.

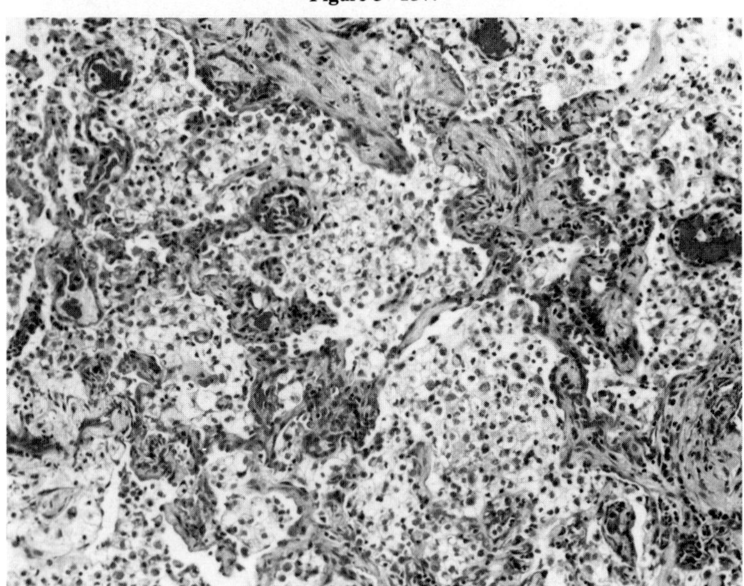

Figure 3-158.

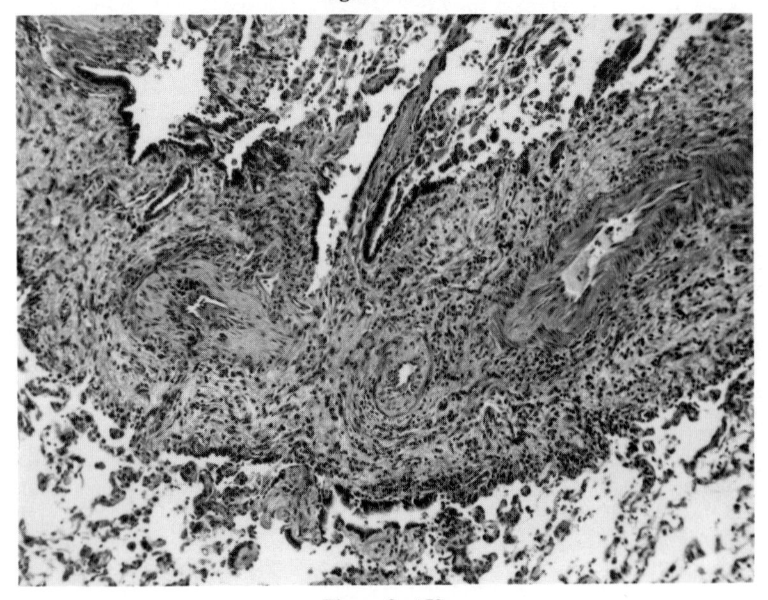

Figure 3-159.

Figures 3-157, 3-158, 3-159. Metastatic renal cell carcinoma. The carcinoma has produced infiltrates of peribronchiolar clear cells, alveolar filling by clear cells, and fusiform expansion around pulmonary arteries without obvious features of malignancy.

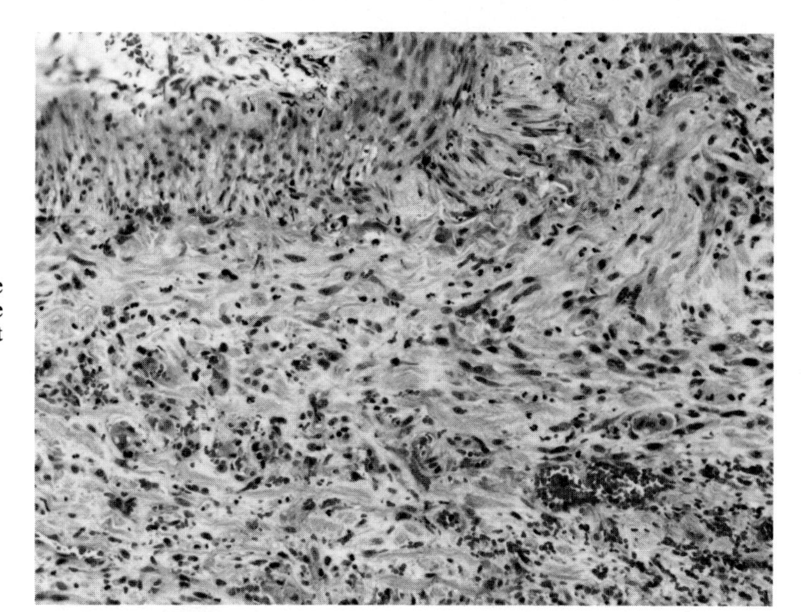

Figure 3–160. Metastatic renal cell carcinoma. A spindle cell infiltrate around a pulmonary artery can be seen. The degree of vascularity and red blood cells might suggest metastatic angiosarcoma.

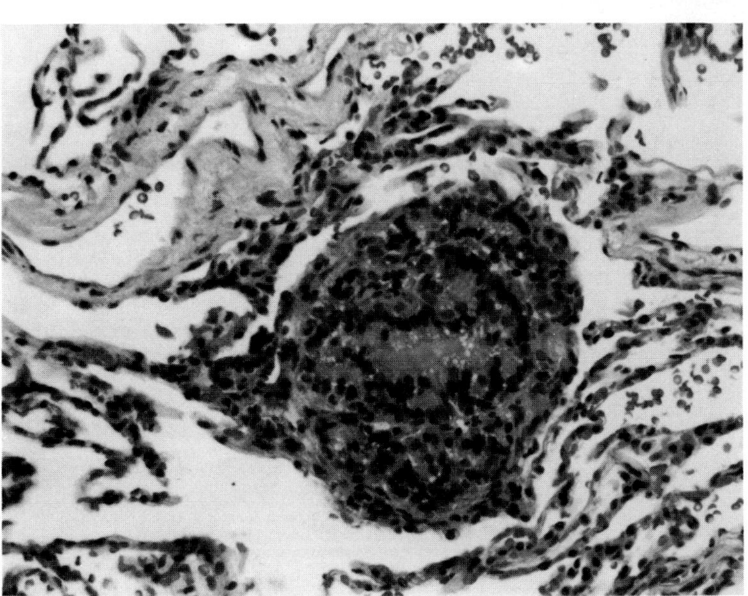

Figure 3–161. Metastatic papillary carcinoma of the thyroid. The tumor is identified as microscopic tumor nodules on transbronchial biopsy.

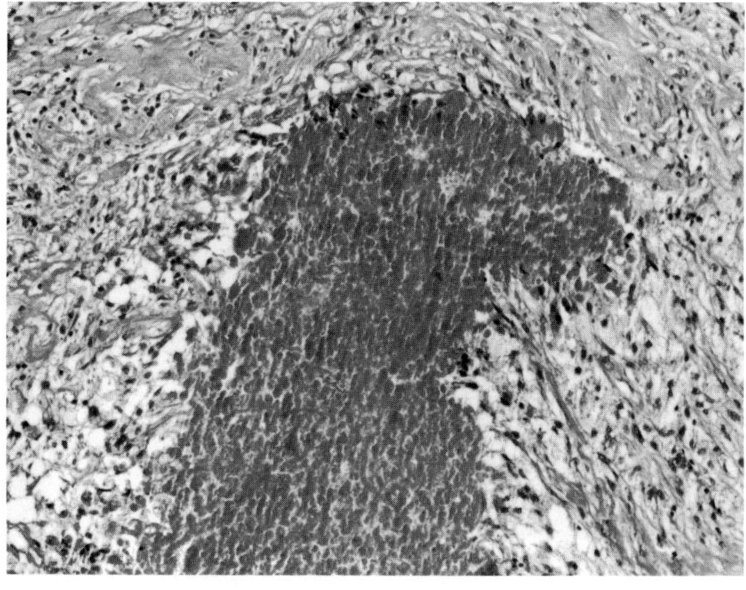

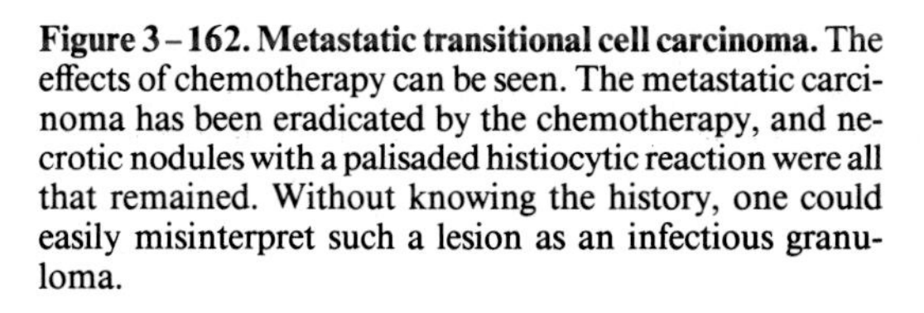

Figure 3–162. Metastatic transitional cell carcinoma. The effects of chemotherapy can be seen. The metastatic carcinoma has been eradicated by the chemotherapy, and necrotic nodules with a palisaded histiocytic reaction were all that remained. Without knowing the history, one could easily misinterpret such a lesion as an infectious granuloma.

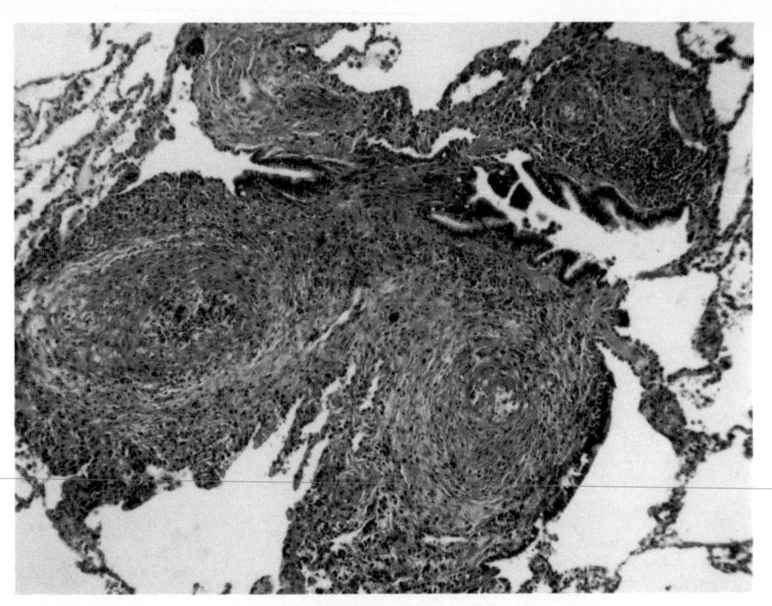

Figure 3-163.

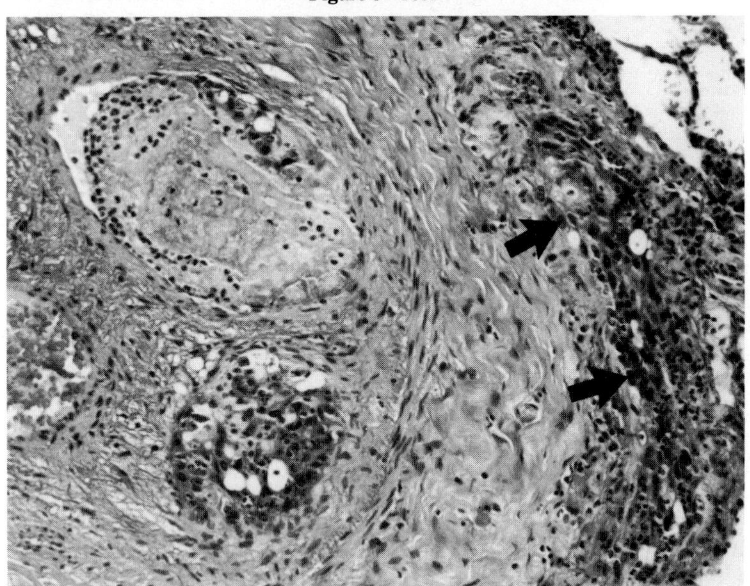

Figure 3-164.

Figures 3-163, 3-164, 3-165. Diffuse intra-arterial metastatic carcinoma. Also known as carcinomatous arteriopathy. There is often associated acute pulmonary hypertension. There is pulmonary arterial intimal and muscular thickening associated with both active and healed thrombi. In a few of the vessels, clusters of mucin-positive tumor cells can be identified (Figs. 3-164, 3-165). Both intralymphatic (arrows) as well as intra-arterial tumor cells may be identified.

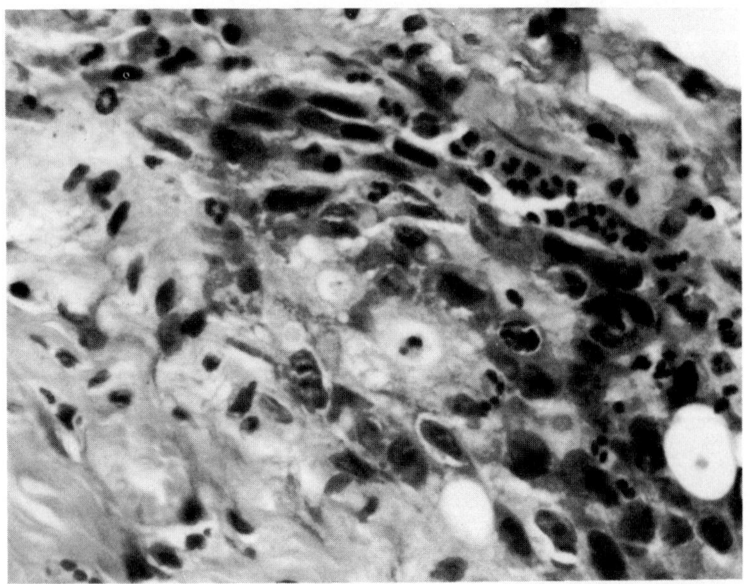

Figure 3-165.

■ Primary Lung Sarcomas

Most of the common sarcomas recognized in the soft tissues occur in the lungs, including fibrosarcoma, malignant fibrous histiocytoma, hemangiopericytoma, chondrosarcoma, osteosarcoma, neurogenic sarcoma, leiomyosarcoma, and rhabdomyosarcoma. These tumors may sometimes be cured, if they can be completely resected; incomplete resection or involvement of the chest wall is a very poor sign.

There is an unusual form of primitive-appearing sarcoma seen in children that may be solid and/or cystic and that contain zones of chondrosarcoma, primitive myxosarcoma, liposarcoma, or rhabdomyosarcoma (Figs. 3–166 to 3–169). The walls of cysts may contain primitive cells showing a cambium layer. Tumors of this type have been called thoracoblastomas, myxosarcomas, rhabdomyosarcomas, and, simply, blastomas. Because of the terminology, they have been confused with classical pulmonary blastomas (discussed later). These tumors are not truly biphasic, although interstitial growth and metaplasia of entrapped alveolar epithelium may simulate a biphasic pattern. Because some are cystic, an origin from congenital cystic disease or adenomatoid malformation has been suggested. Recently, the term pleuropulmonary blastoma has been applied to these primitive sarcomas.

When thinking of a primary lung sarcoma, one should always *consider the possibility of carcinosarcoma* in which the sarcomatous element dominates. The lesion should be adequately sampled, and special techniques such as immunostains, help to identify the epithelial elements. The mere inclusion of a few airspaces at the edge of a sarcoma and the lining of these spaces by metaplastic epithelium is not evidence of biphasic differentiation. Such a pseudobiphasic pattern may be very extensive.

References

Allen BT, Day DL, Dehner LP. Primary pulmonary rhabdomyosarcoma of the lung in children. Cancer 59:1005–1011, 1987.

Carter D, Eggleston JC. Tumors of the Lower Respiratory Tract. AFIP Atlas of Tumor Pathology, Second Series, Fascicle 17. Washington, DC, Armed Forces Institute of Pathology, 1980.

Colby TV, Bilbao JE, Battifora H, Unni KK. Primary osteosarcoma of the lung. Arch Pathol Lab Med. 113:1147–1150, 1989.

Dail DH, Hammer SP (eds). Pulmonary Pathology. New York, Springer-Verlag, 1988.

Guccion GJ, Rosen SH. Bronchopulmonary leiomyosarcoma and fibrosarcoma. A study of 32 cases and review of the literature. Cancer 30:836–847, 1972.

Lee JT, Shelburne JD, Linder J. Primary malignant fibrous histiocytoma of the lung: a clinicopathologic and ultrastructural study of five cases. Cancer 53:1124–1130, 1984.

Lee SH, Rengachary SS, Paramesh J. Primary pulmonary rhabdomyosarcoma. Hum Pathol 12:92–96, 1981.

Manivel JC, Priest JR, Watterson J, et al. Pleuropulmonary blastoma. Cancer 62:1516–1526, 1988.

Martinez JC, Pecero FC, delaPena CG, et al. Pulmonary blastoma: report of a case. J Pediatr Surg 13:93–94, 1978.

Nascimento AG, Unni KK, Bernatz PE. Sarcomas of the lung. Mayo Clin Proc 57:335–359, 1982.

Roth JA, Elguezabal A. Pulmonary blastoma evolving into carcinosarcoma. Am J Surg Pathol 2:407–413, 1978.

Silverman JF, Coalson JJ. Primary malignant myxoid fibrous histiocytoma of the lung: light and ultrastructural examination with review of the literature. Arch Pathol Lab Med 108:49–54, 1984.

Stephanopoulos C, Catsaras H. Myxosarcoma complicating a cystic hamartoma of the lung. Thorax 18:144–145, 1963.

Sumner TE, Phelps CR, Crowe JE, et al: Pulmonary blastoma in a child. AJR 133:147–148, 1979.

Thurlbeck WM (ed). Pathology of the Lung. New York, Thieme, 1988.

Ueda K, Gruppo R, Unger F, et al. Rhabdomyosarcoma of the lung arising in congenital cystic adenomatoid malformation. Cancer 40:383–388, 1977.

Valderrama E, Saluja G, Shende A, et al. Pulmonary blastoma: report of two cases in children. Am J Surg Pathol 2:415–422, 1978.

Weinberg AG, Currarino G, Moore GC, Votteler TP. Mesenchymal neoplasia and congenital pulmonary cysts. Pediatr Radiol 9:179–182, 1980.

Weinblatt ME, Siegel SE, Isaacs H. Pulmonary blastoma associated with cystic lung disease. Cancer 49:669–671, 1982.

Wick MR, Scheithauer BW, Piehler JM, Pairolero PC. Primary pulmonary leiomyosarcomas: a light and electron microscopic study. Arch Pathol Lab Med 106:510–514, 1982.

World Health Organization Monograph: Histologic Typing of Lung Tumors, 2nd ed. Geneva, WHO, 1981.

Yousem SA, Hochholzer L. Malignant fibrous histiocytoma of the lung. Cancer 60:2532–2541, 1987.

Yousem SA, Hochholzer L. Primary pulmonary hemangiopericytoma. Cancer 59:549–555, 1987.

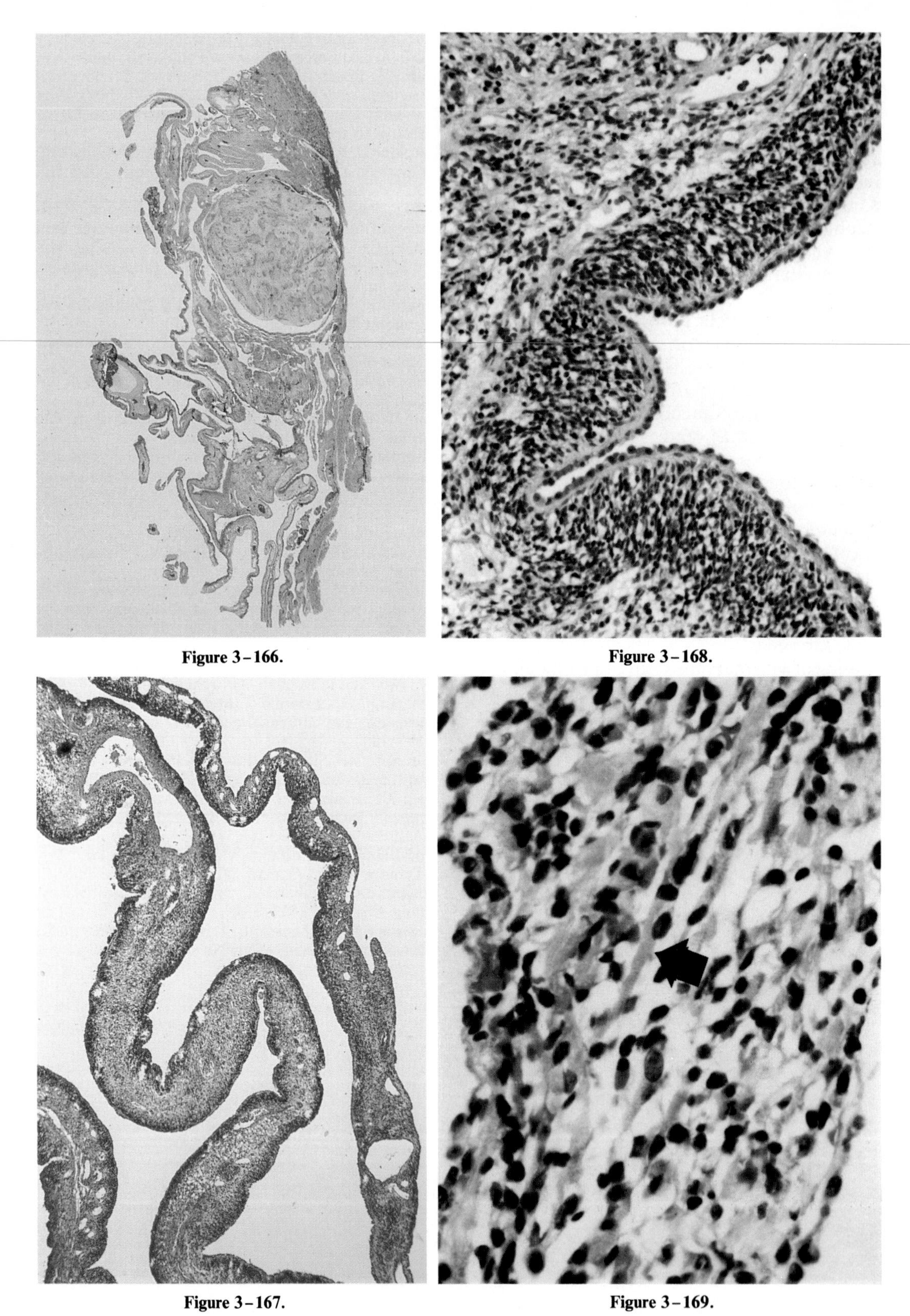

Figure 3–166.

Figure 3–168.

Figure 3–167.

Figure 3–169.

Figures 3–166, 3–167, 3–168, 3–169. Primary multicystic rhabdomyosarcoma of the lung in a child. The walls of the cysts are lined by a cambium layer of primitive cells among which strap cells showing cross striations can be identified (arrow). The epithelial cells lining the cyst walls are metaplastic alveolar lining cells and are not part of biphasic differentiation by the tumor.

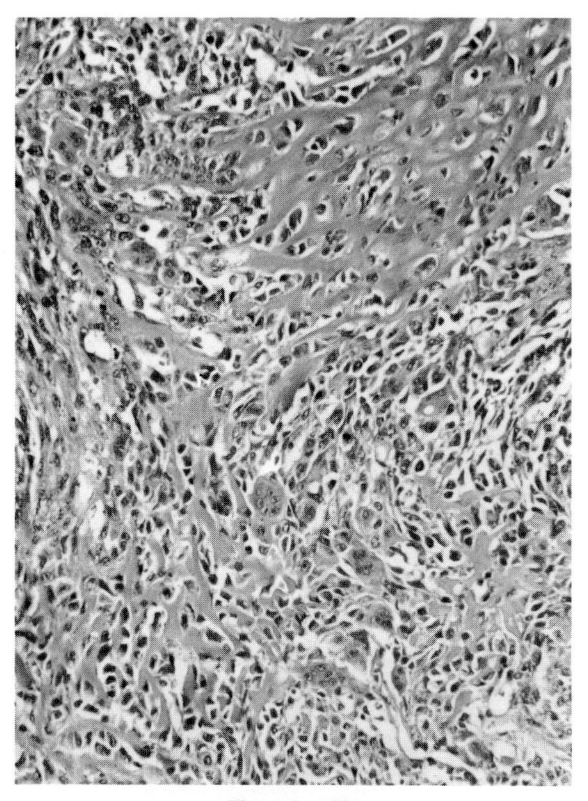

Figure 3-170.

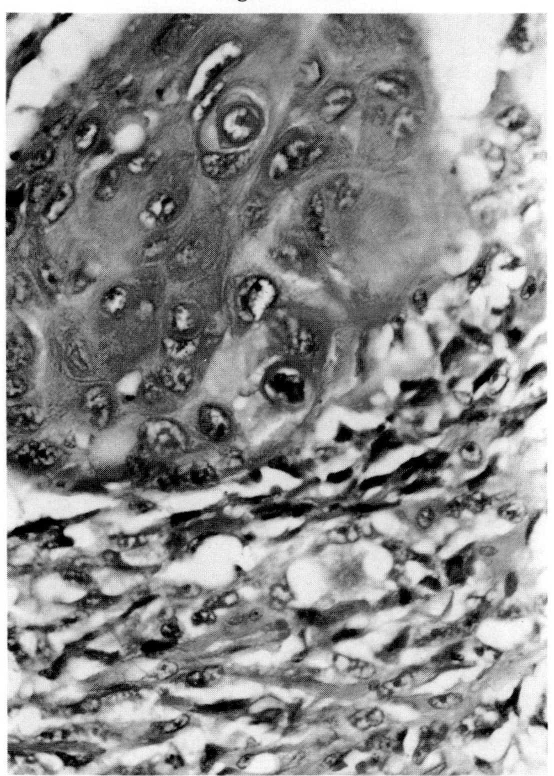

Figure 3-171.

■ **Carcinosarcoma** (Figs. 3-170 to 3-173)

Carcinosarcoma appears as a malignant tumor with carcinomatous and sarcomatous differentiation, typically "mature" carcinoma and "mature" sarcoma. This type of tumor may be parenchymal or endobronchial.

Any combination of adenocarcinoma, small cell undifferentiated carcinoma, squamous cell carcinoma, or large cell undifferentiated carcinoma may be associated with undifferentiated sarcoma, leiomyosarcoma, osteosarcoma, chondrosarcoma, fibrosarcoma, or malignant fibrous histiocytoma. The most frequent combination is squamous or adenocarcinoma associated with fibrosarcoma or malignant fibrous histiocytoma. Immunohistologic studies have suggested that some of these may indeed be metaplastic carcinomas. At present, the term carcinosarcoma can be used for cases recognized by routine histologic examination.

Pathogenetically, collision tumors (carcinoma *and* sarcoma), carcinomas with pseudosarcomatous stromal changes (metaplastic carcinomas), and biphasic differentiation of primitive totipotential cells have all been considered.

Differential diagnosis includes blastoma and spindle cell tumors with interstitial growth with inclusion of alveolar spaces lined by metaplastic cells. In some cases of carcinosarcoma the carcinomatous elements are quite focal.

References

Addis BJ, Corrin B. Pulmonary blastoma, carcinosarcoma and spindle cell carcinoma: an immunohistochemical study of keratin intermediate filaments. J Pathol 147:291-301, 1985.

Carter D, Eggleston JC. Tumors of the Lower Respiratory Tract. AFIP Atlas of Tumor Pathology, Second Series, Fascicle 17. Washington, DC, Armed Forces Institute of Pathology, 1980.

Dail DH, Hammer SP (eds). Pulmonary Pathology. New York, Springer-Verlag, 1988.

Davis PW, Briggs, JC, Seal RME, Storring FK. Benign and malignant mixed tumors of the lung. Thorax 27:657-673, 1972.

Davis MP, Eagan RT, Weiland LH, Pairolero PC. Carcinosarcoma of the lung: Mayo Clinic experience and response to chemotherapy. Mayo Clin Proc 59:598-603, 1984.

Thurlbeck WM (ed). Pathology of the Lung. New York, Thieme, 1988.

World Health Organization Monograph: Histologic Typing of Lung Tumors, 2nd ed. Geneva, WHO, 1981.

Figures 3-170, 3-171. Carcinosarcoma of the lung. This tumor is composed almost entirely of osteosarcoma and undifferentiated sarcoma. Osteoclastic giant cells are relatively numerous. Focally squamous carcinoma was identified (Figure 3-171).

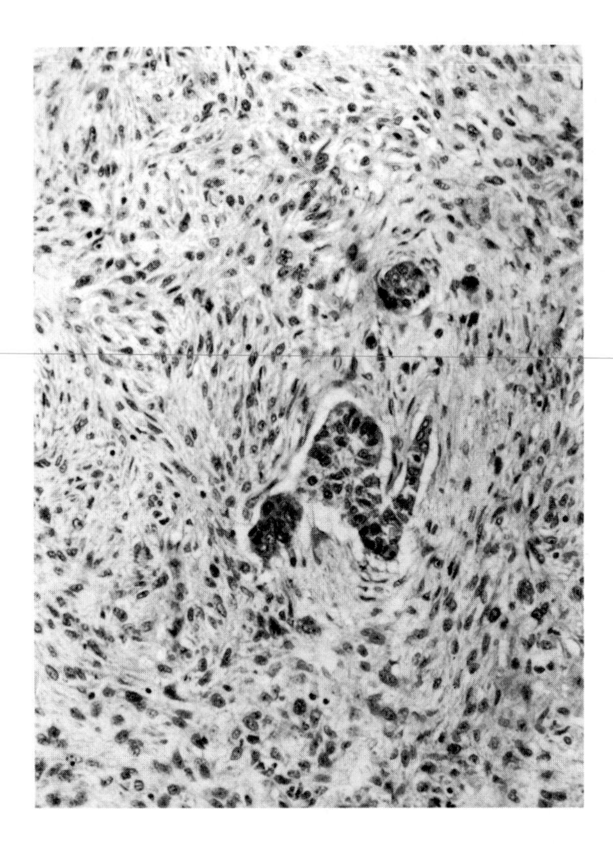

Figure 3–172. Carcinosarcoma associated with small nests of poorly differentiated adenocarcinoma amongst an undifferentiated sarcomatous stroma.

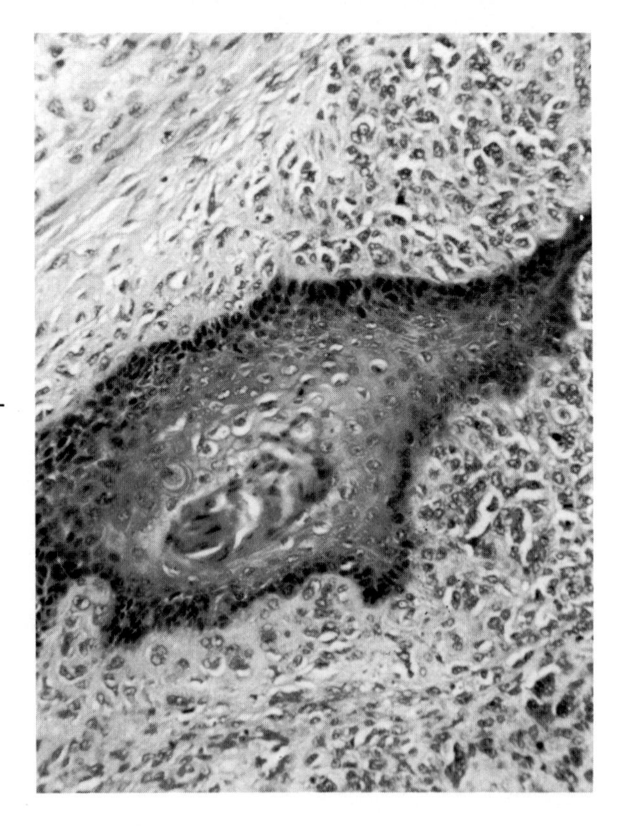

Figure 3–173. Carcinosarcoma of the lung with islands of moderately differentiated squamous carcinoma amongst a fibrosarcomatous stroma.

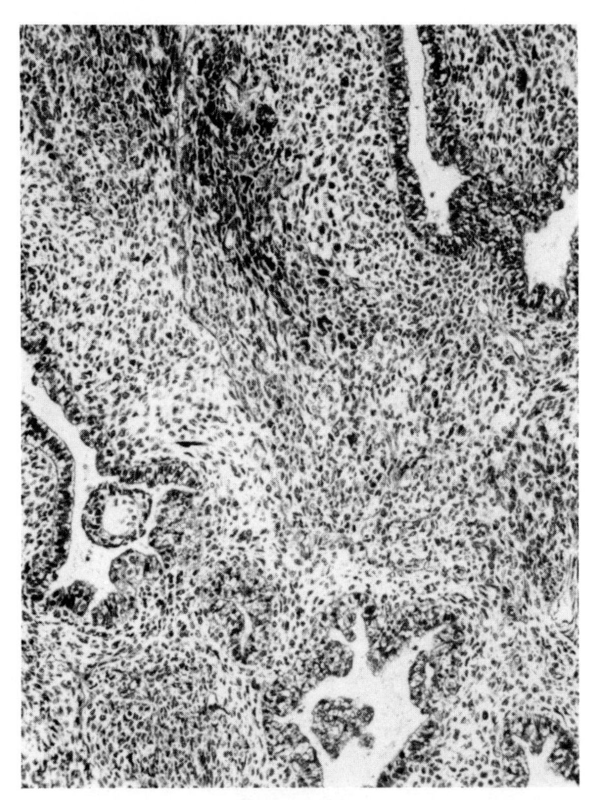

Figure 3-174.

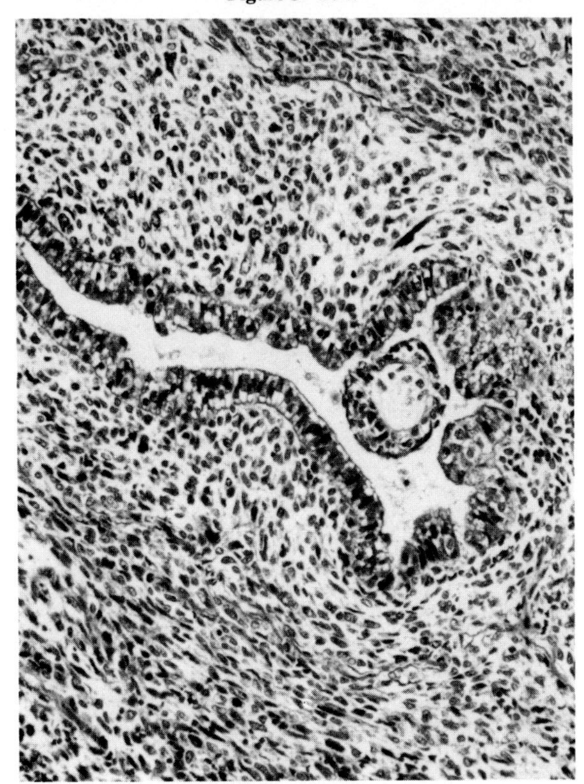

Figure 3-175.

Figures 3-174, 3-175. Pulmonary blastoma. This biphasic tumor is composed of epithelial elements reminiscent of endometrium and intervening primitive blastomatous stroma.

■ Classical Pulmonary Blastoma (Figs. 3-174 to 3-180)

Pulmonary blastoma is a biphasic malignancy of the lung often seen in adults but showing histologic features reminiscent of immature or fetal lung at the pseudoglandular stage of development (Figs. 3-179, 3-180).

The epithelial component often resembles fetal lung or secretory endometrium and one's first thought may be some peculiar endometrioid adenocarcinoma. Special stains show abundant glycogen in the epithelial cells and an absence of mucin. Squamoid nodules (morules) can be found in the center of the glandular elements. The mesenchymal element may have a blastematous feature or a myxoid appearance. The spindle cell foci may be very inconspicuous in some cases, and one may consider only a carcinoma. Likewise, other cases may be dominated by the mesenchymal component. Neuroendocrine cells may be associated with the epithelial elements.

The differential diagnosis is carcinosarcoma, spindle cell tumors with included epithelial clefts at their periphery, and the primitive (often cystic) sarcoma of children described among sarcomas above (see p. 119).

Some blastomas are predominantly epithelial, and when sarcomatous elements are lacking, terms such as well-differentiated adenocarcinoma resembling fetal lung or pulmonary endodermal tumor resembling fetal lung have been used. We prefer to consider these as epithelial-dominant variants of pulmonary blastoma.

In a minority of cases, there is a problem differentiating blastoma from carcinosarcoma; this distinction is somewhat arbitrary, but at either end of the spectrum, these two lesions appear to be quite distinct.

References

Addis BJ, Corrin B. Pulmonary blastoma, carcinosarcoma and spindle cell carcinoma: an immunohistochemical study of keratin intermediate filaments. J Pathol 147:291-301, 1985.

Davis PW, Briggs JC, Seal RME, Storring FK. Benign and malignant mixed tumors of the lung. Thorax 27:657-673, 1972.

Heckman CS, Tryong LD, Cagle PT, Font RL. Pulmonary blastoma with rhabdomyosarcomatous differentiation: an electron microscopic and immunohistochemical study. Am J Surg Pathol 12:35-40, 1988.

Kodama T, Shimosato Y, Watanbe S, Koide T, Naruke T, Shimose J. Six cases of well-differentiated adenocarcinoma simulating fetal lung tissues in pseudoglandular stage: comparison with pulmonary blastoma. Am J Surg Pathol 8:735-744, 1984.

Manning JT, Ordonez NA, Rosenberg HS, Walker WE. Pulmonary endodermal tumor resembling fetal lung. Report of a case with immunohistochemical studies. Arch Pathol Lab Med 109:48-50, 1985.

Spencer H. Pulmonary blastoma. J Pathol Bacteriol 82:161-165, 1961.

Yousem SA, Wick M. Pulmonary blastoma: immunohistologic study. Am J Clin Pathol 93:167-175, 1990.

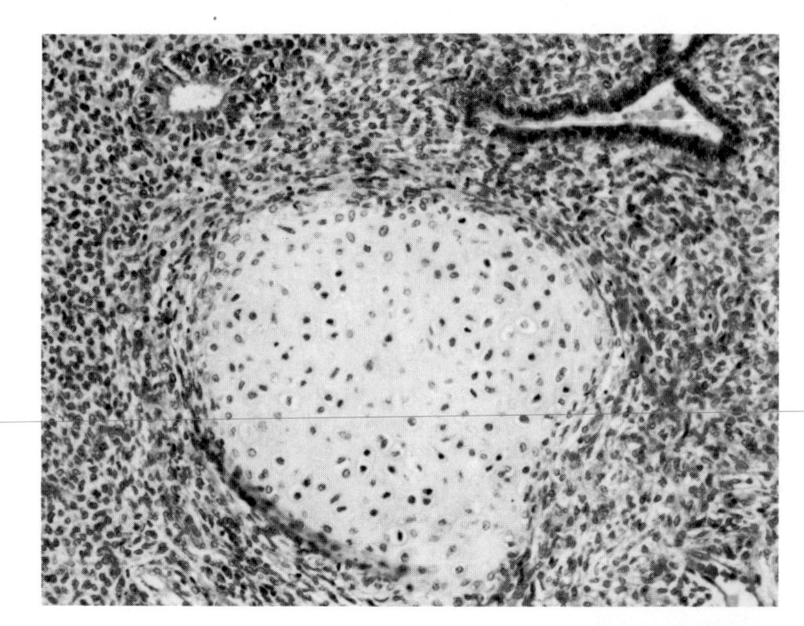

Figure 3–176. Pulmonary blastoma with islands of immature cartilage.

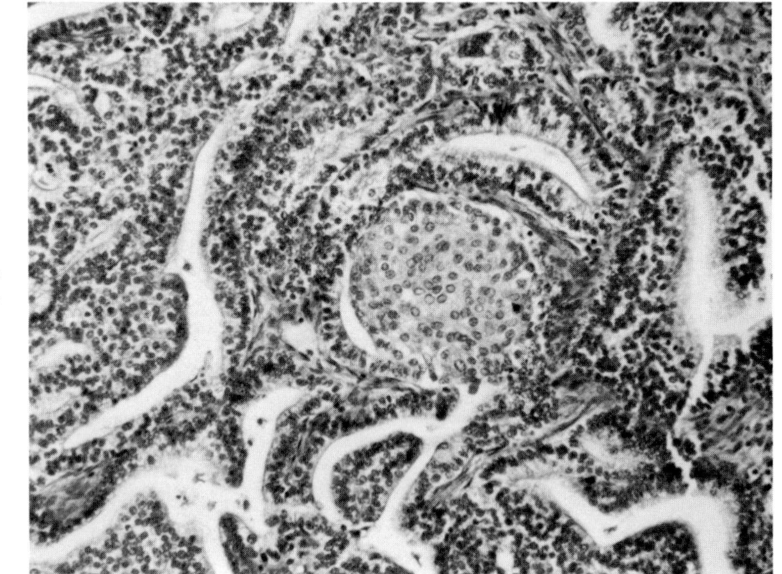

Figure 3–177. Pulmonary blastoma. The blastoma is predominantly epithelial, with a squamous morula-like nodular cluster of cells.

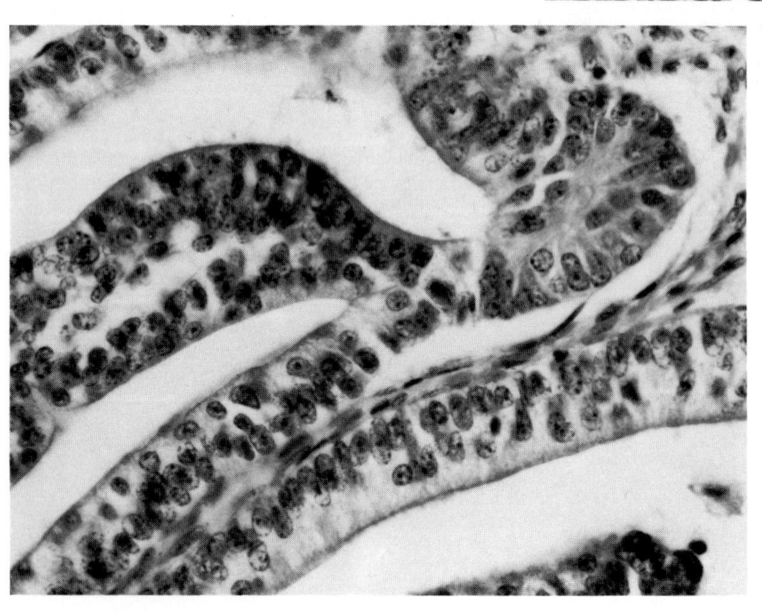

Figure 3–178. Pulmonary blastoma. The epithelial component is reminiscent of endometrial adenocarcinoma as well as fetal lung. The appearance has led to its being called such terms as "fetal adenocarcinoma of the lung."

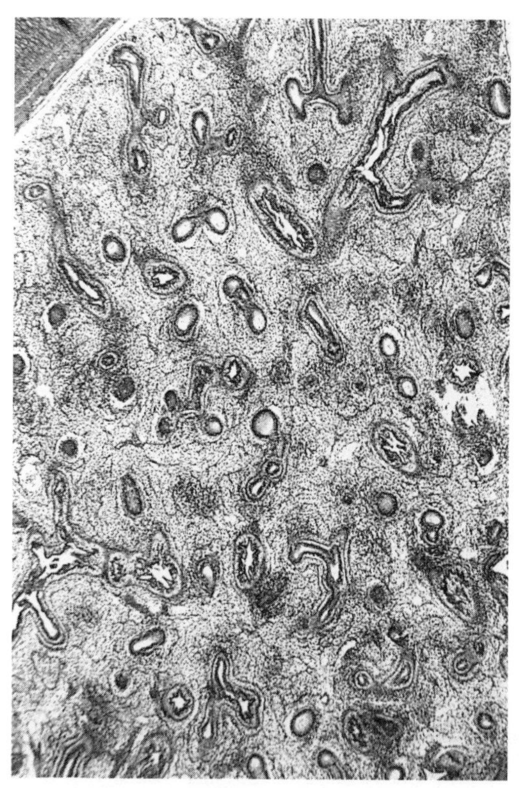

Figure 3-179.

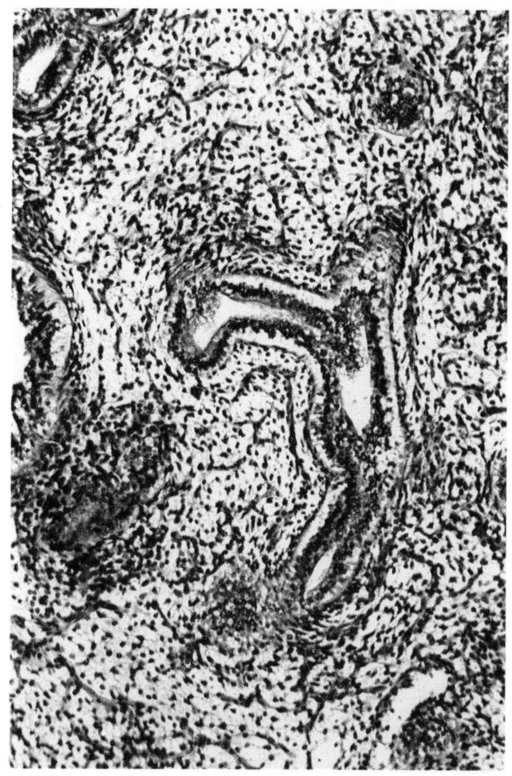

Figure 3-180.

Figures 3-179, 3-180. Fetal lung tissue. Normal fetal lung tissue from an aborted fetus is very similar to that in pulmonary blastoma and shows why the tumor was thus named.

■ Pulmonary Artery Sarcoma (Figs. 3-181 to 3-184)

This rare primary sarcoma of the pulmonary artery and its branches often presents as multiple pulmonary emboli or pulmonary hypertension.

Histologic features of angiosarcoma, malignant fibrous histiocytoma, leiomyosarcoma, chondrosarcoma, rhabdomyosarcoma, mixed or undifferentiated sarcoma may characterize this neoplasm.

These cases often defy diagnosis prior to autopsy because they present as pulmonary emboli and a peripheral lung biopsy shows only infarcted lung tissue or thrombosis and does not sample the tumor unless tumor emboli are seen in small vessels. Computed tomography (CT) scans have been helpful in premortem diagnosis.

References

Bleisch VR, Kraus FT. Polypoid sarcoma of the pulmonary trunk: analysis of the literature and report of a case with ultrastructural features of rhabdomyosarcoma. Cancer 46:314-324, 1980.

McGlennon RC, et al. Pulmonary artery trunk sarcoma: a clinicopathologic, ultrastructural, and immunohistochemical study of four cases. Mod Pathol 2:486-494, 1989.

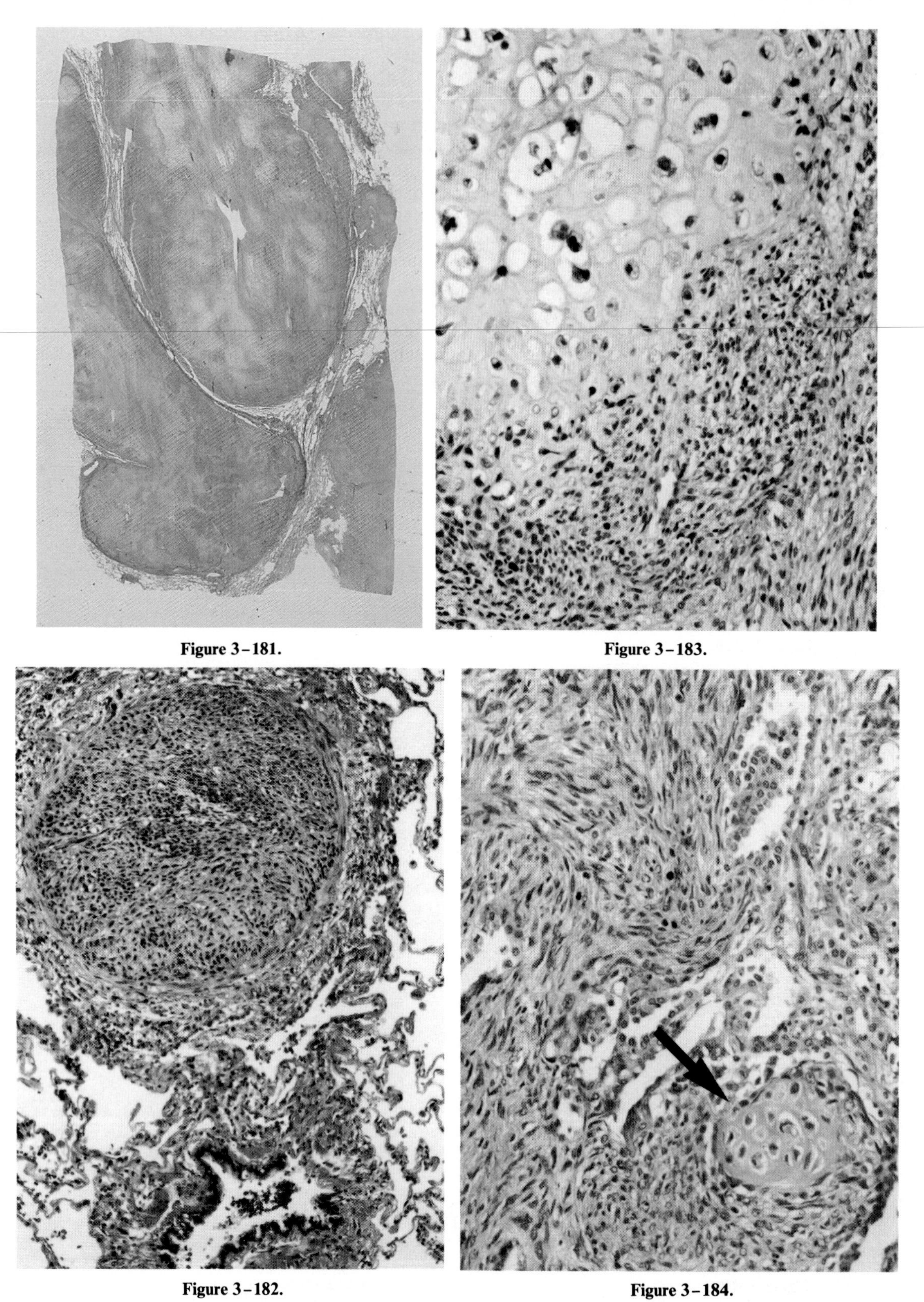

Figure 3-181.

Figure 3-183.

Figure 3-182.

Figure 3-184.

Figures 3-181, 3-182, 3-183, 3-184. Pulmonary artery sarcoma. The tumor nodules represent massive expanded branches of the pulmonary artery in this pneumonectomy specimen. Chondrosarcomatous (Fig. 3-183) and osteosarcomatous elements (arrow) are present. Peripheral small vessels are occluded by metastatic tumor emboli. Not unexpectedly, this patient presented with signs and symptoms of recurrent pulmonary emboli.

■ **Kaposi's Sarcoma** (Figs. 3–185 to 3–189)

This sarcoma of uncertain histogenesis has reached epidemic proportions with the acquired immunodeficiency syndrome (AIDS). The lung may be involved in disseminated disease or, rarely, is the primary site of presentation. Hemoptysis, hemothorax, and pulmonary infiltrates usually develop. At bronchoscopy, there are purple patches and plaques along the airways, particularly at bifurcations.

Kaposi's sarcoma shows a lymphatic distribution with infiltrates in the septa and pleura and along bronchovascular bundles. In the majority of cases, the infiltrates show the classic features of Kaposi's sarcoma, with spindle cells containing clefts with red blood cells, interspersed hemosiderin, and intracellular eosinophilic blobs. Infiltration of vessels and airways is frequent, and the lesions are very distinctive at bronchoscopy. At the periphery of the classic infiltrates, there is often a prominent plasma cell infiltrate with a plump mesenchymal cell proliferation. Early infiltrates of Kaposi's sarcoma may show cuffing of vessels and airways by this mixed "inflammatory" infiltrate.

Figure 3–185.

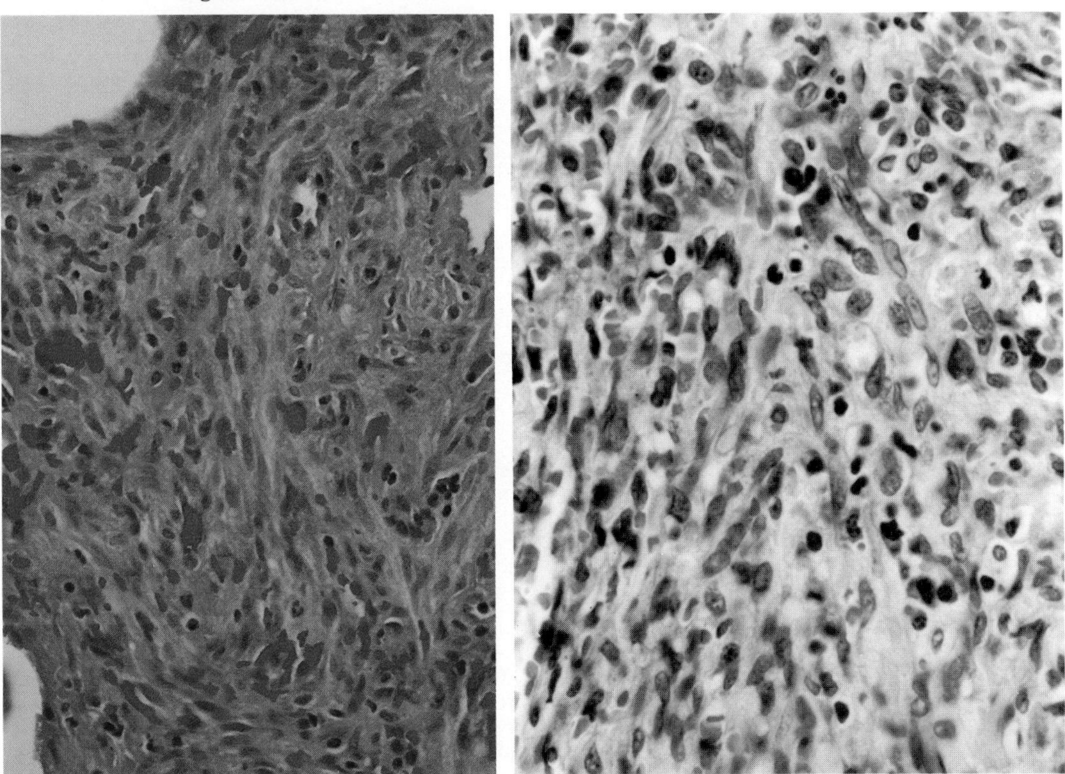

Figure 3–186. **Figure 3–187.**

Figures 3–185, 3–186, 3–187. Kaposi's sarcoma of the lung in acquired immunodeficiency syndrome (AIDS) with massive expansion of bronchovascular bundles. The cytologic features of the infiltrate are typical of Kaposi's sarcoma with spindle cells and interspersed red blood cells and hemosiderin. Plasma cells are also present.

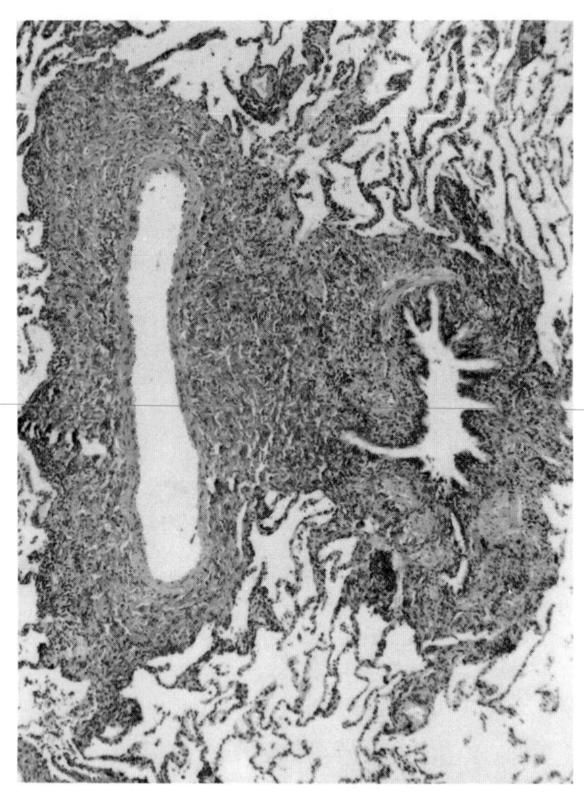

Figure 3-188.

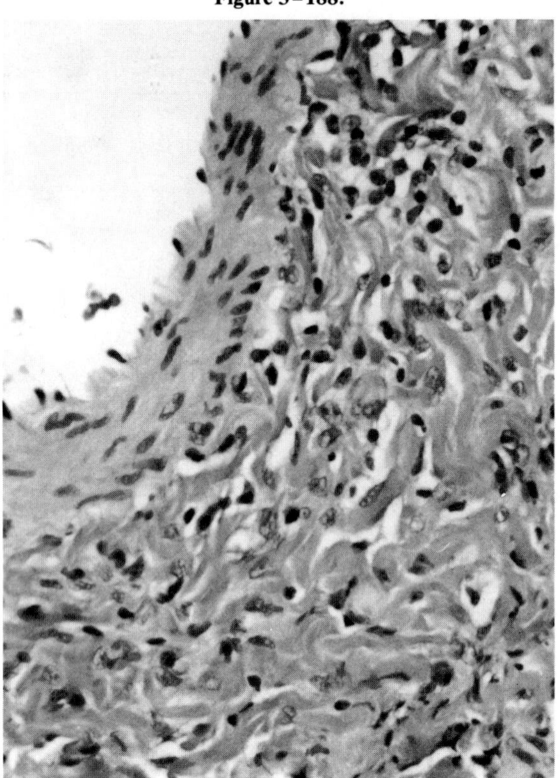

Figure 3-189.

Because of the distribution along airways, diagnosis using transbronchial biopsy findings is possible, if one considers the possibility. Differential diagnosis includes fibrosis and granulation tissue. A lymphatic distribution of Kaposi's sarcoma is one of the most helpful features in differential diagnosis.

References

Moskowitz LB, Hensley GT, Gould EW, Weiss SD. Frequency and anatomic distribution of lymphadenopathic Kaposi's sarcoma in AIDS. Hum Pathol 16:447, 1985.

Purdy LJ, Colby TV, Yousem SA, Battifora H. Pulmonary Kaposi's sarcoma: premortem histologic diagnosis. Am J Surg Pathol 10:301-311, 1986.

Figures 3-188, 3-189. Kaposi's sarcoma of the lung in acquired immunodeficiency syndrome (AIDS). Perivascular and peribronchiolar thickening is due to a mixed infiltrate of spindle cells, plasma cells, and occasional lymphocytes. This infiltrate merged with more characteristic Kaposi's sarcoma elsewhere in the lung.

■ Benign Metastasizing Leiomyoma (Figs. 3–190 to 3–192)

Benign metastasizing leiomyoma (BML) presents as multiple nodules on chest radiographs, usually in women with a history of prior hysterectomy for "leiomyomas."

Histologically, these are *nodular* proliferations of smooth muscle that extend peripherally in the interstitium and surrounding airspaces, which become lined by metaplastic *bland* cuboidal epithelium. The smooth muscle cells lack significant atypia, and mitotic figures are few. The cellularity is mild to moderate.

Whether BML represents a very-low-grade metastatic sarcoma or a peculiar multifocal, smooth muscle cell proliferation is not clear. Some cases are hormonally responsive and either stabilize or regress with antiestrogen therapy. In most cases, the course is one of indolent slow growth of the nodules.

Differential diagnosis includes hamartomas with smooth muscle, lymphangioleiomyomatosis, and primary and metastatic (frankly malignant) spindle cell sarcomas.

References

Wolff M, Kaye G, Silva F. Pulmonary metastases (with admixed epithelial elements) from smooth muscle neoplasms. Report of nine cases, including three males. Am J Surg Pathol 3:325–342, 1979.

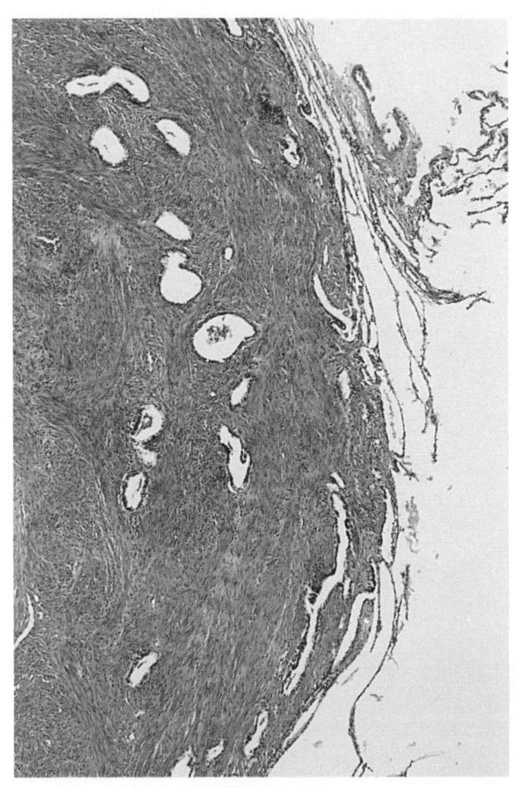

Figure 3–190.

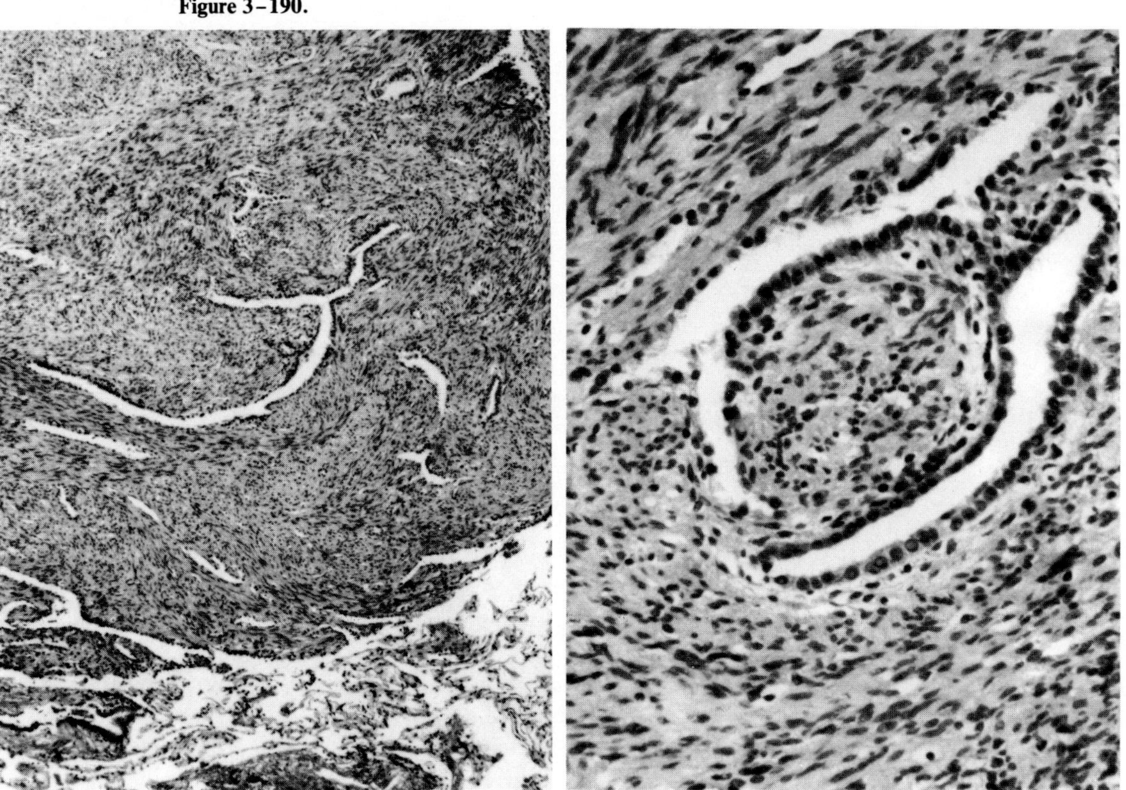

Figure 3–191. **Figure 3–192.**

Figures 3–190, 3–191, 3–192. Benign metastasizing leiomyoma. Multiple discrete nodules are composed of cytologically benign spindle cells with features of smooth muscle cells. The cells grow interstitially and surround the alveoli, which are lined by metaplastic cells.

■ Other Metastatic Sarcomas (Figs. 3–193 to 3–201)

Sarcomas presenting as metastases are unusual. Angiosarcoma and pulmonary artery sarcoma should be considered when sarcomatous cells are seen in pulmonary arteries.

Metastatic endometrial stromal sarcoma produces a distinctive nodular or multicystic mass with short spindly cells that may be deceptively bland and that simulate a benign lesion. One reported case was mistaken for mesenchymal cystic hamartoma.

References

Abrams J, Talcott J, Carson JM. Pulmonary metastases in patients with low-grade endometrial stromal sarcoma: Clinicopathologic findings with immunohistochemical characterization. Am J Surg Pathol 13:133–140, 1989.

■ Miscellaneous Tumors Occurring in the Lung

A number of other tumors may rarely occur in the lung, usually as coin or endobronchial lesions, and they show histologic features identical to these tumors seen elsewhere: hemangiomas, leiomyomas (Fig. 3–51), neurofibromas, neurilemmomas, mixed tumors and other salivary gland tumors, paragangliomas, fibroepithelial polyps of the airways, granular cell tumors of the airways, and lipomas. Miscroscopic nodules of oncocytes representing oncocytic metaplasia and hyperplasia are

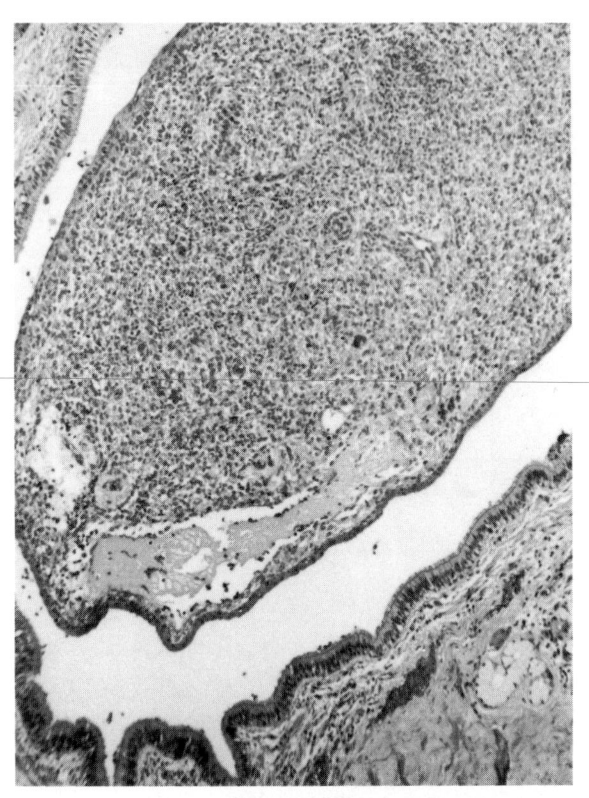

Figure 3–194.

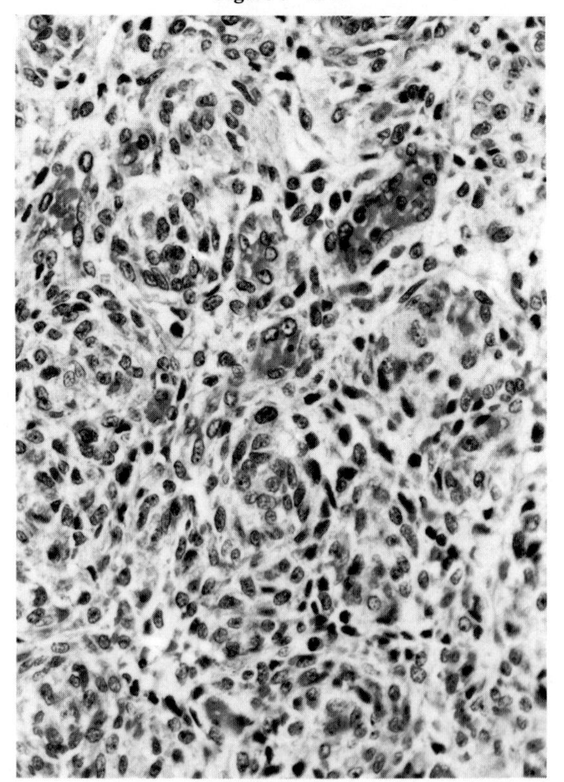

Figure 3–195.

Figures 3–194, 3–195. Metastatic endometrial stromal sarcoma. A large intrabronchiolar polypoid metastasis is present. The tumor is composed of whorled short spindle cells with histologic features typical of low-grade endometrial stromal sarcoma. Some metastatic endometrial stromal sarcomas are multicystic in the lung.

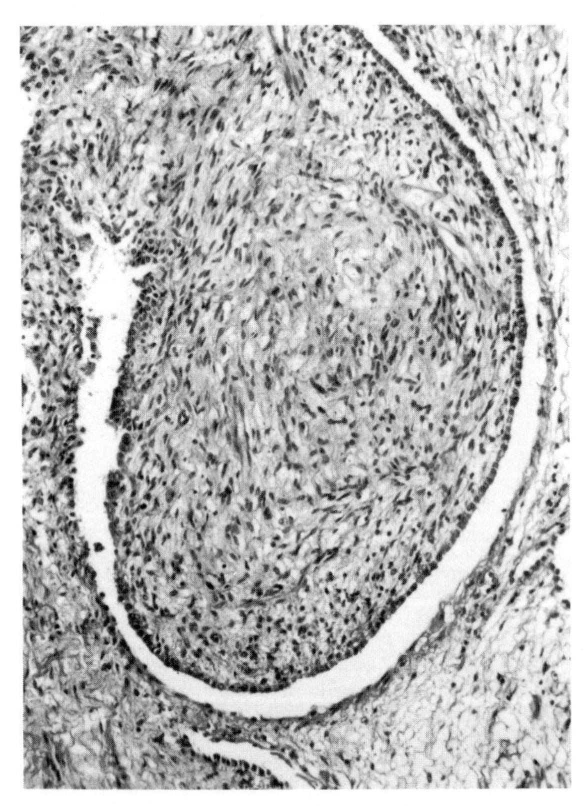

Figure 3–193. Metastatic adenosarcoma. Polyps of tumor grow into airspaces. The tumor polyps are lined by metaplastic epithelium. The spindle cell proliferation is not overtly malignant, but the appearance was identical to the uterine primary resected 12 years earlier.

occasionally seen in older individuals in the tracheobronchial submucosal glands.

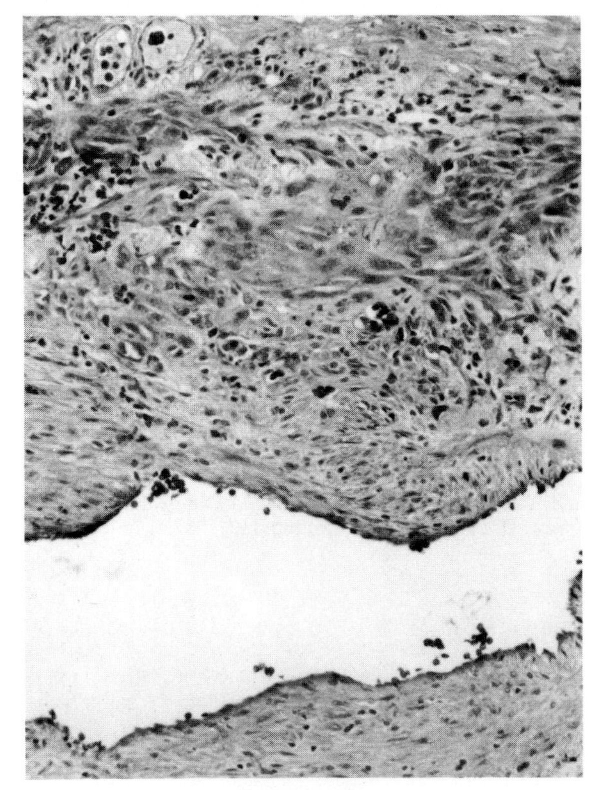

Figure 3-196.

References

Carter D, Eggleston JC. Tumors of the Lower Respiratory Tract. AFIP Atlas of Tumor Pathology, Second Series, Fascicle 17. Washington, DC, Armed Forces Institute of Pathology, 1980.

Dail DH, Hammer SP (eds). Pulmonary Pathology. New York, Springer-Verlag, 1988.

Thurlbeck WM (ed). Pathology of the Lung. New York, Thieme, 1988.

World Health Organization Monograph: Histologic Typing of Lung Tumors, 2nd ed. Geneva, WHO, 1981.

■ Vasotropic Malignancies (Figs. 3-133 to 3-136, 3-157 to 3-159, 3-163 to 3-165, 3-181 to 3-184, 3-196, 3-197)

Vasotropic growth of neoplastic cells is seen in both primary and metastatic carcinomas and sarcomas and lymphomas. Thrombi and infarction may overshadow the tumor. Other cases manifest as pulmonary hypertension or interstitial lung disease. Primary possibilities include breast, kidney, lung, and gastrointestinal tract carcinomas; melanomas; angiosarcomas; venous leiomyosarcomas; pulmonary artery sarcomas; and others. Among occult carcinomas presenting as pulmonary hypertension, primary tumor in the stomach is most common.

The malignant cells within the vessels may or may not

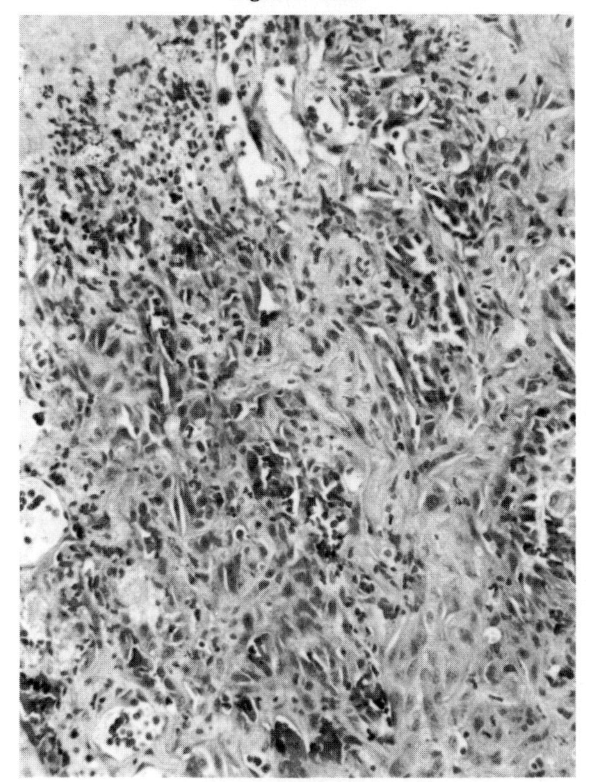

Figure 3-197.

Figures 3-196, 3-197. Metastatic angiosarcoma. Neoplastic vascular channels containing red blood cells are present in the wall of a medium-sized pulmonary artery, which also has prominent intimal thickening. Like pulmonary artery sarcomas, metastatic angiosarcomas often mimic recurrent pulmonary emboli.

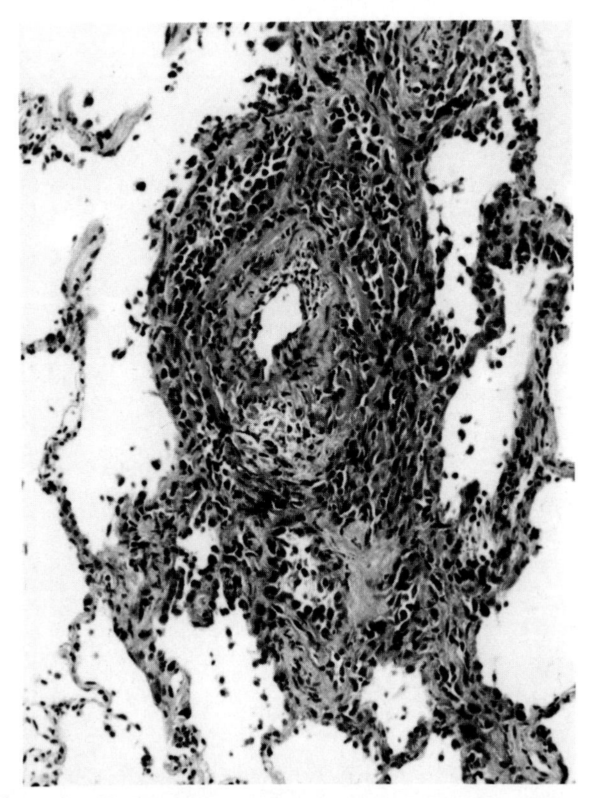

Figure 3-198. Metastatic epithelioid sarcoma. This tumor is associated with diffuse micronodular pulmonary infiltrates. The tumor cells grow in and around a small pulmonary vein and even suggest growth along alveolar walls. Without the history of widely metastatic epithelioid sarcoma, diagnosis in such a case would be extremely difficult.

be obvious. Usually, there is marked intimal proliferation, recent and organizing thrombi, and perivascular scarring with or without parenchymal infarction. Multiple levels may be required to demonstrate tumor cells within the vessels. Lymphatic invasion is also commonly present.

Clues to a vasotropic malignancy include more extensive perivascular scarring than seen in otherwise uncomplicated thromboemboli and the presence of (even a few) atypical cells associated with intimal proliferation or organizing thrombi in the vessel lumen.

References

Case records of the Massachusetts General Hospital. Case 34:1983. N Engl J Med 309:477–487, 1983.

Dail DH, Hammer SP (eds). Pulmonary Pathology. New York, Springer-Verlag, 1988.

Flint A, Colby TV. Surgical Pathology of Diffuse Infiltrative Lung Disease. Orlando, Grune & Stratton, Inc, 1987.

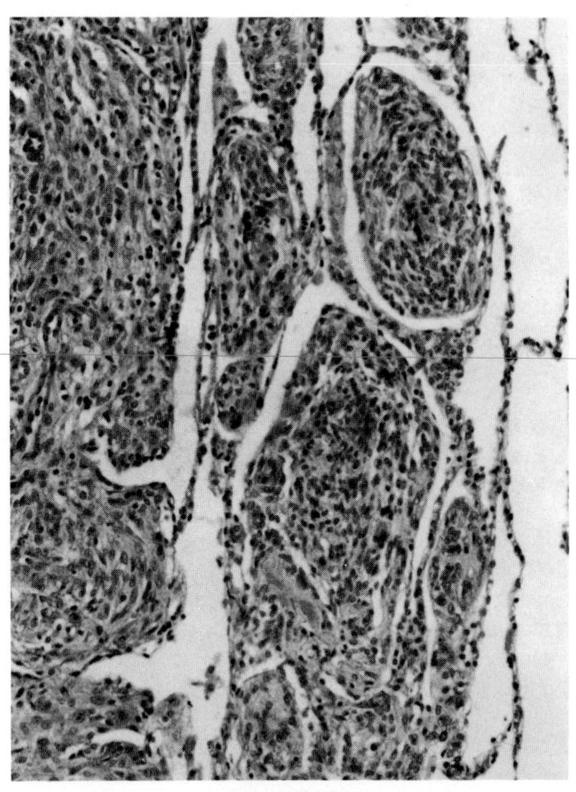

Figure 3–199.

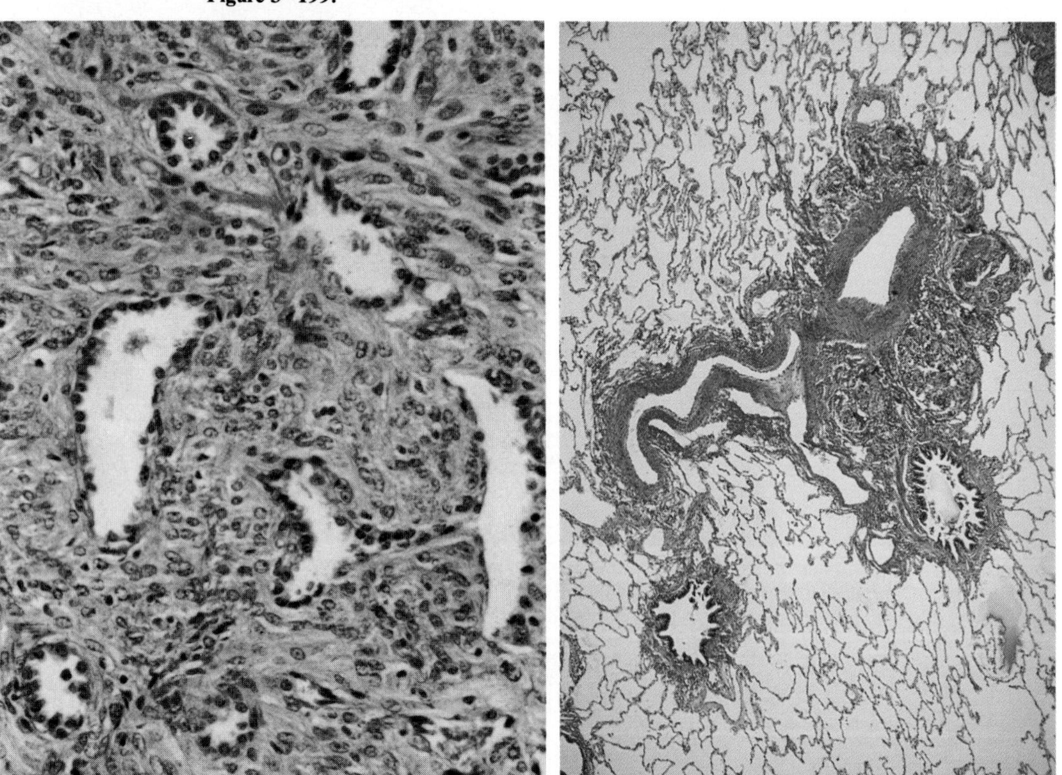

Figure 3–200. **Figure 3–201.**

Figures 3–199, 3–200, 3–201. Metastatic meningioma. This disorder is shown in the lung as the initial clinical manifestation of the intracranial primary tumor. Multiple nodules were found in one lower lobe of the lung. At the edge of the nodules, rounded clusters of cells, cytologically reminiscent of meningioma, extend into alveolar spaces. In the center of the nodule, there is interstitial growth around alveolar spaces, which are lined by metaplastic type II cells. Small airways at some distance from the main nodule showed intralymphatic tumor nodules of meningioma (Fig. 3–201).

CHAPTER 4

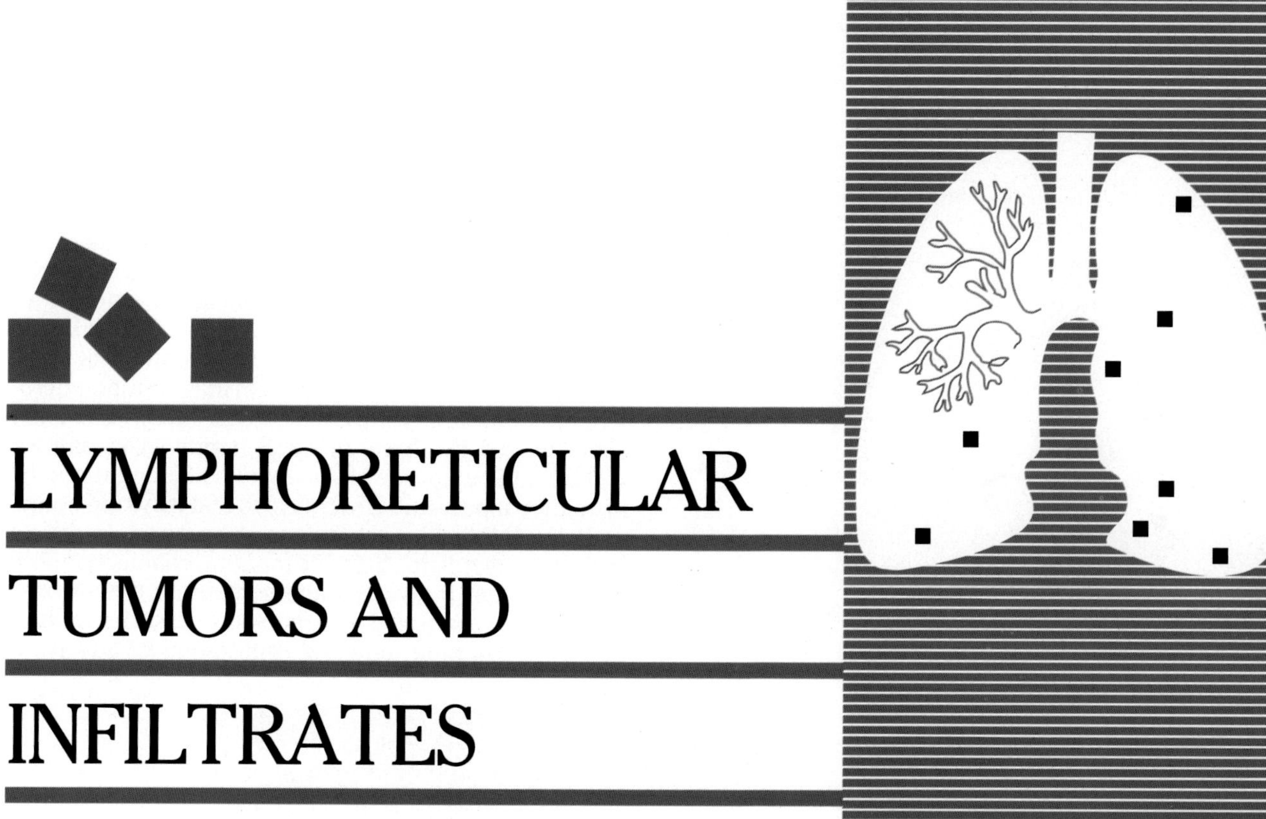

LYMPHORETICULAR TUMORS AND INFILTRATES

Figure 4-1.

■ Well-Differentiated Lymphocytic Lymphoma (Small Lymphocytic Lymphoma) (Figs. 4-1 to 4-11)

Well-differentiated lymphocytic lymphoma is a neoplastic proliferation of small lymphocytes, with or without mild nuclear atypia or plasmacytoid features. Pulmonary involvement may be primary or associated with disseminated disease. These lymphomas may produce a localized mass or diffuse and bilateral infiltrates and/or nodules. The typical lesion is a localized infiltrate or nodule in an asymptomatic patient, in whom there is no history of lymphoma or evidence of extrapulmonary involvement found after evaluation. The majority of patients do well with surgical resection, which is the treatment of choice.

Only a small percentage of cases show an associated serum monoclonal spike, involvement of hilar or other lymph nodes, or evidence of systemic involvement. Pulmonary involvement by chronic lymphocytic leukemia should always be considered in the differential diagnosis.

Involvement may be seen as gross mass lesions, microscopic nodules, or diffuse infiltrates. Mass lesions are characterized by sheets of small lymphocytes with or without mild atypia or plasmacytoid differentiation; the histologic appearance is identical to that in lymph nodes, and pseudofollicular centers may be present. In diffuse infiltrates, there are sheets of monomorphous lymphocytes that cuff the vessels and sometimes the airways, with relative sparing of alveolar walls. Vascular infiltration is uncommon; however, infiltration of airways is

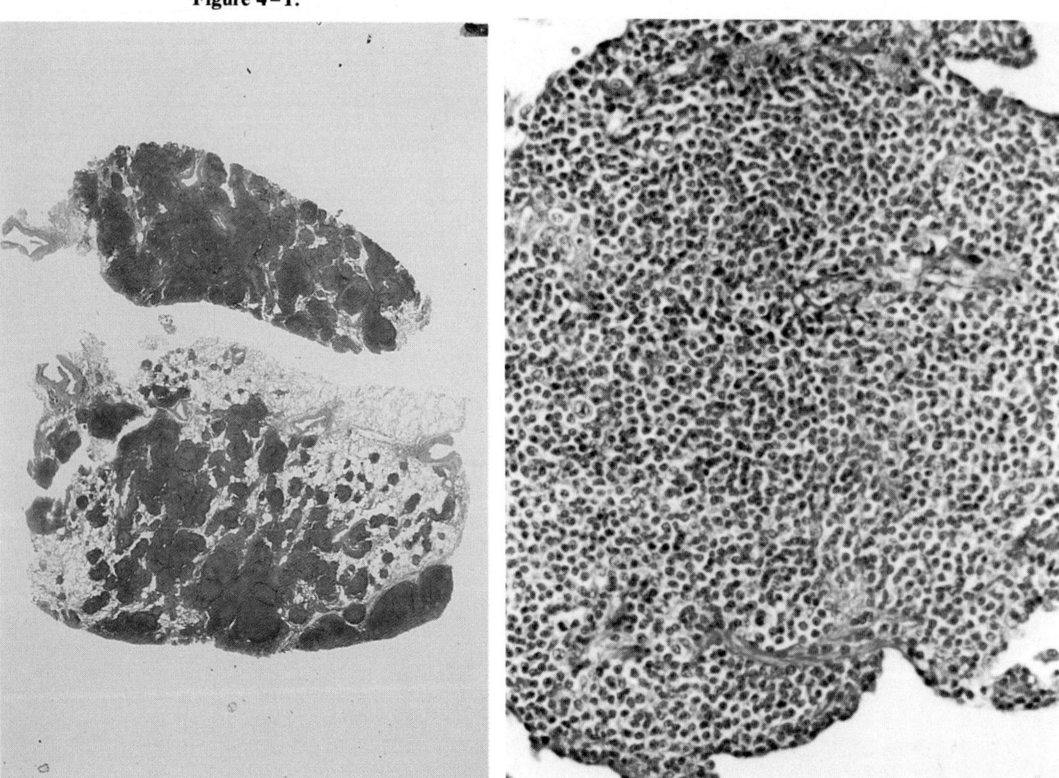

Figure 4-2. Figure 4-3.

Figures 4-1, 4-2, 4-3. Well-differentiated (small) lymphocytic lymphoma. Coalescing sheets of small lymphocytes form masses that show perivascular extension at the edges.

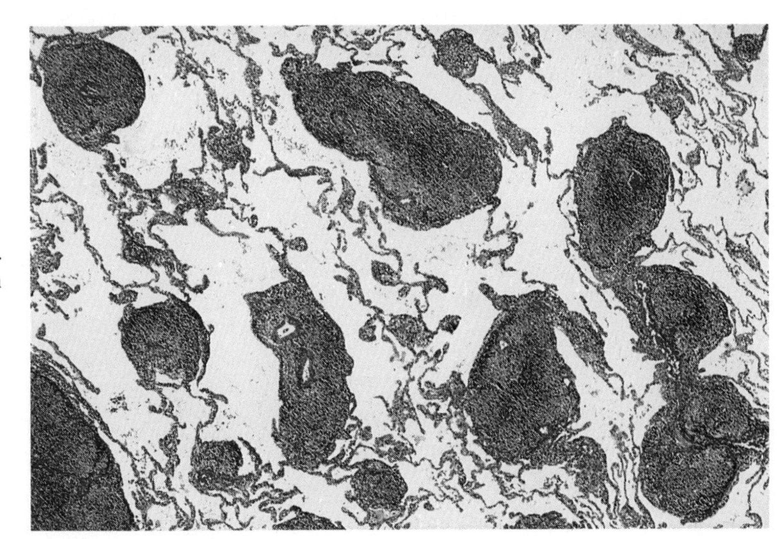

Figure 4-4. Well-differentiated (small) lymphocytic lymphoma. Discrete interstitial nodules are perivascular in distribution.

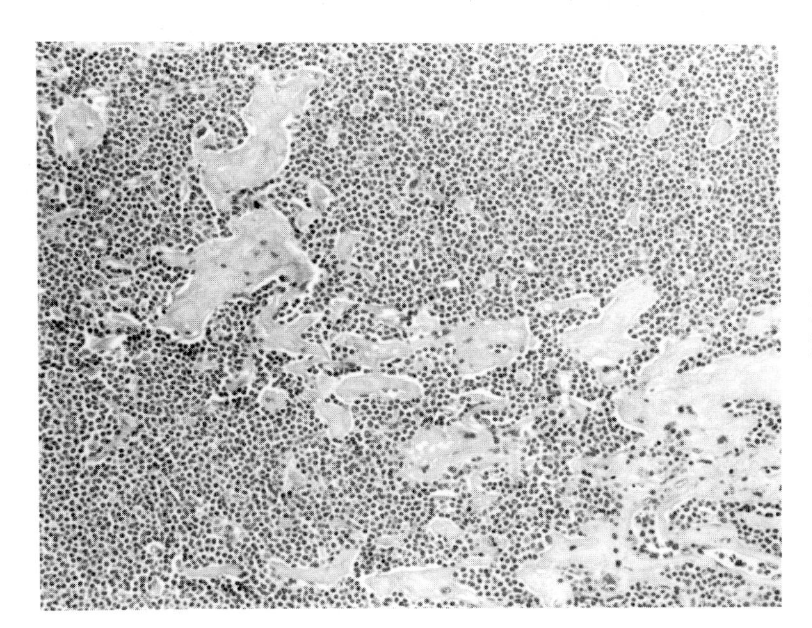

Figure 4-5. Well-differentiated (small) lymphocytic lymphoma associated with relatively acellular hyalinized collagen.

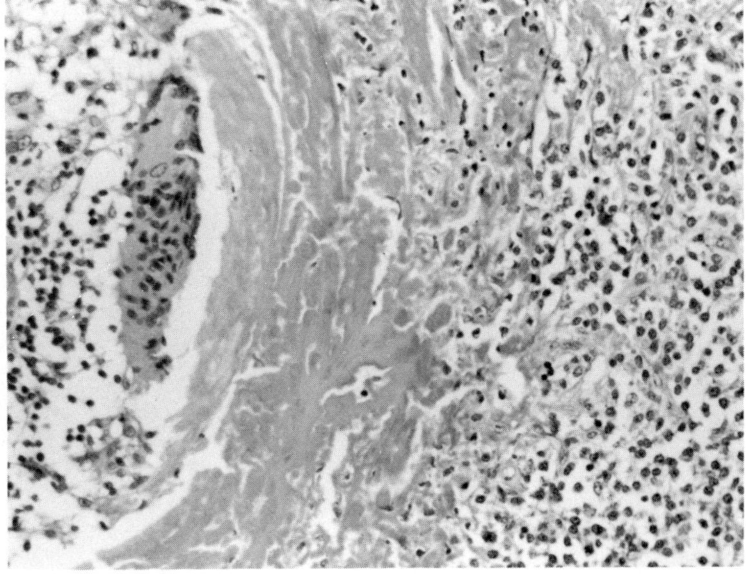

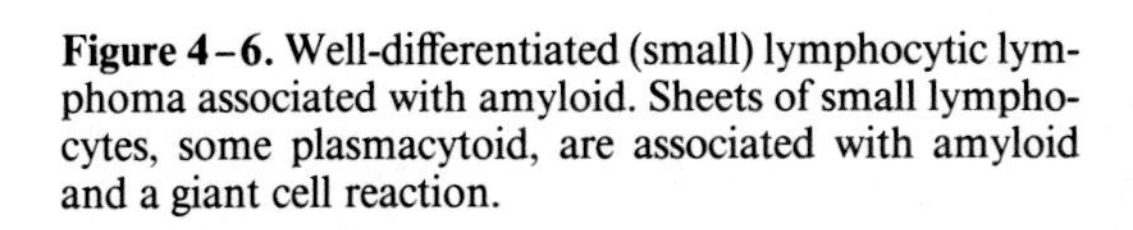

Figure 4-6. Well-differentiated (small) lymphocytic lymphoma associated with amyloid. Sheets of small lymphocytes, some plasmacytoid, are associated with amyloid and a giant cell reaction.

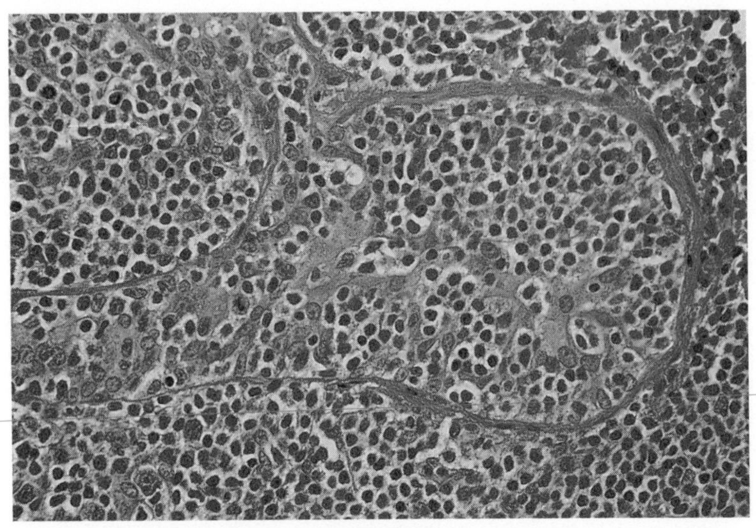

Figure 4-7.

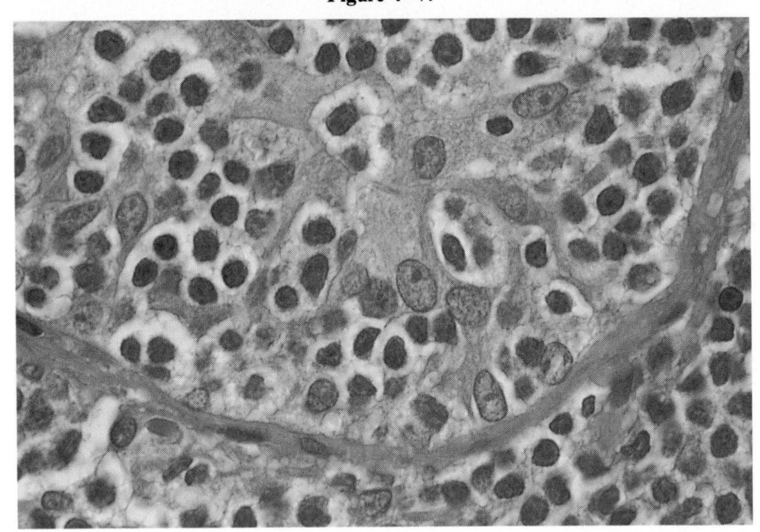

Figure 4-8.

Figures 4-7, 4-8. Well-differentiated (small) lymphocytic lymphoma with a lymphoepithelial lesion. An epithelial nest is infiltrated by lymphocytes producing a lymphoepithelial structure similar to that seen in salivary gland lymphoepithelial lesions.

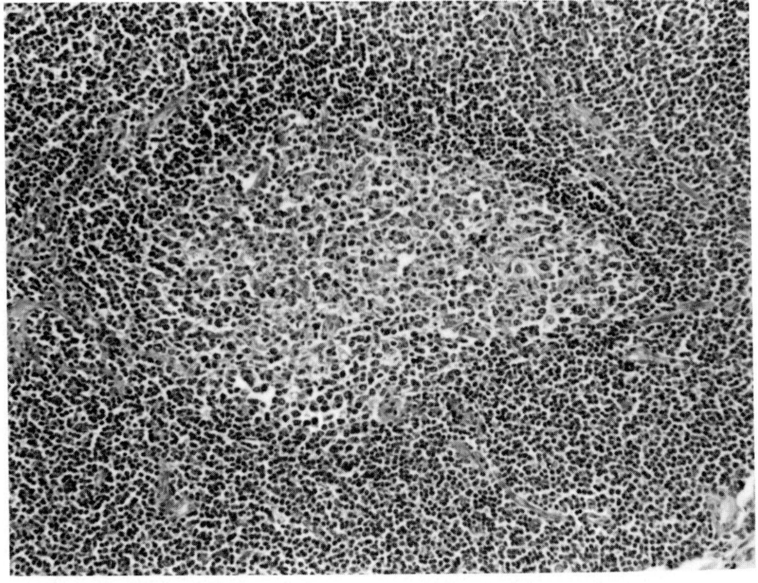

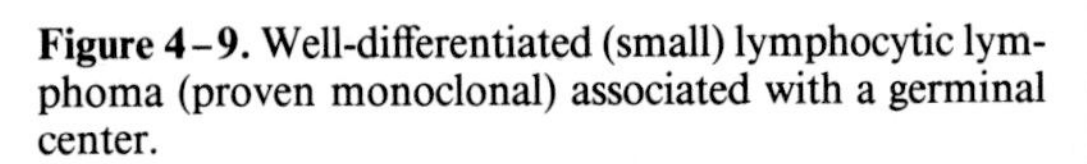

Figure 4-9. Well-differentiated (small) lymphocytic lymphoma (proven monoclonal) associated with a germinal center.

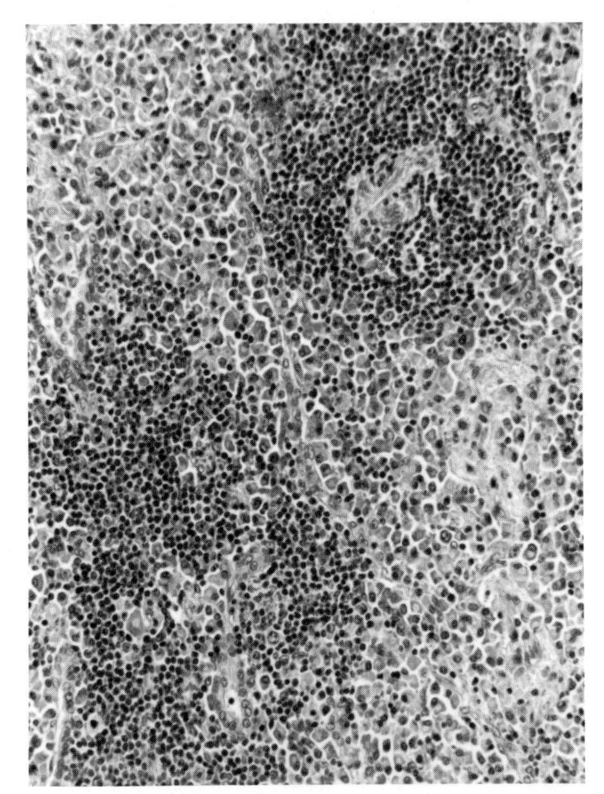

Figure 4–10. Lymphocytic lymphoma. Well-differentiated (small) lymphocytic lymphoma with plasmacytic differentiation; both lymphocytes and plasma cells had the same immunophenotype.

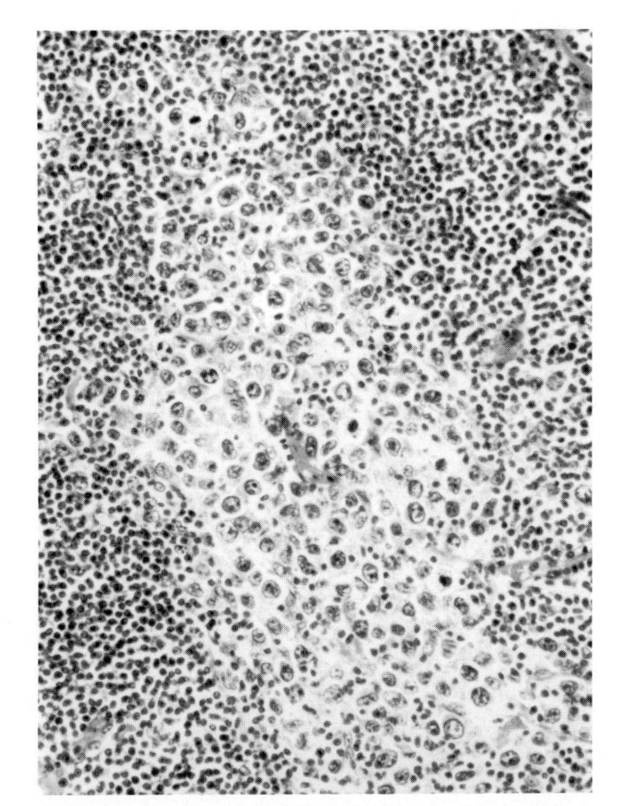

Figure 4–11. Lymphocytic lymphoma will foci of transformation. Well-differentiated (small) lymphocytic lymphoma with foci of transformation to large cell lymphoma. Large zones of large cell lymphoma in this case confirmed that the focus illustrated was not a pseudofollicular center. This is an uncommon occurrence in lymphocytic lymphomas presenting in the lung.

sometimes marked. The septa and pleura are often involved, and extrapleural plaques may be seen.

Well-differentiated lymphocytic lymphomas may have associated germinal centers, granulomas, and amyloid or amyloid-like sclerotic material. At the edge of nodules, there may be a polymorphous cellular infiltrate. Interstitial fibrosis is usually minimal. Infiltration of air-space epithelium may produce a lymphoepithelial lesion.

Differential diagnosis includes pseudolymphoma, when localized, and lymphocytic interstitial pneumonia, when diffuse. Immunologic evaluation of lymphoid tumors of the lung shows the majority to be clonal (i.e., lymphoma), and when confronted with a lung tumor composed of predominantly lymphocytes or dense diffuse interstitial infiltrates of lymphocytes, a lymphoma is usually confirmed with marker studies.

Follicular lymphoma, which, like well differentiated lymphocytic lymphomas are also low grade, involve the lung uncommonly (Figs. 4–12 to 4–14).

References

Colby TV, Yousem SA. Pulmonary lymphoid neoplasms. Semin Diagn Pathol 2:183–196, 1985.

Dail DH, Hammer SP (eds). Pulmonary Pathology. New York, Springer-Verlag, 1988.

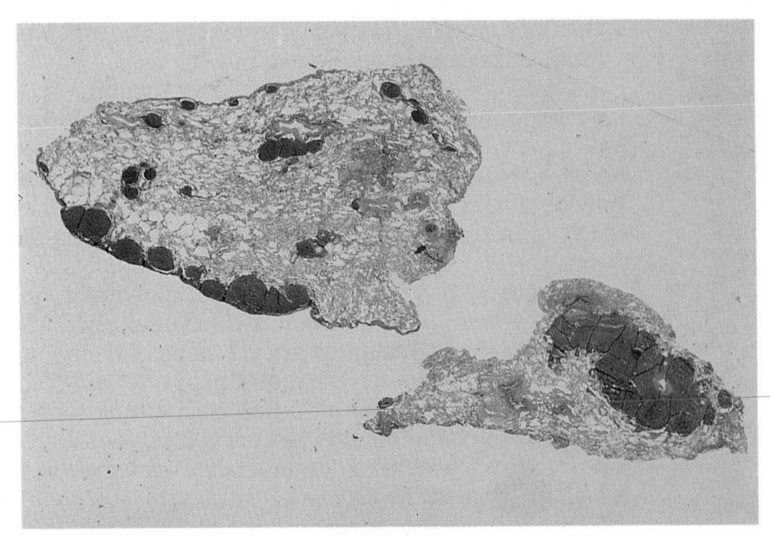

Figure 4–12.

Figures 4–12, 4–13. Follicular lymphoma presenting in the lung and pleura with pleural effusions. Neoplastic lymphoid follicles, which had features of follicular small cleaved cell lymphoma, involve the pleura and interstitial perivascular regions of the lung.

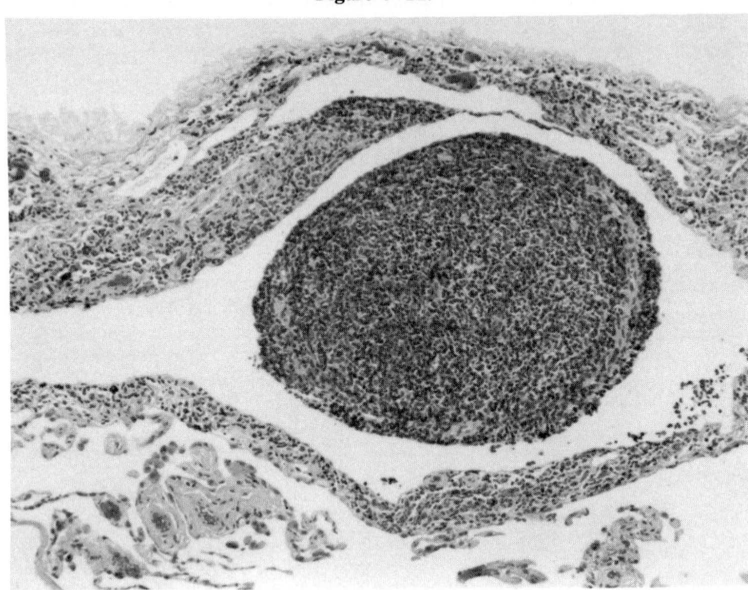

Figure 4–13.

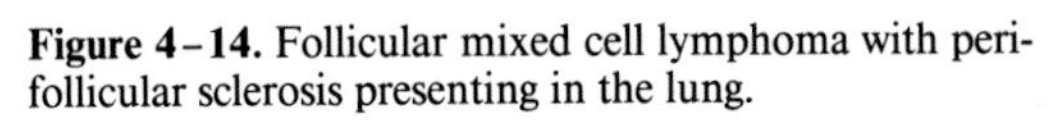

Figure 4–14. Follicular mixed cell lymphoma with perifollicular sclerosis presenting in the lung.

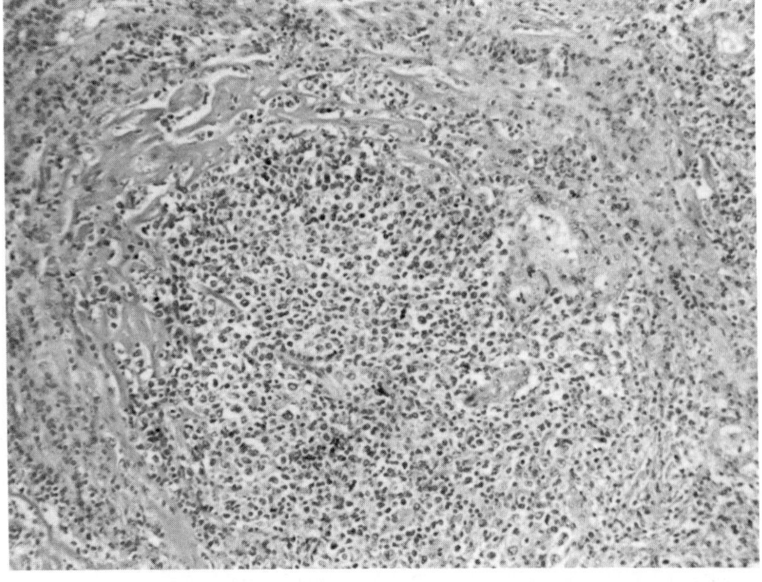

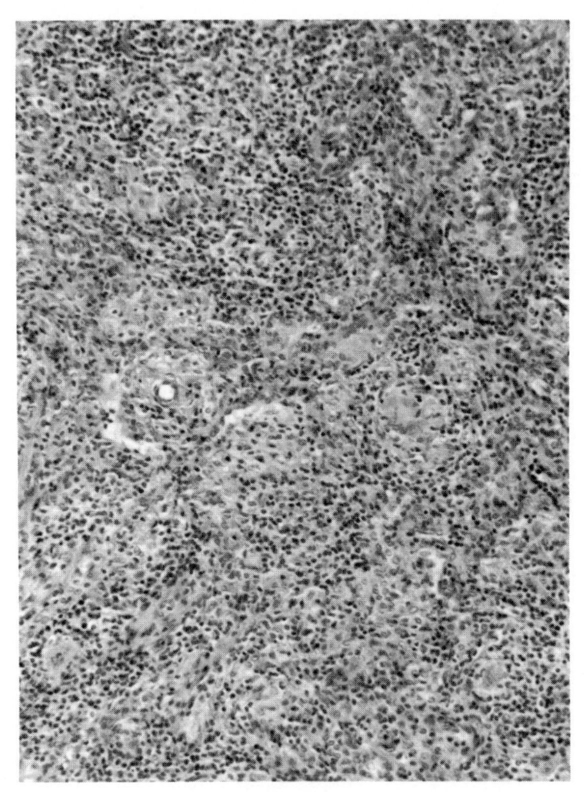

Figure 4-15.

■ Mixed Cell Lymphomas, Lymphomatoid Granulomatosis, Angiocentric Lymphomas (Figs. 4-15 to 4-26, Fig. 4-37)

This group includes lymphoproliferative diseases in the lung composed of a mixed population of atypical lymphoid cells, often with vascular invasion and associated necrosis. The term angiocentric lymphoma is descriptively appropriate, although the vascular infiltration is not always prominent or even present. Secondary involvement of the lung by peripheral nodal mixed cell lymphomas may produce identical pathologic findings. The majority of these lesions are T-cell lymphomas, and cases previously called angioimmunoblastic lymphadenopathy of the lung, polymorphic reticulosis, and benign and malignant angiitis and granulomatosis are included in this group.

These lymphomas are often aggressive and are associated with multiple bilateral nodules or infiltrates. Neurologic and cutaneous findings are relatively frequent.

Histologically, these lesions manifest as nodular and/or diffuse infiltrates of mixed lymphoid cells that show a propensity to perivascular distribution and vascular in-

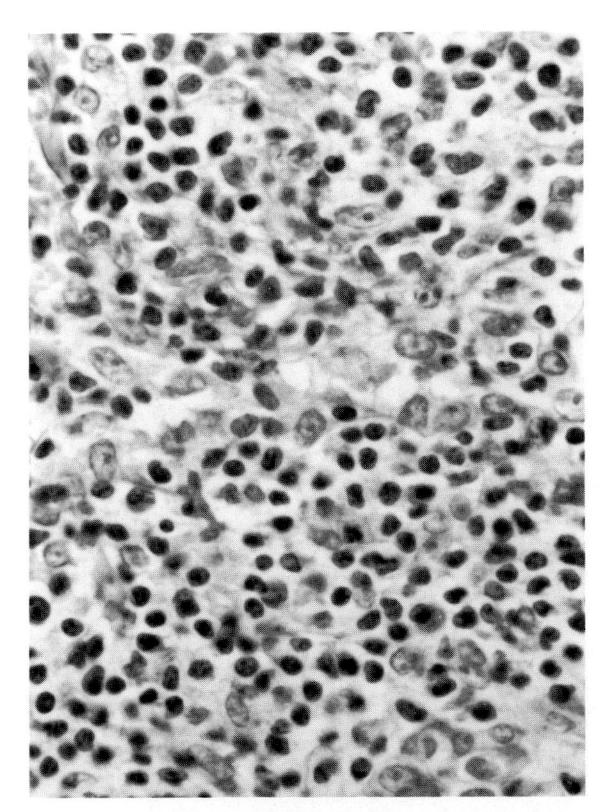

Figure 4-16.

Figures 4-15, 4-16. Diffuse mixed cell lymphoma (low-grade angiocentric immunoproliferative lesion; lymphomatoid granulomatosis). The lesion is composed of a mixed population of cells, including the small lymphocytes with minimal cytologic atypia, a few large lymphoid cells, and numerous histiocytes. In this case, there was only focal vascular infiltration. Immunophenotyping revealed predominantly T cells.

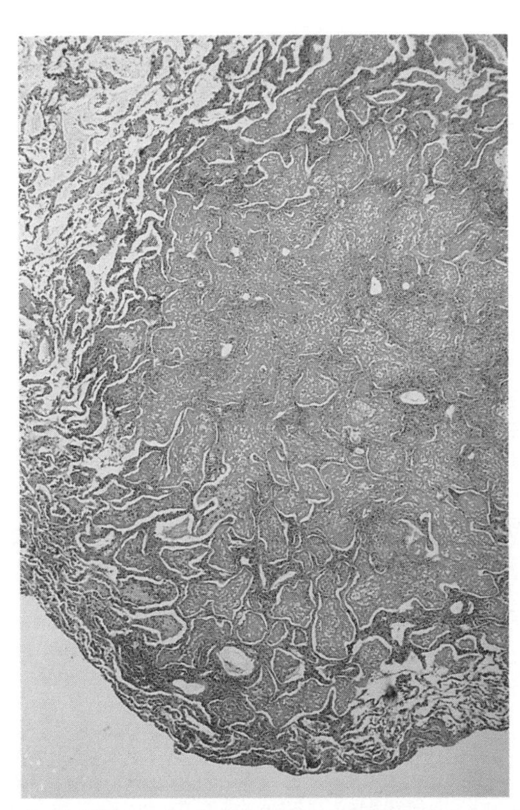

Figure 4-17. Diffuse mixed cell lymphoma (angiocentric lymphoma, intermediate grade; lymphomatoid granulomatosis). Marked central fibrinous exudate and early necrosis overshadow the lymphoid infiltrate.

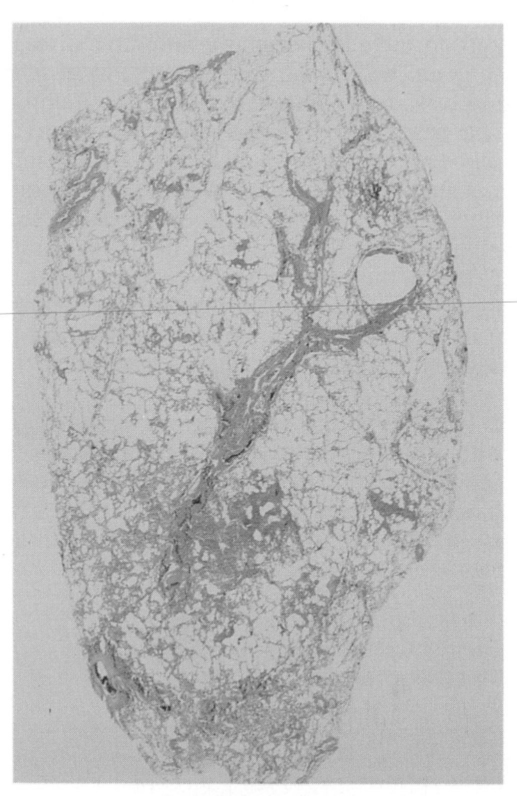

Figure 4-18.

vasion. Larger nodules often show central necrosis. Cytologically, they are very heterogeneous with numerous histiocytes, small lymphocytes, plasmacytoid cells, eosinophils, and variable numbers of atypical small lymphocytes and large lymphoid cells. Obstructive changes, fibrinous exudates, inflammation, and organization can be seen in the adjacent parenchyma.

These lymphomas should be graded as low-grade or high-grade, based on the cytologic atypia, mitotic figures, and number of large cells.

References

Colby TV, Yousem SA. Pulmonary lymphoid neoplasms. Semin Diagn Pathol 2:183-196, 1985.

Dail DH, Hammer SP (eds). Pulmonary Pathology. New York, Springer-Verlag, 1988.

Jaffe ES. Pathologic and clinical spectrum of post-thymic T cell malignancies. Cancer Invest 2:413-426, 1984.

Lipford E, Margolick J, Longo D, Fauci A, Jaffe E. Angiocentric immunoproliferative lesions: a clinicopathologic spectrum of post-thymic T cell proliferations. Blood 72:1674-1681, 1988.

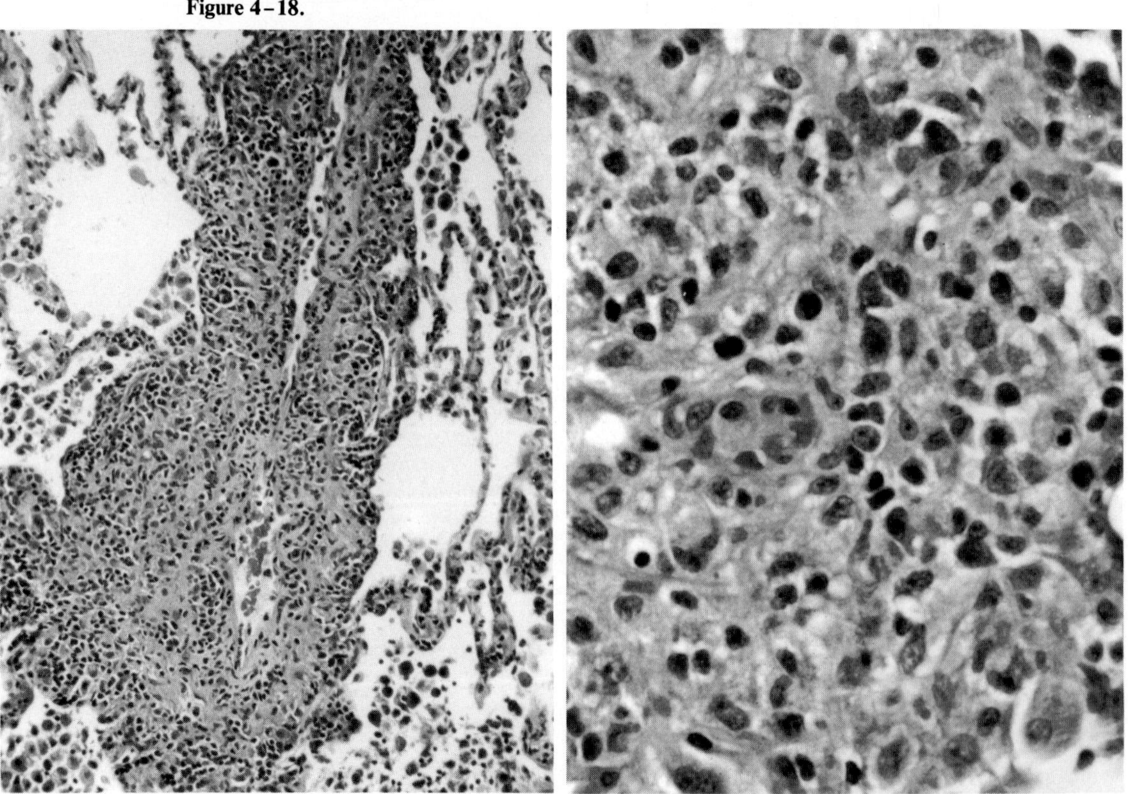

Figure 4-19. Figure 4-20.

Figures 4-18, 4-19, 4-20. Diffuse mixed cell lymphoma. This case presented as diffuse vascular and perivascular infiltrates without the formation of discrete nodules. Atypical small and large lymphoid cells show prominent infiltration of vessels.

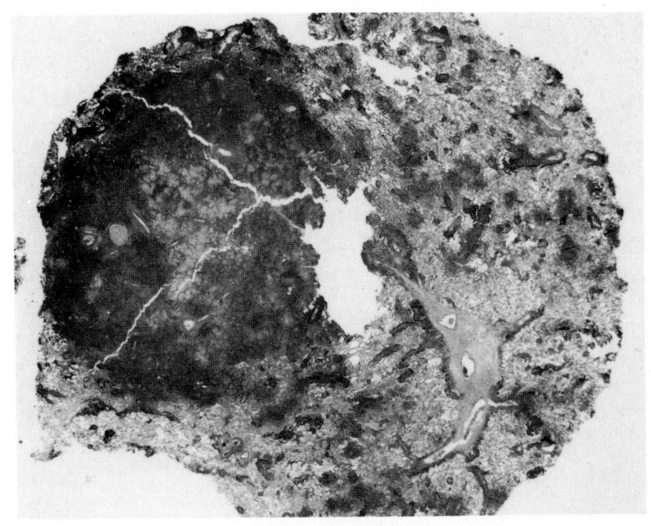

Figure 4–21.

Figures 4–21, 4–22, 4–23. Diffuse mixed cell lymphoma (angiocentric lymphoma, intermediate to high grade; lymphomatoid granulomatosis). In this case, there are large nodules with central fibrinous necrosis and satellite perivascular infiltrates. Small nodules form adjacent to bronchovascular structures. There are atypical small and large lymphoid cells, and mitotic figures are relatively numerous. The variation in histologic appearance from field to field shows how important adequate sampling is.

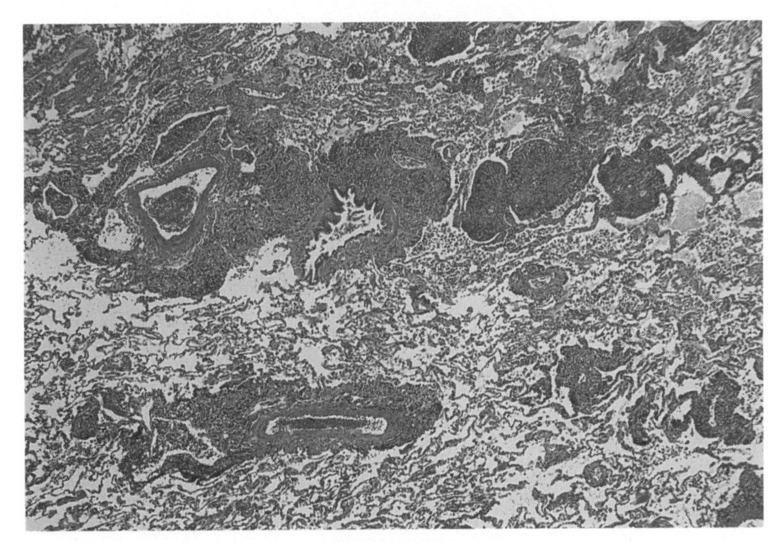

Figure 4–22.

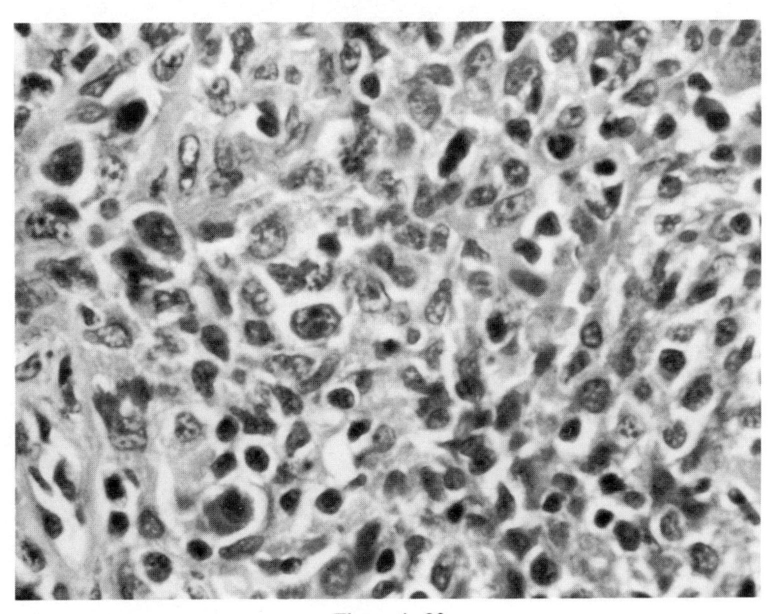

Figure 4–23.

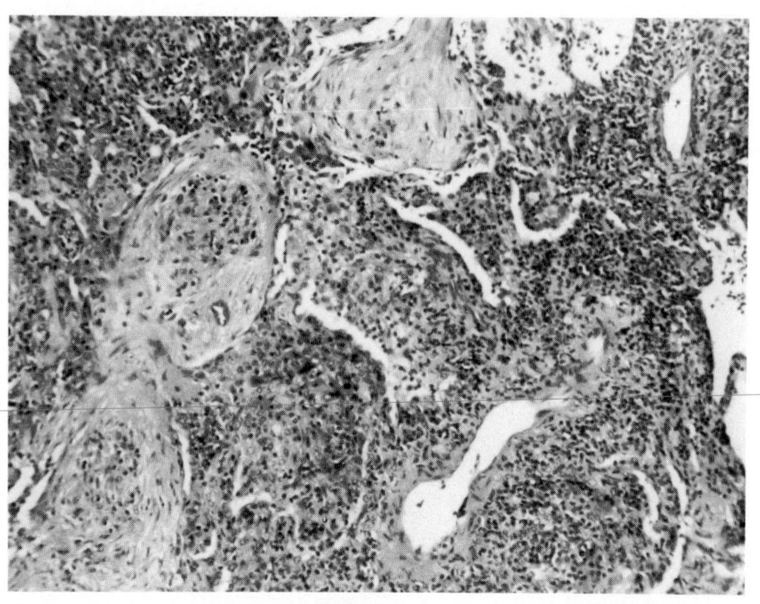

Figure 4-24.

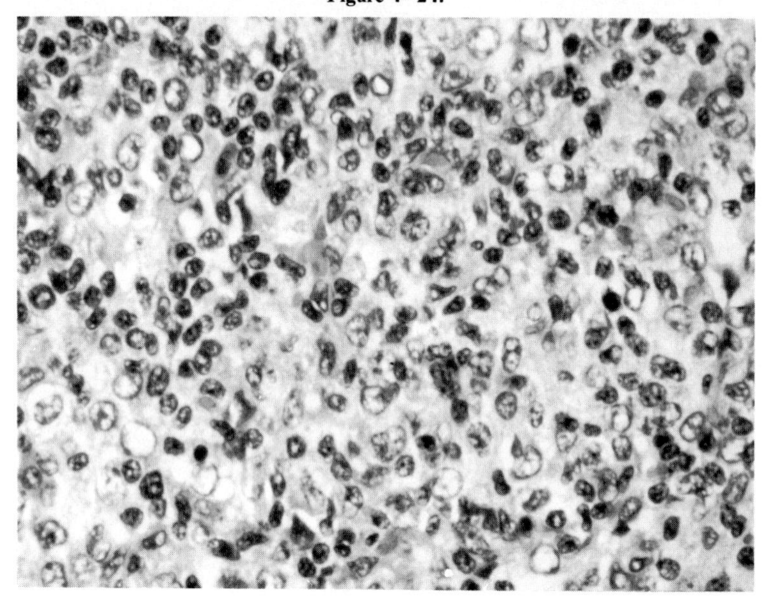

Figure 4-25.

Figures 4-24, 4-25. Diffuse mixed cell lymphoma associated with organization. Multiple nodules composed of relatively dense lymphoid infiltrates have interspersed organization resembling organizing pneumonia. The cytologic features of the infiltrate are those of a diffuse mixed cell lymphoma with atypical small and large lymphoid cells.

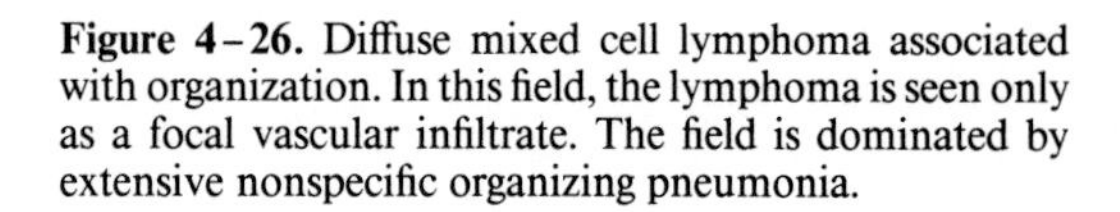

Figure 4-26. Diffuse mixed cell lymphoma associated with organization. In this field, the lymphoma is seen only as a focal vascular infiltrate. The field is dominated by extensive nonspecific organizing pneumonia.

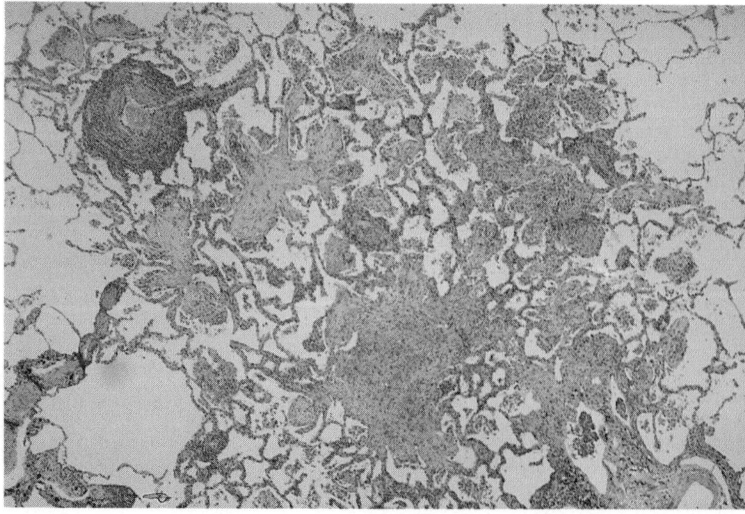

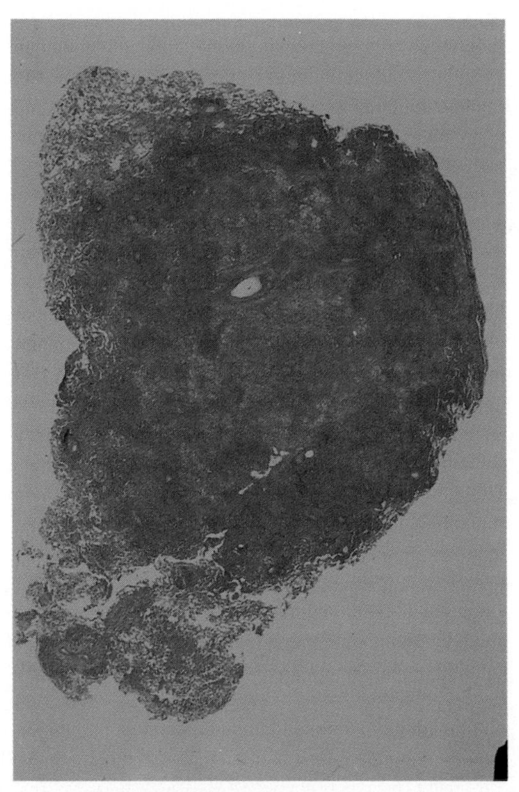

Figure 4-27. Large cell lymphoma presenting as multiple pulmonary nodules. The resected nodule shows central necrosis that descriptively is angiocentric and angiodestructive, although quite simply it is necrosis in the center of a tumor nodule that also happens to contain a vessel.

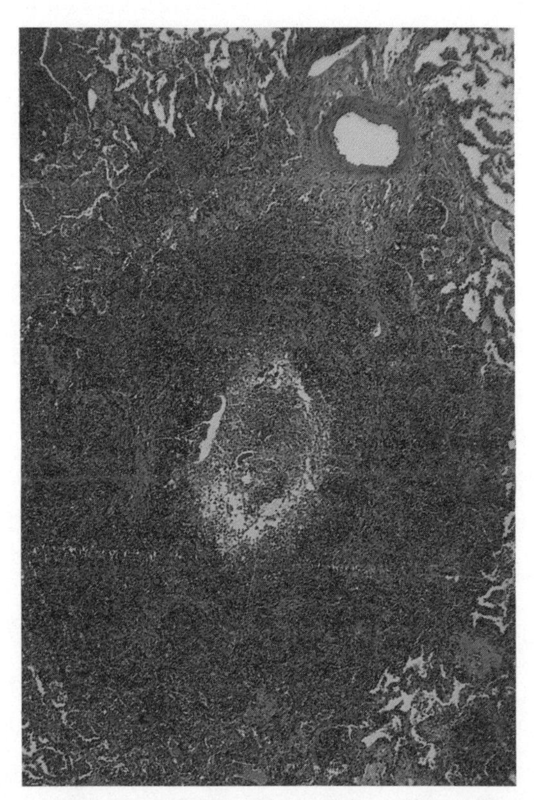

Figure 4-28. Large cell lymphoma presenting as bilateral lower lobe infiltrates. In this case, there is marked infiltration of airways with sparing of vessels. This T-cell lymphoma by immunophenotype was predominantly mixed cell in composition around the airways; however, the infiltrate around septal veins was a large cell lymphoma.

■ Large Cell Lymphomas (Figs. 4-27 to 4-37)

Large cell lymphomas may be primary in the lung or may involve the lung as part of disseminated disease. They present as single or multiple masses or infiltrates.

Mass lesions are most common and show the same cytologic variations as do large cell lymphomas in lymph nodes. Diffuse lesions are associated with lymphangitic infiltrates along bronchovascular structures and in the pleura and septa. Vascular infiltration may be marked. Central necrosis imparting a necrotizing angiocentric appearance is typical of larger nodules. Secondary changes of obstruction, inflammation, and organizing pneumonia are often found in the adjacent lung parenchyma.

The diagnosis of malignancy is usually no problem in these cases. Sometimes one must employ special studies to exclude the possibility of poorly differentiated carcinoma and leukemic infiltrates.

References

Colby TV, Yousem SA. Pulmonary lymphoid neoplasms. Semin Diagn Pathol 2:183-196, 1985.

Dail DH, Hammer SP (eds). Pulmonary Pathology. New York, Springer-Verlag, 1988.

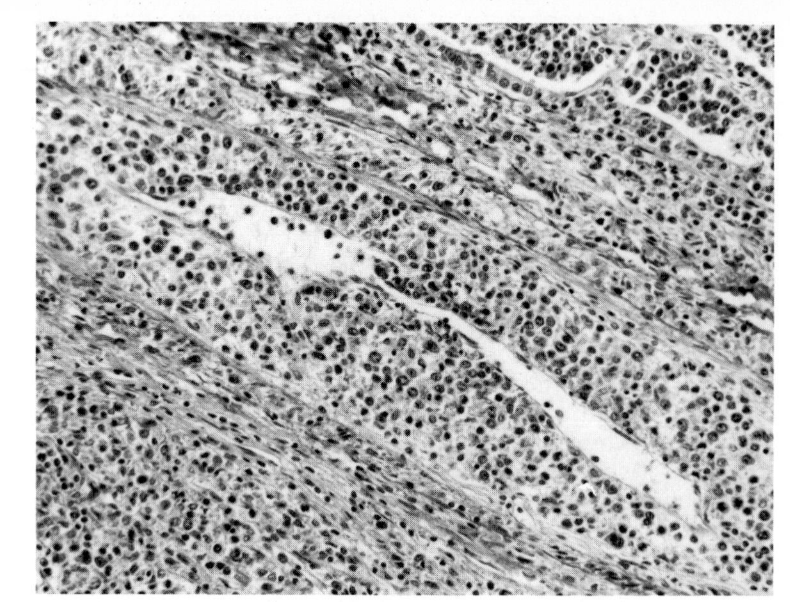

Figure 4–29.

Figure 4–29. Large cell lymphoma with marked vascular infiltration. As is characteristic of the vast majority of lymphomas, there is little vascular necrosis despite the impressive degree of mural and intimal infiltration.

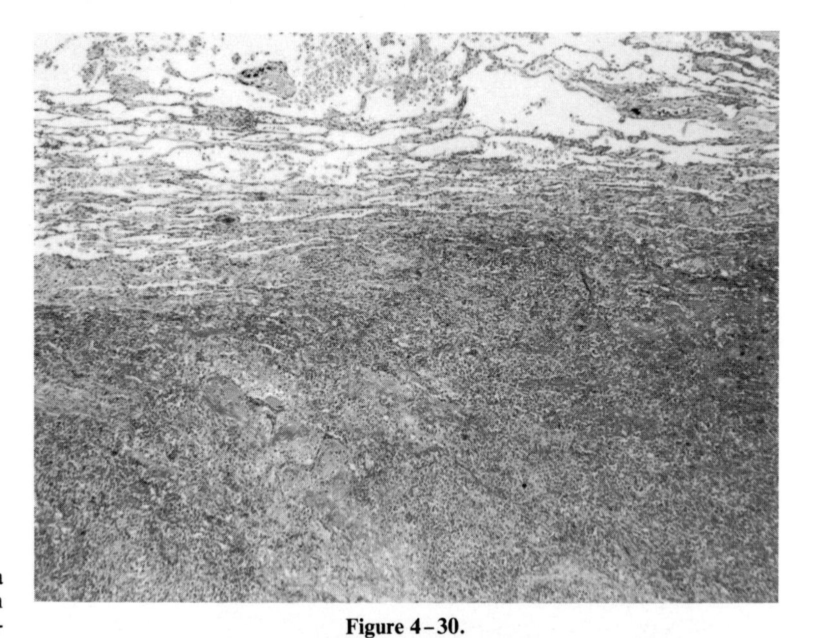

Figure 4–30.

Figures 4–30, 4–31. Large cell lymphoma presenting as a single large mass. The lesion is well circumscribed from the surrounding lung tissue, and it does not show perilesional lymphatic tracking. Cytologic features are those of a large cell lymphoma.

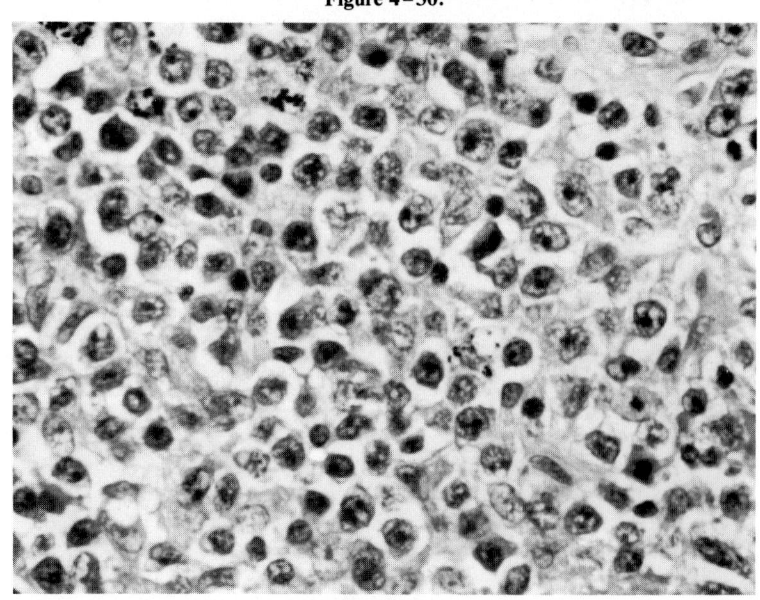

Figure 4–31.

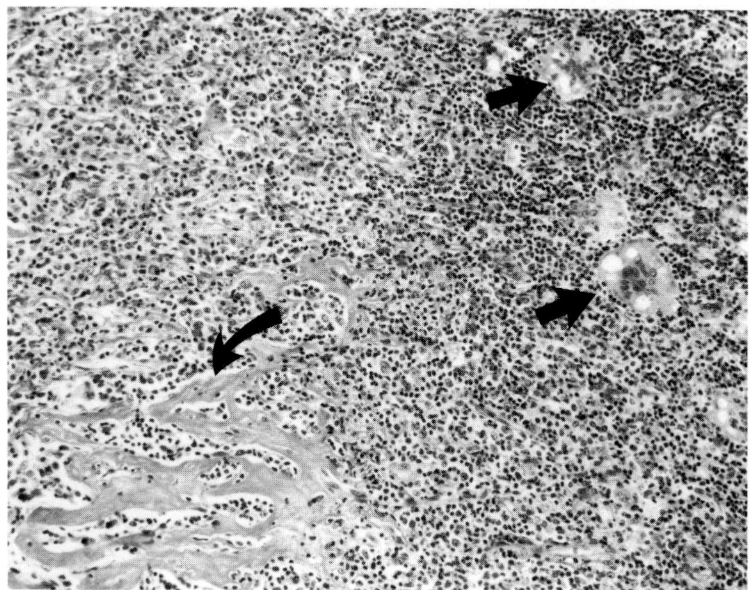

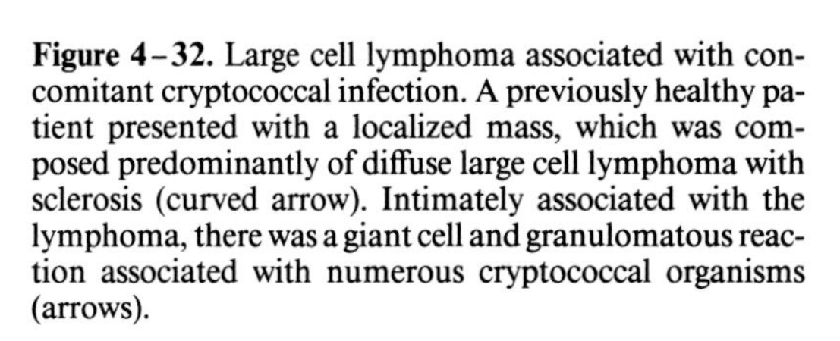

Figure 4–32. Large cell lymphoma associated with concomitant cryptococcal infection. A previously healthy patient presented with a localized mass, which was composed predominantly of diffuse large cell lymphoma with sclerosis (curved arrow). Intimately associated with the lymphoma, there was a giant cell and granulomatous reaction associated with numerous cryptococcal organisms (arrows).

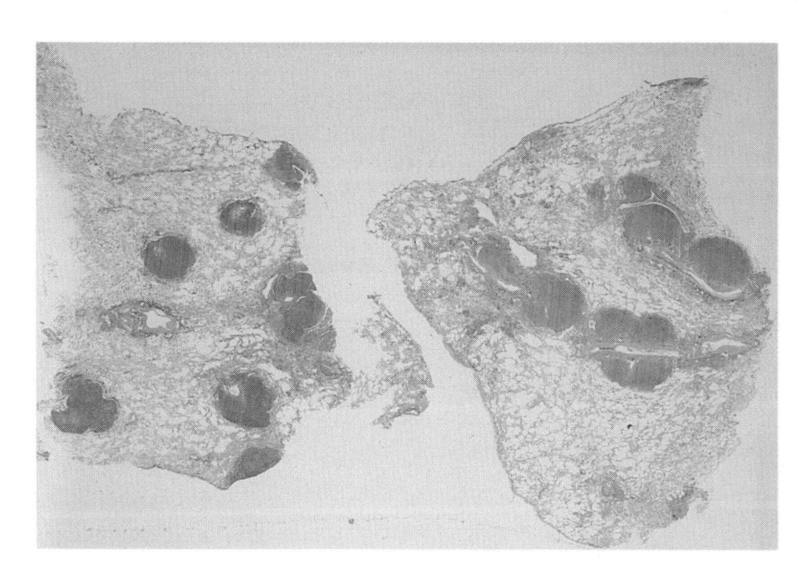

Figure 4–33. Pulmonary relapse of large cell lymphoma manifests as multiple perivascular lymphomatous nodules. Vessel infiltration in this case was minimal.

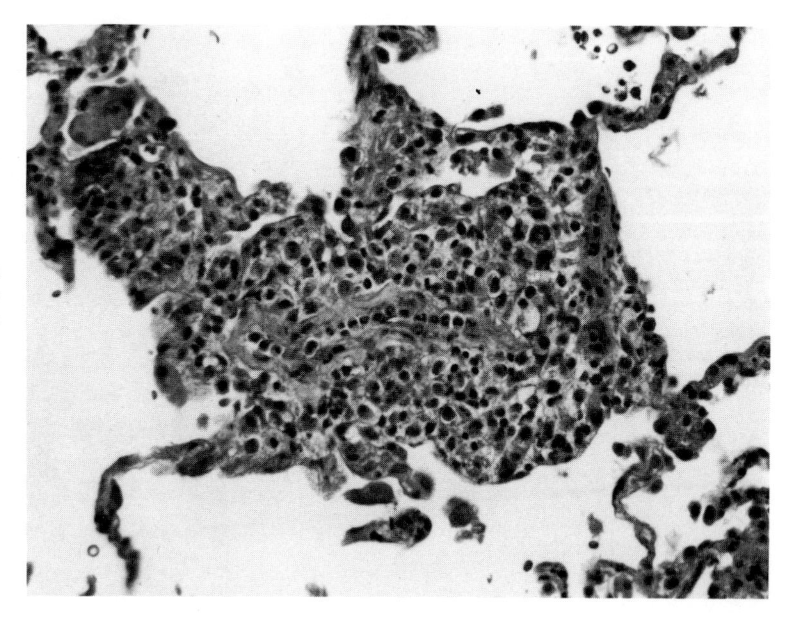

Figure 4–34. Pulmonary relapse of large cell lymphoma manifests as perivascular infiltrates of atypical large lymphoid cells. Some infiltration of vessel walls was also present.

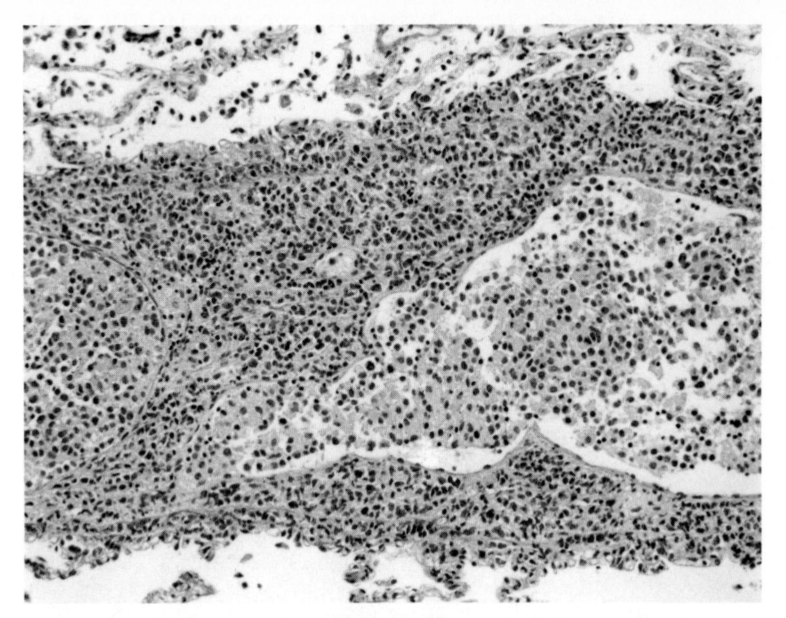

Figure 4-35.

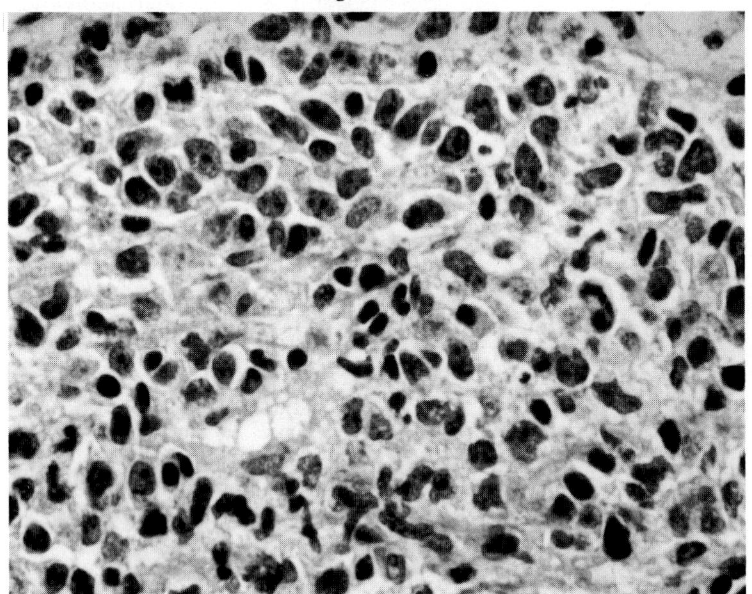

Figure 4-36.

Figures 4-35, 4-36. Pulmonary relapse of large cell lymphoma manifests as septal infiltrates of atypical large lymphoid cells. In this case, septal lymphatics are dilated and filled with tumor cells in addition to soft tissue infiltration of the septum itself.

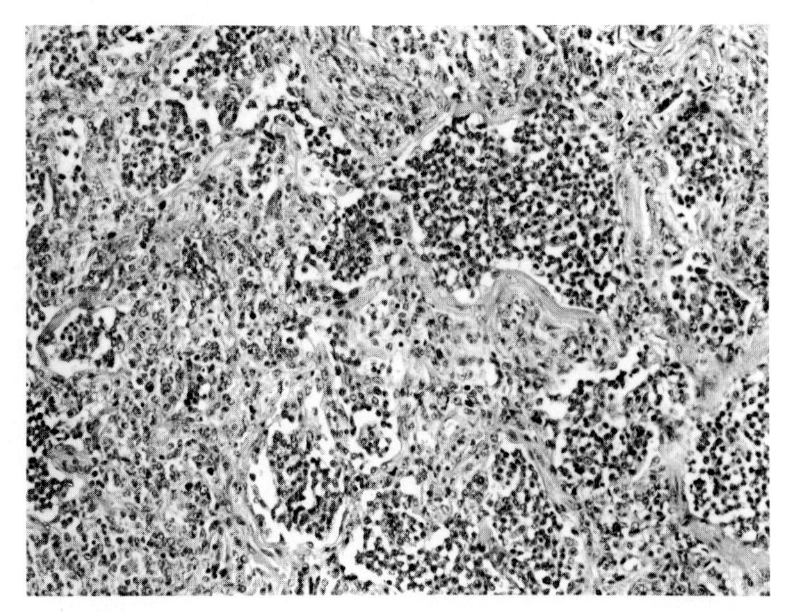

Figure 4-37. Relapse of mixed cell lymphoma. This case of pulmonary relapse of mixed cell lymphoma illustrates the unusual pattern of diffuse consolidation. Both the alveolar spaces and the alveolar walls are diffusely infiltrated by atypical large lymphoid cells. A discrete lymphatic distribution was not appreciated.

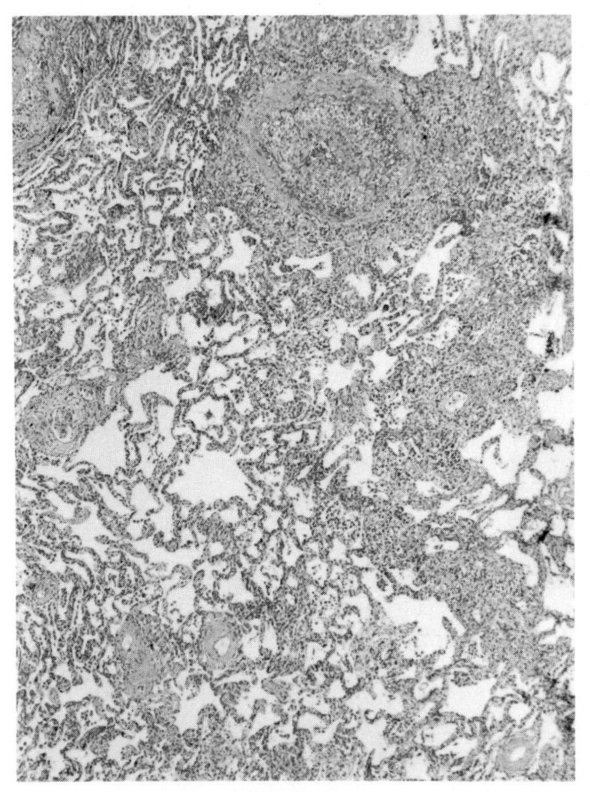

Figure 4–38.

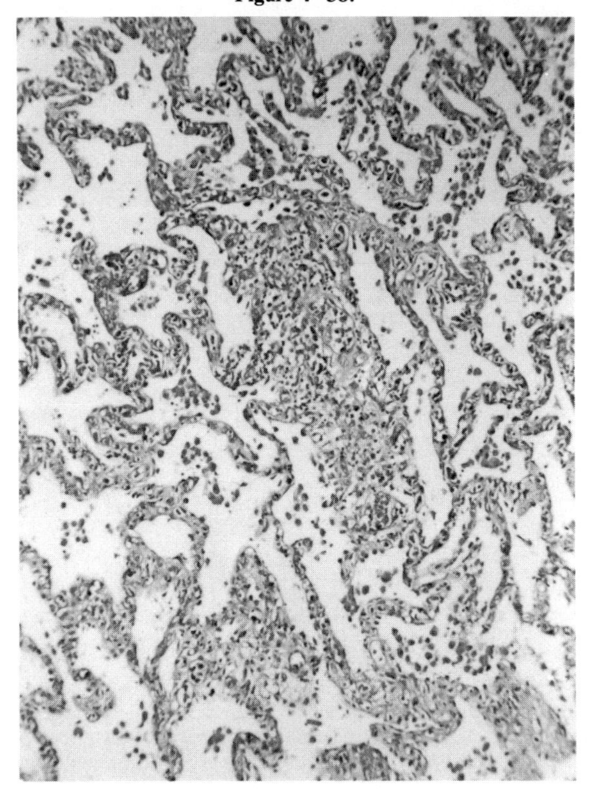

Figure 4–39.

■ Intravascular Lymphomatosis (Angiotropic Lymphoma, Malignant Angioendotheliomatosis, Proliferative Angioendotheliomatosis) (Figs. 4–38 to 4–41)

Intravascular lymphomatosis (angiotropic lymphoma) is a peculiar lymphoreticular malignancy with extensive intravascular tumor cells. Pulmonary involvement may be primary or part of systemic disease and at autopsy is almost universal. Clinically, skin and central nervous system involvement are frequent.

Neoplastic cells, which have the features of large lymphoid cells, show a patchy intravascular distribution, although some perivascular infiltration may also be present. Intimal thickening is seen. The lymphoid origin of these cells can be confirmed with immunologic marker studies (usually they are of B-cell origin), although the routine histologic examination is usually diagnostic.

This histologic abnormality may be relatively subtle and, at first glance, may be mistaken for interstitial infiltrates of inflammatory cells; however, the size and cytologic features of the cells and their presence within vessels (including capillaries) should alert one to the diagnosis. Intravascular carcinomas and metastatic sarcomas, especially angiosarcoma, should be included in the differential diagnosis.

References

Ferry JA, Harris NL, Picker LJ, Weinberg DS, Rosales RK, Tapia J, Richardson EP. Intravascular lymphomatosis (malignant angioendotheliomatosis). Mod Pathol 1:444–452, 1988.

Wick MR, Mills SE, Scheithauer BW, et al. Reassessment of malignant angioendotheliomatosis: Evidence in favor of its reclassification as intravascular lymphomatosis. Am J Surg Pathol 10:112–123, 1986.

Yousem SA, Colby TV. Intravascular lymphomatosis presenting in the lung. Cancer 65:349–353, 1990.

Figures 4–38, 4–39. Intravascular lymphomatosis (angiotropic lymphoma). Despite the extensive intravascular infiltrate in small and large vessels, there is a distinct resemblance to an interstitial pneumonia.

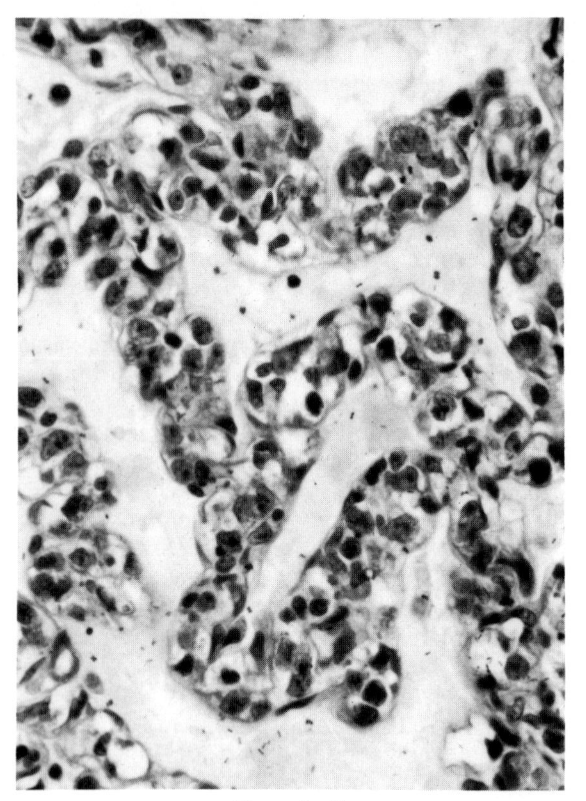

Figure 4-40.

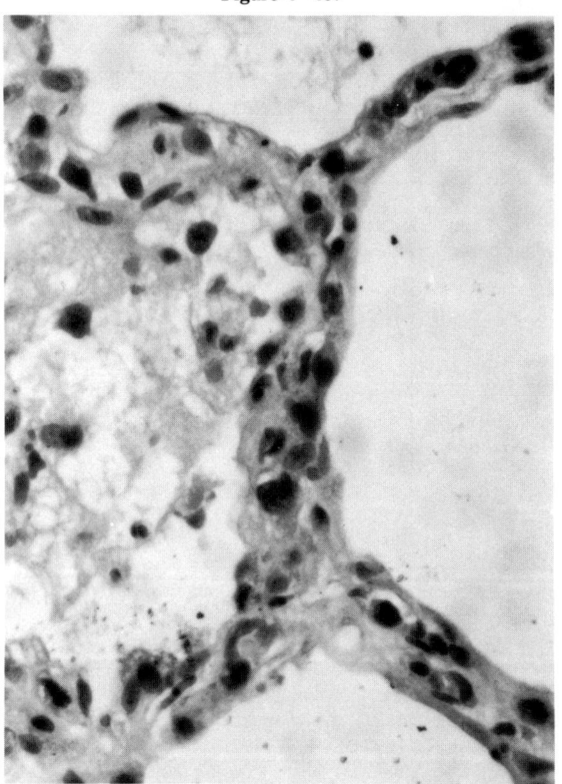

Figure 4-41.

■ Pulmonary Hodgkin's Disease (Figs. 4-42 to 4-48)

Hodgkin's disease may involve the lung primarily, may be part of systemic disease at presentation, or may involve the lung at relapse. Primary pulmonary Hodgkin's disease is rare, whereas pulmonary involvement in disseminated disease or at relapse is relatively common.

Histologic features are similar to Hodgkin's disease in lymph nodes with a mixed cell composition in which Reed-Sternberg cells and Reed-Sternberg cell variants are identified. In large masses, the histologic appearance is virtually identical to that in lymph nodes, whereas in more diffuse infiltrates the cytologic features are best appreciated in small nodules showing a lymphatic distribution, usually along vessels. Vascular infiltration may be seen in both primary and secondary pulmonary Hodgkin's disease, and the necrosis may at times suggest a granulomatous process or an angiocentric (mixed cell) non-Hodgkin's lymphoma.

Relapse of Hodgkin's disease in the lung may be markedly pleomorphic and raise the possibility of a de novo non-Hodgkin's lymphoma. Immunologic markers and other studies may be necessary for definitive diagnosis.

The differential diagnosis also includes infectious and noninfectious granulomatous lesions, including Wegener's granulomatosis.

References

Yousem SA, Weiss L, Colby TV. Primary pulmonary Hodgkin's disease. Cancer 57:1217-1224, 1986.

Figures 4-40, 4-41. Intravascular lymphomatosis (angiotropic lymphoma). The diffuse capillary infiltrates of atypical large lymphoid cells may be obvious or relatively subtle, and it may be somewhat difficult to separate the lymphoma cells from other interstitial nuclei, particularly those of type II cells and endothelial cells.

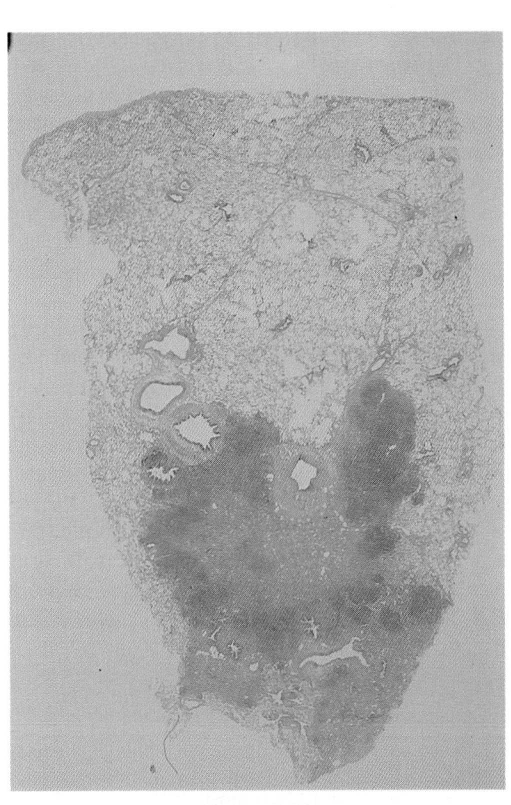

Figure 4–42.

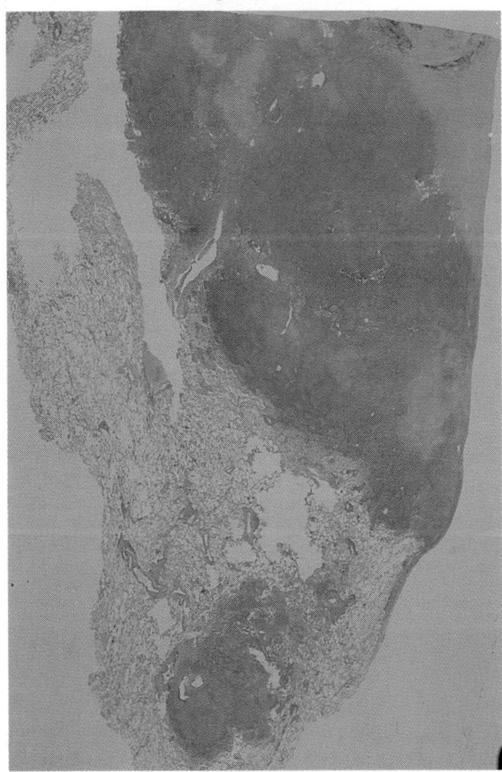

Figure 4–43.

Figures 4–42, 4–43. Hodgkin's disease presenting in the lung. These two cases are examples of nodular infiltrates that are perivascular in distribution. One shows typical sclerosis and nodularity of nodular sclerosing Hodgkin's disease, whereas the other is more cellular and is characterized by necrosis and a satellite nodule.

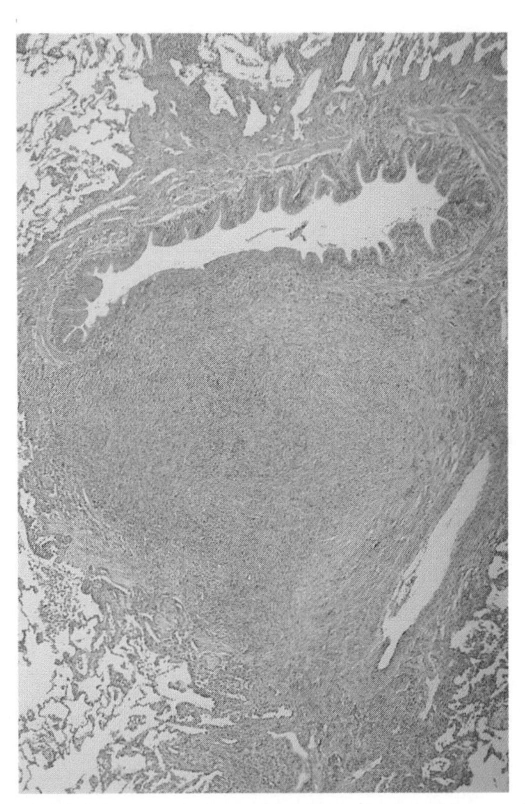

Figure 4–44. Primary pulmonary Hodgkin's disease with a neoplastic nodule along (and splaying apart) a bronchovascular bundle.

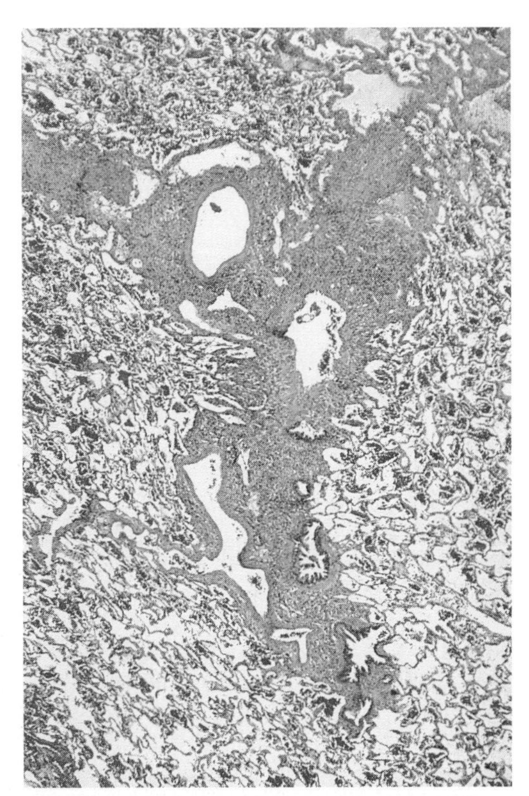

Figure 4–45. Hodgkin's disease in the lung at presentation. The patient presented with lymphadenopathy and pulmonary infiltrates. Lymph node biopsy showed nodular sclerosing Hodgkin's disease, and open lung biopsy findings showed perivascular polymorphous lymphoid infiltrates containing Reed-Sternberg cells and their mononuclear variants.

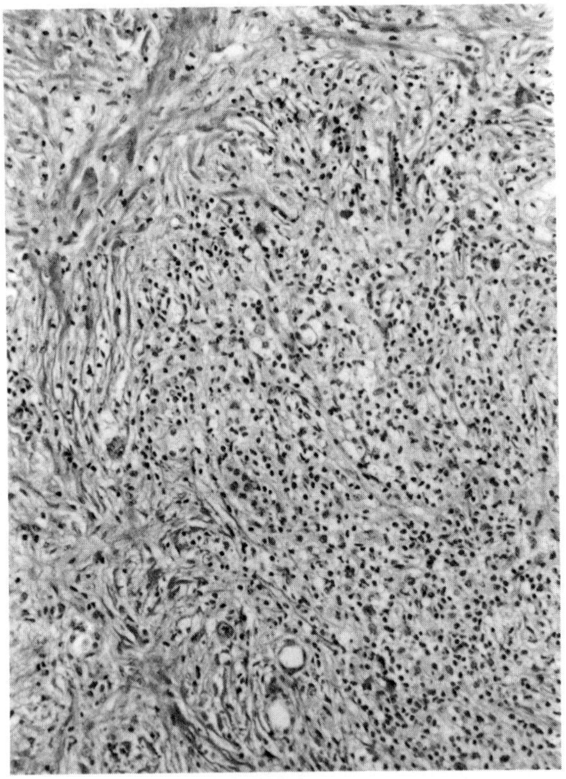

Figure 4-46.

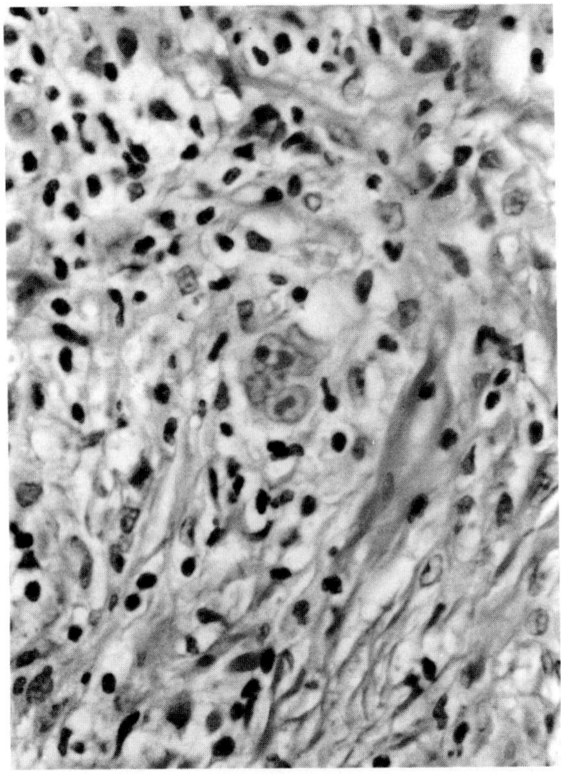

Figure 4-47.

Figures 4-46, 4-47. Hodgkin's disease presenting in the lung. Cytologic features in this case are identical to those seen in lymph nodes with nodular sclerosing Hodgkin's disease.

■ Leukemic Infiltrates of the Lung (Figs. 4-49 to 4-60)

The lung is rarely the site of presentation for either myelogenous (usually acute) or lymphocytic (chronic) leukemia. A somewhat more common occurrence is pulmonary involvement in patients who have already been diagnosed as having leukemia; even then, however, *clinically significant pulmonary infiltrates of leukemia during life are uncommon.* At autopsy, pulmonary involvement is relatively frequent. In general, pulmonary problems should not be accepted as being due to leukemia until other possible causes, notably infection and leukostasis, have been excluded.

The histologic pattern is that of a hematolymphoid infiltrate along the lymphatic routes or diffusely involving the interstitium, showing histologic and cytologic features of the leukemia. Infiltration of the alveolar walls themselves is usually inconspicuous in comparison with the perivascular and peribronchiolar infiltrates. In chronic lymphocytic leukemia (CLL), marked infiltration of small bronchioles has been associated with wheezing and evidence of airway obstruction. A granulomatous reaction for which no infectious etiology can be found may also accompany the infiltrates of chronic lymphocytic leukemia.

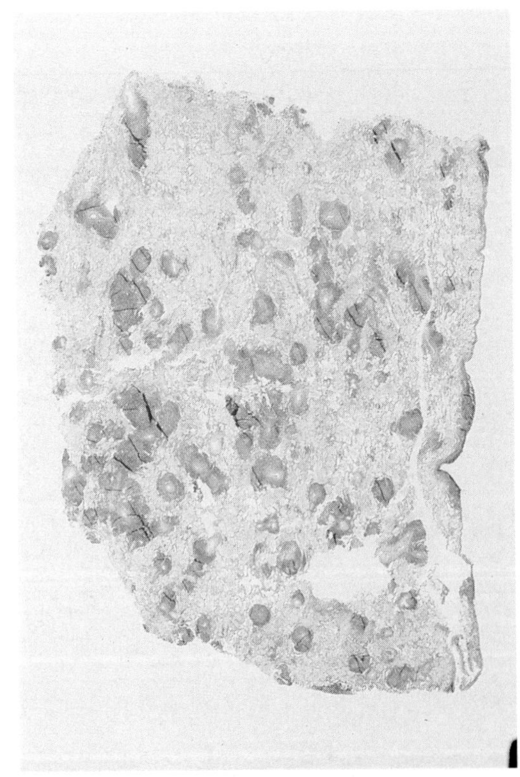

Figure 4-48. Relapse of Hodgkin's disease. In a patient with known Hodgkin's disease, an isolated relapse developed, manifesting as a localized pulmonary infiltrate. Histologically, the lymphoid infiltrate is restricted to the perivascular regions. The infiltrate had the cytologic features of Hodgkin's disease.

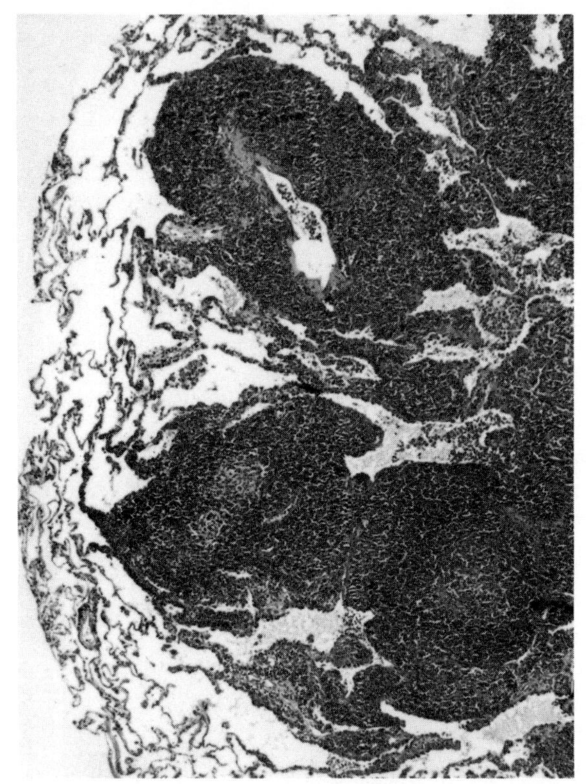

Figure 4-49. Chronic lymphocytic leukemia involving the lung with dense perivascular infiltrates of small lymphocytes.

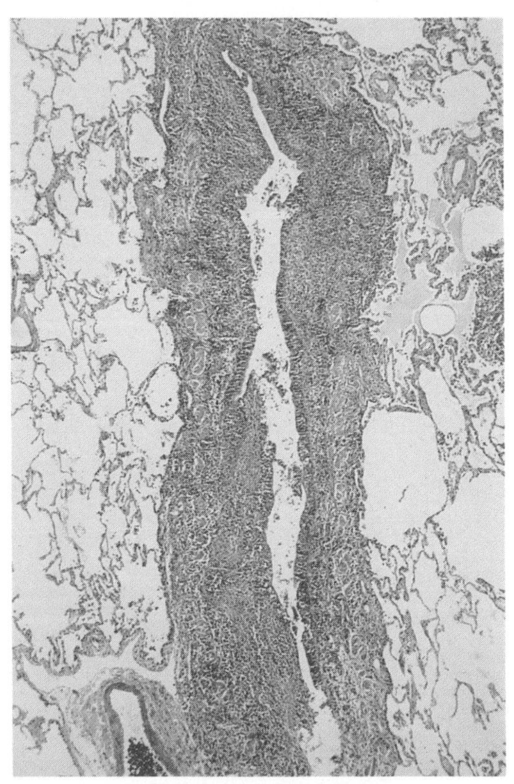

Figure 4-50. Chronic lymphocytic leukemia presenting in the lung. There is a dense infiltrate of lymphocytes forming a thick cuff around a bronchiole and splaying apart the smooth muscle. The patient was experiencing wheezing, and diffuse pulmonary infiltrates that were steroid-responsive were present.

The diagnosis of clinically significant leukemic infiltrates is one of exclusion. Because chronic lymphocytic leukemia is a relatively common condition, its finding as an incidental lesion on a lung biopsy is not unexpected. Likewise, in the case of myelogenous leukemia, the possibility that the leukemic cells may be chemotactically attracted to a site of infection should always be kept in mind. Chemotherapy in patients with very high peripheral blast counts may result in pulmonary leukostasis (see p. 311).

Infiltrates of myelogenous leukemia also may occur as an incidental finding to some other more significant lesion, particularly an infection.

References

Dail DH, Hammer, SP (eds). Pulmonary Pathology. New York, Springer-Verlag, 1988.

Rollins SD, Colby TV. Lung biopsy in chronic lymphocytic leukemia. Arch Pathol Lab Med 112:607-611, 1988.

■ Plasmacytoma and Myeloma

Primary plasmacytomas of the lung are quite rare, and they may or may not be associated with a systemic plasma cell dyscrasia. The lung may also be secondarily affected in patients with established multiple myeloma, either as localized or diffuse bilateral infiltrates.

Histologic findings include localized nodules composed of plasma cells showing varying degrees of differentiation and/or diffuse interstitial infiltrates with a predisposition for lymphatic routes. Amyloid is sometimes present.

References

Carter D, Eggleston JC. Tumors of the Lower Respiratory Tract. AFIP Atlas of Tumor Pathology, Second Series, Fascicle 17. Washington, DC, Armed Forces Institute of Pathology, 1980.

Dail DH, Hammer, SP (eds). Pulmonary Pathology. New York, Springer-Verlag, 1988.

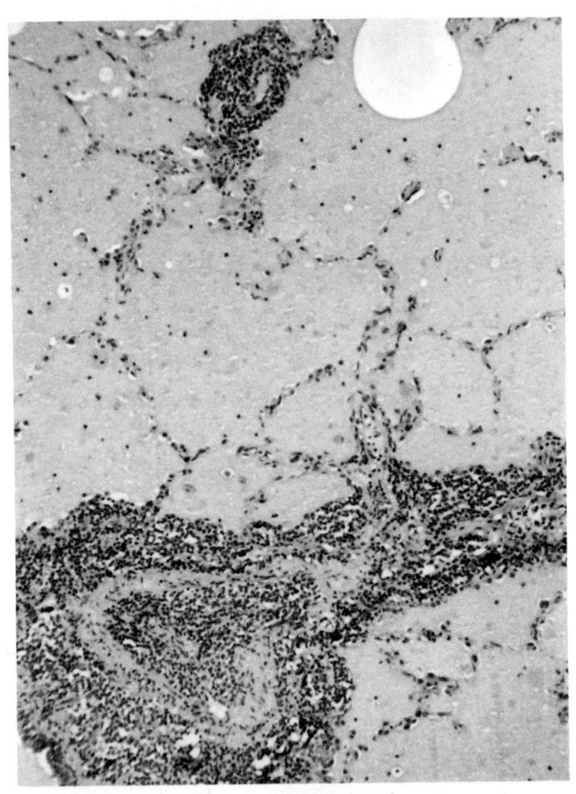

Figure 4–51.

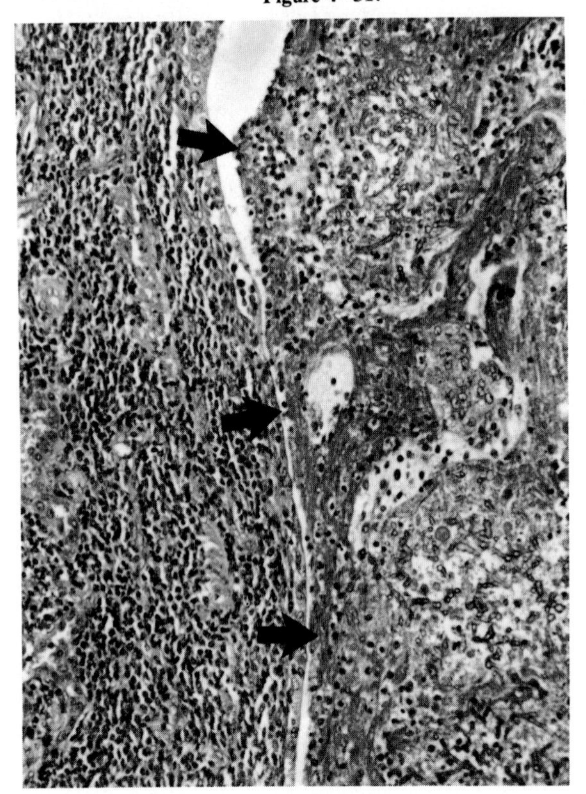

Figure 4–52.

Figures 4–51, 4–52. Chronic lymphocytic leukemia. There was lymphocytic cuffing of vessels and airways, and many of the airways had colonies of *Aspergillus* (arrows) growing in their lumens. The patient eventually died 6 months later with an *Aspergillus* empyema. In some fields, the alveoli showed a pseudoproteinosis reaction (Fig. 4–51).

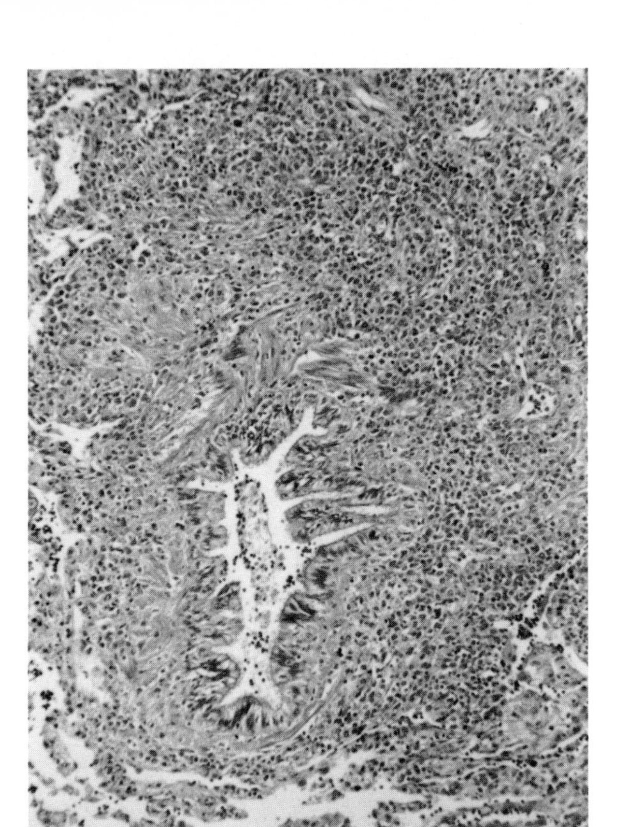

Figure 4-53.

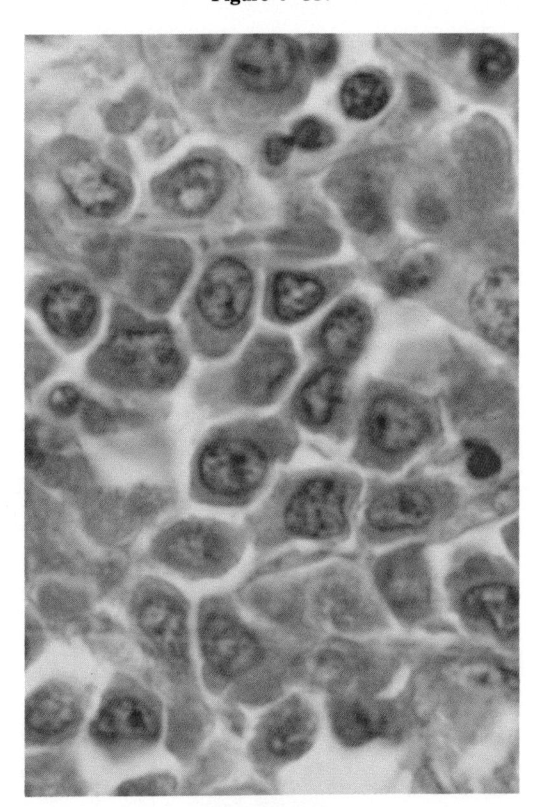

Figure 4-54.

Figures 4-53, 4-54. Acute myelogenous leukemia presenting in the lung. Persistent pulmonary infiltrates were evident. Open biopsy shows a dense infiltrate of large, promyelocytoid cells around airways and vessels. Chloroacetate esterase stain was strongly positive, and subsequent examination of the bone marow and autopsy confirmed the presence of myelogenous leukemia.

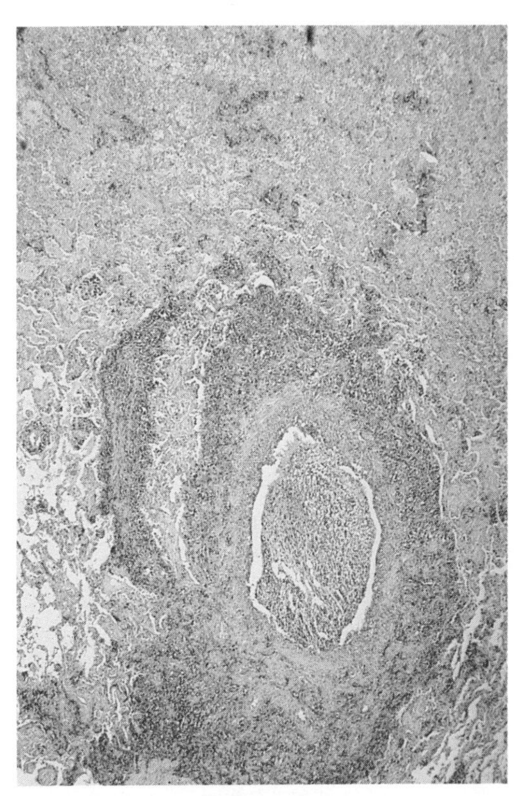

Figure 4-55.

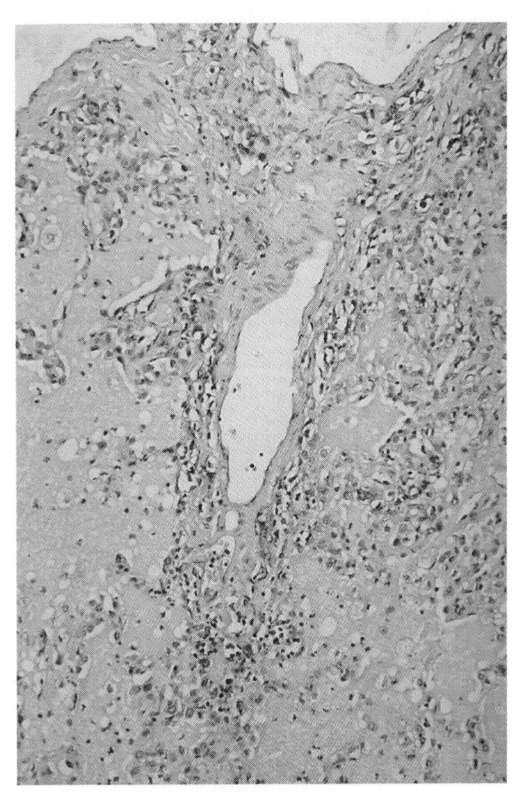

Figure 4-56.

Figures 4-55, 4-56. Relapse of acute myelogenous leukemia in the lung. Chloroacetate esterase stains show dense infiltrates of positive-staining cells around airways and vessels. The alveoli show diffuse alveolar damage, which was thought to be the explanation for the patient's clinical pulmonary signs and symptoms. The leukemic infiltrate was considered incidental, although it was the initial manifestation of relapse in this patient.

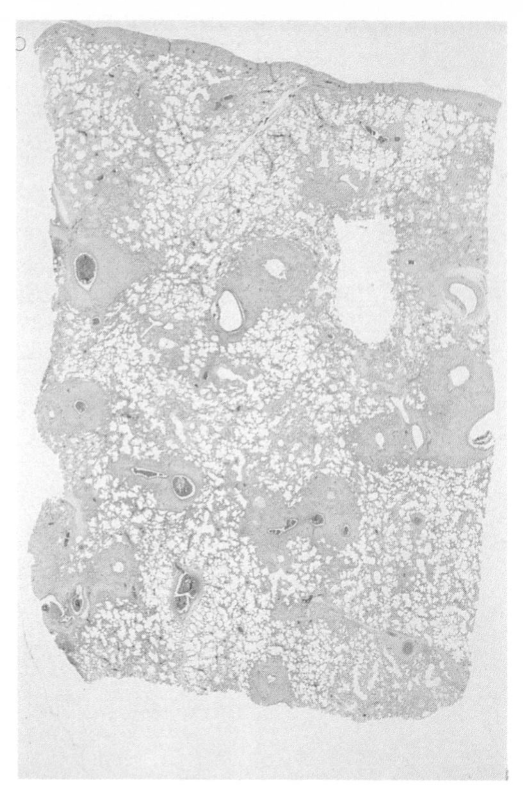

Figure 4–57. Acute myelogenous leukemia (acute myelosclerosis) involving the lung. This patient had rapidly fatal acute myelosclerosis, and fibrotic changes can be seen around bronchovascular structures, septa, and pleura. Cytologically, these foci contained immature myeloid cells and megakaryocytic forms.

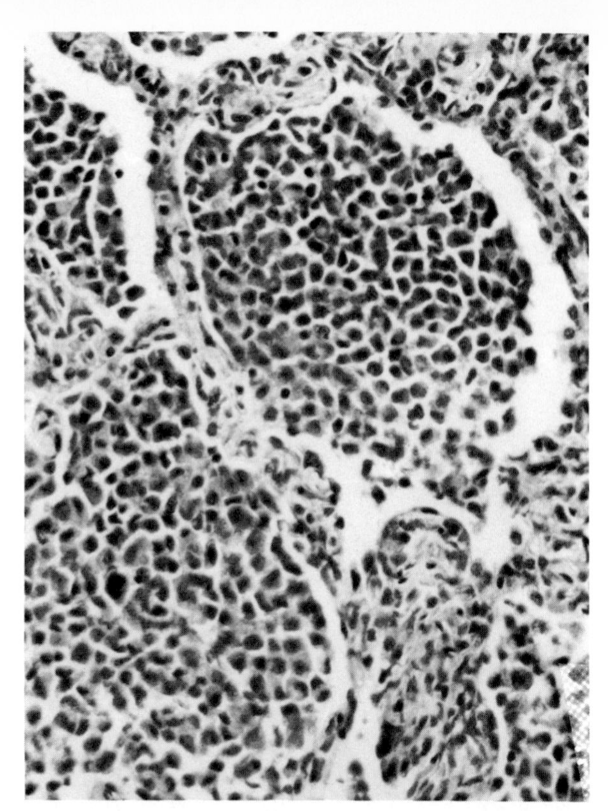

Figure 4–59. Acute myelomonocytic leukemia involving the lung at presentation. In a previously untreated patient with acute myelomonocytic leukemia, pulmonary infiltrates were evident at the time of presentation. Open lung biopsy showed interstitial and alveolar infiltrates of chloroacetate esterase–positive myelomonocytoid cells identical to those replacing the bone marrow.

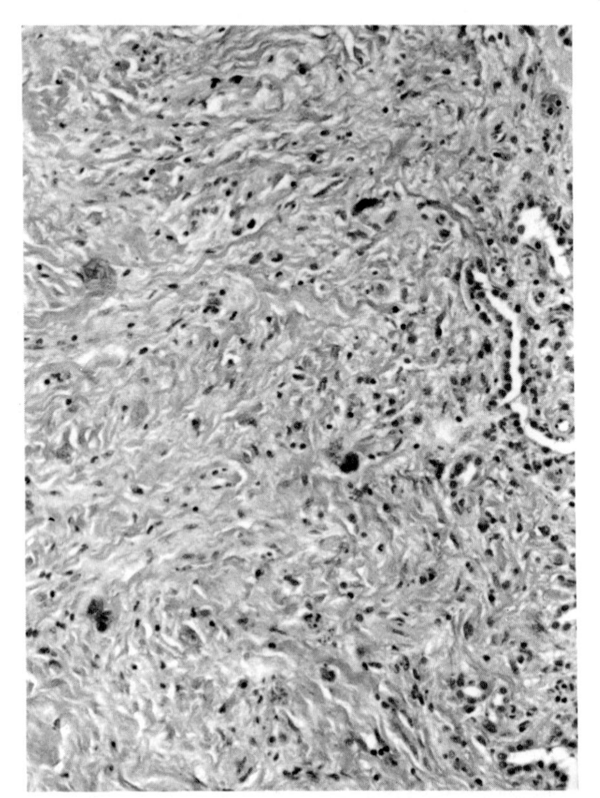

Figure 4–58. Myelofibrosis involving the pleura. The patient, who had long-standing myelofibrosis (proven on bone marrow biopsy several years previously), presented with pleural and parenchymal infiltrates on chest radiograph. Pleural biopsy findings showed dense fibrous tissue in which scattered large megakaryocytes could be identified.

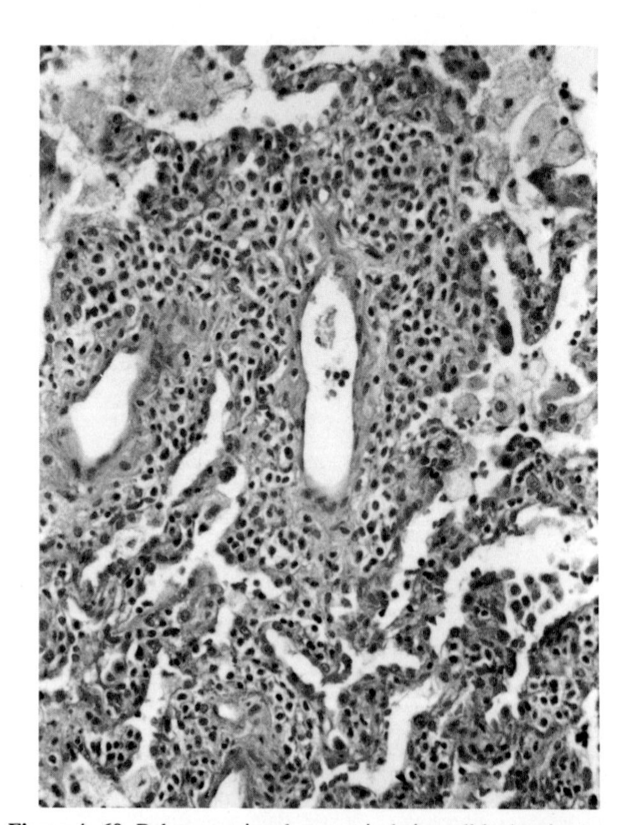

Figure 4–60. Pulmonary involvement in hairy cell leukemia. A patient with long-standing hairy cell leukemia underwent an open lung biopsy for pulmonary infiltrates. The only finding was a moderate interstitial and perivascular infiltrate of hairy cell leukemia cells.

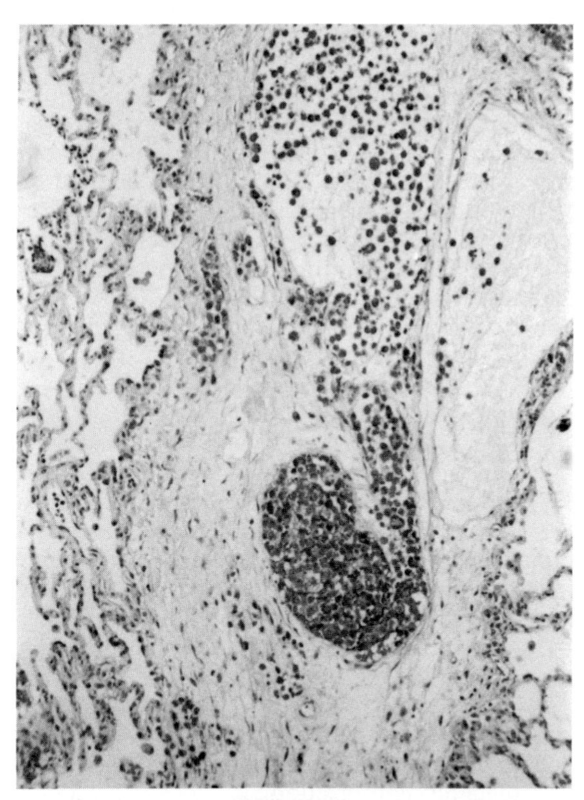

Figure 4-61.

■ Miscellaneous Lymphoreticular Infiltrates in the Lung—Mycosis Fungoides, Malignant Histiocytosis, Angioimmunoblastic Lymphadenopathy (Figs. 4-61 to 4-65)

The lung is frequently involved in disseminated mycosis fungoides, malignant histiocytosis, and angioimmunoblastic lymphadenopathy. The histogenesis of these lesions has been recently reevaluated and a significant portion of cases represent T cell lymphomas. The infiltrates show a predisposition for the lymphatic routes, and the histologic features reflect the underlying disease process. Localized, nodular, and diffuse infiltrates may be seen.

References

Dail DH, Hammer SP (eds). Pulmonary Pathology. New York, Springer-Verlag, 1988.

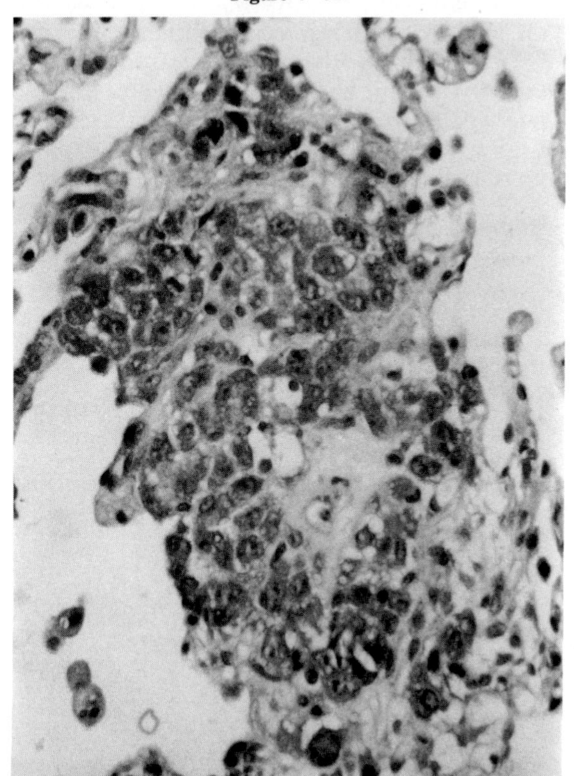

Figure 4-62.

Figures 4-61, 4-62. Malignant histiocytosis involving the lung. Open lung biopsy showed atypical cells infiltrating the septa and forming pools within the lymphatic spaces. Cytologically, the cells have the features of a large cell lymphoreticular malignancy.

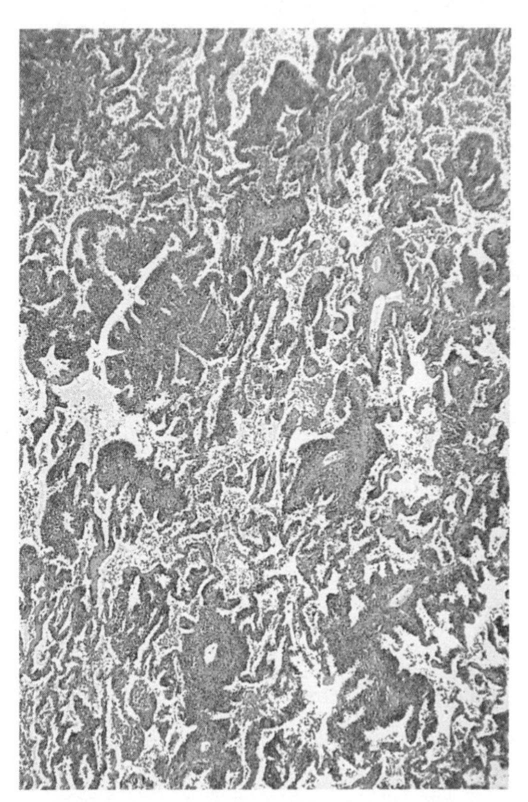

Figure 4-63. Mycosis fungoides involving the lung. Prominent perivascular interstitial infiltrates of lymphoid cells are present in a patient with known extracutaneous involvement by mycosis fungoides. Cytologically, the cells were identical to those infiltrating the skin and lymph nodes.

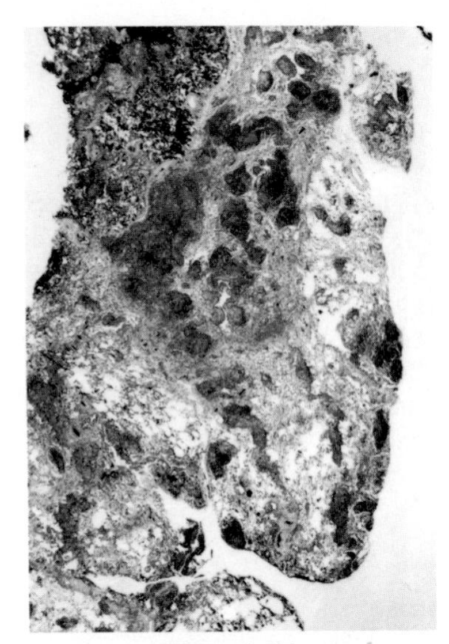

Figure 4–64.

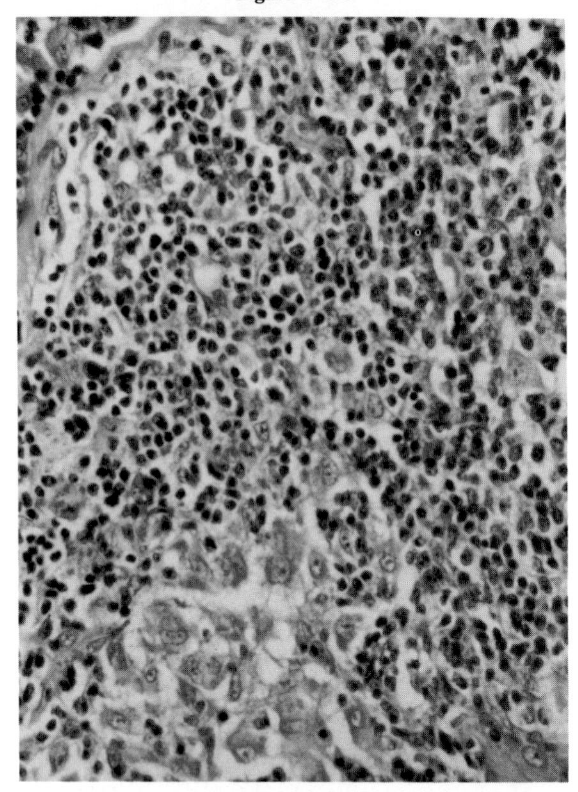

Figure 4–65.

Figures 4–64, 4–65. Angioimmunoblastic lymphadenopathy involving the lung. This biopsy specimen was taken from a patient with lymph node biopsy diagnosis of angioimmunoblastic lymphadenopathy, in whom pulmonary infiltrates had developed. There is a cellular infiltrate along lymphatic routes with numerous plasma cells, immunoblasts, and clusters of histiocytes. Most cases of angioimmunoblastic lymphadenopathy are now recognized as variants of T-cell lymphomas.

■ Post-transplantation Lymphoproliferative Disorders (See Figs. 1–30 to 1–33)

In transplant recipients in general, there is an increased incidence of lymphoproliferative disease, particularly at extranodal sites. With the introduction of cyclosporine into the transplant drug regimen, there has been an even greater increase in this occurrence. Many of these lymphoproliferative lesions have been found to be associated with the Epstein-Barr virus (EBV) genome in the proliferating cells, and, consequently, the conceptual difference between reactive and neoplastic proliferations in these individuals has become blurred.

Post-transplant lymphoproliferations usually develop within a year or so after transplant. By evaluation, they may be monoclonal or polyclonal and may have the EBV genome in the proliferating cells. Clonality does not always predict behavior, since some patients with monoclonal processes recover when immunosuppression is decreased and some patients with polyclonal processes have progressive disease. Follow-up is the only way to determine for certain the clinical behavior. In general, the following are true:

- The prognosis for patients with high-grade-appearing lesions is worse than for those with lesions of a more heterogenous composition.
- Patients with primary EBV infection fare worse than those with prior EBV infection and the development of reactivation EBV lymphoproliferations.
- Patients with monoclonal lesions fare worse than those with polyclonal processes.
- Mitoses, necrosis, vascular invasion, and atypical immunoblasts are *not specifically helpful* in prognosis.

Note: These lesions look like lymphomas with vascular infiltration and necrosis. The clinical history must be known in order to avoid a diagnosis of lymphoma.

References

Starzl TE, Nalesnik MA, Porter KE, et al. Reversibility of lymphoproliferative lesions developing under cyclosporin-steroid therapy. Lancet 1:583, 1984.

Yousem SA, Randhawa P, Nalesnik MA, et al. Post-transplant lymphoproliferative disorders in heart-lung transplant recipients: primary presentation in the allograft. Hum Pathol 20:361–369, 1989.

CHAPTER 5

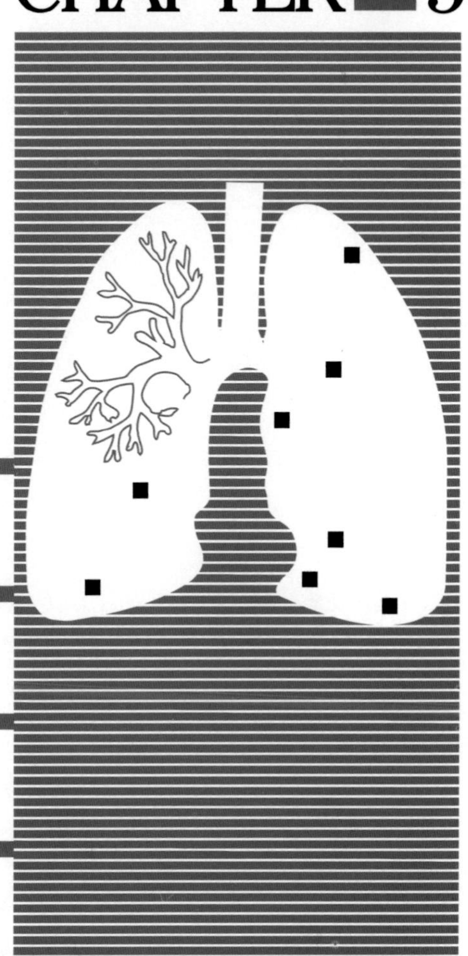

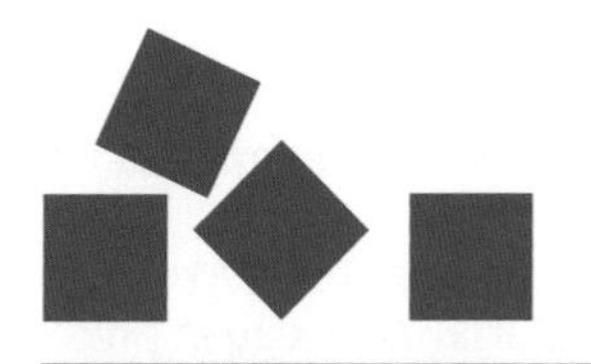

INFECTIONS

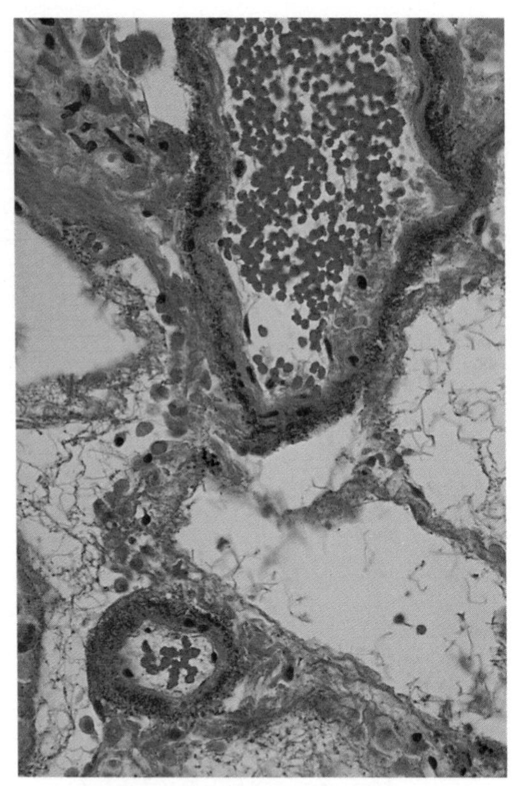

Figure 5-1. *Pseudomonas aeruginosa* pneumonia. Basophilic staining of vessel walls is due to massive numbers of bacteria.

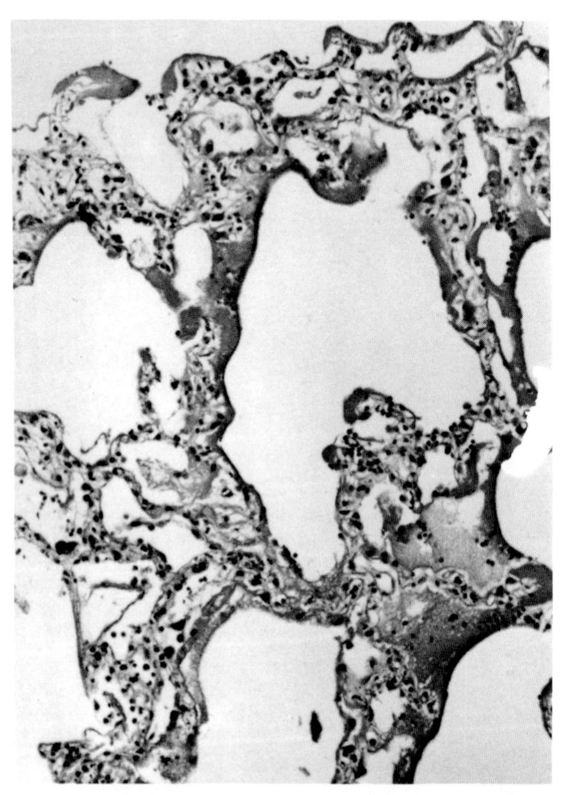

Figure 5-2. Legionnaires' disease. This biopsy specimen of early legionnaires' disease shows hyaline membranes with scant interstitial inflammation. Histologically, there is acute diffuse alveolar damage.

■ Common Bacterial Infections (Figs. 5-1 to 5-5)

The more common bacterial pneumonias are rarely diagnosed by the surgical pathologist; diagnosis is usually made by sputum evaluation or bronchoalveolar lavage and cultures.

Histologically, bacterial infection includes acute pneumonia with fibrinous exudate (with or without hemorrhage) and neutrophils, nonspecific organizing pneumonia, and a nonspecific chronic inflammatory infiltrate. Sometimes acute and/or chronic cellular bronchiolitis are prominent.

Note: Gram-stained smears, cultures, serologic tests, and clinical correlation are usually needed for specific diagnosis.

■ Aspiration With Secondary Bacterial Pneumonia

A prior aspiration event may or may not have been clinically apparent. Infected material may cause pneumonia directly, or pneumonia may develop distal to an aspirated foreign body.

Location is important because the regions of the lung that are dependent at the time of aspiration are the ones most often affected.

Localized lesions may be resected for diagnosis or treatment.

Histologically, bronchiolocentricity is sometimes apparent; early on there is an acute exudative pneumonia, later an abscess cavity with chronic inflammation, fibrosis, and organization in the wall can be seen. The center of a localized lesion is often necrotic and contains neutrophils and large numbers of histiocytes, some of which are foamy. Organisms are not commonly seen in surgical material; a foreign body reaction to aspirated material (often periodic acid-Schiff [PAS]-positive) may or may not be present. Calcified debris is seen in late cases and should also raise suspicion of an aspirated broncholith.

Chronic and recurrent aspiration may occur in patients with gastric reflux and may lead to chronic and recurring pneumonias or to insidious interstitial lung disease. A histologic diagnosis or chronic (granulomatous) bronchiolitis, bronchiolitis obliterans, or usual interstitial pneumonia may be considered.

References

Dail DH, Hammer SP (eds). Pulmonary Pathology. New York, Springer-Verlag, 1988.

Thurlbeck WM (ed). Pathology of the Lung. New York, Thieme, 1988.

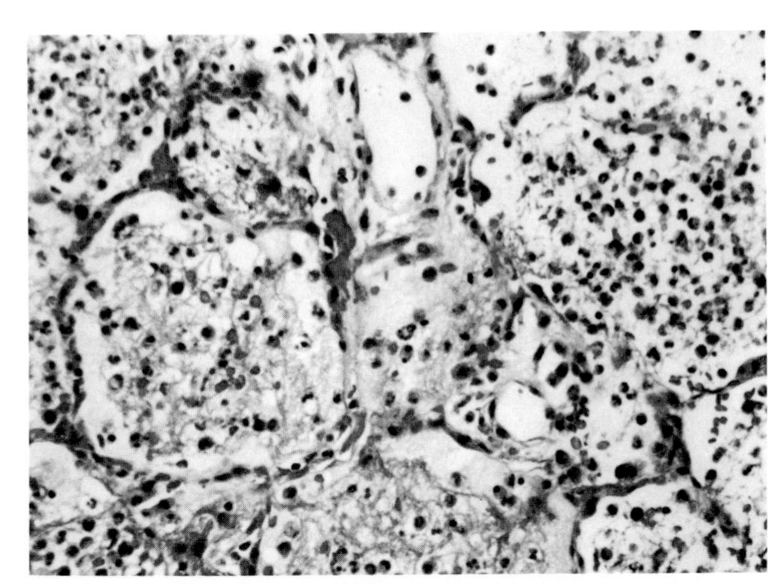

Figures 5–3, 5–4. Legionnaires' disease. There is consolidation with large numbers of neutrophils, fibrin, and macrophages. In this stage, silver stains will usually be positive for legionnaires' bacilli, as illustrated in a Dieterle stain (Fig. 5–4). Fluorescent studies on smears and scrapes of lung tissue are much more reliable, if they are available, and silver stains need not be performed.

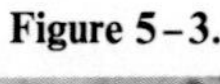

Figure 5–3.

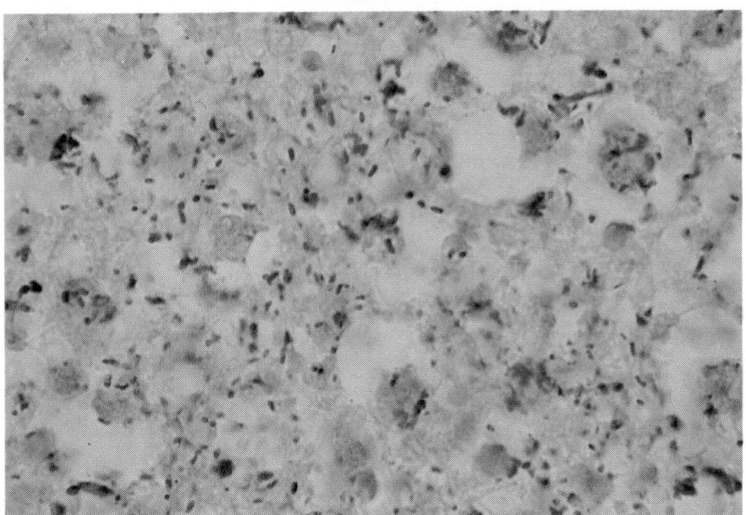

Figure 5–4.

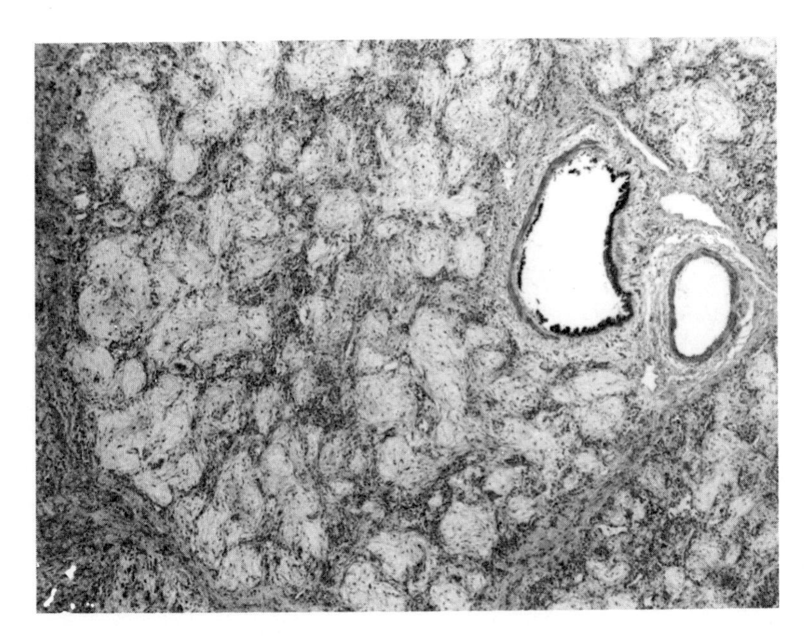

Figure 5–5. Organizing legionnaires' disease. There is a nonspecific organizing pneumonia with edematous granulation tissue filling airspaces adjacent to a terminal bronchiole. In this stage, special stains for organisms would be negative. The diagnosis in this case was confirmed by specific immunofluorescent studies.

■ Abscess

An abscess appears as a mass or infiltrate on a chest radiograph, which may be resected for diagnosis or, rarely, for therapy.

Histologically, a purulent center is surrounded by fibrosis, organizing pneumonia, and a mixed inflammatory infiltrate. A few nonspecific granulomas can be seen, but their presence should raise the possibility of granulomatous infection.

A chronic abscess may mimic an old granuloma with a necrotic center and a somewhat palisaded histiocytic wall, but there is an absence of satellite non-necrotizing granulomas. Extensively necrotic tumors may simulate an abscess.

■ **Pulmonary Nocardiosis** (Figs. 5–6 to 5–9)

Nocardia may involve the lung as a localized abscess or as a miliary bilateral infection.

Histologically, there is generally a mixture of acute and chronic inflammation with a purulent microabscess surrounded by a chronic inflammatory and often granulomatous reaction, although the well-formed granulomas seen in sarcoid or tuberculosis are lacking. This histologic appearance is seen in both localized and diffuse lesions. A reaction resembling pulmonary alveolar proteinosis may be seen in immunocompromised hosts. Nocardia can be best seen with a silver stain as fine filamentous organisms; *sometimes, however, they are relatively inconspicuous and must be sought very carefully.* They are also weakly acid-fast (Fite's stain) and gram-positive; however, in our experience, the silver stain is usually the best stain for identifying the organism. Colonies of organisms ("sulfur granules") are not seen in the lung.

It is sometimes extremely difficult to identify the organisms; if there is a strong suspicion for nocardiosis, performing special stains on multiple levels and a very careful search may provide confirmation.

References

Dail DH, Hammer SP (eds). Pulmonary Pathology. New York, Springer-Verlag, 1988.

Thurlbeck WM (ed). Pathology of the Lung. New York, Thieme, 1988.

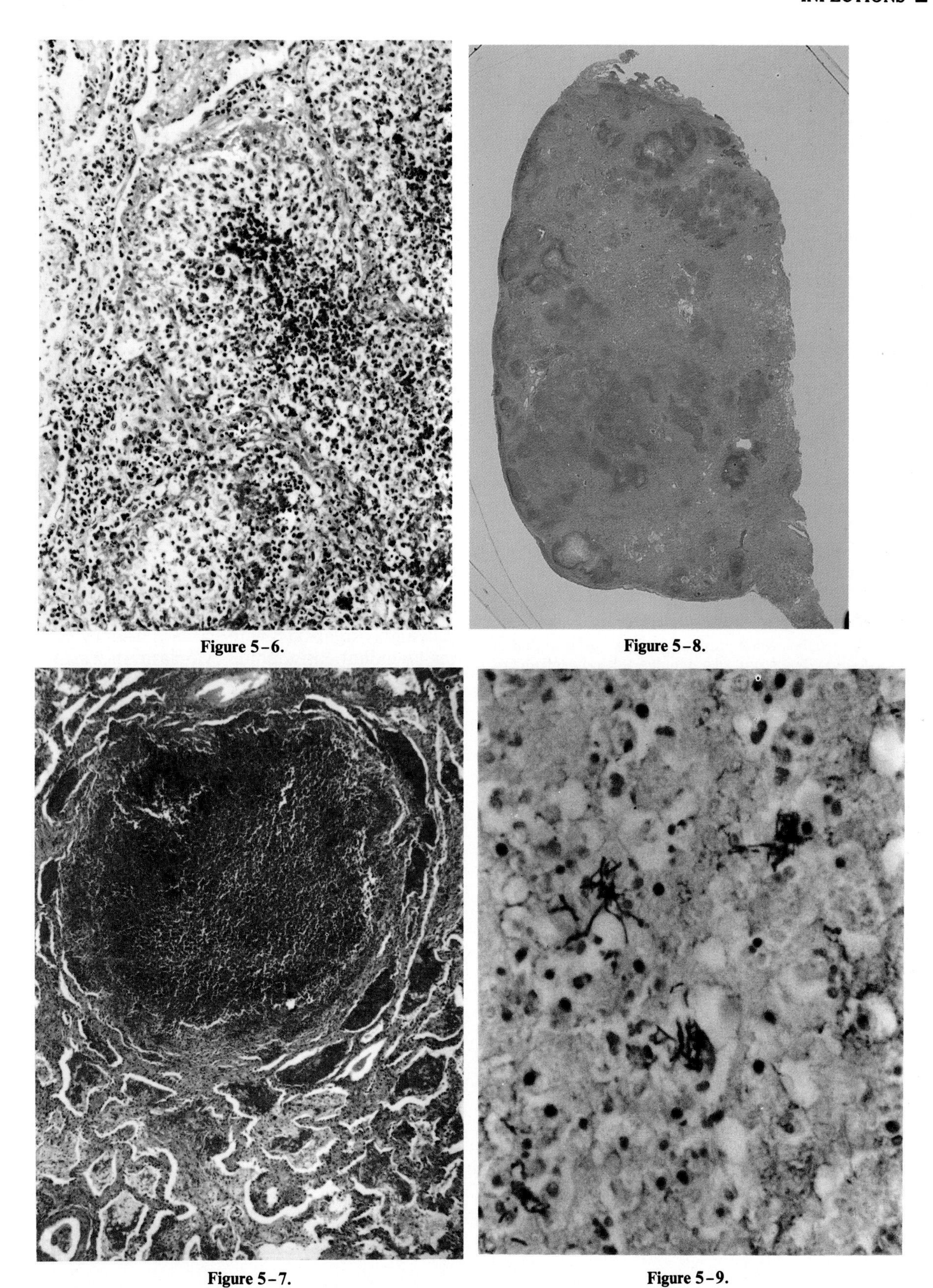

Figure 5-6.

Figure 5-8.

Figure 5-7.

Figure 5-9.

Figures 5-6, 5-7, 5-8, 5-9. Pulmonary nocardiosis. The necrotizing granulomas of nocardiosis begin as small inflammatory foci with acute inflammation and exudation into alveolar spaces (Fig. 5-6). These expand to form single (Fig. 5-7) or confluent (Fig. 5-8) necrotizing granulomas with central purulent abscesses surrounded by a cuff of chronic inflammatory and granulomatous reaction. The fine filamentous organisms may be found only focally and are best appreciated with silver stains (Fig. 5-9).

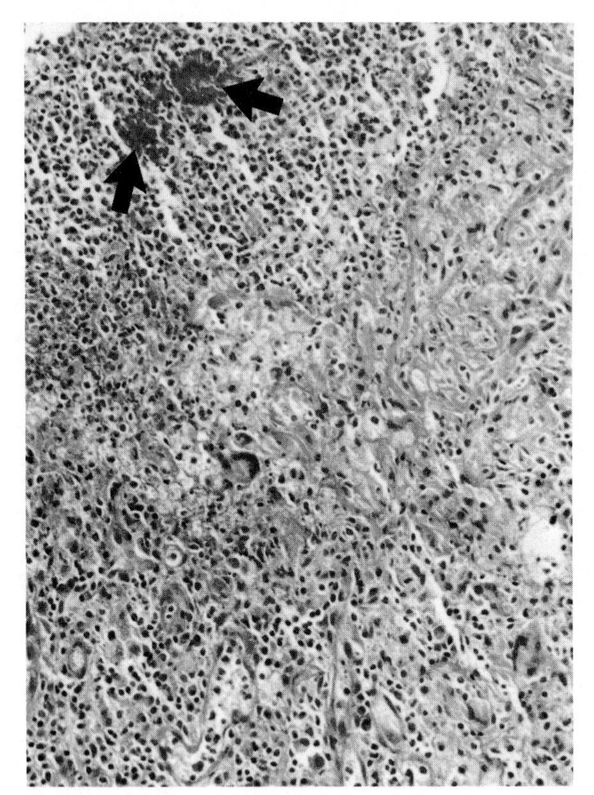

Figure 5-10. Pulmonary actinomycosis. A mass resected to exclude a neoplasm was found to be a necrotizing granulomatous and inflammatory process. Microabscesses contained a few small sulfur granules within the purulent debris (arrows). Scattered giant cells can be seen in the fibrotic wall.

■ Pulmonary Actinomycosis (Fig. 5-10)

Actinomyces infection of the lung is thought to follow aspiration of oral or tonsillar *actinomyces*. This disorder is more common in individuals with poor dentition or repeated tonsillitis.

There may be an inflammatory mass in the lung or mediastinum. The pulmonary lesion takes the form of large abscesses with a peripheral rim of granulation tissue and fibrosis; within the purulent center sulfur granules are found. These are basophilic in appearance and have a granular character. They may be surrounded by a radiating eosinophilic proteinaceous halo, the Splendore-Hoeppli reaction. Sulfur granules vary from microscopic to a few millimeters in size. The organism is gram-positive, silver-positive, and acid-fast-negative.

Treatment is resection or intravenous penicillin. Actinomycosis should be distinguished from pulmonary botryomycosis and nocardiosis.

References

Thurlbeck WM (ed). Pathology of the Lung. New York, Thieme, 1988.

■ Malakoplakia of the Lung (Figs. 5-11 to 5-13)

Malakoplakia represents an abnormal response to a chronic infection with the accumulation of characteristic histiocytes. It is usually seen in the genitourinary system, although many other sites of involvement have been described, including the lung. Most of the patients described with lung involvement have been immunosuppressed, and most have had nodular lesions, which on biopsy show the typical features of malakoplakia: background chronic inflammatory infiltrate of plasma cells and lymphocytes with sheets of histiocytes containing abundant eosinophilic cytoplasm in which numerous lysosomes and occasional classical Michaelis-Gutmann bodies can be found. Typically, there are scattered small microabscesses of neutrophils among the histiocytes.

The diagnosis of malakoplakia should be restricted to cases in which Michaelis-Gutmann bodies can be identified. A xanthogranulomatous reaction is relatively common in chronic abscesses, in obstructive pneumonia, in legionellosis, and in some cases of chronic bronchitis.

References

Colby TV, Pelzmann K, Carrington CB. Malakoplakia of the lung: a report of two cases. Respiration 39:295-299, 1980.

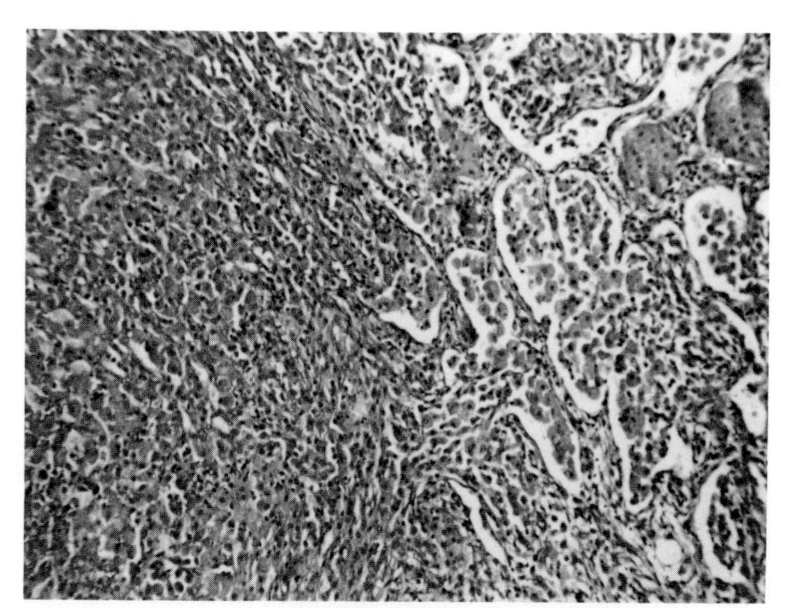

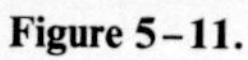

Figure 5–11.

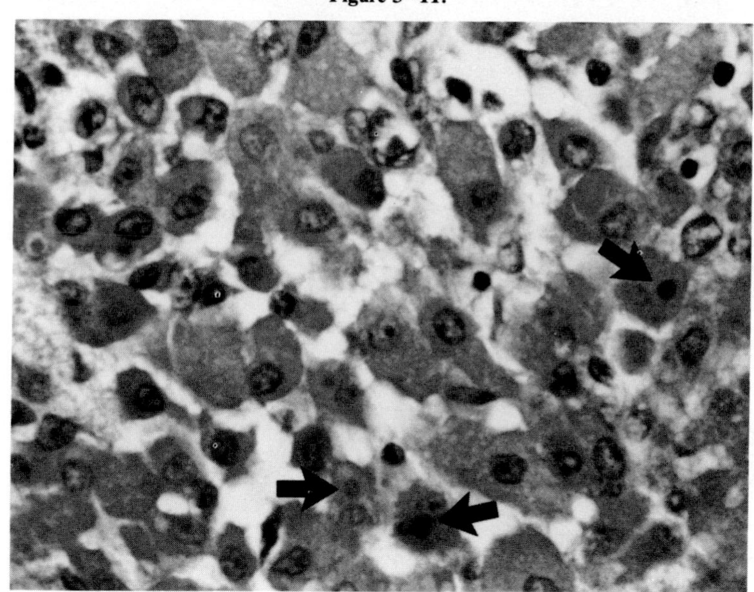

Figure 5–12.

Figures 5–11, 5–12. Malakoplakia. Pulmonary malakoplakia in a patient with acquired immunodeficiency syndrome (AIDS). There are multiple nodules composed entirely of histiocytes, some of which showed central abscess formation. At the edge of the nodules, the histiocytes spill into alveolar spaces. The histiocytes have abundant eosinophilic cytoplasm, and in many of them, typical Michaelis-Gutmann bodies (arrows) can be identified. These bodies are calcified phagolysosomes. Phagolysosomes are generally numerous and are stained with periodic acid–Schiff (PAS) stain. Small colonies of bacteria (*Rhodococcus equi* in this case) could be identified in tiny foci of acute inflammation.

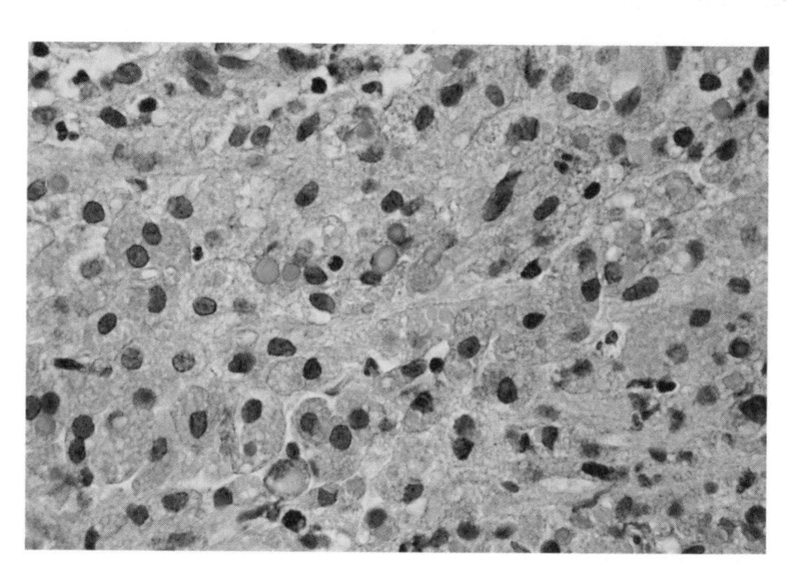

Figure 5–13. Malakoplakia. Pulmonary malakoplakia in a patient with a history of Hodgkin's disease. Transbronchial biopsy showed sheets of eosinophilic histiocytes containing grayish Michaelis-Gutmann bodies.

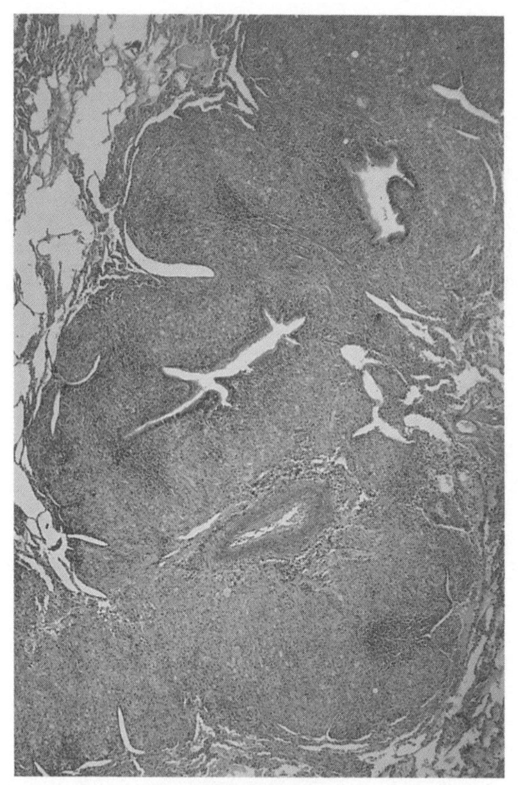

Figure 5-14.

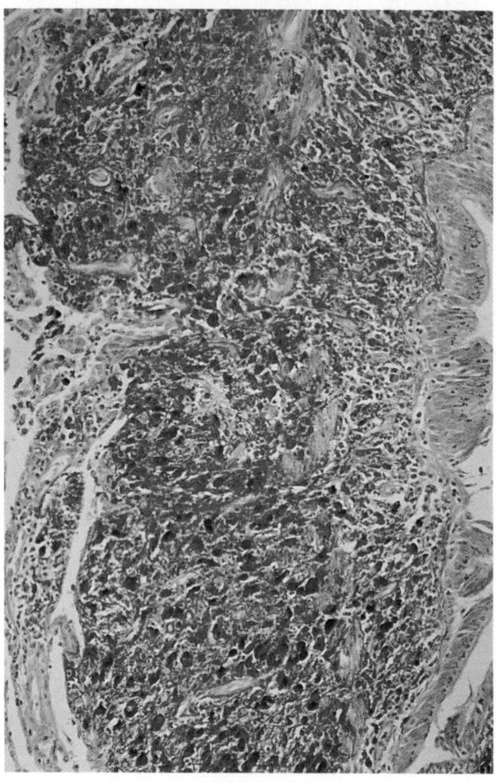

Figure 5-15.

■ Whipple's Disease of the Lung (Figs. 5-14 and 5-15)

Whipple's disease usually affects the gastrointestinal tract. Although rare, pulmonary involvement has been reported. Histologically, there are sheets of histiocytes that contain PAS-positive granules along bronchovascular bundles. The histiocytes are somewhat more granular and foamy in appearance than in malakoplakia. The diagnosis can be confirmed by electron microscopy, clinical correlation, or biopsy of more typical gastrointestinal lesions.

References

Winberg CD, Rose M, Rappaport H. Whipple's disease of the lung. Am J Med 65:873-880, 1978.

Figures 5-14, 5-15. Whipple's disease. There is a thick peribronchiolar and perivascular cuff of histiocytes containing abundant periodic acid-Schiff (PAS)-positive material. Intestinal involvement was confirmed both histologically and ultrastructurally.

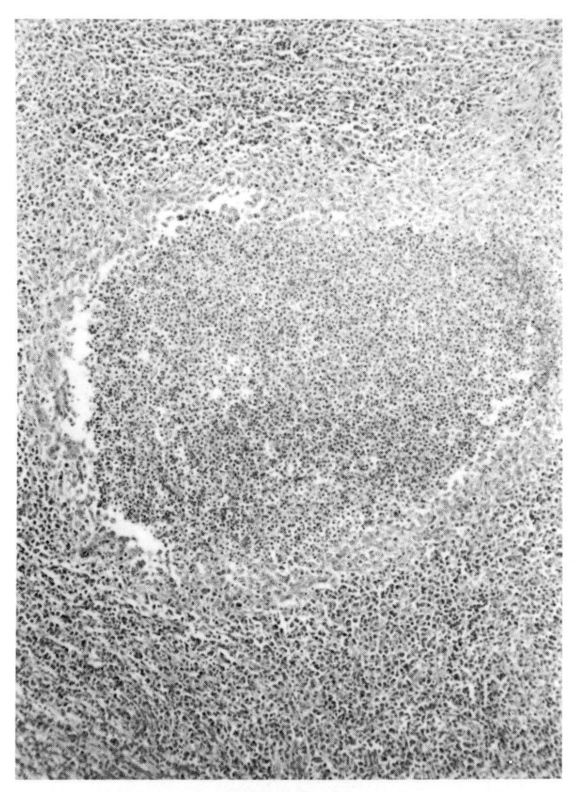

Figure 5–16.

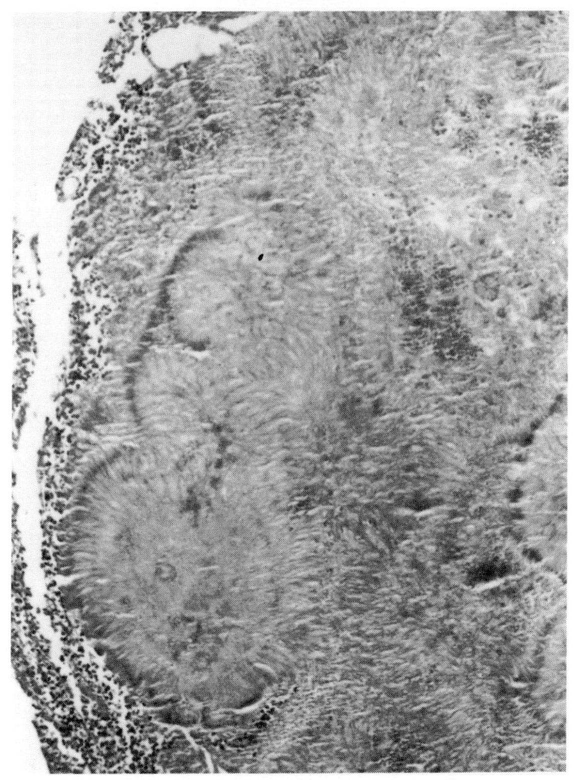

Figure 5–17.

■ Pulmonary Botryomycosis (Figs. 5–16 and 5–17)

Pulmonary botryomycosis is a chronic granulomatous and suppurative bacterial infection of the lung associated with abscesses and scarring. Immunologically intact hosts and patients with cystic fibrosis may be affected.

Histologically, there is acute and chronic inflammation with abscesses and granulomatous reaction. Sulfur granules resembling those seen in actinomycosis can be found, and they are composed of the causative bacteria. *Staphylococcus aureus* is most often implicated. Other causative organisms include *Pseudomonas aeruginosa, Proteus* sp., and *Streptococcus* sp.

References

Dail DH, Hammer SP (eds). Pulmonary Pathology. New York, Springer-Verlag, 1988.

Thurlbeck WM (ed). Pathology of the Lung. New York, Thieme, 1988.

Figures 5–16, 5–17. Pulmonary botryomycosis (bacterial pseudomycosis). A necrotizing granulomatous process with central neutrophilic microabscess is surrounded by a histiocytic and chronic inflammatory infiltrate. From another case, a colony of gram-positive cocci resembles a sulfur granule.

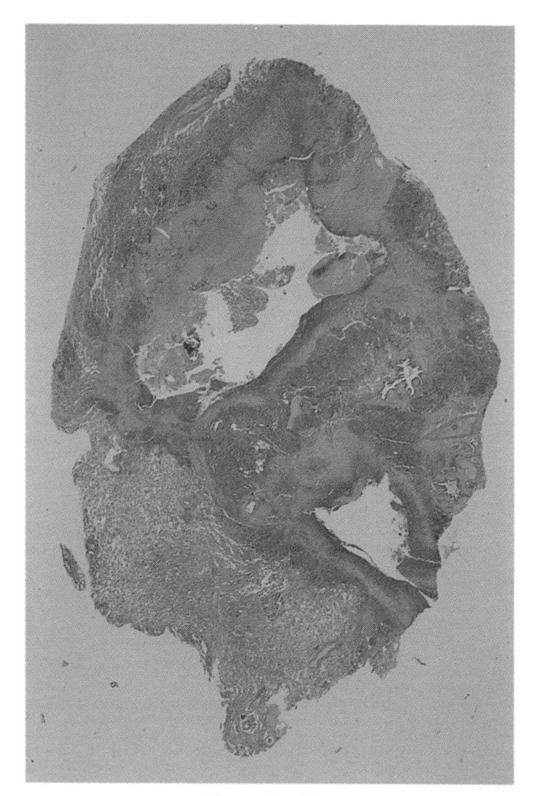

Figure 5-18.

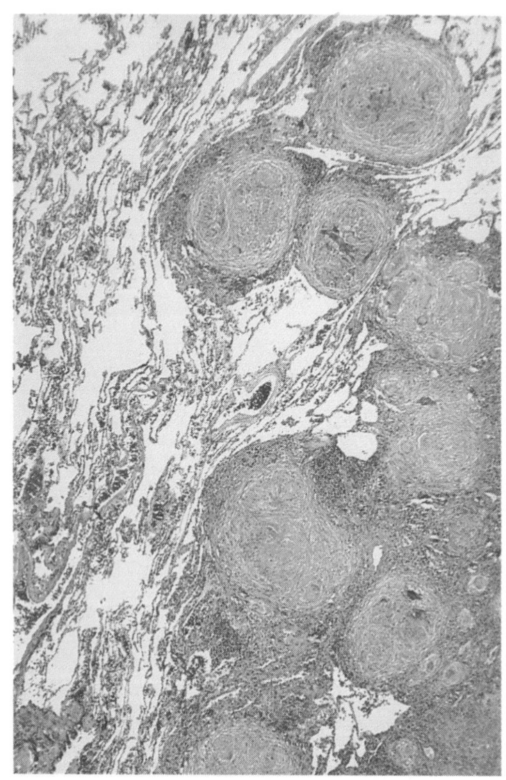

Figure 5-19.

Figures 5-18, 5-19. Pulmonary tuberculosis. Upper lobe expansile cavities are lined by necrotizing granulomatous inflammation associated with marked chronic inflammation and scarring.

■ Mycobacterial Infections (Including Atypical Mycobacteria) (Figs. 5-18 to 5-23)

Mycobacterial infections are generally seen in a biopsy specimen taken for specific diagnosis or as a resection in a patient with known infection that is refractory to treatment. Infections occur in both normal and immunosuppressed hosts.

Usually, single upper-lobe masses with or without cavitation are apparent; occasionally, the infection presents as a miliary process with scattered granulomatous nodules with or without necrosis.

The histologic appearance is generally similar for all mycobacteria: necrotizing (caseous) granulomatous inflammation, sometimes with a variable amount of acute inflammation; and small satellite granulomas with or without necrosis. Identification of organisms may necessitate a long and careful search and the staining of multiple levels with special stains. Poor granuloma formation should raise the possibility of immunodeficiency.

Uncommon histologic patterns seen in atypical mycobacterial infections have included eosinophilic pneumonia, diffuse interstitial fibrosis, organizing pneumonia, and a desquamative interstitial pneumonia (DIP)-like reaction.

Note: A lack of organisms on special stains is common and does not exclude a diagnosis of infection. Negative cultures are much more important than negative special stains in excluding mycobacterial infection. Needless to say, no method of confirming or excluding a diagnosis is foolproof. Finally, some nonpathogenic mycobacteria occur in tap water and may contaminate slides.

Turning down the light intensity of the microscope facilitates screening for and recognition of acid-fast organisms.

References

Dail DH, Hammer SP (eds). Pulmonary Pathology. New York, Springer-Verlag, 1988.

Farhi DC, Mason UG, Horsburgh CR. Pathologic findings in disseminated *Mycobacterium avium-intracellulare* infection. Am J Clin Pathol 85:67-72, 1986.

Marchevsky A, Damsker B, Gribetz A, et al. The spectrum of pathology of nontuberculous mycobacterial infections in open lung biopsy specimens. Am J Clin Pathol 78:695-700, 1982.

Thurlbeck WM (ed). Pathology of the Lung. New York, Thieme, 1988.

Wright JL, Pare PD, Hammond M, Donevan RE. Eosinophilic pneumonia and atypical mycobacterial infection. Am Rev Respir Dis 127:497-499, 1983.

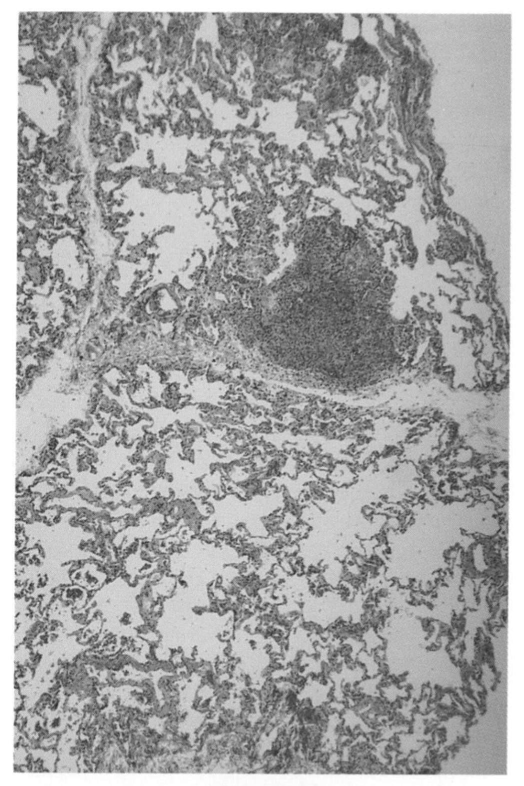

Figure 5-20.

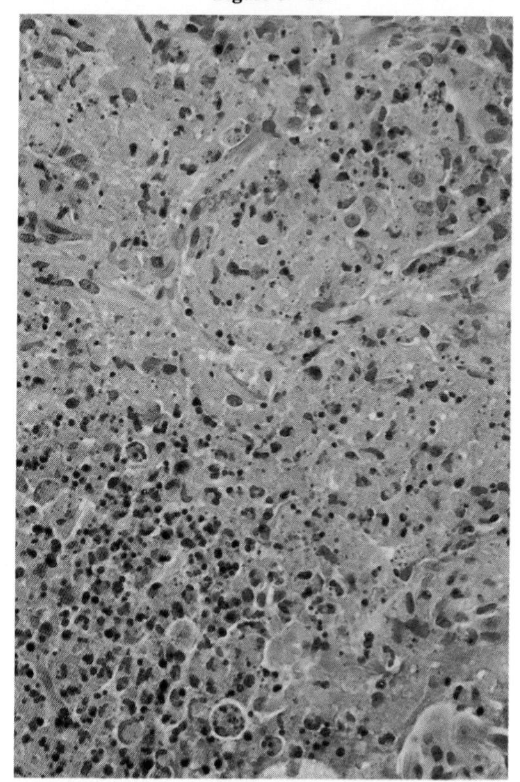

Figure 5-21.

Figures 5-20, 5-21. Miliary tuberculosis in an immunosuppressed host. There are scattered necrotizing nodules composed of neutrophils and necrotic debris. A true granulomatous reaction is not present. Special stains showed relatively numerous acid-fast organisms.

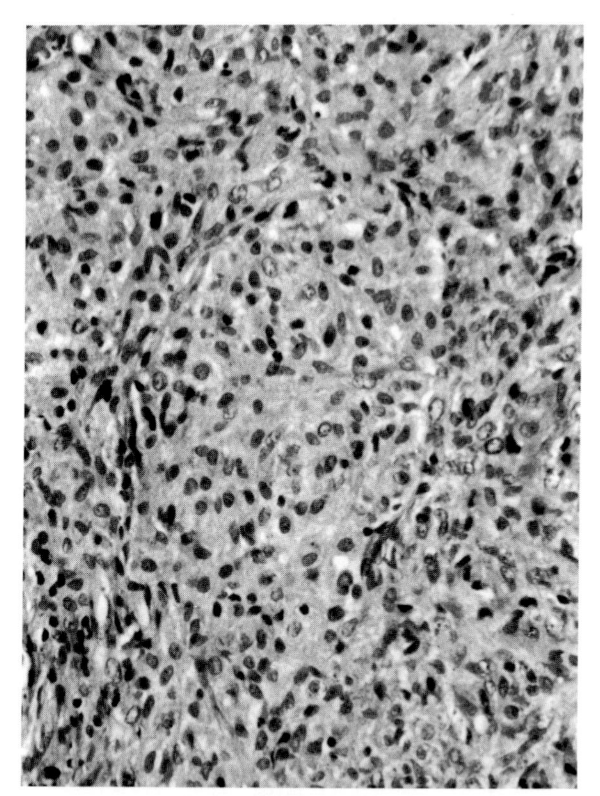

Figure 5-22.

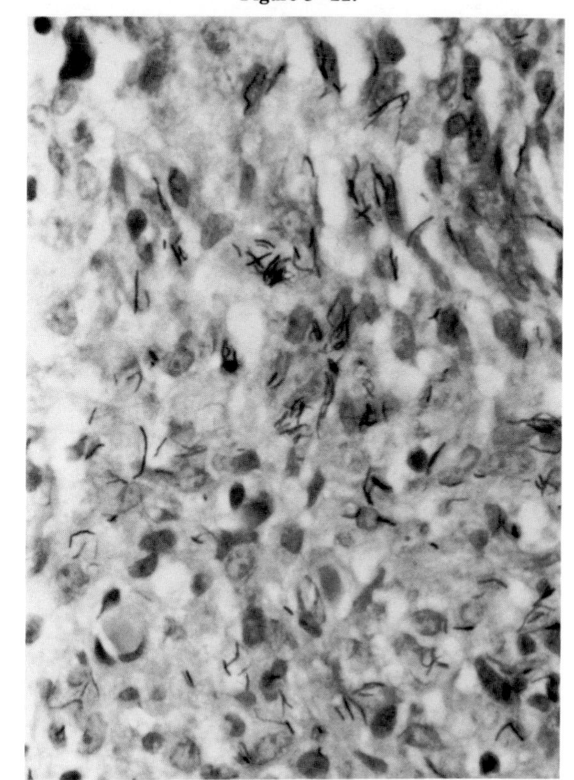

Figure 5-23.

Figures 5-22, 5-23. *Mycobacterium avium intracellulare.* *Mycobacterium avium intracellulare* infection in the lung in acquired immunodeficiency syndrome (AIDS). Large nodules of histiocytes have only a vaguely granulomatous character to them. Giant cells, necrosis, and purulent inflammation are absent. Acid-fast stain shows large numbers of organisms in the histiocytes.

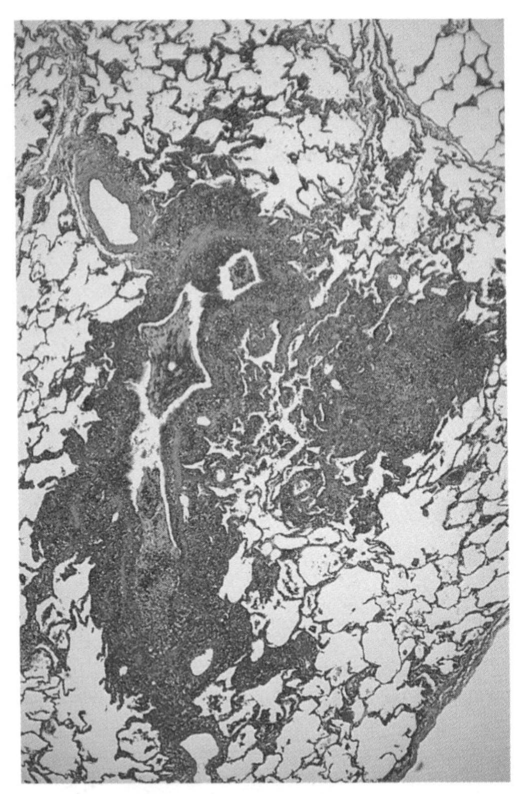

Figure 5-24.

■ Mycobacterial and Fungal Infections Producing Clinical Diffuse Interstitial Lung Disease

Miliary mycobacterial or fungal infections may produce an acute diffuse interstitial lung disease. Chest radiographic findings show a typical miliary distribution of small nodules.

Histologically one sees miliary granulomatous inflammation in the lung parenchyma manifesting as small granulomatous nodules with or without necrosis without any specific distribution (a helpful feature in the distinction from sarcoid). Vessels and/or airways, however, may be affected and some cases suggest perivascular predilection. Organisms are usually seen on special stains. In occasional cases, one must rely on cultures, serologic tests, or both for the diagnosis.

Differential diagnosis includes sarcoidosis; allergic alveolitis, which generally lacks necrosis; and noninfectious granulomas, including Wegener's granulomatosis, necrotizing sarcoid, and bronchocentric granulomatosis.

References

Dail DH, Hammer SP (eds). Pulmonary Pathology. New York, Springer-Verlag, 1988.

Flint A, Colby TV. Surgical Pathology of Diffuse Infiltrative Lung Disease. Orlando, Grune & Stratton, Inc, 1987.

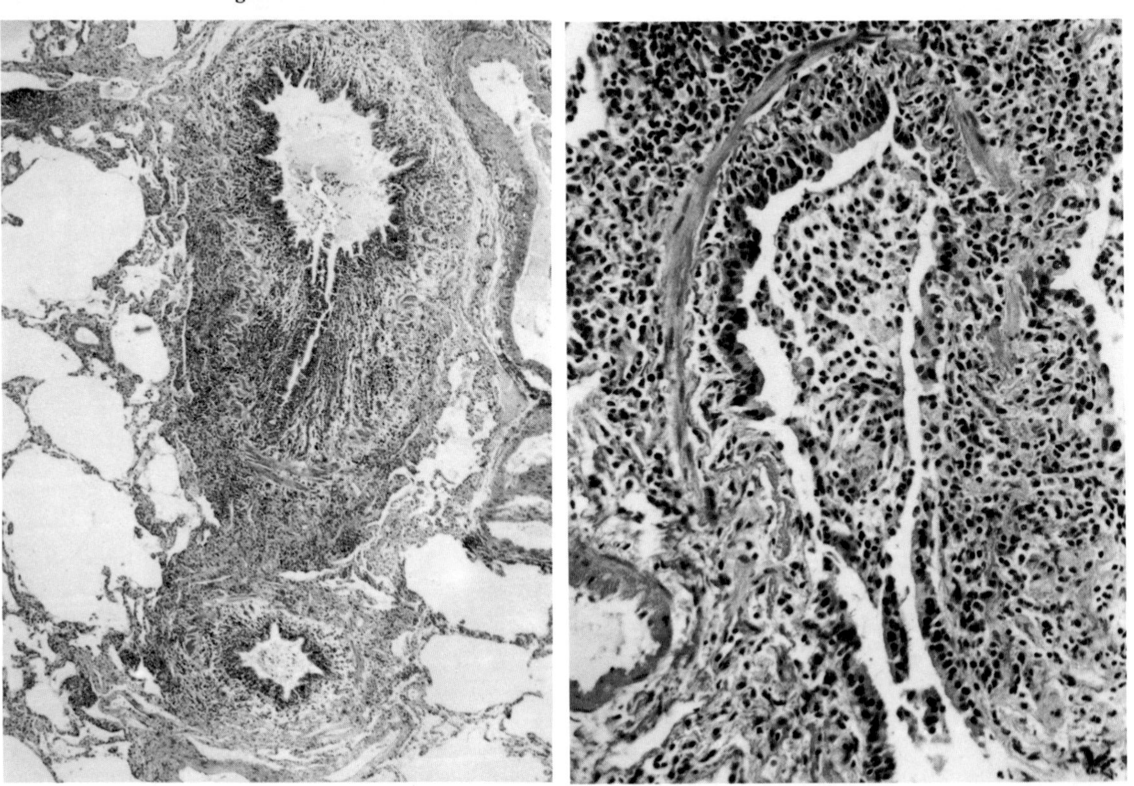

Figure 5-25. Figure 5-26.

Figures 5-24, 5-25, 5-26. *Mycoplasma pneumoniae* pneumonia. Mycoplasma pneumonias affect primarily the small airways and are best visualized at scanning power microscopy. One sees an acute inflammatory exudate in the lumen and chronic inflammation in the wall with numerous plasma cells. Characteristically, metaplastic epithelium lines the airway because the organism preferentially attacks the ciliated cells.

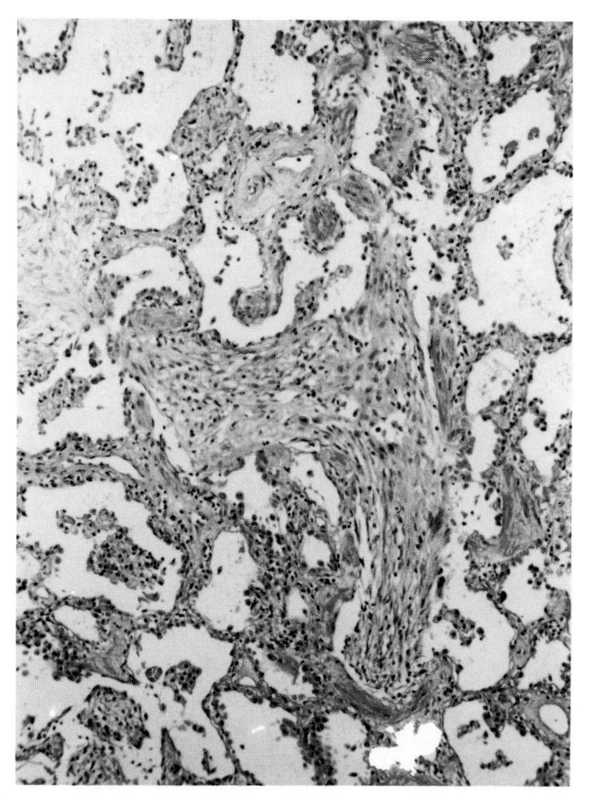

Figure 5-27. Organizing *Mycoplasma pneumoniae* pneumonia. The histologic features are those of a nonspecific organizing pneumonia. The diagnosis of mycoplasma infection was confirmed serologically.

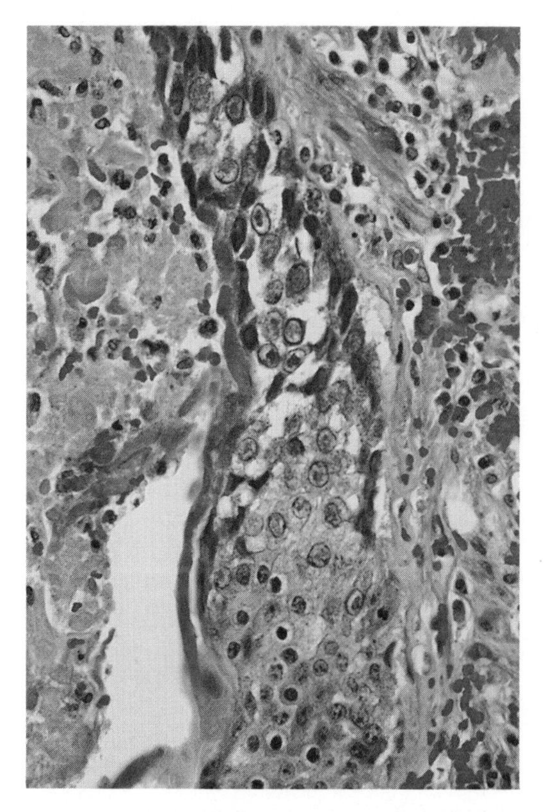

Figure 5-28. Herpetic bronchitis. Adjacent to metaplastic squamoid bronchiolar epithelium there are cells with intranuclear inclusions typical of herpes.

■ *Mycoplasma pneumoniae* Pneumonia (Figs. 5-24 to 5-27)

There is a cellular bronchiolitis with acute inflammatory exudate within the bronchioles and a chronic inflammatory infiltrate rich in plasma cells in bronchiolar walls. Bronchiolar epithelium is replaced by metaplastic cells lacking cilia (the organism attacks ciliated cells). Rarely, a pattern of diffuse alveolar damage is seen. Healed lesions may be associated with constrictive bronchiolitis.

Ultrastructural studies show organisms adherent to ciliated bronchiolar epithelium. Such studies, however, are not practical in diagnostic work.

Diagnosis is usually made on the basis of serologic data, rarely on the basis of culture. Histologic features are characteristic but nonspecific.

References

Rollins S, Colby TV. Open lung biopsy in *Mycoplasma pneumoniae* pneumonia. Arch Pathol Lab Med 110:34-41, 1986.

Thurlbeck WM (ed). Pathology of the Lung. New York, Thieme, 1988.

■ Herpes Simplex Pneumonia (Figs. 5-28 to 5-35, 5-44, and 5-45)

Herpes simplex may involve the lung by either airway or blood-borne dissemination. Blood-borne dissemination occurs almost exclusively in the severely immunocompromised patient. Spread of herpes through the airway also occurs in the immunocompromised patient, but in addition it may occur in patients with inhalation injuries (burn victims) or in those with chronic obstructive pulmonary disease (COPD). Morphologic diagnosis depends on recognition of herpes virus cytopathic changes in infected cells.

Herpetic cytopathic changes include:

1. Mild nucleomegaly (nuclear sizes up to 1.25 to 1.5 times normal size).
2. Dispersion of nuclear chromatin.
3. Condensation of nuclear chromatin on nuclear membrane.
4. Formation of intranuclear viral particles that coalesce, forming eosinophilic viral inclusion surrounded by a clear zone (Cowdry type A inclusion).

Absence of multinucleation of infected cells is common in the lung. Cytoplasmic inclusions are absent, and epithelial cells are affected primarily in contrast to cytomegalovirus (CMV), which often affects *both* epithelial and mesenchymal elements.

The airway pattern of dissemination in herpes pneumonia includes (1) *laryngotracheobronchitis* with purulent necrotizing bronchitis, healing with squamous metaplasia and herpetic intranuclear inclusions; and (2) *bronchopneumonia* with herpetic bronchitis, and necrotizing bronchopneumonia with coagulative necrosis, nuclear debris, and hemorrhage. Herpetic intranuclear inclusions may be hard to find. In severe cases, diffuse alveolar damage is an accompanying feature.

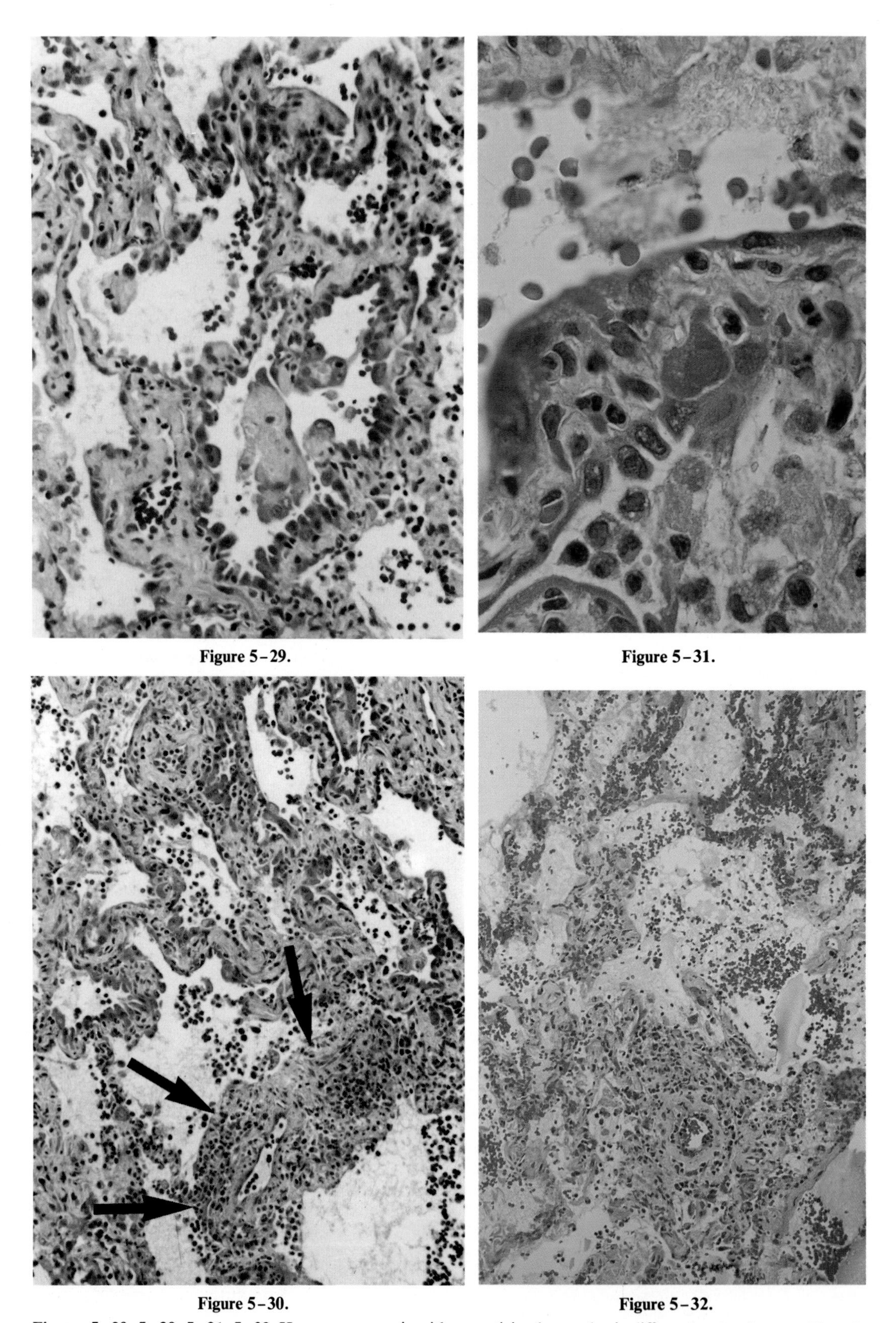

Figure 5-29.

Figure 5-31.

Figure 5-30.

Figure 5-32.

Figures 5-29, 5-30, 5-31, 5-32. Herpes pneumonia with necrotizing hemorrhagic diffuse alveolar damage. There is edema and mild inflammation of alveolar walls, which are lined by reactive type II cells. Around a small vein, an acute and chronic inflammatory infiltrate (arrows) was identified. Occasional cells with intranuclear inclusions typical of herpes were found (Fig. 5-31). Previously, herpes was found in a sputum cytology specimen. Elsewhere in the lung, there was extensive hemorrhagic necrosis attributed to the herpes infection (Fig. 5-32).

Herpes simplex pneumonia from hematogenous dissemination includes (1) a *miliary pattern,* with small inflammatory nodules centered on alveolar septa; mixed acute and chronic inflammation; variable necrosis, coagulative in type; and cells with herpetic intranuclear inclusions; and (2) *diffuse alveolar damage* (DAD), with diffuse interstitial thickening with edema, chronic inflammation, and fibroblasts, hyaline membranes, reactive type II alveolar lining cells, and variable numbers of cells with herpetic inclusions.

Specific diagnosis may require culture or immunostaining.

References

Dail DH, Hammer SP (eds). Pulmonary Pathology. New York, Springer-Verlag, 1988.

Flint A, Colby TV. Surgical Pathology of Diffuse Infiltrative Lung Disease. Orlando, Grune & Stratton, Inc, 1987.

Graham BS, Snell JD Jr. Herpes simplex virus infection of the adult lower respiratory tract. Medicine (Baltimore) 62:384–393, 1983.

Nash G. Necrotizing tracheobronchitis and bronchopneumonia consistent with herpetic infection. Hum Pathol 3:283–291, 1972.

Ramsey PG, Fife KH, Hackman RC, Meyers JD, Corey L. Herpes simplex virus pneumonia: clinical, virologic, and pathologic features in 20 patients. Ann Intern Med 97:813–820, 1982.

Thurlbeck WM (ed). Pathology of the Lung. New York, Thieme, 1988.

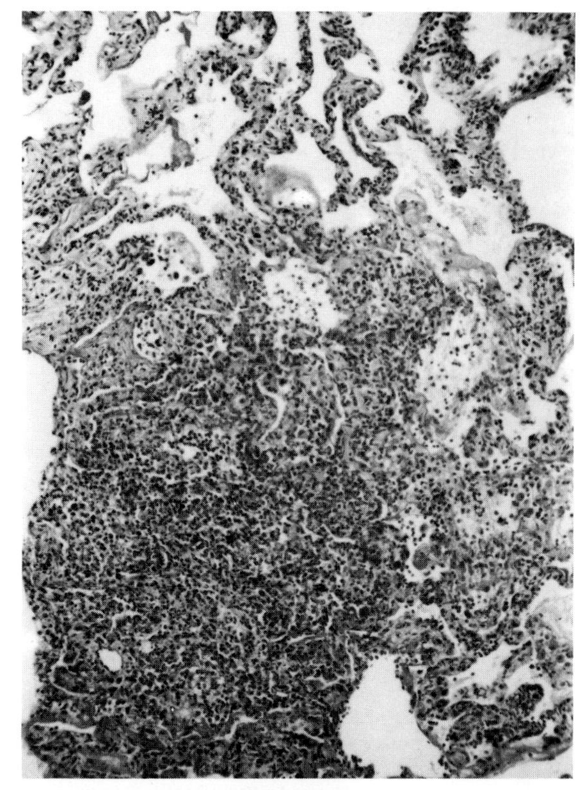

Figure 5–34.

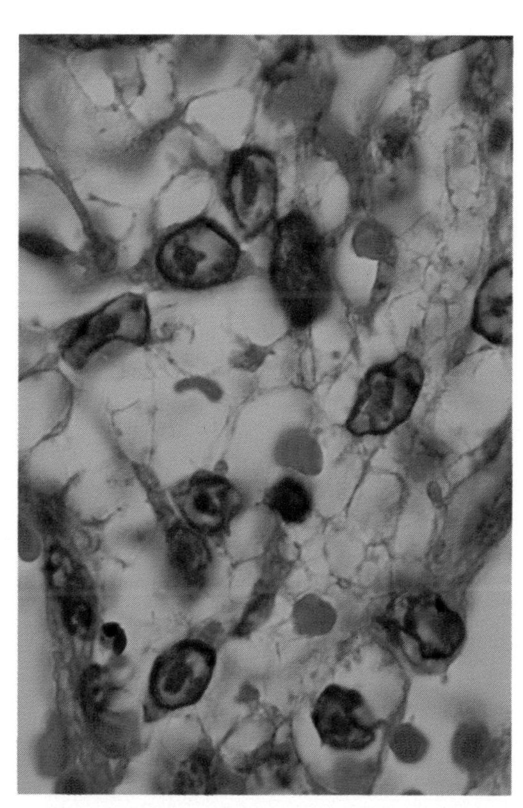

Figure 5–33. Congenital herpes pneumonia. Congenital herpes pneumonia with large numbers of cells showing intranuclear inclusions typical of herpes infection.

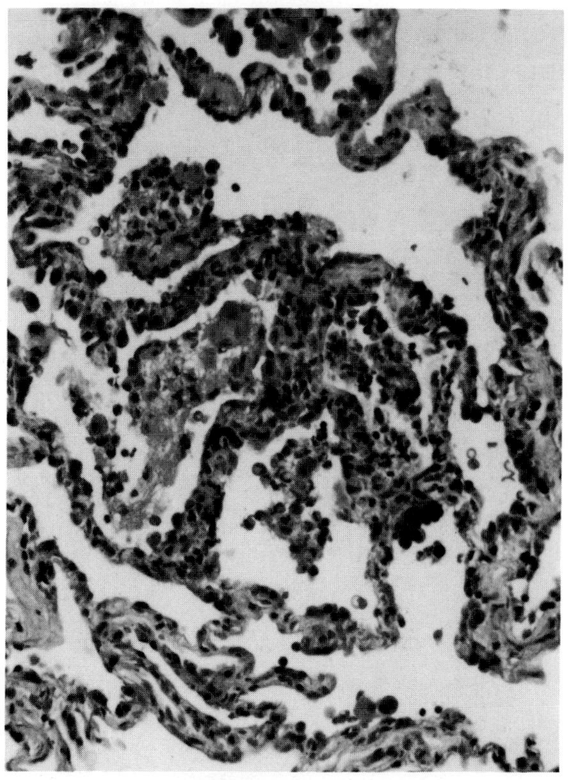

Figure 5–35.

Figures 5–34, 5–35. Miliary herpes pneumonia. Palpable inflammatory nodules (Fig. 5–34) arise from microscopic foci of capillaritis and associated alveolar exudate (Fig. 5–35). In these foci, occasional virally infected epithelial cells were identified. Cultures and immunofluorescence were positive for herpes in this case.

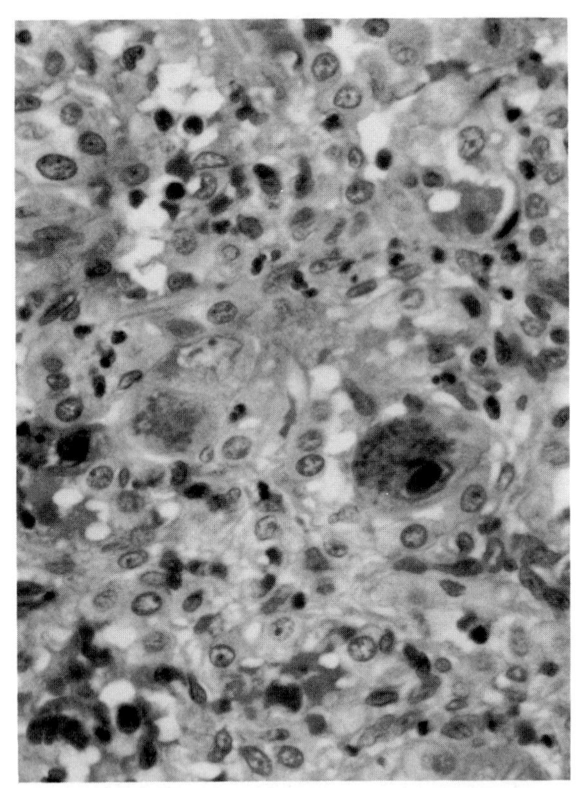

Figure 5–36. Congenital cytomegalovirus (CMV) pneumonia. Congenital cytomegalovirus infection was detected in a neonate, who underwent open biopsy for diagnosis of pulmonary infiltrates. There was extensive airspace and interstitial inflammation associated with numerous virally infected cells. The cell illustrated has the typical features of CMV with cytomegaly, large intranuclear inclusion with surrounding halo and thick nuclear membrane, and irregular basophilic cytoplasmic inclusions.

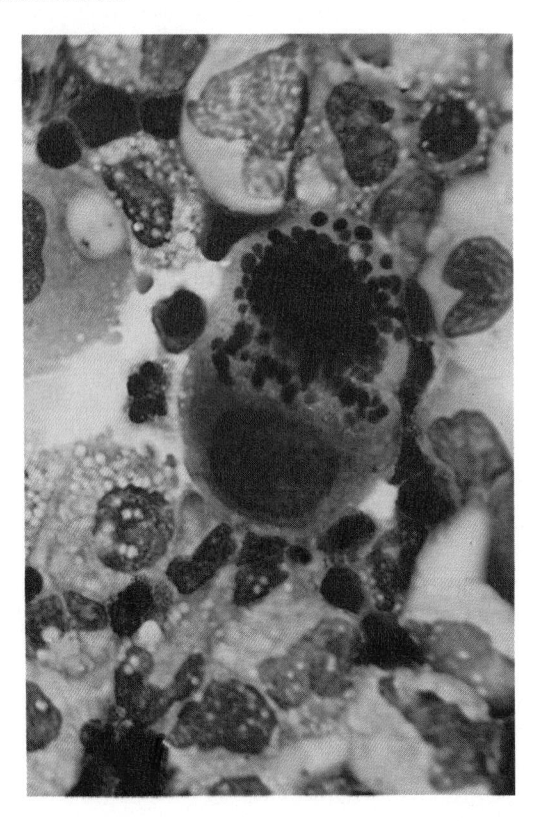

Figure 5–37. CMV-infected cell with both intranuclear and cytoplasmic inclusions as seen in a stain of bronchoalveolar lavage fluid from a patient with acquired immunodeficiency syndrome (AIDS).

■ Cytomegalovirus Pneumonia (Figs. 5–36 to 5–45)

CMV pneumonia occurs almost exclusively in the immunocompromised host. There are two patterns of disease associated with CMV pneumonitis: (1) diffuse interstitial pneumonitis and (2) miliary (nodular) pneumonitis. Histologic diagnosis of CMV is dependent on the recognition of CMV-type cytopathic change in infected cells. Immunostaining is diagnostically helpful and probably more sensitive than routine histology.

CMV cytopathic changes include (1) cytomegaly (two to three times larger than normal size, with both the nucleus and the cytoplasm enlarged); (2) amphophilic to basophilic nuclear inclusion with a peripheral halo; and (3) basophilic granular cytoplasmic inclusion bodies, which are PAS-positive and Grocott-positive.

Note: CMV-infected cells may be seen in uninflamed lung, since cytomegalovirus is known to occur as a commensal organism in immunosuppressed individuals.

CMV interstitial pneumonitis is within the spectrum of diffuse alveolar damage and includes:

1. Interstitial widening by edema and mononuclear inflammation;
2. Alveolar fibrinous exudates;
3. Variable numbers of hyaline membranes;
4. Variable interstitial and airspace organization by fibroblasts and macrophages; and
5. CMV-type inclusions in pneumocytes, histiocytes, and endothelial cells.

CMV miliary pneumonitis (hematogenous dissemination) includes:

1. Numerous small, scattered, inflammatory nodules centered on alveolar capillaries, which are composed of collections of mononuclear cells and neutrophils associated with a fibrinous alveolar exudate, hemorrhage, patchy necrosis, and reactive hyperplastic alveolar lining cells; and
2. CMV cytopathic change.

(*Note:* This change may affect only a few cells and may be difficult to identify.)

In any case in which CMV is identified in the lung, the distinction between pathogenic CMV and commensal CMV is important. Cases must be individualized with clinical correlation and exclusion of other organisms and noninfectious causes of lung disease.

Some CMV-infected cells may resemble those seen in herpes and adenovirus infections, and specific diagnosis may require culture or immunostaining.

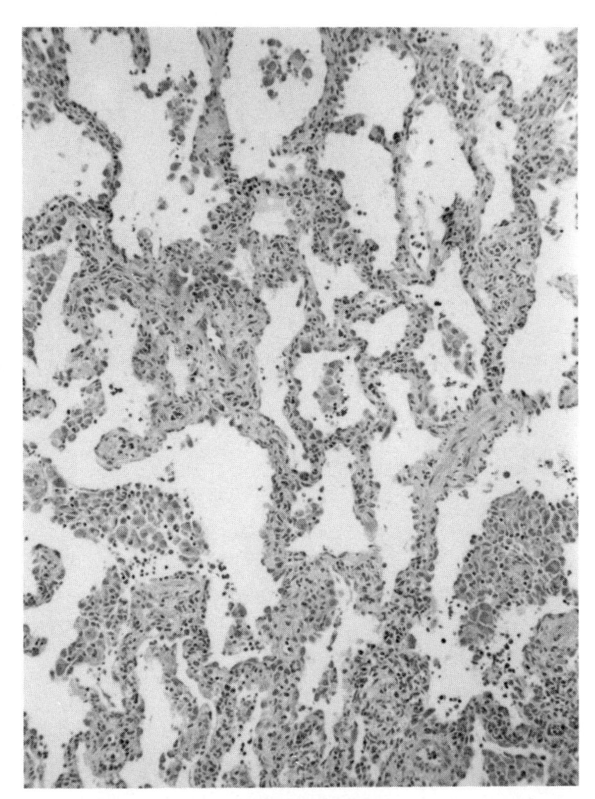

Figure 5-38.

References

Beschorner WE, Hutchins GM, Burns WH, Saral R, Tutschka PJ, Santos GW. Cytomegalovirus pneumonia in bone marrow transplant recipients: miliary and diffuse patterns. Am Rev Respir Dis 122:107-114, 1980.

Craighead, JE. Cytomegalovirus pulmonary disease. Pathobiol Annu 5:197-220, 1975.

Dail DH, Hammer SP (eds). Pulmonary Pathology. New York, Springer-Verlag, 1988.

Flint A, Colby TV. Surgical Pathology of Diffuse Infiltrative Lung Disease. Orlando, Grune & Stratton, Inc, 1987.

Myerson D, Hackman RC, Nelson JA, Ward DC, McDougall JK. Widespread presence of histologically occult cytomegalovirus. Hum Pathol 15:430-439, 1984.

Thurlbeck WM (ed). Pathology of the Lung. New York, Thieme, 1988.

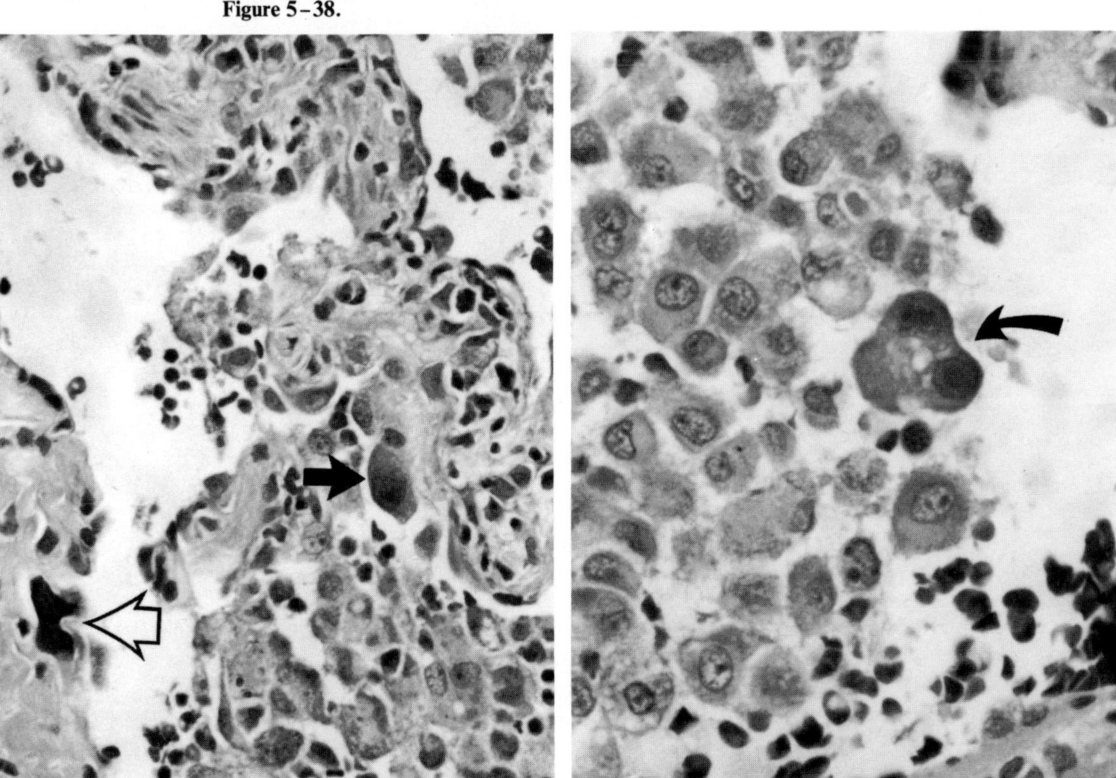

Figure 5-39. Figure 5-40.

Figures 5-38, 5-39, 5-40. CMV pneumonia in a heart transplant patient. There is a diffuse mild interstitial infiltrate associated with edema of the alveolar walls and prominent type II cells, some of which were large and bizarre in appearance (arrow); although virally infected cells occurred only rarely, they could be identified morphologically (curved arrow). Immunofluorescent studies of smears from tissue showed numerous positive cells, many more than could be appreciated on the histologic slides. An incidental megakaryocyte is present (hollow arrow).

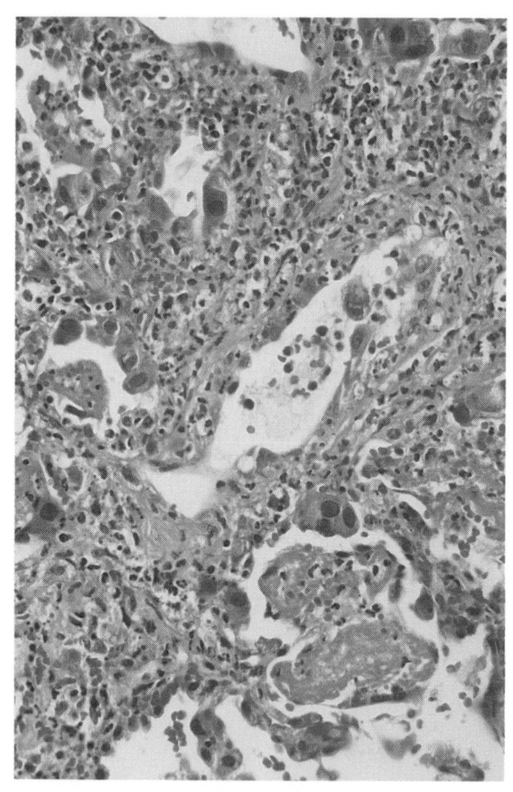

Figure 5-41.

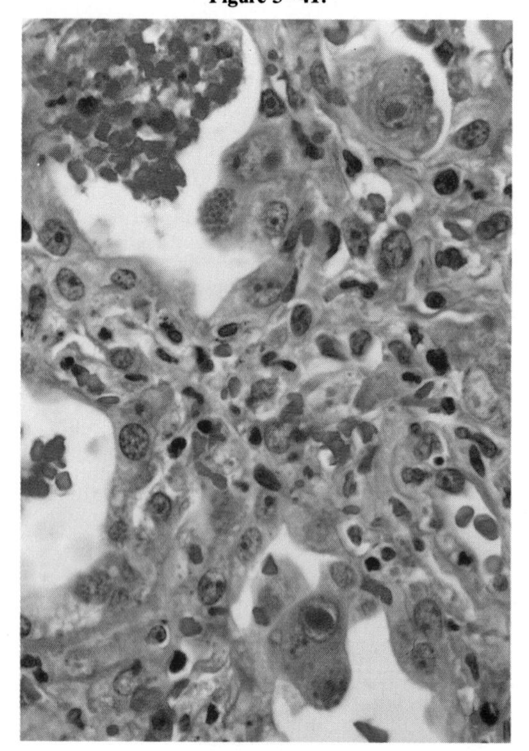

Figure 5-42.

Figures 5-41, 5-42. CMV pneumonia in a liver transplant patient with diffuse interstitial pneumonia and large numbers of infected cells in the air spaces.

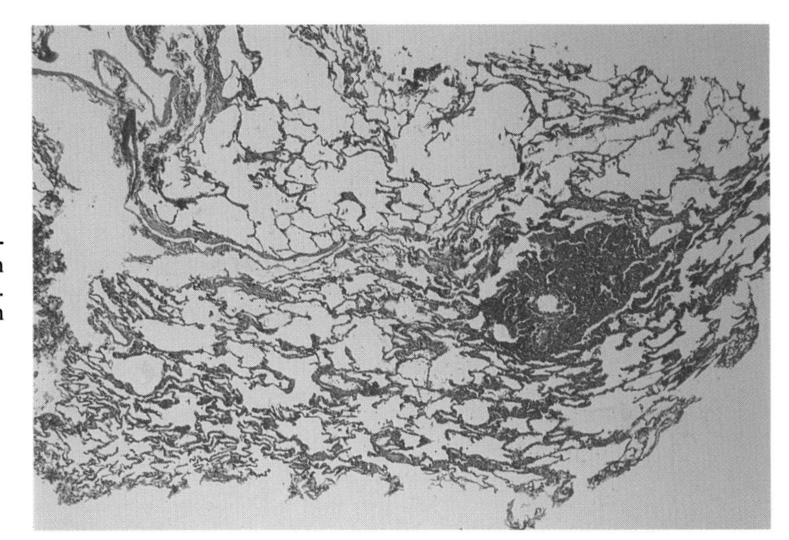

Figure 5-43. Miliary cytomegalovirus (CMV) pneumonia. Discrete inflammatory nodules identical to those seen in miliary herpes pneumonia at low power are shown. Large numbers of CMV-infected cells were found within the nodules.

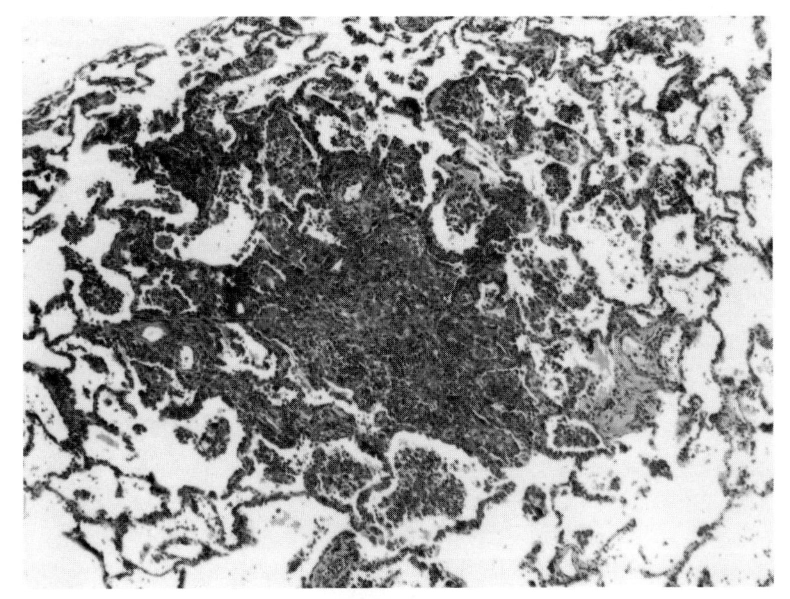

Figure 5-44.

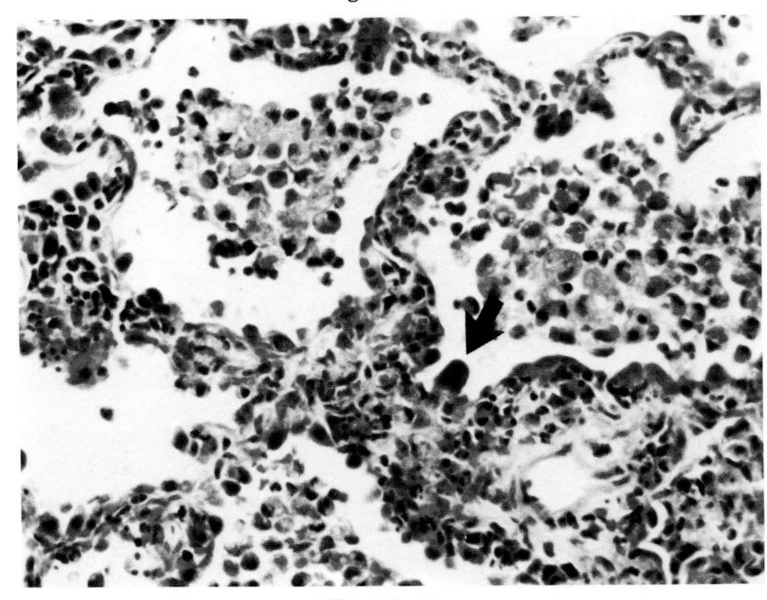

Figure 5-45.

Figures 5-44, 5-45. Mixed herpes and cytomegalovirus (CMV) miliary pneumonia. Sections show inflammatory nodules composed of interstitial and airspace inflammation and exudation with central necrosis. At the periphery of these nodules, there is capillaritis, and virally infected cells were easy to find. Some of the infected cells showed basophilic cytoplasmic inclusions typical of CMV, whereas others were smaller and suggestive of a herpes virus. Cultures and immunofluorescent studies confirmed the presence of both viruses. It would be impossible to determine by purely morphologic features which virus caused the inclusion illustrated (arrow).

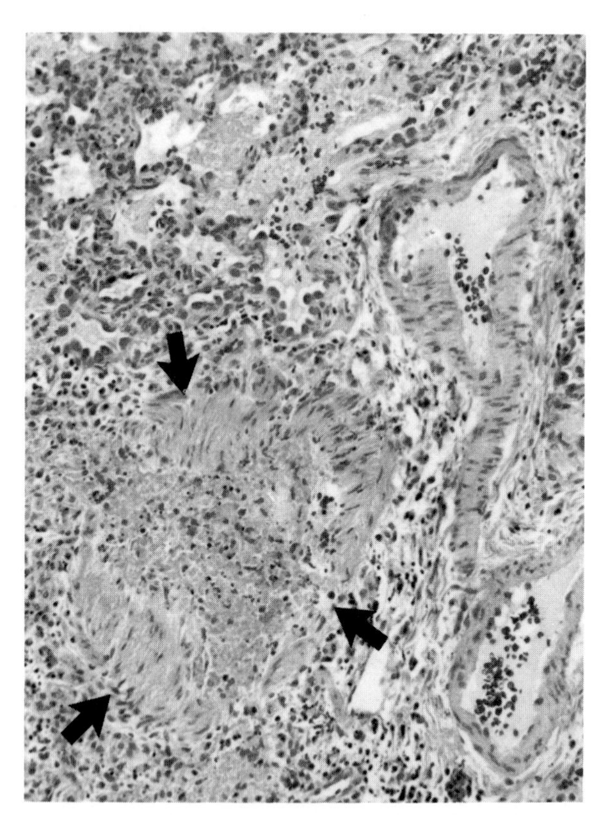

Figure 5-46. Adenovirus pneumonia in a child. Open biopsy material shows a complete necrosis and sloughing of bronchiolar epithelium (arrows) with reactive changes in the surrounding alveoli. No inclusions were seen, and the diagnosis was confirmed ultrastructurally and by culture.

■ Adenovirus Pneumonia (Figs. 5-46 to 5-51)

Adenovirus pneumonia is an infection generally found in children, and biopsy is rarely performed. It may cause fulminant pneumonia in the immunosuppressed, leading to a biopsy.

The histologic findings in the acute phase are a cellular bronchiolitis with necrosis of bronchiolar walls; viral inclusions may be recognized as either smudge cells or Cowdry type A inclusions. DAD, particularly in immunosuppressed patients, also occurs. A late healed phase, producing constrictive bronchiolitis with obstruction, is seen.

Adenovirus cytopathic changes include:

1. Herpetic-type alterations with intranuclear eosinophilic inclusions, halo surrounding the inclusion, and chromatin condensation on nuclear membrane; and
2. Smudge cell alteration with basophilic nuclear inclusions with no clear chromatinic rim around the inclusion.

The electron microscopic findings of crystalline hexagonal viral particles are typical of adenovirus. The diagnosis may also be made by culture, by serologic studies, or by immunostaining.

References

Becroft DMO. Histopathology of fatal adenovirus infection of the respiratory tract in young children. J Clin Pathol 20:561-569, 1967.

Dail DH, Hammer SP (eds). Pulmonary Pathology. New York, Springer-Verlag, 1988.

Flint A, Colby TV. Surgical Pathology of Diffuse Infiltrative Lung Disease. Orlando, Grune & Stratton, Inc, 1987.

Katzenstein ALA, Askin FB. Surgical Pathology of Non-Neoplastic Lung Disease, 2nd ed. Philadelphia, WB Saunders, Co, 1990.

Mark EJ. Lung Biopsy Interpretation. Baltimore, Williams & Wilkins, 1984.

Thurlbeck WM (ed). Pathology of the Lung. New York, Thieme, 1988.

Zahradnik JM, Spencer MJ, Porter DD. Adenovirus infection in the immunocompromised patient. Am J Med 68:725-732, 1980.

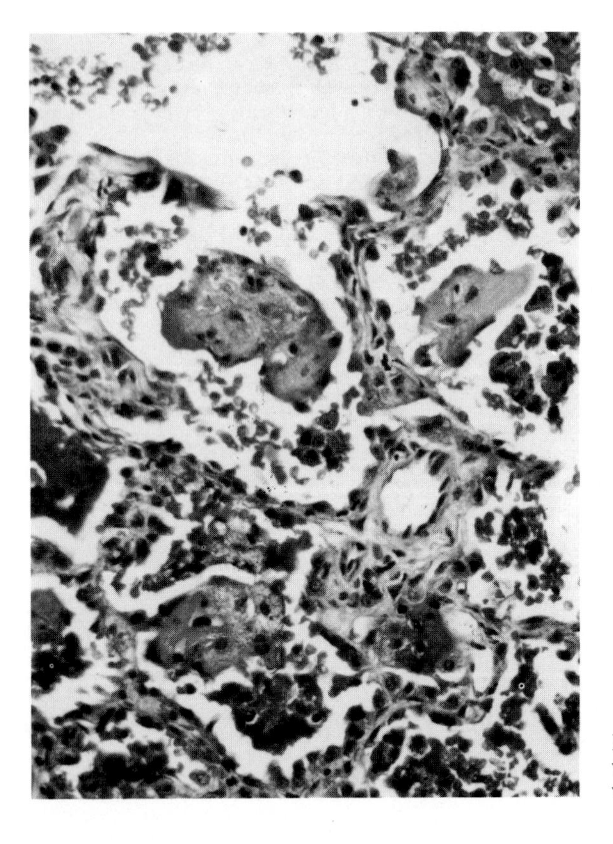

Figure 5-47. Adenovirus pneumonia with diffuse alveolar damage in a patient with systemic lupus erythematosus (SLE) on steroid therapy. No inclusions were seen, and the diagnosis was made by electron microscopy.

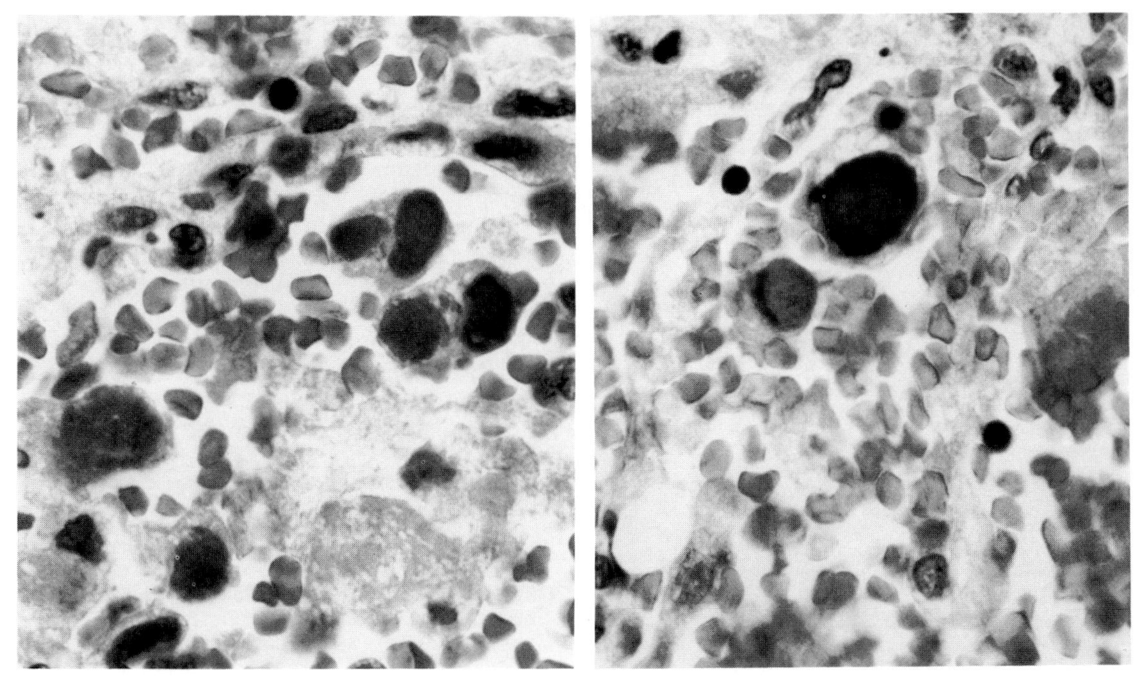

Figure 5-48.

Figure 5-50.

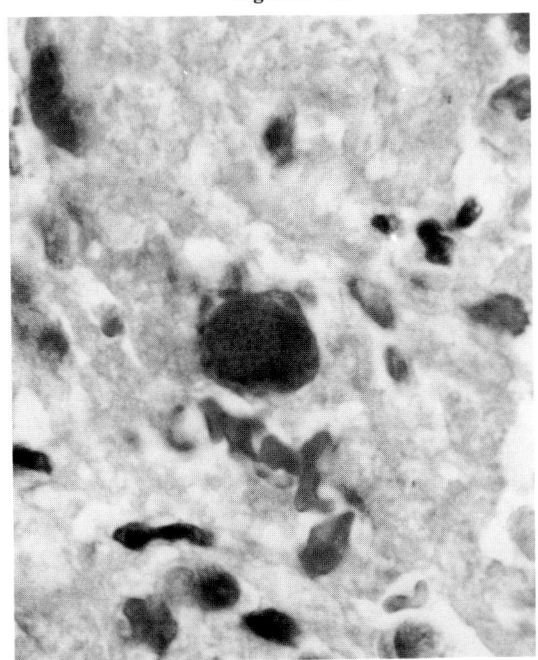

Figure 5-49.

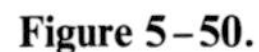

Figures 5-48, 5-49, 5-50. Adenovirus. Fatal adenovirus pneumonia in a bone marrow transplant recipient. The variety of cytopathic effects of adenovirus is illustrated, including a "ground glass" change in the nuclei with peripheral chromatin clumping, a suggestion of crystalline arrays, and a smudge cell change with markedly hyperchromatic forms.

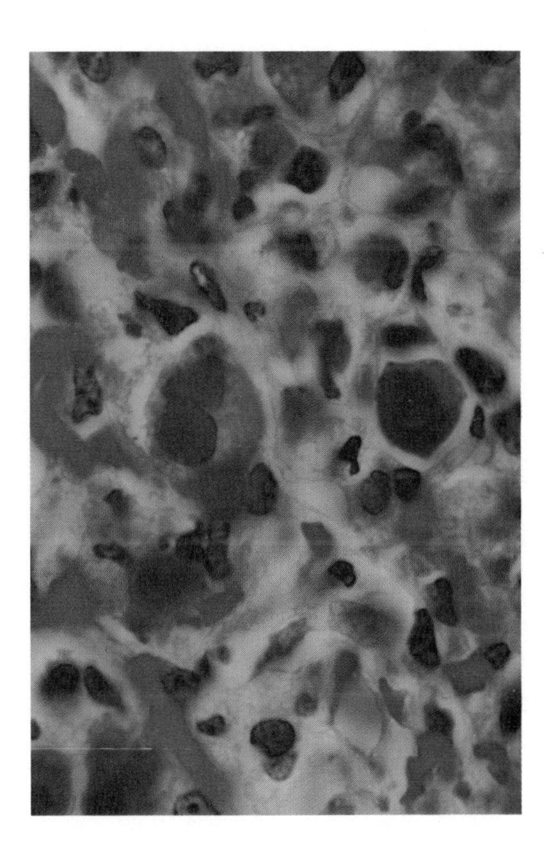

Figure 5-51. Adenovirus pneumonia showing a smudge cell adjacent to a binucleate cell containing eosinophilic intranuclear inclusions.

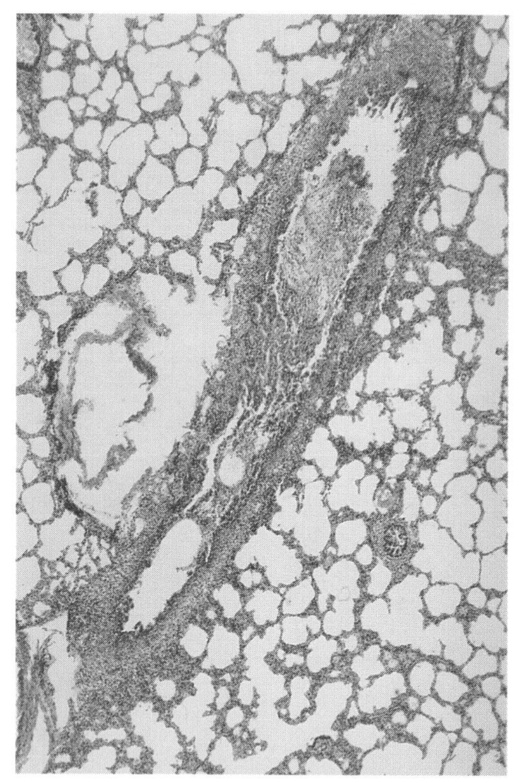

Figure 5-52.

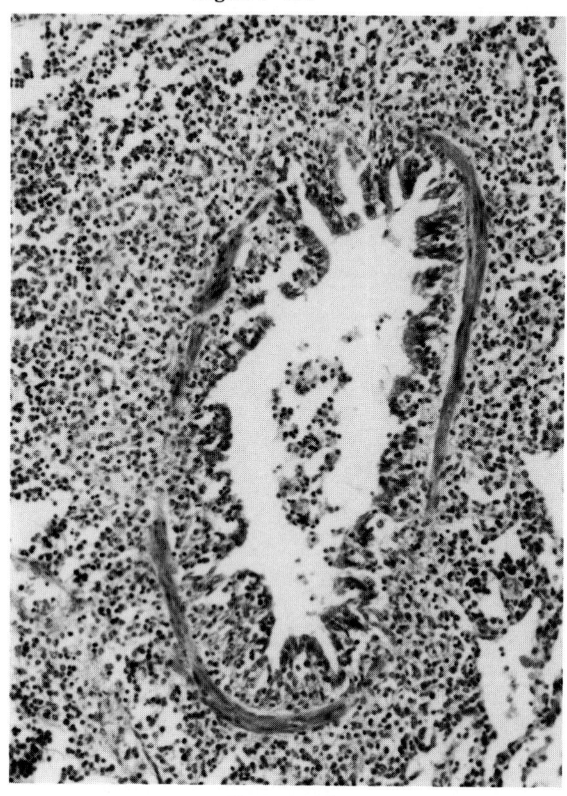

Figure 5-53.

■ Respiratory Syncytial Virus Pneumonia (Figs. 5-52 to 5-56)

Respiratory synctial virus (RSV) pneumonia is usually seen in babies and young children and a biopsy is rarely performed. Immunosuppressed individuals may also develop RSV pneumonia.

Histologically, there is a cellular, predominantly lymphocytic, bronchiolitis, with acute inflammation in the lumen and metaplastic bronchiolar epithelium (sometimes with cellular syncytia). Small inconspicuous eosinophilic cytoplasmic inclusions may occasionally be appreciated in the metaplastic bronchiolar cells.

Diagnosis is made by serologic studies, by culture, or by immunologic detection of the agent.

References

Dail DH, Hammer SP (eds). Pulmonary Pathology. New York, Springer-Verlag, 1988.

Flint A, Colby TV. Surgical Pathology of Diffuse Infiltrative Lung Disease. Orlando, Grune & Stratton, Inc, 1987.

Thurlbeck WM (ed). Pathology of the Lung. New York, Thieme, 1988.

■ Parainfluenza Virus Pneumonia

Parainfluenza virus is usually seen in children. A biopsy is rarely performed.

Histologic findings are those of a cellular bronchiolitis, or more rarely, a cellular interstitial pneumonia, sometimes with giant cells.

The diagnosis is usually made by culture or serologic study. Rarely, electron microscopy may suggest the diagnosis.

References

Dail DH, Hammer SP (eds). Pulmonary Pathology. New York, Springer-Verlag, 1988.

Flint A, Colby TV. Surgical Pathology of Diffuse Infiltrative Lung Disease. Orlando, Grune & Stratton, Inc, 1987.

Thurlbeck WM (ed). Pathology of the Lung. New York, Thieme, 1988.

Figures 5-52, 5-53. Fatal respiratory syncytial virus (RSV) pneumonia. There is a cellular bronchiolitis with modest numbers of acute inflammatory cells in the lumen and a prominent mural infiltrate of chronic inflammatory cells.

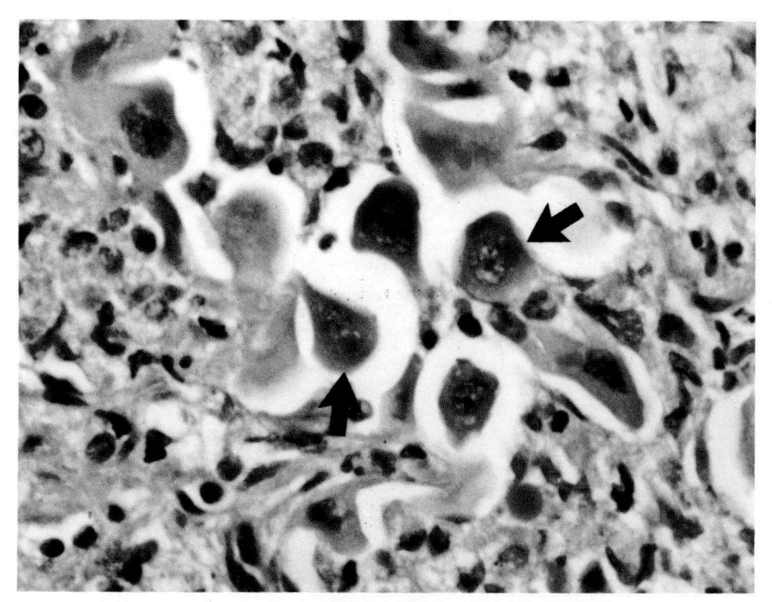

Figure 5-54.

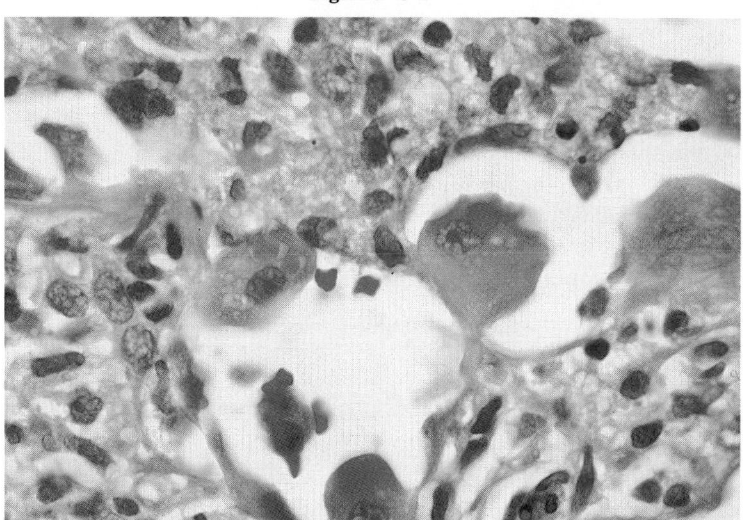

Figure 5-55.

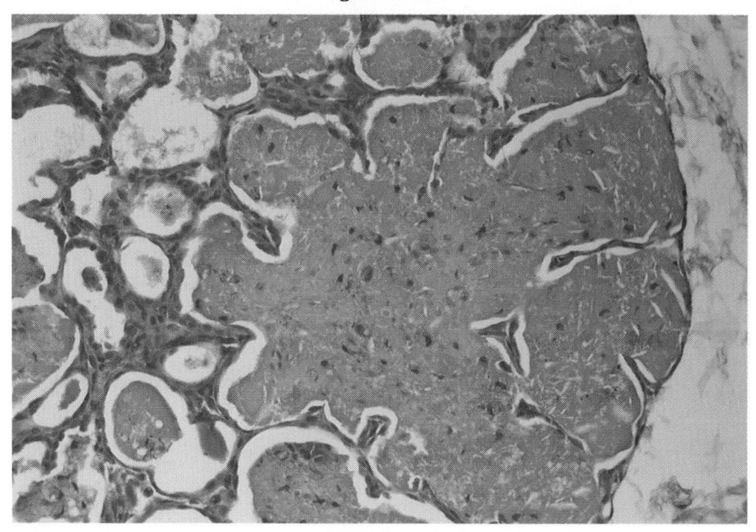

Figure 5-56.

Figures 5-54, 5-55, 5-56. Fatal RSV pneumonia in congenital combined immunodeficiency syndrome. Type II alveolar lining cells are transformed into large bizarre forms, some of which are multinucleated and many of which contain small eosinophilic cytoplasmic inclusions (arrows). Many of the adjacent airspaces showed a pseudoproteinosis reaction (Fig. 5-56).

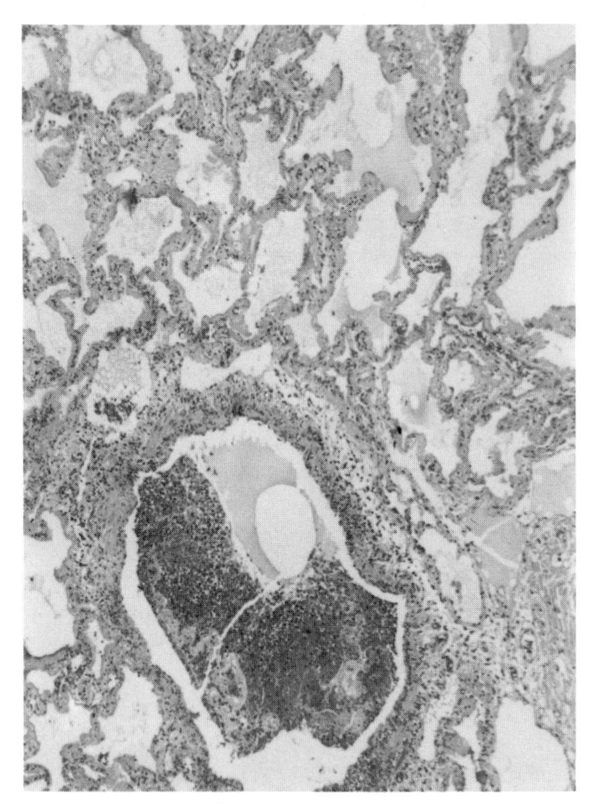

Figure 5-57.

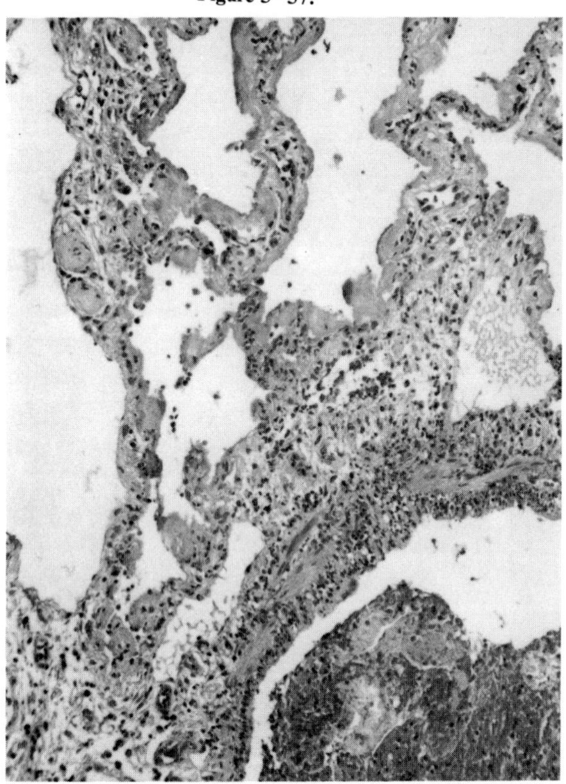

Figure 5-58.

■ Influenza Pneumonia (Figs. 5-57 to 5-60)

Occasionally, influenza pneumonia is seen at autopsy, but biopsy specimens are rarely submitted in suspected cases.

In mild cases, a chronic pulmonary infiltrate appears in the airway walls corresponding to the laryngotracheobronchitis seen clinically. In more severe cases, necrosis of airway epithelium is associated with diffuse hemorrhagic alveolar damage. Healing phases may be identical to bronchiolitis obliterans organizing pneumonia (BOOP), whereas healed cases may be associated with interstitial scarring and a variable degree of cellular infiltrate.

The diagnosis is usually made by culture or serologic findings.

References

Dail DH, Hammer SP (eds). Pulmonary Pathology. New York, Springer-Verlag, 1988.

Oseasohn R, Adelson L, Kaji M. Clinicopathologic study of 33 fatal cases of Asian influenza. N Engl J Med 260:509-518, 1959.

Thurlbeck WM (ed). Pathology of the Lung. New York, Thieme, 1988.

Figures 5-57, 5-58. Acute influenza B pneumonia. Open biopsy findings show a necrotizing bronchiolitis with loss of bronchiolar mucosa and acute inflammatory exudate in the lumen. Surrounding alveoli show diffuse alveolar damage with hyaline membranes.

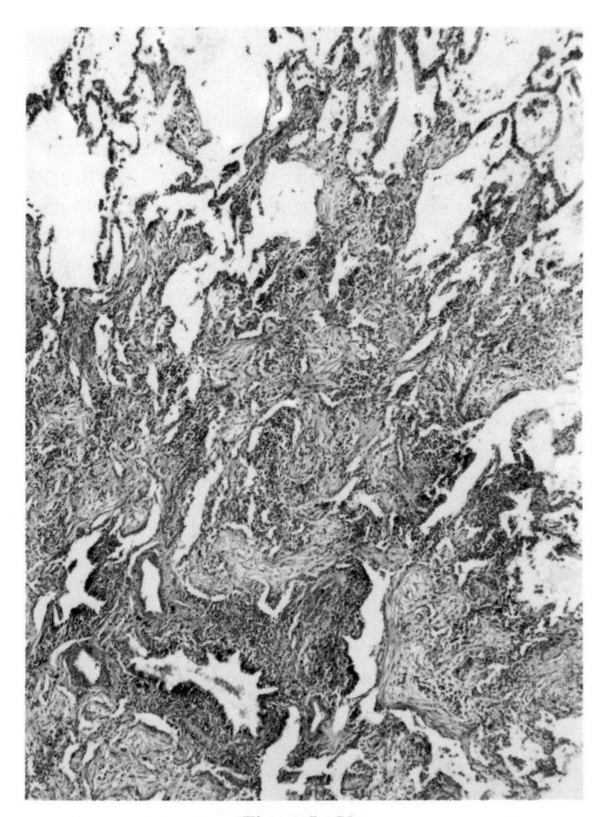

Figure 5-59.

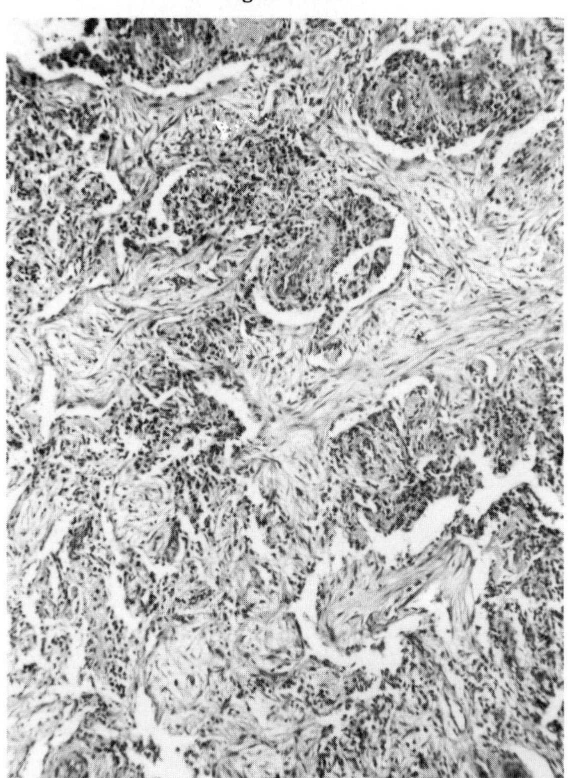

Figure 5-60.

Figures 5-59, 5-60. Organizing influenza A pneumonia. Shown here is a nonspecific proliferative bronchiolitis obliterans and organizing pneumonia that centers on small airways. The diagnosis of influenza A was confirmed by serologic studies. Nevertheless, the patient showed a dramatic response to steroid therapy.

■ Epstein-Barr Virus Pneumonia (Fig. 5-61)

In Epstein-Barr virus (EBV) pneumonia, biopsy is rarely performed, although up to 10 percent of the patients with mononucleosis show signs, symptoms, or chest radiographic evidence of mild pulmonary involvement. The agent has been recognized in immunocompromised organ transplant recipients as a cause of lymphoproliferative lesions which commonly affect the lung.

Histologically, perivascular (especially perivenular) chronic inflammatory infiltrates with plasmacytoid and/or immunoblastic features, cellular bronchiolitis, and interstitial infiltrates are seen.

References

Fermaglich DR. Pulmonary involvement in infectious mononucleosis. J Pediatr 86:93-95, 1975.

Myers JL, Peiper SC, Katzenstein ALA. Pulmonary involvement in infectious mononucleosis: histopathologic features and detection of Epstein-Barr virus-related DNA sequences. Mod Pathol 2:444-448, 1989.

Natvig J. Infectious mononucleosis with multiple organ involvement complicated by pseudomembranous laryngotracheitis: an autopsy report. Acta Pathol Microbiol Scand 56:353-361, 1962.

Timbury MC, Edmond E. Herpes viruses. J Clin Pathol 32:859-881, 1979.

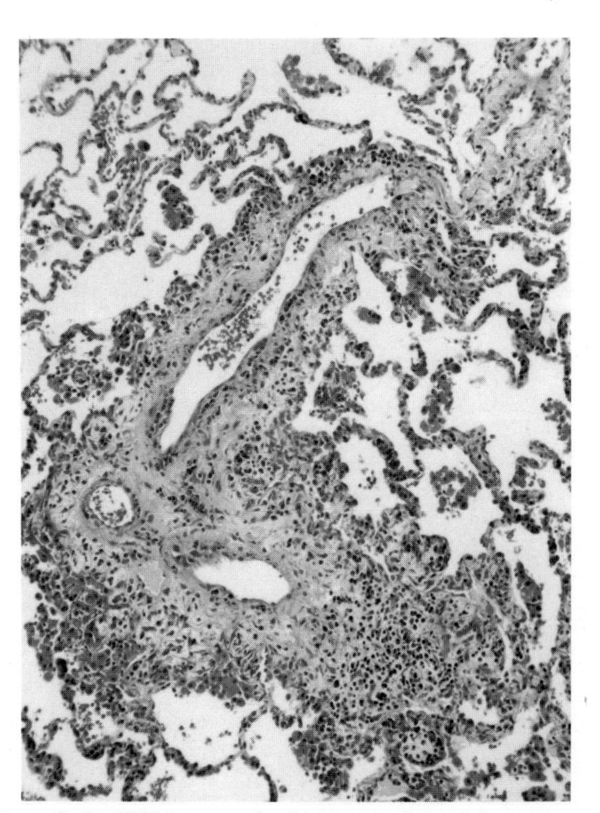

Figure 5-61. EBV (mononucleosis) pneumonia in an immunocompetent individual. Serologic and lymph node biopsy findings were typical of infectious mononucleosis. Because of pulmonary infiltrates, open lung biopsy was performed. The major changes were perivascular infiltrates of lymphocytes, plasma cells, and immunoblasts. Subendothelial infiltration by the cells is seen in this pulmonary vein and is reminiscent of the changes seen in the splenic veins in splenectomy specimens from patients with infectious mononucleosis.

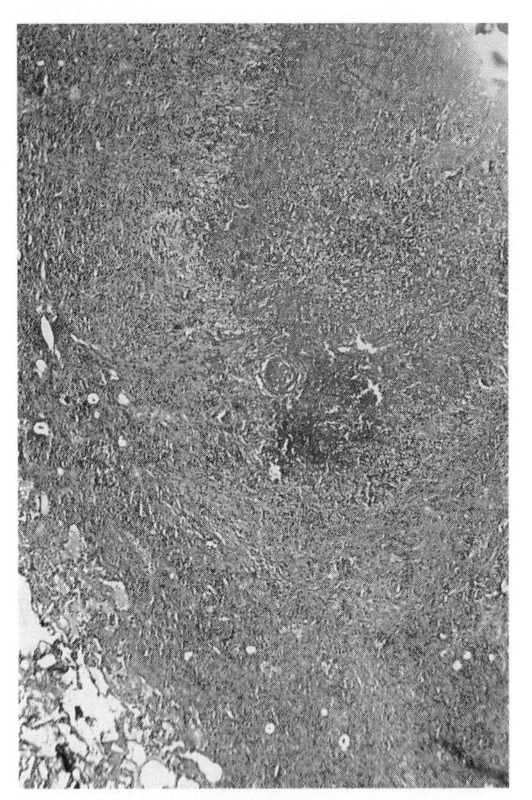

Figure 5-62.

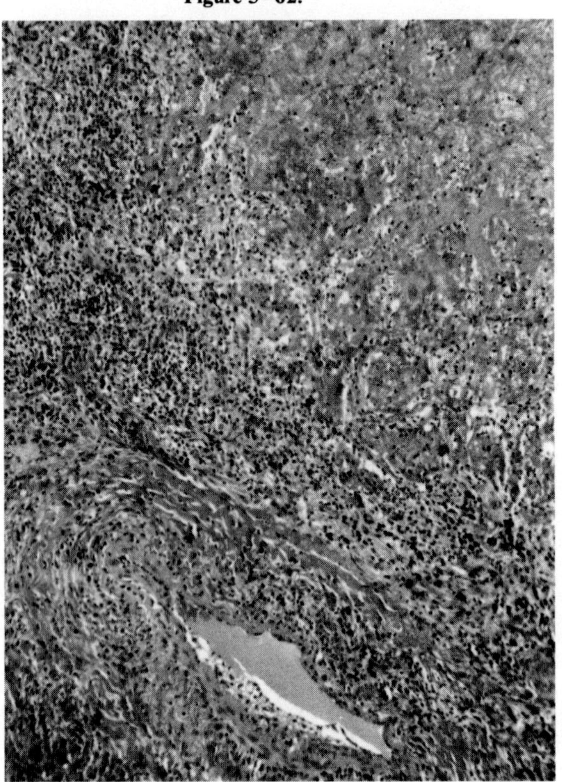

Figure 5-63.

■ Varicella, Measles, Other Viral Infections (Figs. 5-62 to 5-71)

These infections are rarely seen in normal hosts. Varicella produces miliary foci of necrosis, which may become visible radiographically. Inclusions are found at the edge of the necrosis. Measles produces diffuse alveolar damage with multinucleated virally infected type II cells, which are draped over part of the alveolar wall. Eosinophilic intranuclear and intracytoplasmic inclusion 2 to 10 μm (microns) in size are seen.

In many viral syndromes, mild lung involvement may occur. These cases are rarely seen histologically. A few examples are illustrated (Figs. 5-67 to 5-71).

Other agents, including *Chlamydia* and Q fever, represent curiosities for the surgical pathologist. The histologic appearance in these is rarely specific. The diagnosis is usually made by culture, serologic study, or immunohistologic findings.

References

Flint A, Colby TV. Surgical Pathology of Diffuse Infiltrative Lung Disease. Orlando, Grune & Stratton, Inc, 1987.

Figures 5-62, 5-63. Varicella pneumonia. Disseminated varicella pneumonia in a child with small nodules seen on chest radiograph. There is central necrosis with surrounding chronic inflammatory infiltrate. On low-power microscopy, there is a resemblance to a lymphoma. When such lesions heal, they may result in miliary calcified nodules on the chest radiograph.

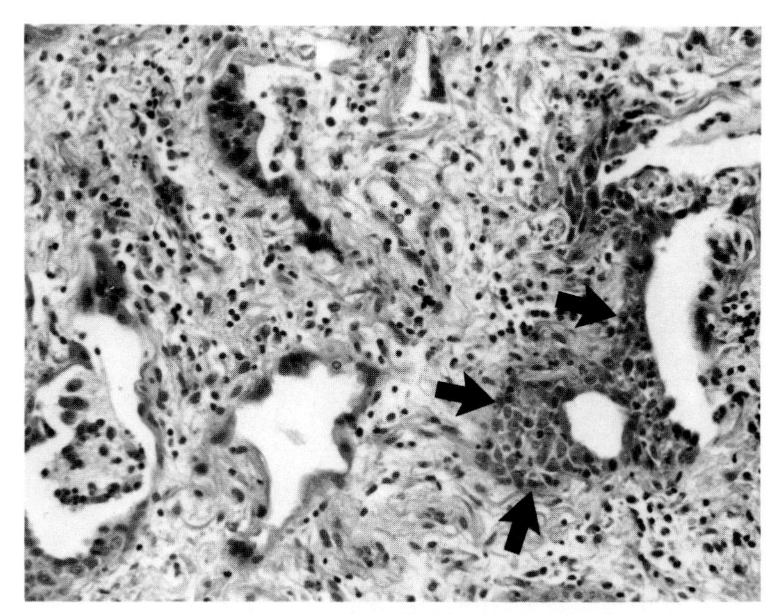

Figure 5–64.

Figures 5–64, 5–65, 5–66. Measles pneumonia in an immunosuppressed patient. The biopsy specimen shows diffuse alveolar damage with squamous metaplasia in the airways extending into some of the surrounding alveolar spaces (arrows). In some of the adjacent alveolar spaces, multinucleated virally infected forms can be contrasted with the squamous metaplasia. The virally infected cells show both eosinophilic nuclear and cytoplasmic inclusions, and they are draped over the alveolar walls.

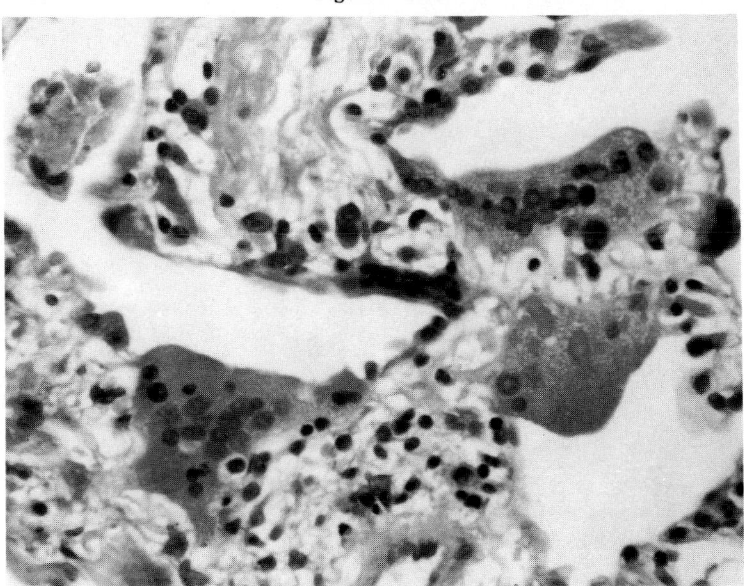

Figure 5–65.

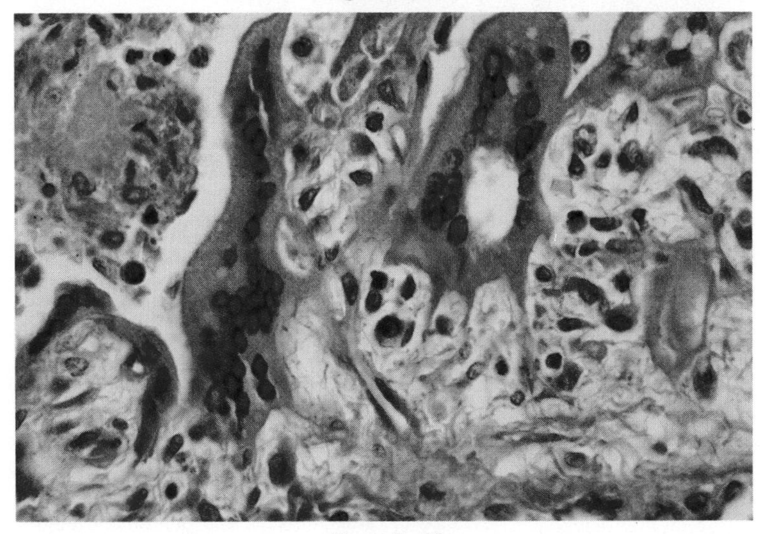

Figure 5–66.

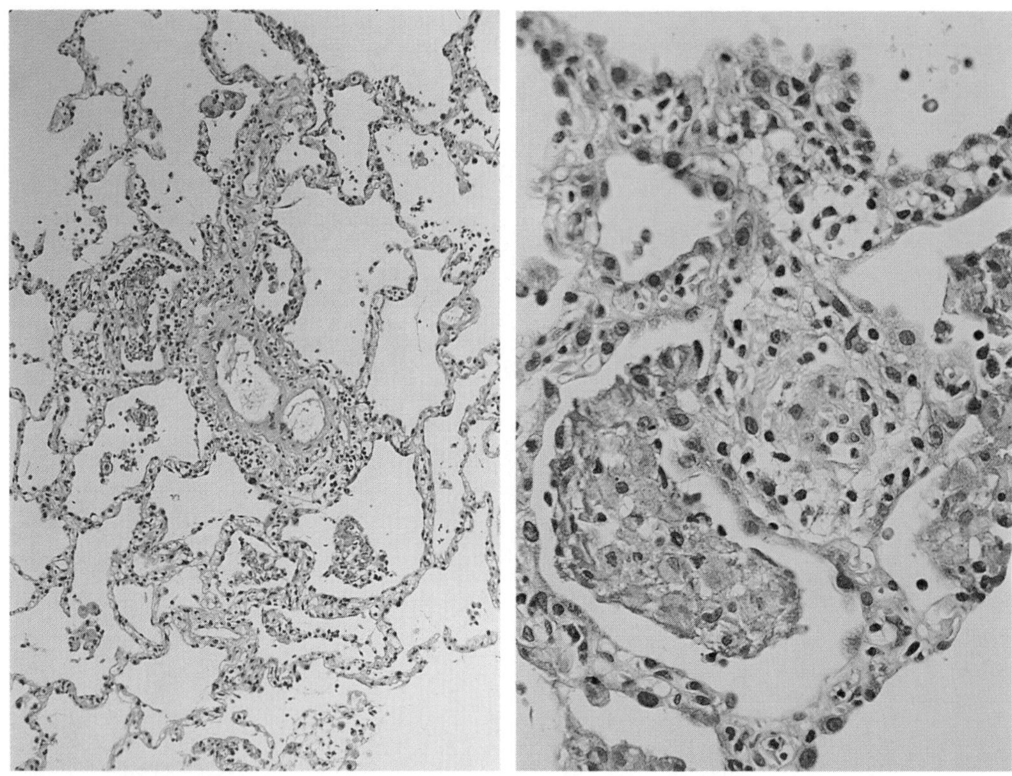

Figure 5-67.

Figure 5-68.

Figures 5-67, 5-68, 5-69. Echo-7 pneumonia. Culture-proven enteric cytopathogenic human orphan virus (Echo-7) virus pneumonia. Biopsy was performed because the patient was immunosuppressed. Pulmonary infiltrates resolved without therapy. Histologic findings included perivascular inflammatory infiltrates and exudation into alveolar spaces. In some foci, there was prominent reactive type II cell metaplasia, which in a single high-power field might raise the possibility of bronchioloalveolar carcinoma (Fig. 5-69).

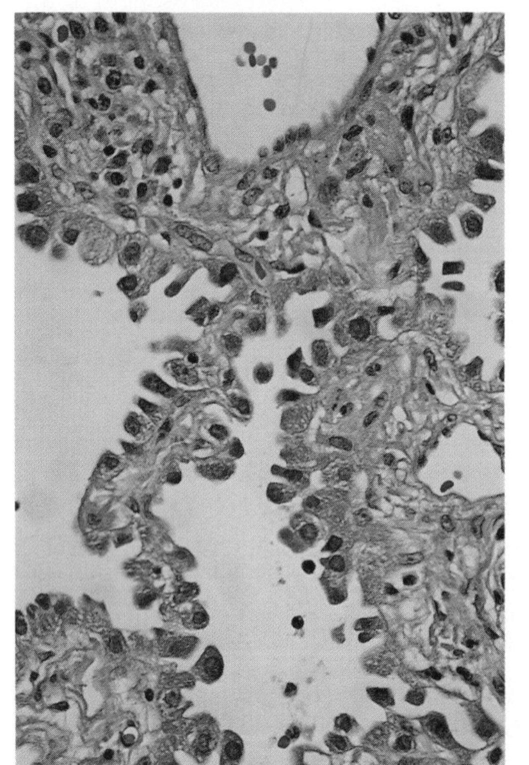

Figure 5-69.

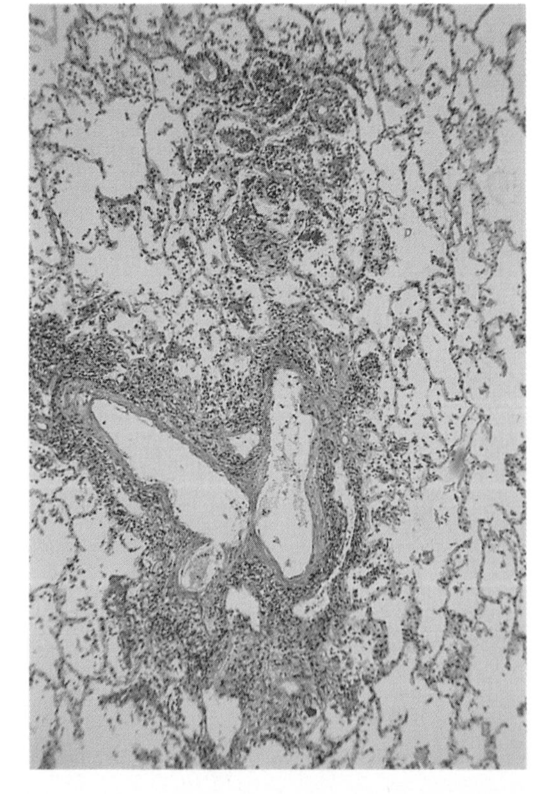

Figure 5-70. Coxsackie B pneumonitis. Pulmonary infiltrates in a patient with Coxsackie B myocarditis. The patient died of cardiac disease, and pulmonary infiltrates were noted prior to death. Histologic study shows perivascular chronic inflammatory infiltrates with some exudation into airspaces.

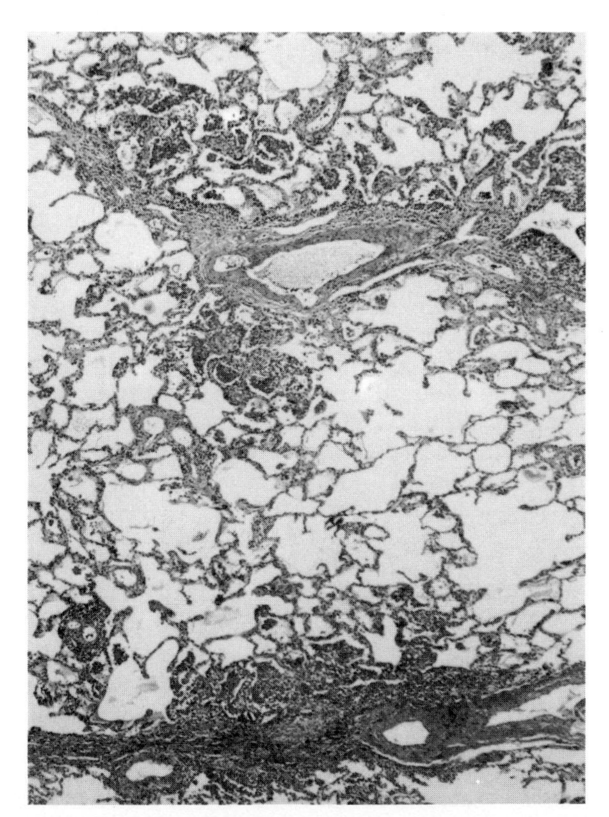

Figure 5-71. Viral pneumonia. Perivascular infiltrates and airspace exudates consistent with viral pneumonia. This patient had a clinical syndrome typical of a viremia but was immunosuppressed and underwent biopsy to exclude opportunistic infection. The biopsy specimen shows only perivascular lymphoid infiltrates with some airspace exudation in the perivascular alveolar spaces. The patient's symptoms cleared spontaneously, and a clinical diagnosis of a mild viral pneumonia (etiology unknown) was made. Such a perivascular distribution of infiltrates is similar to that seen in Epstein-Barr virus (EBV) pneumonia as well as those cases illustrated in Figures 5-67 through 5-70.

■ Fungal Infections Usually Seen in Normal Hosts (Figs. 5-72 to 5-79)

The following are examples of fungal infections found in normal hosts:

- Histoplasmosis
- Coccidioidomycosis
- Blastomycosis
- Cryptococcosis
- Chronic necrotizing aspergillosis
- Sporotrichosis

These infections may mimic tuberculosis with upper-lobe cavitary disease, or they may present as a nodule, or a localized infiltrate anywhere in the lungs. Patients may be asymptomatic.

These infections are characterized by a necrotizing or non-necrotizing granulomatous inflammation with a variable amount of acute inflammation. Microabscess-type inflammation is sometimes more common than in mycobacterial infections. Histoplasmosis and coccidioidomycosis are more like tuberculosis with caseation, whereas blastomycosis and cryptococcosis more often feature microabscesses with granulomatous inflammation. Although chronic necrotizing aspergillosis may look like an aspergilloma with erosion and superficial invasion of the cavity wall and a secondary palisaded histiocytic reaction, it occurs in a lung without pre-existing cavitary or fibrotic disease and fewer hyphae are generally present than in aspergillomas. Chronic necro-

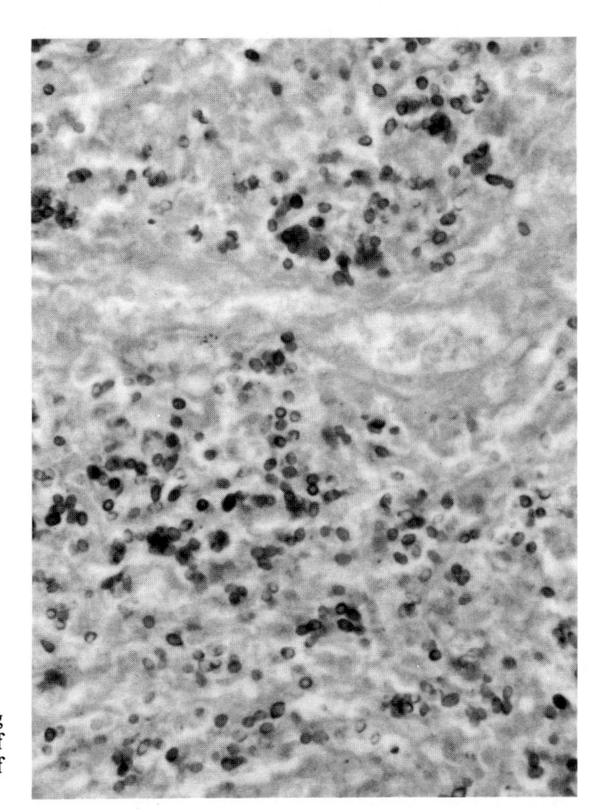

Figure 5-72. Pulmonary histoplasmosis. The center of a solitary necrotizing granuloma on silver stain shows numerous small yeast organisms, some of which are budding. Even in ancient healed granulomas, a small number of degenerate yeast forms are often identifiable by means of silver stains.

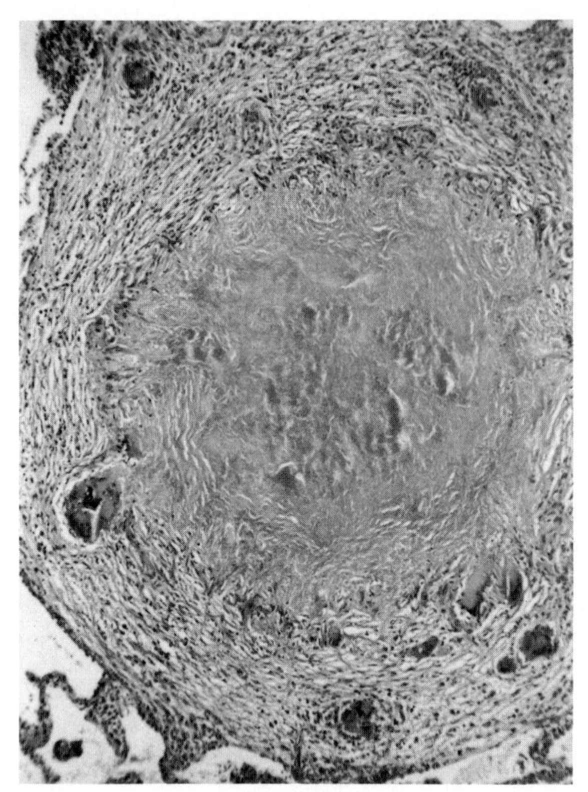

Figure 5-73.

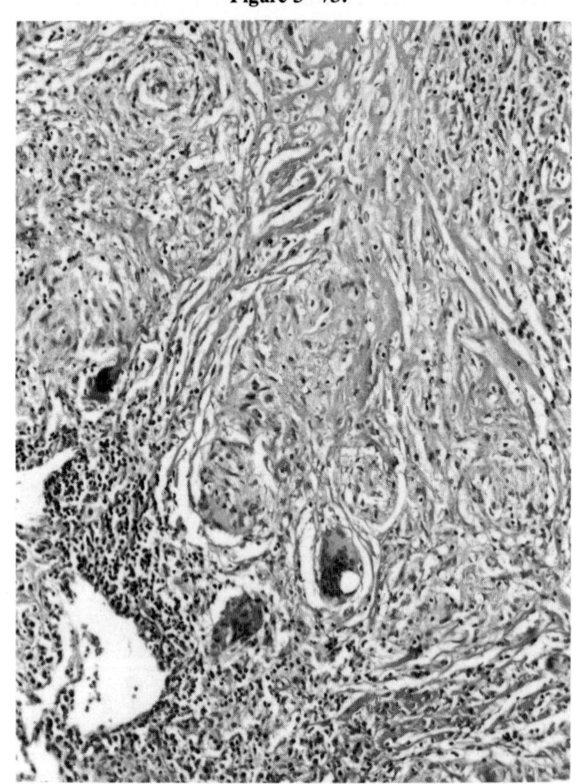

Figure 5-74.

Figures 5-73, 5-74. Slowly resolving histoplasmosis. An asymptomatic patient had multiple nodules that eventually resulted in the need for open lung biopsy. Some of the granulomatous inflammation suggested a healing granulomatous infection, whereas others were associated with lamellar fibrosis and raised the possibility of sarcoidosis. Cultures and special stains were negative, although follow-up and seriologic studies over the next year confirmed a diagnosis of histoplasmosis.

tizing aspergillosis should not be equated with invasive aspergillosis.

Organisms are usually easier to find than in mycobacterial infection; however, in any of these conditions, organisms may be few. Negative reactions to special stains do not rule out a fungal infection, and in some cases causative organisms are identified only by culture and/or serologic tests.

Note: Although the morphologic features of the fungal organisms usually allow presumptive diagnosis, a specific diagnosis should await culture results because the yeast forms in these infections may be considerably pleomorphic and difficult to distinguish from one another. Occasionally, cultures remain negative, even when unequivocal organisms are seen morphologically.

References

Dail DH, Hammer SP (eds). Pulmonary Pathology. New York, Springer-Verlag, 1988.

Drutz DJ, Catanzaro A. Coccidioidomycosis. Part I. Am Rev Respir Dis 117:559-585, 1978.

Drutz DJ, Catanzaro A. Coccidioidomycosis. Part II. Am Rev Respir Dis 117:727-771, 1978.

Goodwin RA, Des Prez RM. Histoplasmosis: state of the art. Am Rev Respir Dis 117:929-956, 1978.

Wheat LJ, Slama TH, Zeckel ML. Histoplasmosis in the acquired immune deficiency syndrome. Am J Med 78:203-210, 1985.

Hutton JP, Durham JB, Miller DP, Everett ED. Hyphal forms of histoplasma capsulatum: a common manifestation of intravascular infections. Arch Pathol Lab Med 109:330-332, 1985.

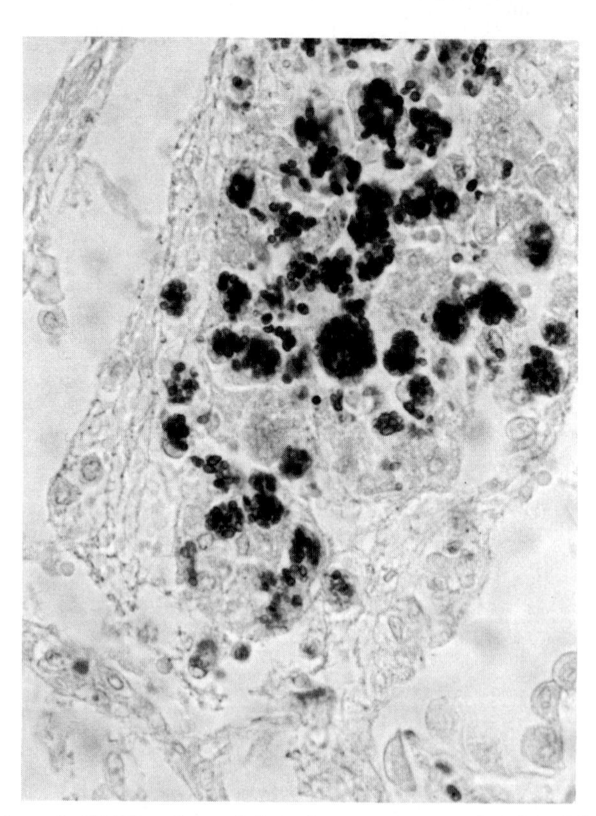

Figure 5-75. Histoplasmosis in an immunosuppressed patient. Massive numbers of yeasts, 2 to 4 microns in size, stuff alveolar macrophages, which fill alveoli (histoplasmosis histiocytic pneumonia). The patient had been receiving high-dose steroids because of an erroneous diagnosis of sarcoidosis.

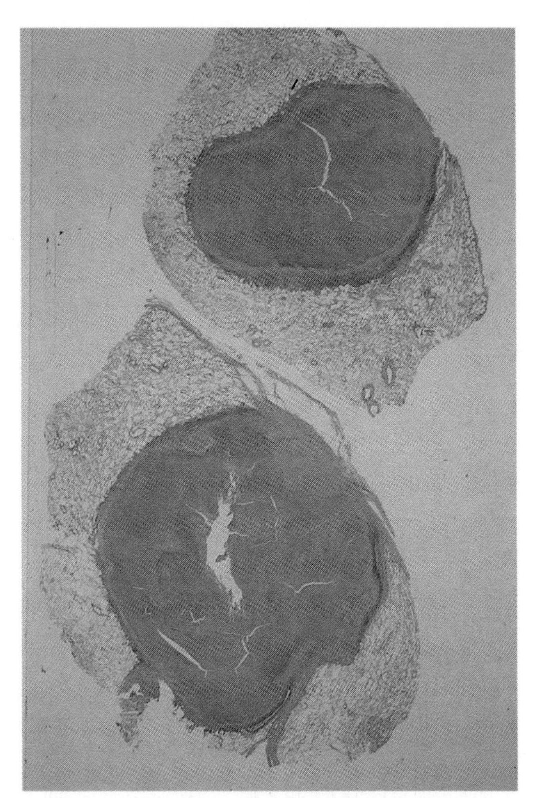

Figure 5-76. Coccidioidomycosis. Solitary necrotizing granuloma due to coccidioidomycosis. The rounded contour and thin inflammatory wall around the necrotic center are characteristic.

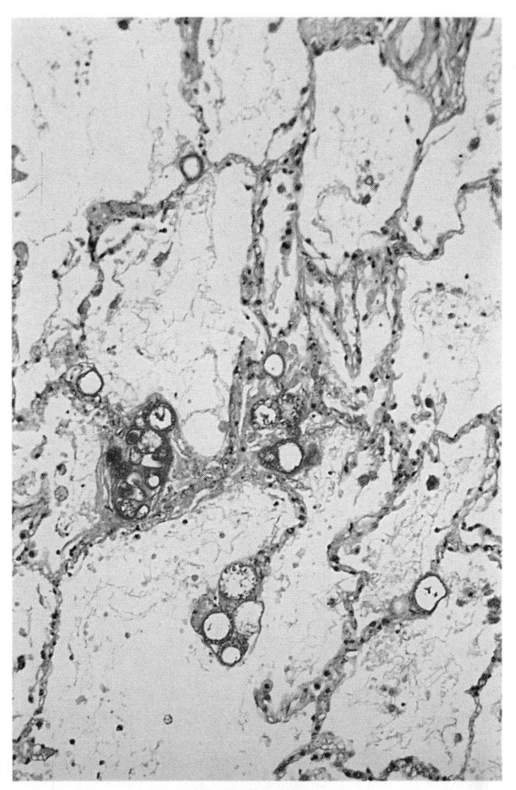

Figure 5-78.

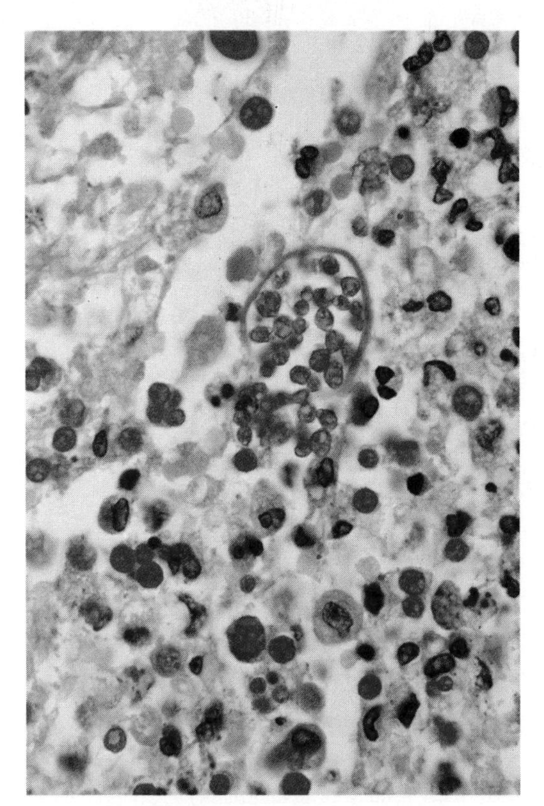

Figure 5-77. Coccidioidomycosis. Digested periodic acid-Schiff (PAS) stain shows a central spherule that has recently ruptured and released its endospores. Other organisms, somewhat larger than the endospores, are seen in the surrounding tissue.

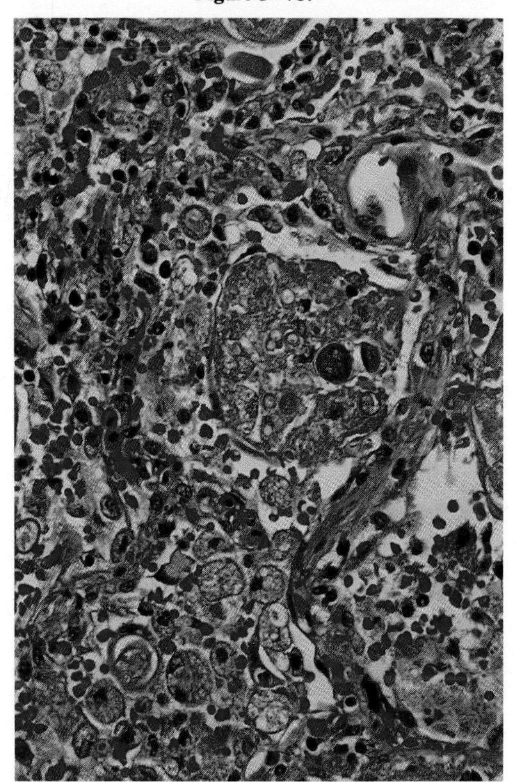

Figure 5-79.

Figures 5-78, 5-79. Coccioidomycosis. Disseminated coccidioidomycosis in an immunosuppressed transplant patient manifesting as large numbers of spherules within the pulmonary microvasculature (Fig. 5-78) and as massive numbers of organisms in the alveoli (Fig. 5-79). At this magnification, the differential diagnosis includes fat emboli (Fig. 5-78).

■ Aspergillosis (Figs. 5–80 to 5–90)

Pathologic changes associated with aspergillosis in the lung are seen in a variety of patterns, including:

1. Allergic bronchopulmonary aspergillosis (ABPA).
2. Aspergilloma (mycetoma or fungus ball).
3. Chronic necrotizing aspergillosis.
4. Fulminant invasive aspergillosis.

Allergic bronchopulmonary aspergillosis is usually associated with mucoid impaction, bronchocentric granulomatosis, and/or eosinophilic pneumonia in asthmatics, or it is a syndrome resembling extrinsic allergic alveolitis (hypersensitivity pneumonitis).

An aspergilloma is a mass of fungal hyphae growing as a fungus ball in a pre-existing cavity that is usually caused by some other pathologic condition. Aspergilloma is discussed later.

Fulminant invasive necrotizing aspergillosis is usually restricted to significantly immunocompromised patients who present with massive zones of consolidation corresponding to septic infarcts related to massive vascular occlusion. Less commonly, an invasive bronchocentric form or a miliary form from hematogenous spread is seen in immunocompromised patients.

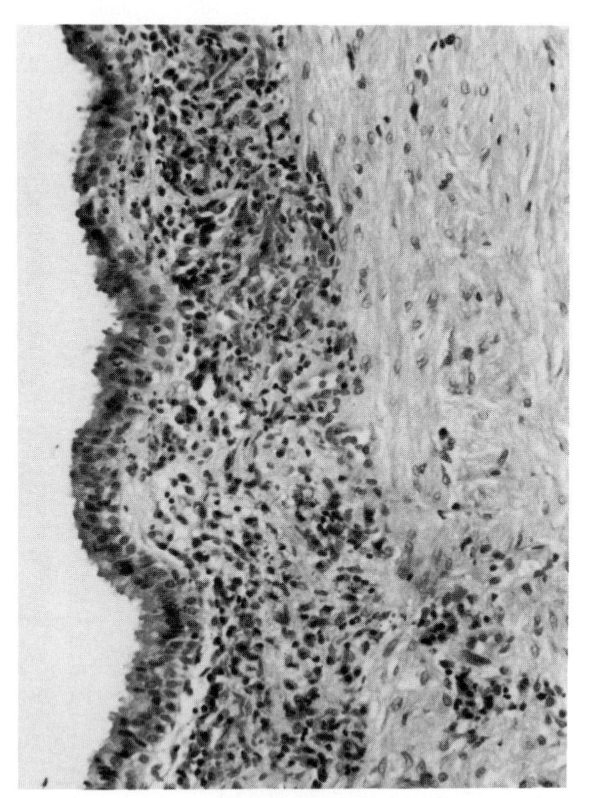

Figure 5–80.

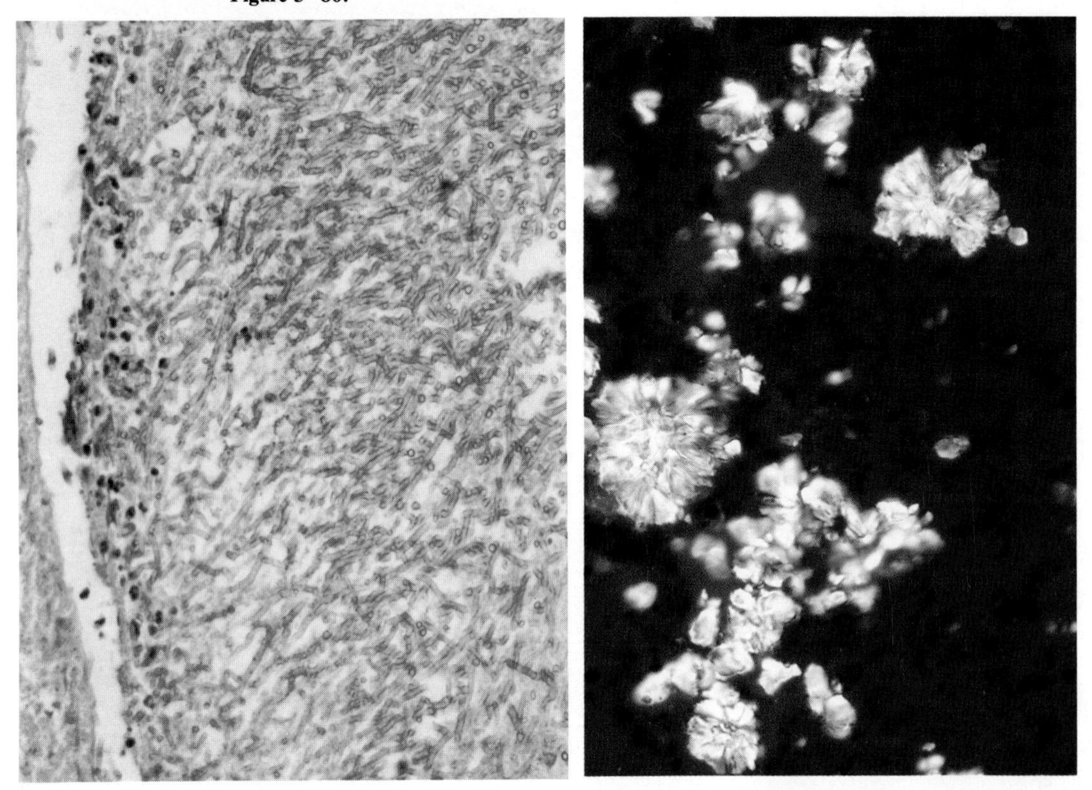

Figure 5–81. Figure 5–82.

Figures 5–80, 5–81, 5–82. Pulmonary aspergilloma (mycetoma). A fibrous-walled cavity from prior inflammatory disease (Fig. 5–80) contains a mass of hyphae with features of *Aspergillus.* The hyphae are generally so numerous that they are easily seen with hematoxylin and eosin stains (Fig. 5–81). The wall of the cavity shows fibrosis, chronic inflammation, and an intact lining of metaplastic bronchiolar epithelium. Tissue around an aspergilloma is often rich in oxalate crystals, here shown with polarization (Fig. 5–82).

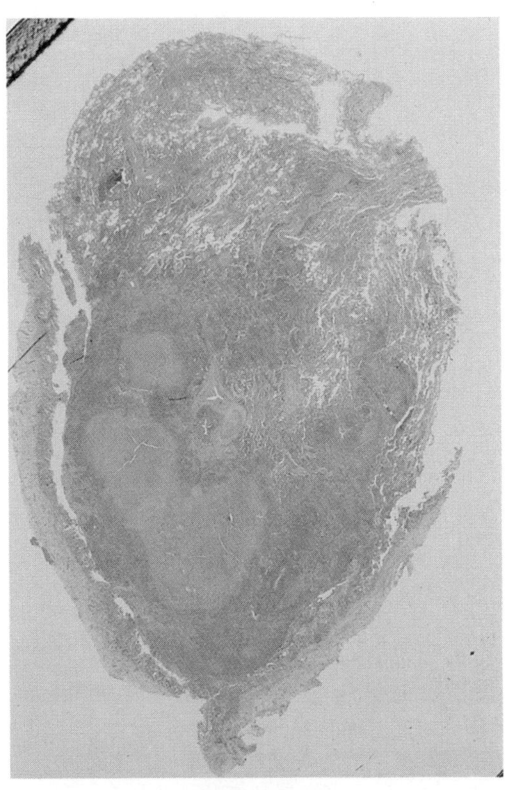

Figure 5-83.

Chronic necrotizing aspergillosis is usually associated with a single lesion (often in the upper lobes), identified in the patient as an incidental radiologic finding or associated with relatively mild pulmonary symptoms. The tissue is usually resected for diagnosis and shows a necrotic granuloma in which the hyphae are identified, occurring in a background of relatively normal lung tissue. The inflammatory reaction is usually chronic and granulomatous, although caseation and large numbers of non-necrotizing granulomas in the wall are unusual. Eosinophils may occasionally be prominent in the wall. Vascular invasion should be absent, and large numbers of hyphae occurring in a starburst array, which is typical of invasive aspergillosis in immunosuppressed individuals, should be lacking.

Invasive aspergillosis in immunocompromised individuals is a severe and often fulminant infection. It is associated with extensive vascular invasion, secondary thrombosis, necrosis of large zones of lung parenchyma (large septic infarcts), and nodular, segmental, or lobar infiltrates on chest radiograph. A less common bronchocentric form occurs, as does a miliary hematogenous form associated with small necrotic nodules in which the hyphae can be seen. The inflammatory reaction in invasive aspergillosis in immunocompromised hosts is usually neutrophilic, although cells may be lacking in patients with severe cytopenias. In such cases, hemorrhage, infarction, and fibrinous exudates dominate.

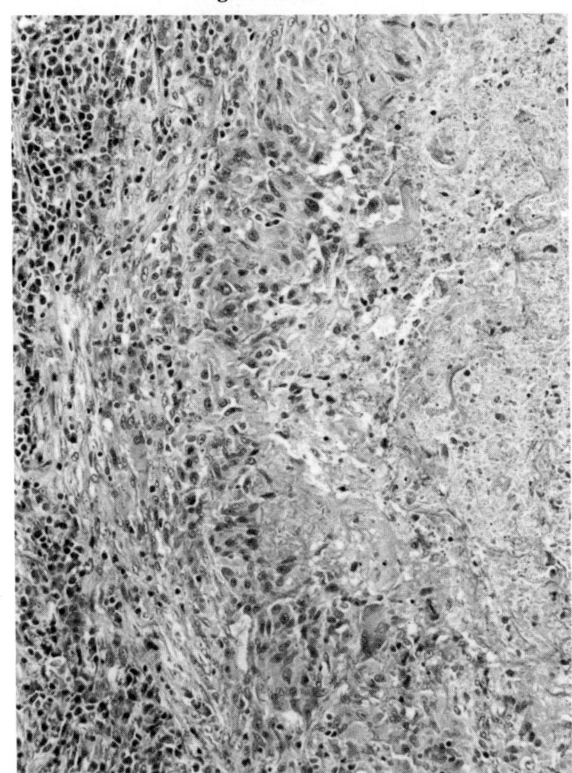

Figure 5-84.

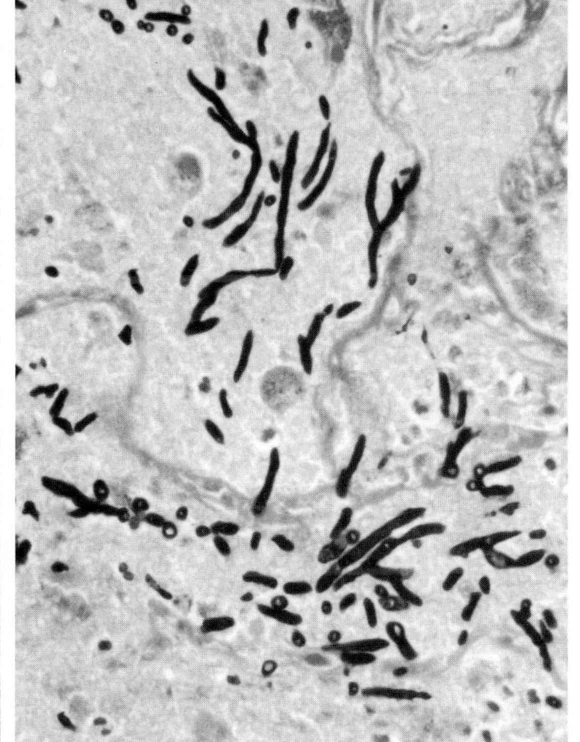

Figure 5-85.

Figures 5-83, 5-84, 5-85. Chronic necrotizing aspergillosis. An immunocompetent individual was found to have a coin lesion on chest radiograph. The excised lung tissue showed a focal necrotic granuloma arising in otherwise normal lung tissue. Within the necrosis, degenerating hyphae typical of *Aspergillus* were found.

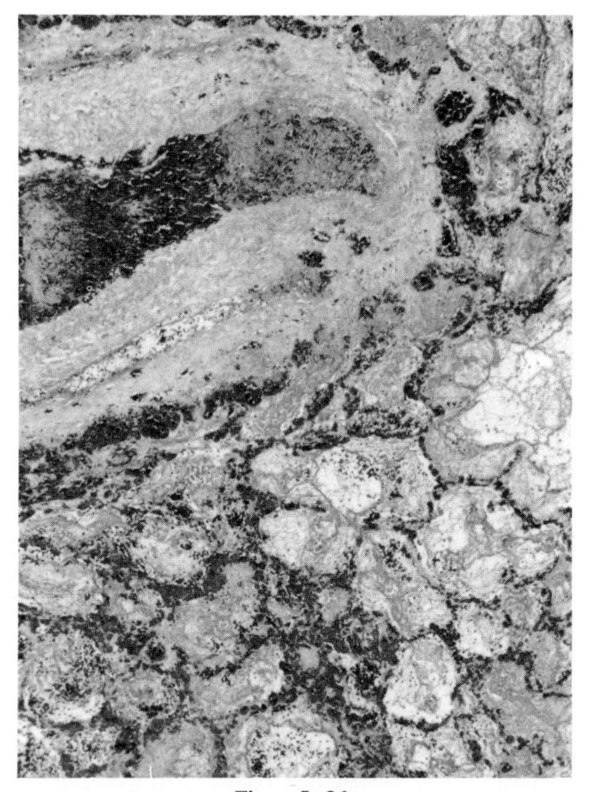

Figure 5-86.

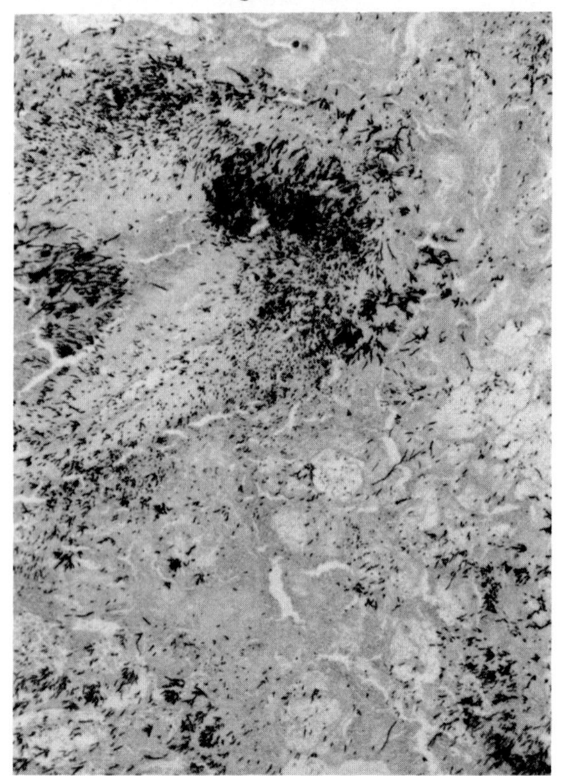

Figure 5-87.

Figures 5-86, 5-87. Invasive aspergillosis in an immunosuppressed patient. This biopsy specimen from a hemorrhagic infarcted zone of lung tissue shows alveolar hemorrhage and exudate as well as thrombosis of a medium-sized pulmonary artery. Silver stain from the same region shows permeation of the vessel wall and surrounding parenchyma by hyphae typical of *Aspergillus.*

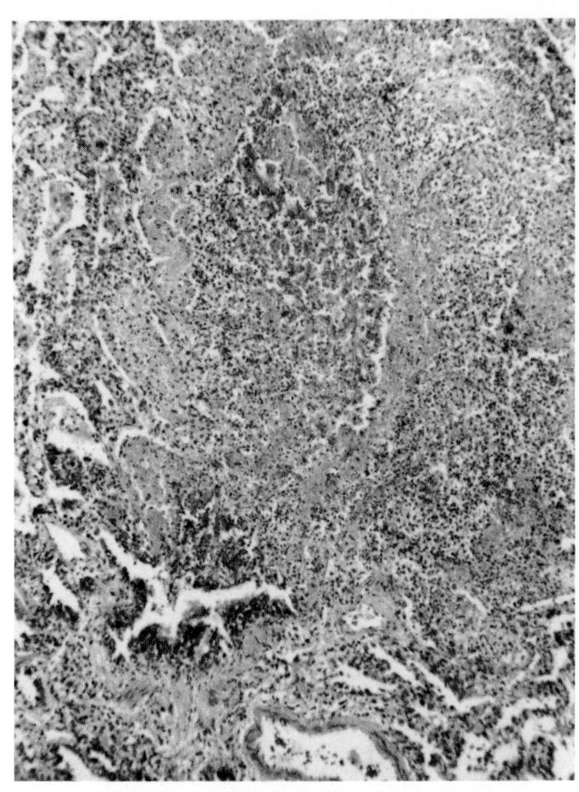

Figure 5-88.

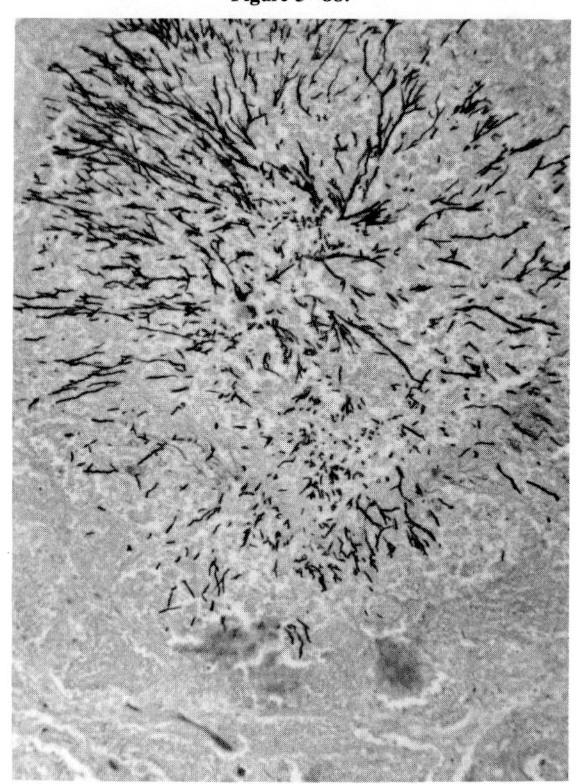

Figure 5-89.

Figures 5-88, 5-89. Invasive bronchocentric aspergillosis in an immunosuppressed individual. There is a necrotic granuloma involving a small bronchiole, and all the lesions in this case were airway-centered. Silver stain shows the typical starburst array of invasive aspergillosis.

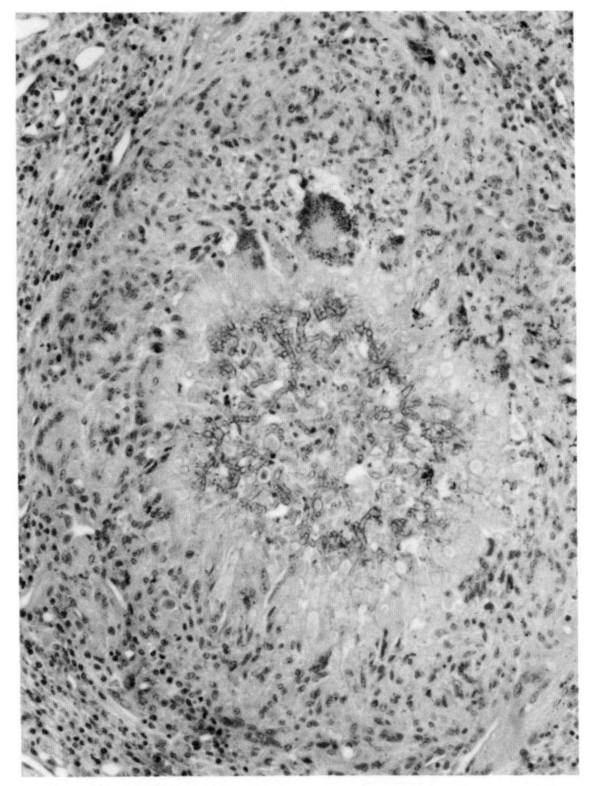

Figure 5-90. Miliary aspergillosis in an immunosuppressed individual. Biopsy material shows scattered nodules composed of hyphae (with fruiting bodies) surrounded by a granulomatous reaction.

Some overlap exists between the various clinical forms of aspergillosis, and definitive separation is not always possible. For example, a cavity associated with bronchocentric granulomatosis in allergic bronchopulmonary aspergillosis may be colonized by organisms to produce a fungus ball, or a fungus ball may erode the epithelial lining of the cavity in which it resides and share some features of chronic necrotizing aspergillosis.

The hyphae in *Aspergillus* infection are 3 to 6 μm wide, septate, and show dichotomous branching with acute (45°) angle branching. The walls of the hyphae are parallel, and the hyphae often are seen in radiating starburst arrays in invasive aspergillosis in immunosuppressed hosts. Smaller numbers of hyphae, some of which show degenerative changes, are characteristic of chronic necrotizing aspergillosis. In aspergillomas (described later), a tangled mass of hyphae without tissue invasion produces the fungus ball. In allergic bronchopulmonary aspergillosis, only small fragments of hyphae are identified, sometimes with some difficulty, in the inspissated mucus.

In damaged or poorly preserved tissues, the hyphae in *Aspergillus* infection may become swollen and much more irregular in size and shape, lacking the typical parallel walls. Such changes make *Aspergillus* infection difficult to separate from mucormycosis. Culture is usually required for the final diagnosis.

References

Binder RE, Faling LJ, Pugatch RD, Mahasaen C, Snider GL. Chronic necrotizing pulmonary aspergillosis: a discrete clinical entity. Medicine (Baltimore) 61:109-124, 1982.

Dail DH, Hammer SP (eds). Pulmonary Pathology. New York, Springer-Verlag, 1988.

Flint A, Colby TV. Surgical Pathology of Diffuse Infiltrative Lung Disease. Orlando, Grune & Stratton, Inc, 1987.

Katzenstein AL, Liebow AA, Friedman PF. Bronchocentric granulomatosis, mucoid impaction, and hypersensitivity reactions to fungi. Am Rev Respir Dis 111:497-537, 1975.

Orr DP, Myerowitz RL, Dubois PJ. Patho-radiologic correlation of invasive pulmonary aspergillosis in the compromised host. Cancer 41:2028-2039, 1978.

Thurlbeck WM (ed). Pathology of the Lung. New York, Thieme, 1988.

■ Mycetoma (Fungus Ball) (Figs. 5-80 and 5-81)

Mycetomas represent tangled masses of fungal hyphae growing in cavities caused by some prior pathologic condition such as healed tuberculosis or sarcoidosis. The most common cause of a mycetoma is *Aspergillus* (aspergilloma), but many other fungi may occasionally grow as saprophytes in cavities, including coccidiodomycosis and others. When the fungus grows in this fashion, fruiting bodies may develop and simulate yeast forms, particularly in aspergillomas. When erosion of the epithelium lining the cavity occurs, an appearance resembling chronic cavitary aspergillosis results and the differential diagnosis becomes somewhat difficult.

Pseudallescheria boydii is a fungus commonly found in soil. It is an increasingly significant cause of infection in immunosuppressed or otherwise debilitated individuals. The morphologic appearance of the fungus is quite similar to that of *Aspergillus,* and *P. boydii* has been linked to the development of mycetomas in the lungs as well as other organs. It has been suggested that the mycetomas related to this organism may be the result of invasive disease, resulting in necrosis and infarction of the host tissue, which then separates from the surrounding viable tissue, simulating the appearance of a mycetoma. Similar events may take place in immunosuppressed patients with mycetomas caused by other fungi, such as *Aspergillus.*

References

Schwartz DA. Organ-specific variation in the morphology of the fungomas (fungus balls) of *Pseudallescheria boydii.* Arch Pathol Lab Med 113:476-480, 1989.

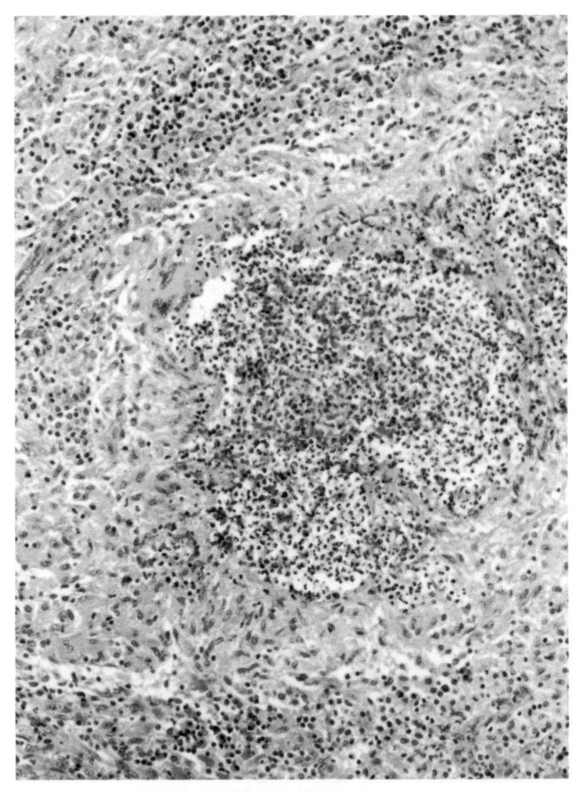

Figure 5-91.

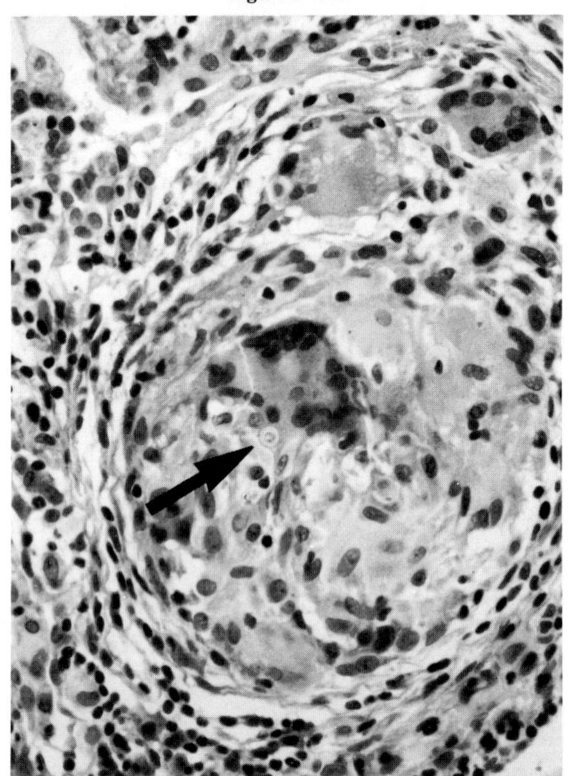

Figure 5-92.

Figures 5-91, 5-92. Pulmonary blastomycosis in an immunologically normal host. Large necrotizing granulomas contain abundant purulent material surrounded by a thick cuff of epithelioid histiocytes. The adjacent lung tissue shows organization, chronic inflammation, and scattered non-necrotizing granulomas. A thick-walled organism is seen in a non-necrotizing granuloma (arrow).

■ Blastomycosis (Figs. 5-91 to 5-94)

This fungal infection occurs in both immunocompetent and immunocompromised hosts with similar pathologic features. Cutaneous or genitourinary findings may accompany the lung disease.

Blastomycosis manifests with 5 to 15 μm yeast forms with a nucleus seen easily on hematoxylin and eosin (H & E) slides with a thick wall, which is PAS-positive and faintly mucicarminophilic. Yeast forms show single broad-based budding. Both intracellular and extracellular organisms can be found.

Blastomycosis usually is a suppurative and granulomatous pneumonia with intra-alveolar exudates of fibrin, neutrophils, histiocytes, scattered eosinophils, and microabscess formation. There are variable numbers of organisms, and granuloma formation with both necrotizing and non-necrotizing features. Large numbers of histiocytes may simulate a lipoid pneumonia. A miliary pattern and diffuse alveolar damage may also be seen.

References

Atkinson JB, McCurley TL. Pulmonary blastomycosis: filamentous forms in an immunocompromised patient with fulminating respiratory failure. Hum Pathol 14:186-188, 1983.

Dail DH, Hammer SP (eds). Pulmonary Pathology. New York, Springer-Verlag, 1988.

Sarosi GA, Davies SF. Blastomycosis. Am Rev Respir Dis 120:911-938, 1979.

Thurlbeck WM (ed). Pathology of the Lung. New York, Thieme, 1988.

■ *Candida* Infections (Figs. 5-95 to 5-97)

Pulmonary infection by *Candida* is found in patients with suppressed cell-mediated immunity and also in other patients with skin and mucosal surface abnormalities, such as result from burns, trauma, catheters, and gastrointestinal surgery. Broad-spectrum antibiotics, steroids, and neutropenia are also important predisposing factors. Pulmonary candidiasis may take one of two forms: (1) bronchopneumonia, and (2) embolic. Diagnosis depends on identification of the fungal organism in diseased tissue.

The features of *Candida* include (1) spheroidal-oval yeast forms, 2 to 6 μm in diameter; and (2) mycelial (pseudohyphae) forms ("sausages and meatballs"); the pseudohyphae are 3 to 5 μm in width.

Candidal bronchopneumonia features airway colonization by *Candida,* neutrophilic bronchopneumonia, vascular invasion, and frequently other associated infections (i.e., bacterial or fungal).

Candidal embolic (hematogenous) pneumonia manifests as small necrotic nodules associated with vascular invasion, neutrophilic inflammation, and hemorrhage.

Note: In neutropenic patients the inflammatory response may be limited.

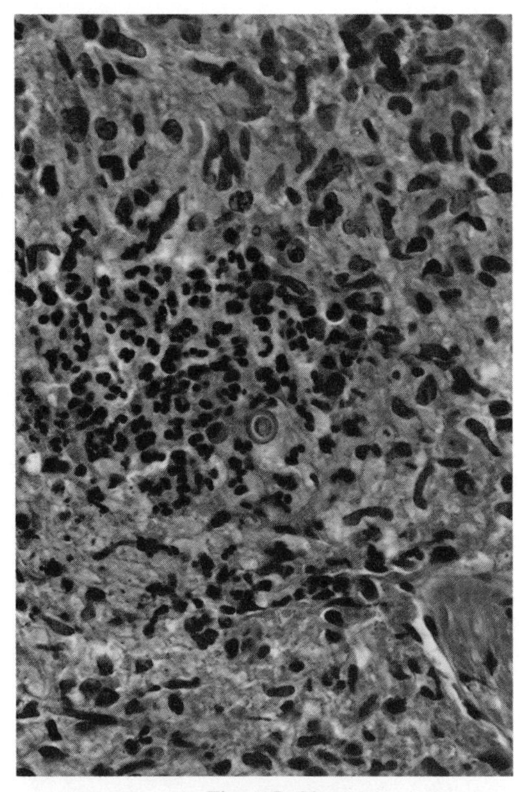

Figure 5-93.

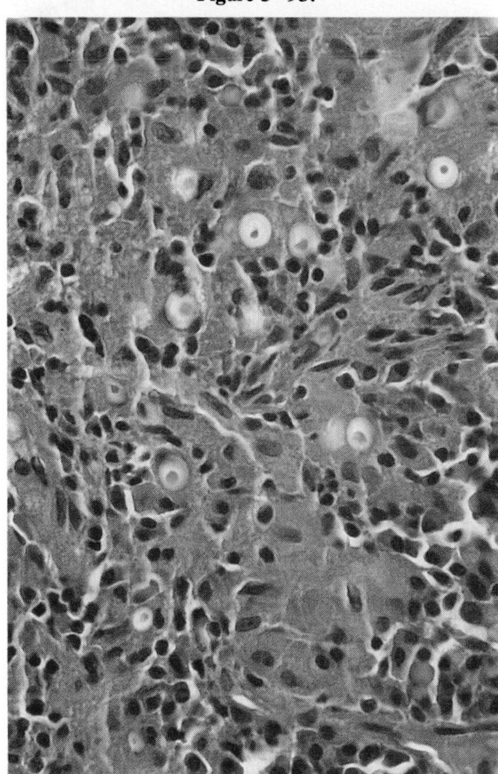

Figure 5-94.

Figures 5-93, 5-94. Blastomycosis with isolated organisms seen on routine stains in a microabscess of neutrophils and as multiple organisms with halos within epithelioid histiocytes. The organisms in Figure 5-94 could easily be confused with cryptococcal organisms. The culture was positive for blastomycosis.

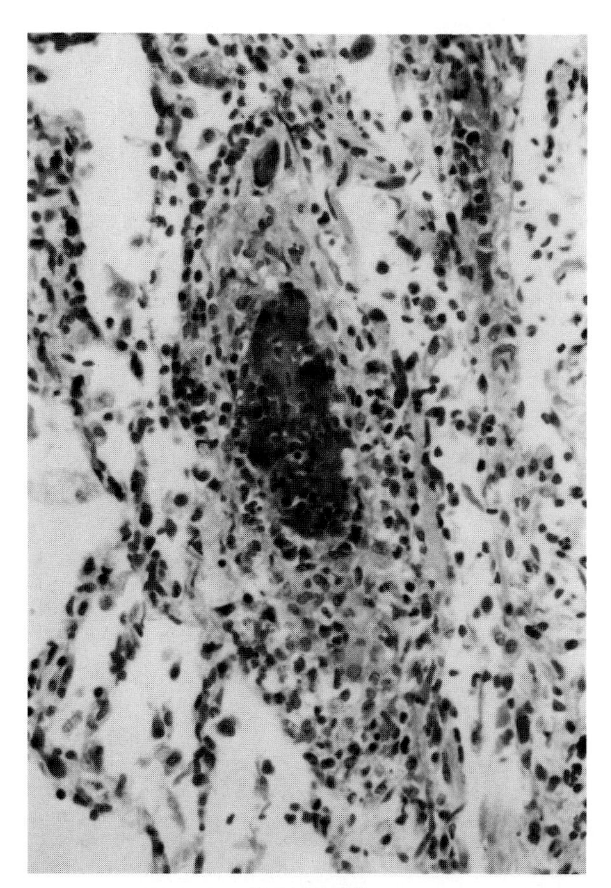

Figure 5-95.

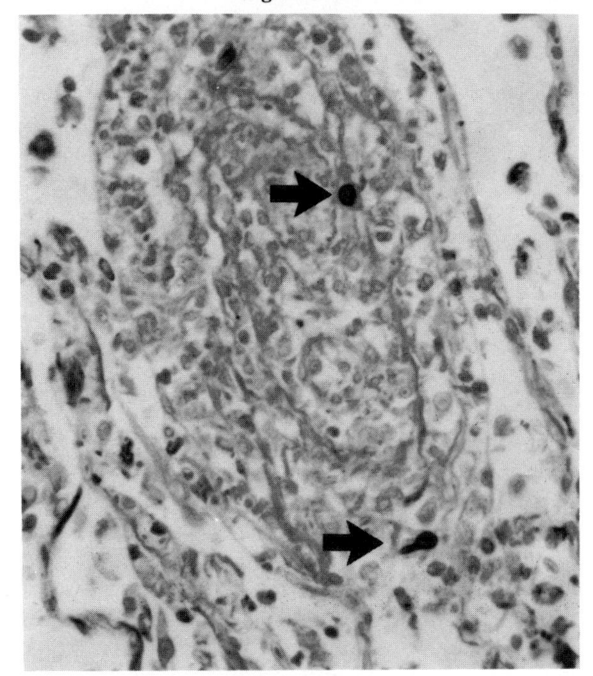

Figure 5-96.

Figures 5-95, 5-96. Candidemia with vascular involvement in an immunosuppressed individual. A small pulmonary vein is thrombosed and shows a modest inflammatory infiltrate in the wall. Silver stain shows occasional yeast forms, one budding, in the vessel. Blood cultures grew *Candida albicans.*

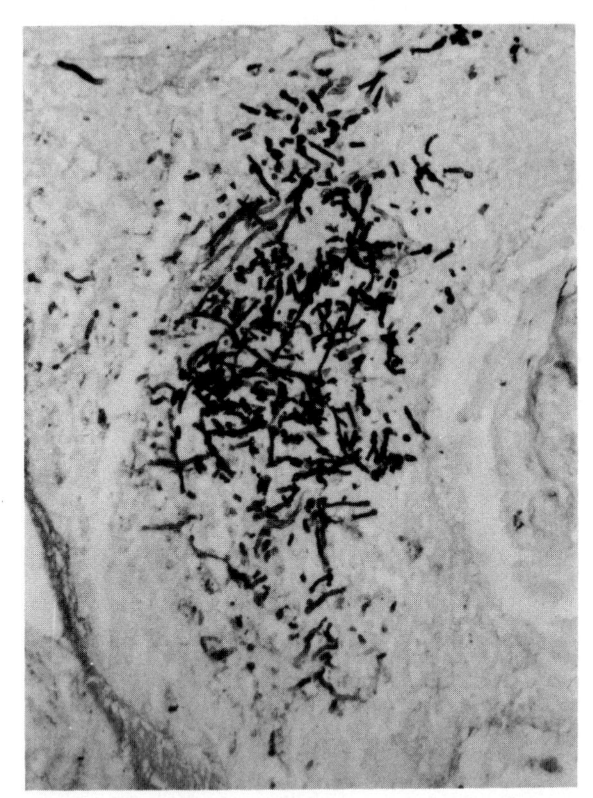

Figure 5-97. Disseminated candidiasis in a heart transplant patient. *Candida* pseudohyphae strongly resemble *Aspergillus,* and this emphasizes the importance of culture in the definitive diagnosis of fungal infections.

References

Dail DH, Hammer SP (eds). Pulmonary Pathology. New York, Springer-Verlag, 1988.

Marsh PK, Tally FP, Kellum J, et al. Candida infections in surgical patients. Ann Surg 198:42-47, 1983.

Myerowitz RL, Pazin GJ, Allen CM. Disseminated candidiasis: changes in incidence, underlying diseases, and pathology. Am J Clin Pathol 68:29-38, 1977.

Thurlbeck WM (ed). Pathology of the Lung. New York, Thieme, 1988.

■ **Cryptococcosis** (Figs. 5-98 to 5-104)

This fungal infection may cause disease in immunocompetent hosts, and not uncommonly it is asymptomatic; however, most clinically significant cases occur in immunocompromised hosts. The pattern of disease varies, depending on the immunocompetence of the host. In normal and mildly immunocompromised patients, there is a granulomatous response to the organism. Mixed granulomatous and suppurative inflammation with necrosis and organizing pneumonia is common. In more severely immunocompromised hosts, there is a histiocytic response to the organism without granuloma formation. In these cases, there are usually few other inflammatory cells. In profoundly immunocompromised patients, the alveoli are filled with cryptococcal organisms with virtually no inflammatory reaction ("mucoid pneumonia").

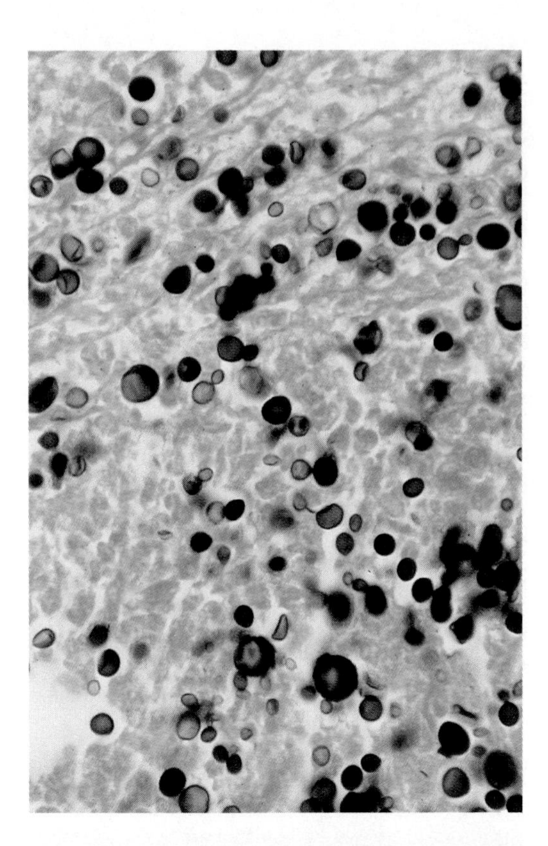

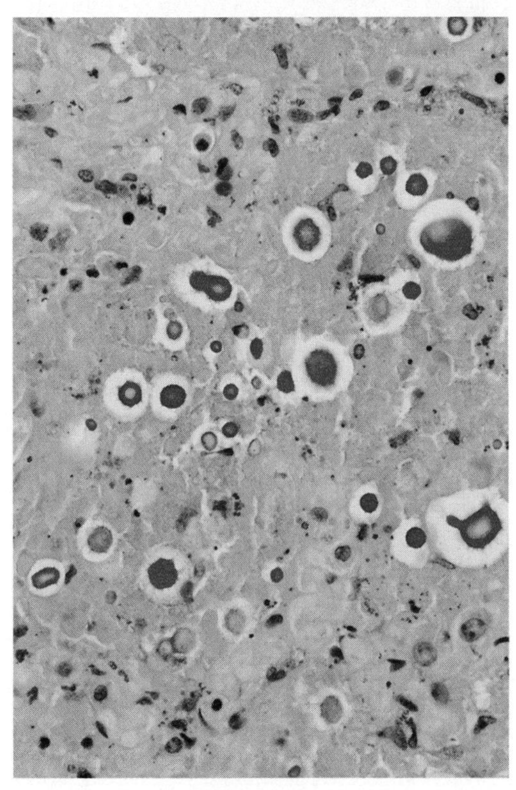

Figure 5-99.

Figures 5-98, 5-99. *Cryptococcus* as seen with silver and mucicarmine stains.

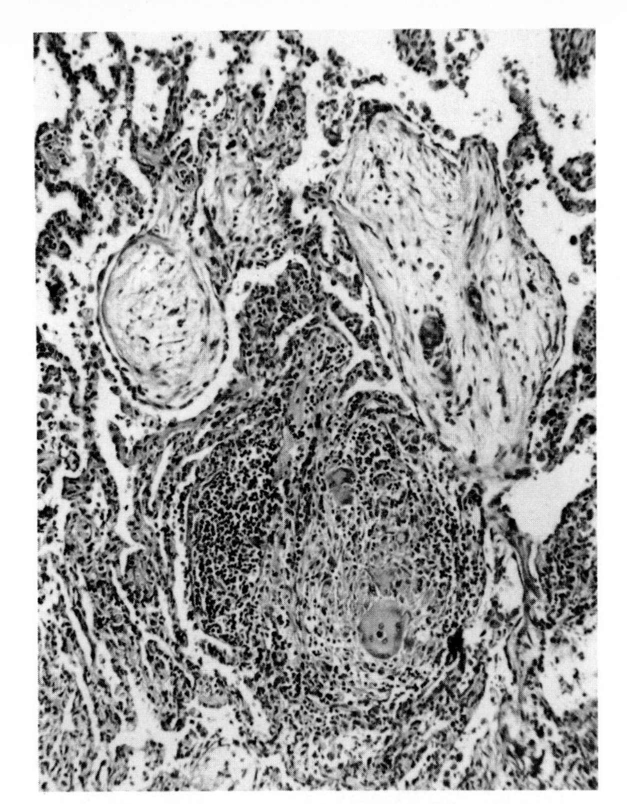

Figure 5-100. Organizing cryptococcal pneumonia. Organizing cryptococcal pneumonia in an immunocompetent patient. A localized infiltrate had developed and was resected. Histologic sections showed granulomatous inflammation and extensive organizing pneumonia. Cultures were positive for *Cryptococcus,* although no organisms were ever seen with special stains.

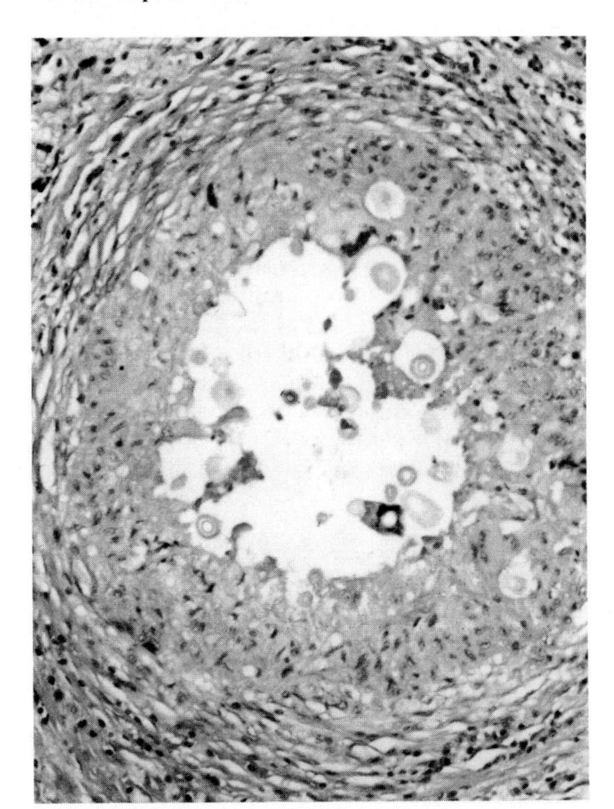

Figure 5-101. Cryptococcal pneumonia. Cryptococcal pneumonia in an immunologically normal host. There are granulomas containing vacuolated histiocytes, and within some of the vacuoles the pleomorphic yeast forms of *Cryptococcus* can be identified. Granulomas containing microabscesses may also be seen in cryptococcal pneumonia.

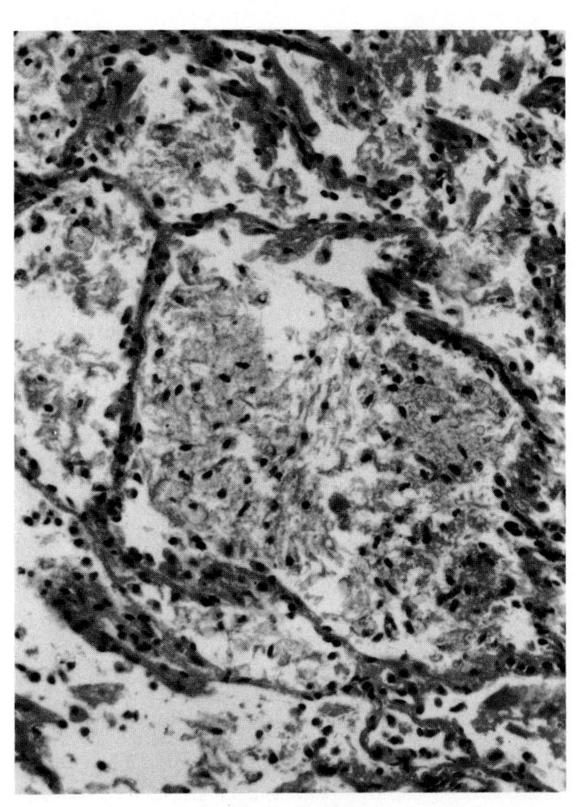

Figure 5-102.

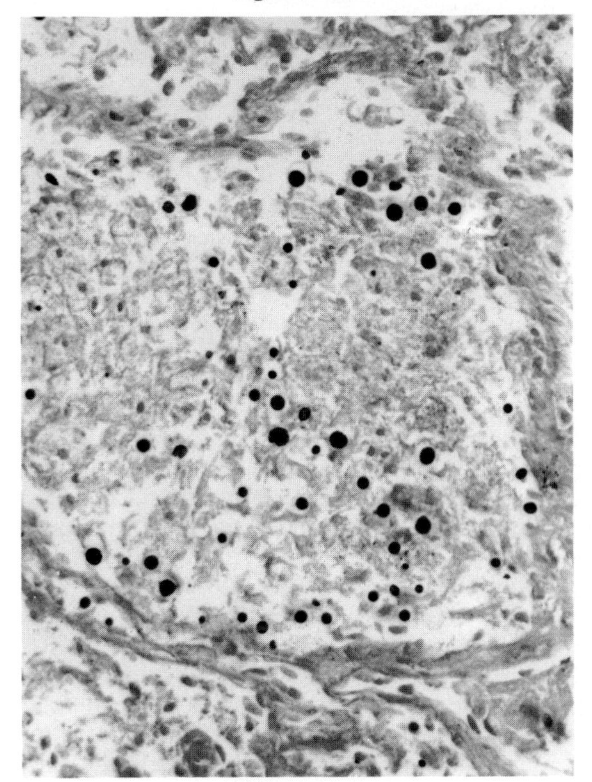

Figure 5-103.

Figures 5-102, 5-103. Cryptococcal ("histiocytic") pneumonia in an immunosuppressed patient. The alveoli contain only histiocytes with foamy cytoplasm. The pleomorphic yeast forms of *Cryptococcus* are seen on silver stain.

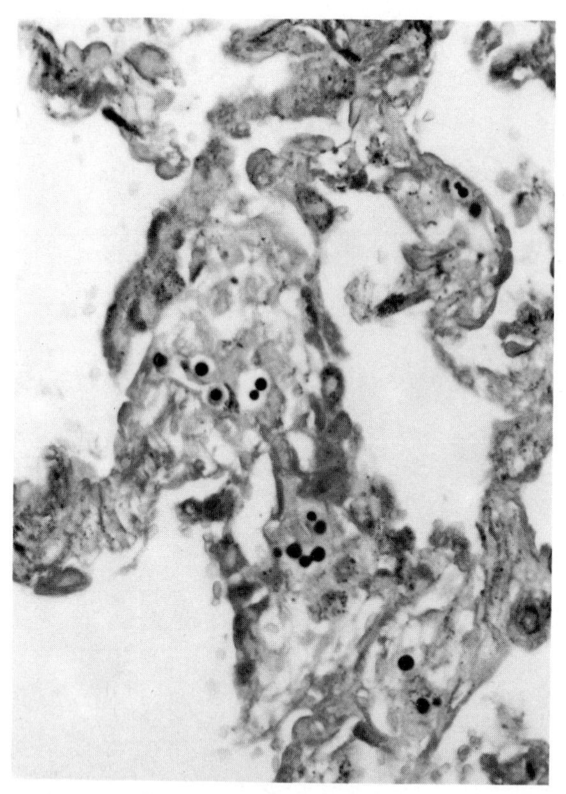

Figure 5–104. Diffuse intracapillary cryptococcosis in an immunosuppressed patient. The alveolar walls are thickened and edematous, and special stains show numerous yeast forms, some with budding, within the capillary lumens.

Cryptococcus is recognized as a yeast form 3 to 8 μm in diameter. The organism has a thick, gelatinous capsule that is mucicarmine-positive, and shows single, narrow-based budding. Intracellular or extracellular forms may be appreciated. *Cryptococcus* may be quite pleomorphic on silver stains. Capsule-deficient forms can be seen in the immunosuppressed patient.

Cryptococcosis with granulomatous inflammation manifests as mixed neutrophilic and histiocytic inflammation, necrosis with pallisading histiocytes and peripheral xanthoma cells (some containing organisms), multinucleate giant cells, and variable numbers of free organisms. Some cases manifest only as non-necrotizing granulomas. The giant cells and histiocytes may appear vacuolated as a result of the presence of organisms.

Cryptococcosis with histiocytic pneumonia shows large numbers of intra-alveolar histiocytes containing organisms, minimal lymphocytic inflammation, and a large number of free organisms in alveoli and capillaries; this form resembles obstructive pneumonia.

Cryptococcal infection with a pauci-inflammatory response typically includes intracapillary organisms and a mucoid pneumonia without inflammatory reaction; this is seen especially in acquired immunodeficiency syndrome (AIDS).

References

Dail DH, Hammer SP (eds). Pulmonary Pathology. New York, Springer-Verlag, 1988.

Feigin DS. Pulmonary cryptococcosis: radiologic-pathologic correlates of its three forms. AJR 141:1262–1272, 1983.

Harding SA, Scheld WM, Feldman PS, Sande MA. Pulmonary infection with capsule-deficient *Cryptococcus neoformans*. Virchows Arch (A) 382:113–118, 1979.

Kerkering TM, Duma RJ, Shadomy S. The evolution of pulmonary cryptococcosis: clinical implications from a study of 41 patients with and without compromising host factors. Ann Intern Med 94:611–616, 1981.

Thurlbeck WM (ed). Pathology of the Lung. New York, Thieme, 1988.

■ Mucormycosis (Phycomycosis, Zygomycosis) (Figs. 5–105 to 5–107)

Mucormycosis occurs almost exclusively in immunocompromised hosts and those with predisposing factors, including leukemia, lymphoma, neutropenia, immunosuppressive chemotherapy, antibiotic therapy, concurrent bacterial infection, severe uncontrolled diabetes, acidotic renal failure, and severe burn injury.

Mucormycotic lung infections usually have two overlapping patterns: (1) pulmonary infarction and (2) necrotizing bronchopneumonia. Diagnosis of each requires recognition of the fungal forms in diseased tissue. Sinus involvement may be an accompanying finding. An uncommon pattern is a chronic bronchocentric mycosis.

The features of mucormycosis include nonseptate hyphae 10 to 25 μm wide, with irregular right angle branching, pleomorphic, collapsing, nonparallel walls, and rare chlamydoconidia and sporangia.

The typical histologic findings of mucormycosis in the lung include (1) fungal vascular invasion with pulmonary infarction (nodular infarcts [small], wedge-shaped infarcts [large and peripheral]), (2) pulmonary hemorrhage and edema, and (3) an acute necrotizing bronchopneumonia.

References

Dail DH, Hammer SP (eds). Pulmonary Pathology. New York, Springer-Verlag, 1988.

Marchevsky AM, Bottone EJ, Geller SA, Giger DK. The changing spectrum of disease, etiology, and diagnosis of mucormycosis. Hum Pathol 11:457–464, 1980.

Thurlbeck WM (ed). Pathology of the Lung. New York, Thieme, 1988.

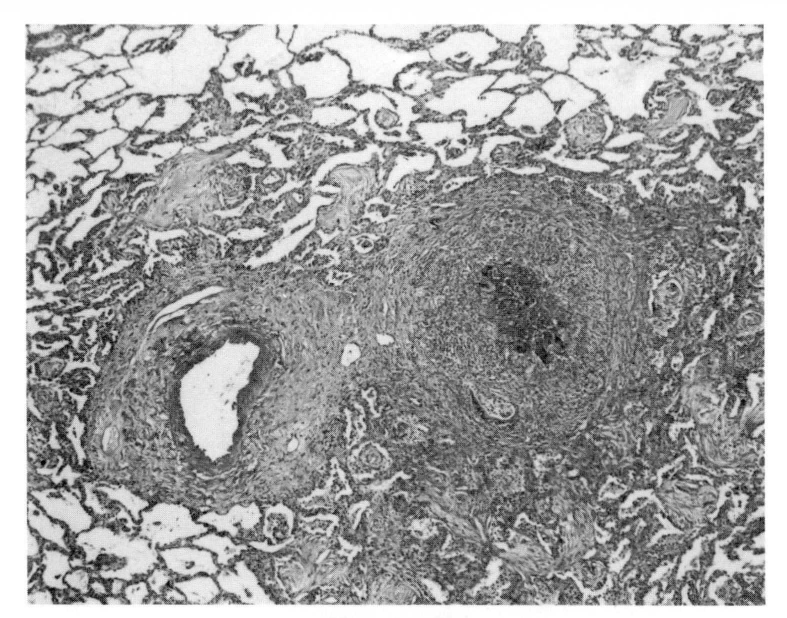

Figure 5-105.

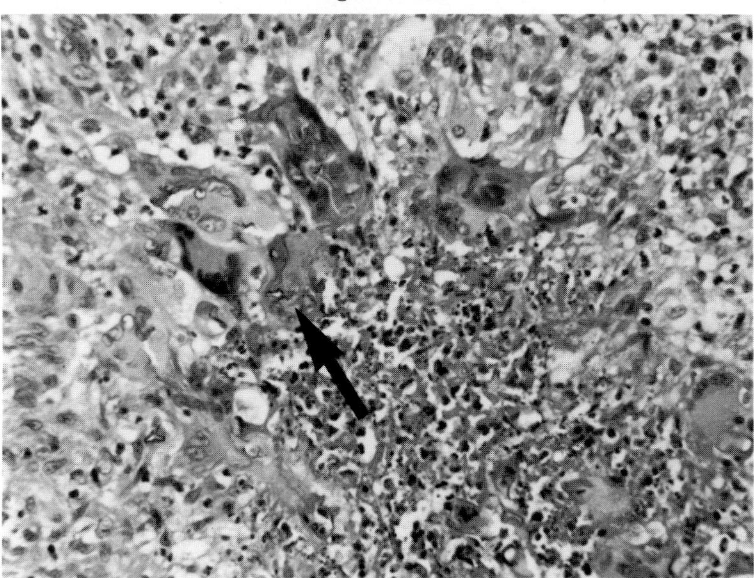

Figure 5-106.

Figures 5-105, 5-106, 5-107. Chronic bronchocentric mucormycosis in a bone marrow transplant patient. There is inflammation and granulomatous destruction of the bronchiolar wall. Fat, irregular, somewhat degenerative-appearing hyphal fragments can be identified on both hematoxylin and eosin (H & E), and silver-stained sections (arrows).

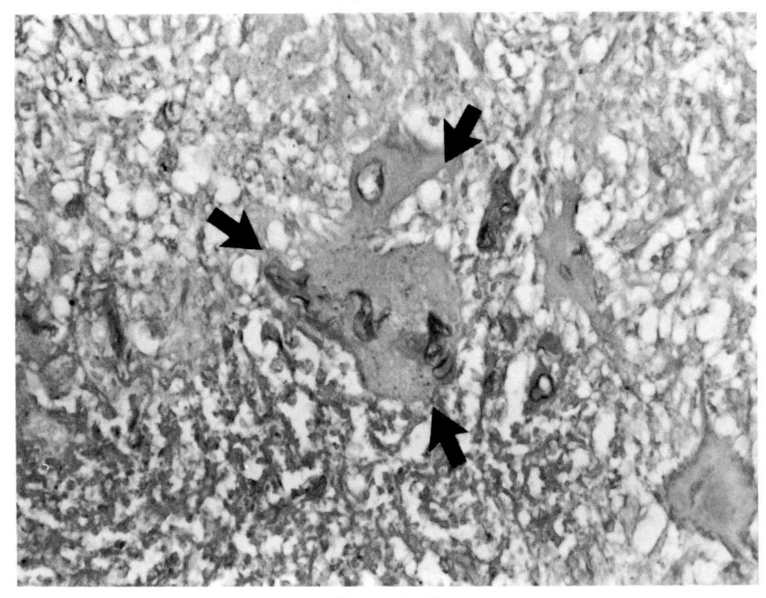

Figure 5-107.

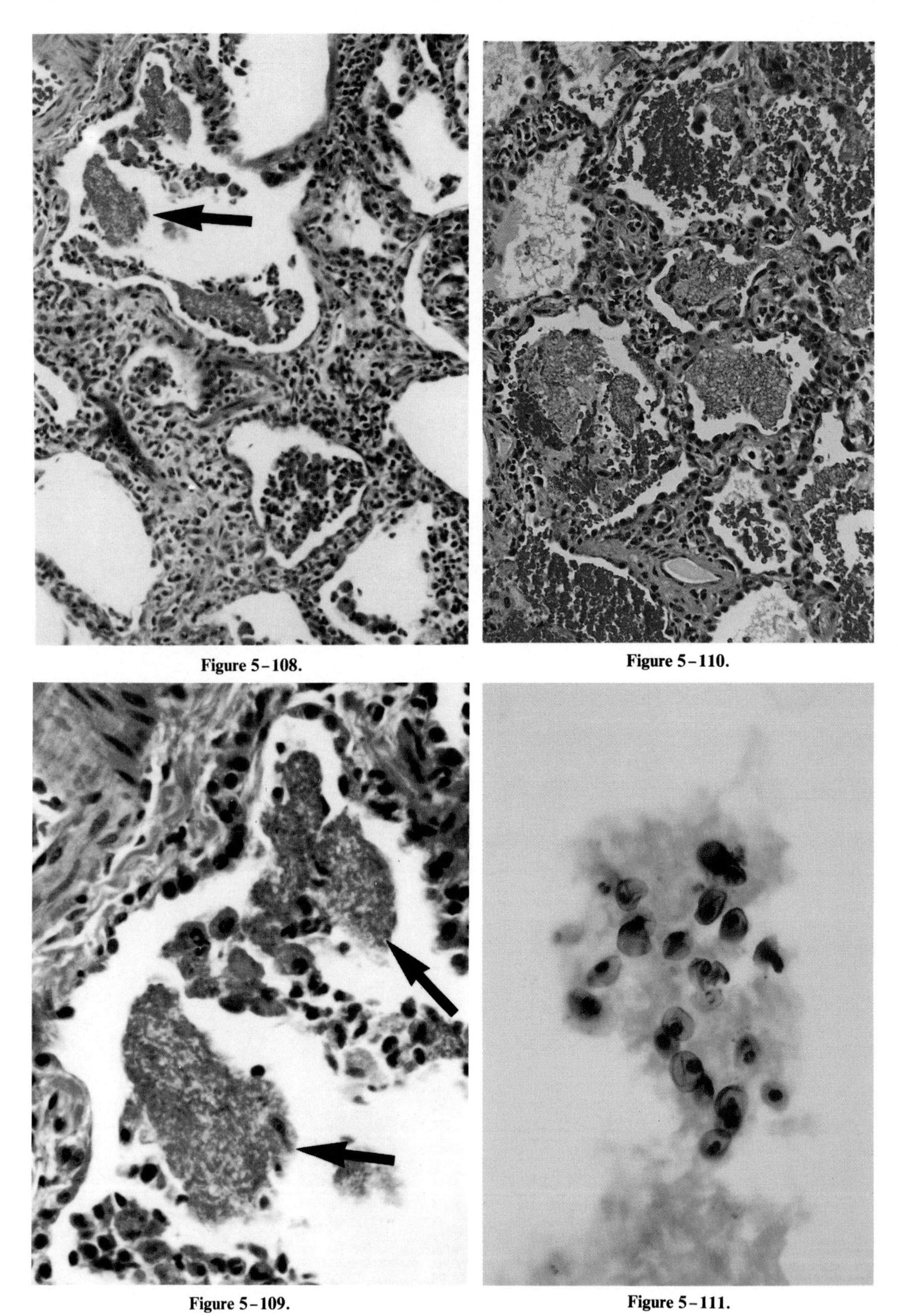

Figure 5-108.

Figure 5-110.

Figure 5-109.

Figure 5-111.

Figures 5-108, 5-109, 5-110, 5-111. ***Pneumocystis carinii*** **pneumonia.** Biopsy material shows the typical airspace exudate of pneumocystis with surrounding inflammatory changes in alveolar walls. This pink, frothy material is composed of colonies of organisms that appear as small bluish dots on hematoxylin and eosin (H & E) slides. The presence of this frothy material in a lung biopsy specimen should be considered pneumocystis until proven otherwise. Silver stains (Fig. 5-111) show staining of the cyst wall.

■ *Pneumocystis carinii* Pneumonia (Figs. 5–108 to 5–119)

Pneumocystis carinii was initially described in malnourished infants following World War II as plasma cell interstitial pneumonia. More recently, it has become an extremely common infection in immunosuppressed patients, particularly patients with AIDS. There may be an acute fulminant bilateral infiltrate, or the patient may experience a more insidious shortness of breath that increases over months or weeks. The latter is characteristic of AIDS. In such cases, the clinician may even be considering a chronic interstitial pneumonia and may be surprised by the diagnosis of pneumocystosis. Rarely, *Pneumocystis* infection has been associated with localized infiltrates and even localized necrotizing granulomas, with the organisms identified in the center.

Classically, *Pneumocystis* is seen as a frothy, eosinophilic intra-alveolar exudate in which tiny blue dots (probably corresponding to the nucleoprotein of the organism) can be barely discerned on routine H & E stains. The interstitial reaction in such cases is generally mild, consisting of few chronic inflammatory cells and prominent type II alveolar lining cells. This classical pattern has become the exception rather than the rule, as any number of other patterns may be seen, including nearly normal pulmonary histologic appearance with numerous organisms seen by special stains; cellular interstitial pneumonia, often rich in plasma cells, which may be dense enough to suggest a lymphoreticular neoplasm; diffuse alveolar damage with hyaline membranes; gran-

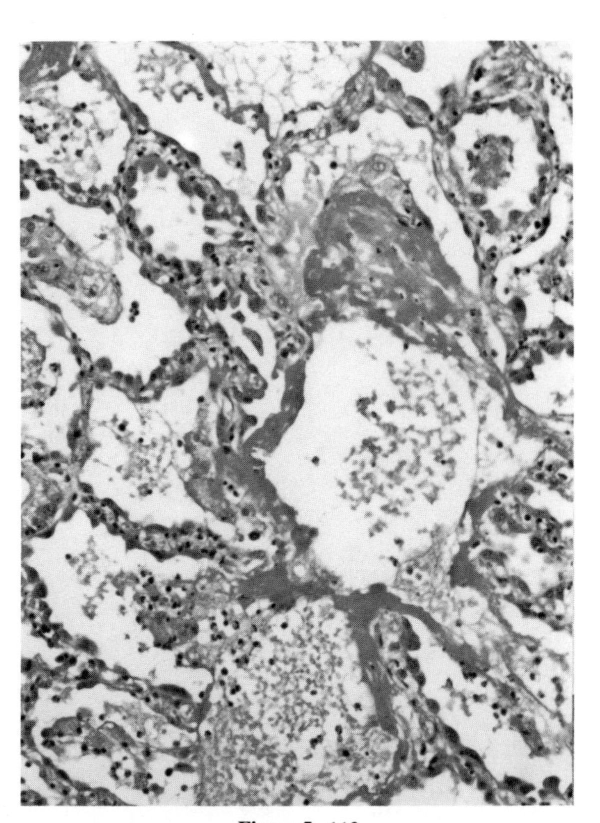

Figure 5–113.

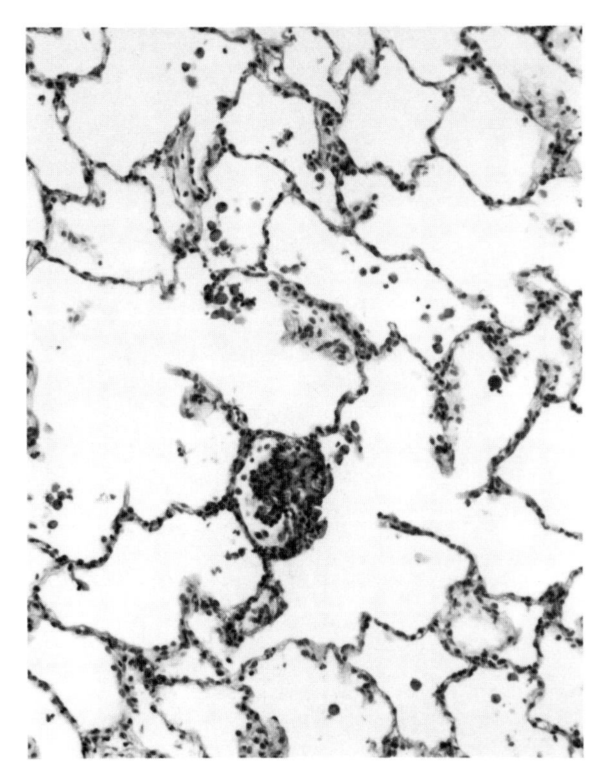

Figure 5–112. *P. carinii* pneumonia in a patient with acquired immunodeficiency syndrome (AIDS). There is minimal inflammatory reaction and absence of the characteristic airspace exudate of *Pneumocystis.* Silver stain showed large numbers of organisms lining the alveolar walls.

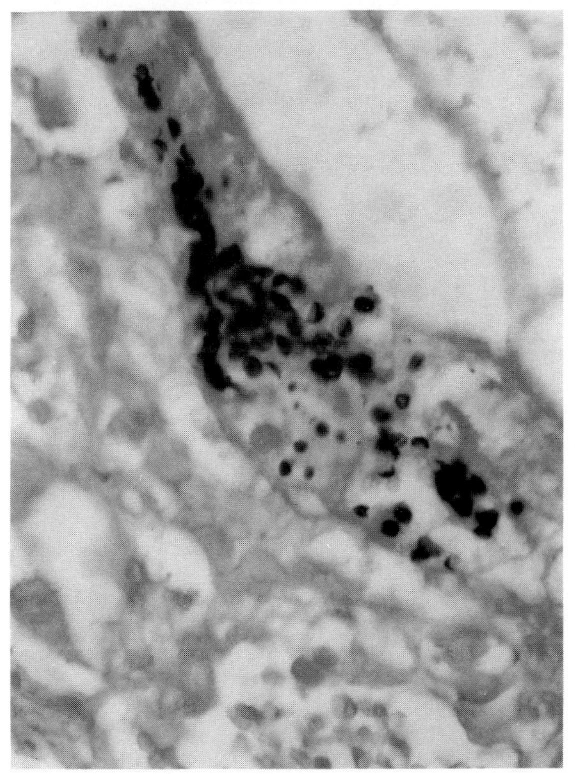

Figure 5–114.

Figures 5–113, 5–114. *P. carinii* pneumonia with hyaline membranes and features of diffuse alveolar damage. There is an absence of the characteristic exudate of *Pneumocystis.* Special stains show large colonies of organisms within the hyaline membranes.

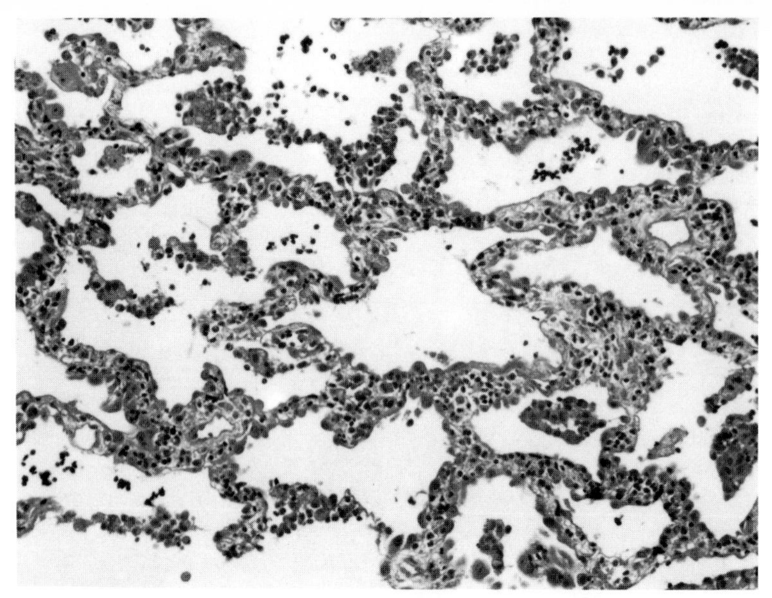

Figure 5–115.

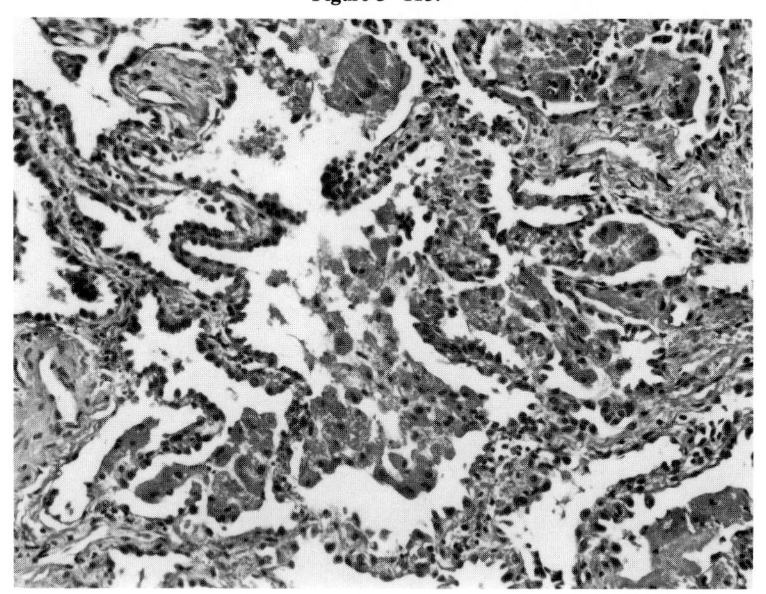

Figure 5–116.

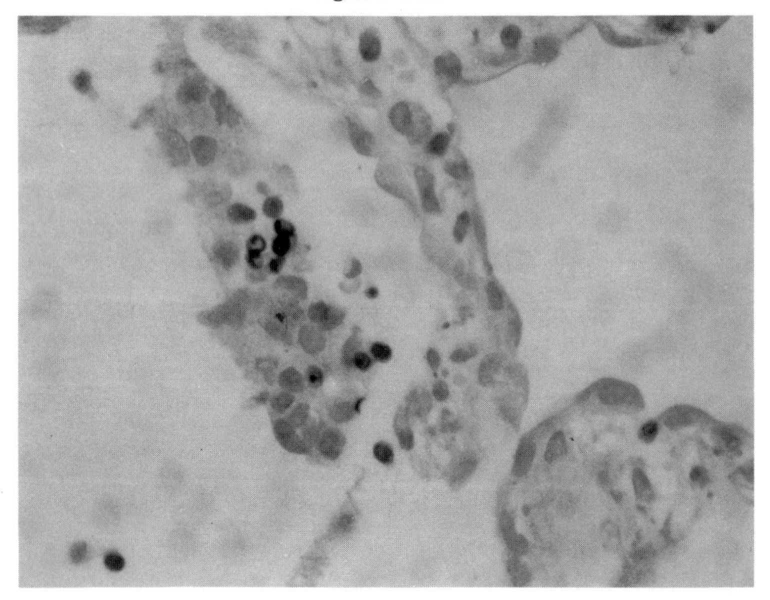

Figure 5–117.

Figures 5–115, 5–116, 5–117. *P. carinii* pneumonia in acquired immunodeficiency syndrome (AIDS) with nonspecific cellular interstitial pneumonia and foci resembling desquamative interstitial pneumonia. There are prominent type II alveolar lining cells, and the characteristic exudate of *Pneumocystis* is lacking. Organisms were found associated with macrophages in the alveoli (Fig. 5–117).

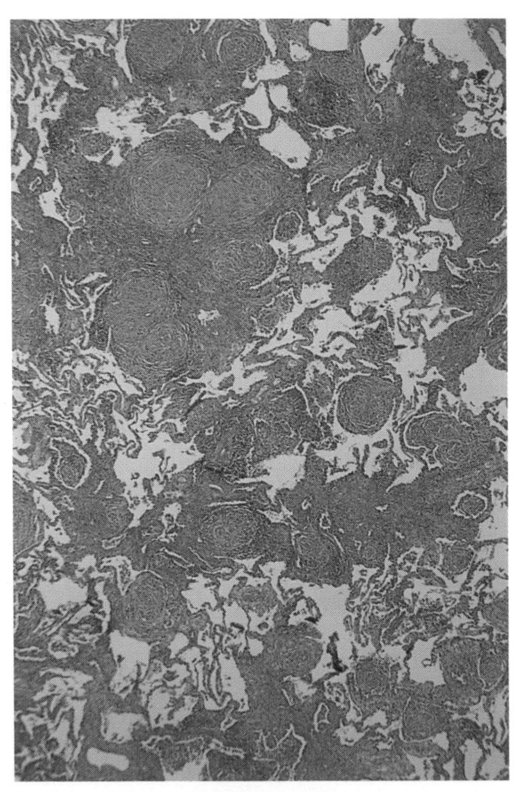

Figure 5–118.

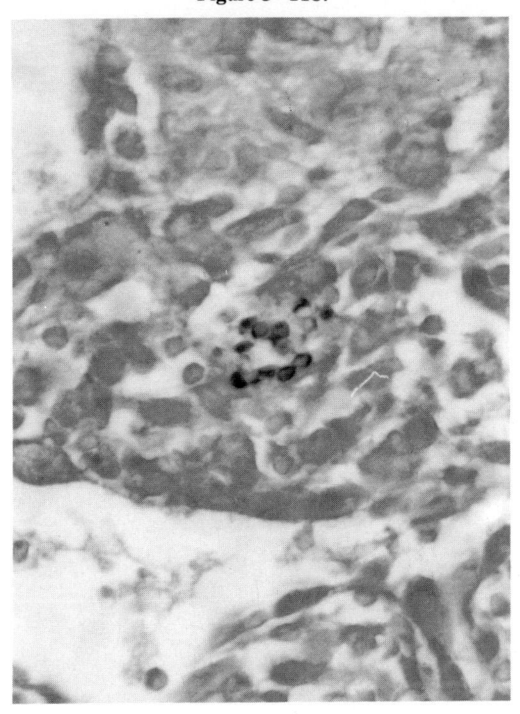

Figure 5–119.

Figures 5–118, 5–119. *P. carinii* pneumonia with granulomatous reaction. Numerous non-necrotizing granulomas reminiscent of those seen in sarcoidosis characterize this open lung biopsy specimen. Moderate numbers of organisms could be identified within the granulomas.

ulomatous interstitial pneumonia; a pattern resembling desquamative interstitial pneumonia; a pattern of alveolar hemorrhage; and necrotic nodules.

The diagnosis of *P. carinii* pneumonia is dependent on morphologic identification of the organism, which is usually best accomplished with a methenamine silver stain that highlights the cyst wall. A number of other special stains have been employed, including Gram-Weigert, Giemsa, and Papanicolaou. The cyst wall is approximately the size of a red blood cell and commonly shows cup-shaped, helmet-shaped, and crinkled forms that may have a small silver-positive dot in the center. The organisms typically occur in clusters. The characteristic foamy exudate can be identified on Papanicolaou-stained material, Wright-Giemsa–stained lavage material, and even H & E slides. Identification of the characteristic foamy exudate is *virtually diagnostic* of the organism. When the typical foamy exudate is seen and the special stains are "negative," it is usually due to a technical problem as there is no other pulmonary condition that causes the *classic* pulmonary alveolar exudate, which represents a colony of organisms.

Occasionally, *Pneumocystis* organisms are incidental findings in autopsy lung specimens and as such are not necessarily indicative of infection. It appears as though they may exist as a saprophyte, but with immunosuppression *Pneumocystis* often becomes a significant infection. The histologic features of pneumocystosis are so protean that *any lung biopsy from an immunosuppressed patient should be carefully evaluated for the presence of* Pneumocystis. It is an organism that is not to be underestimated. *Pneumocystis* should also be sought in lung biopsy specimens that show a rather nondescript cellular interstitial infiltrate (without much fibrosis) in a patient who has some history of immunosuppression or who is presumed to have a chronic interstitial pneumonia.

References

Dail DH, Hammer SP (eds). Pulmonary Pathology. New York, Springer-Verlag, 1988.

Flint A, Colby TV. Surgical Pathology of Diffuse Infiltrative Lung Disease. Orlando, Grune & Stratton, Inc, 1987.

Katzenstein ALA, Askin FB. Surgical Pathology of Non-Neoplastic Lung Disease, 2nd ed. Philadelphia, WB Saunders, Co, 1990.

Thurlbeck WM (ed). Pathology of the Lung. New York, Thieme, 1988.

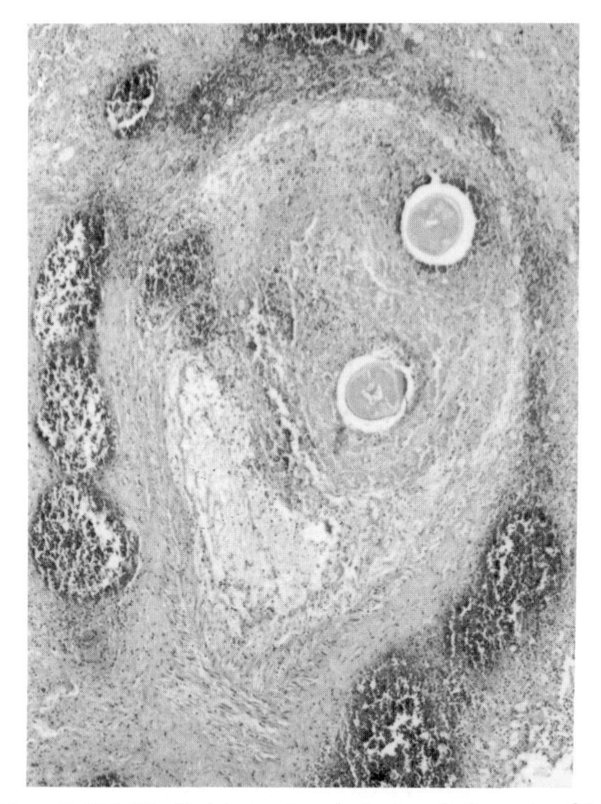

Figure 5-120. Dirofilarial granuloma in the lung. In the center of the necrotic granuloma, two cross sections of the necrotic organism can be seen within a thrombosed and partially necrotic pulmonary artery.

■ Dirofilarial (Dog Heartworm) Granulomas (Fig. 5-120)

Humans are incidental hosts for *Dirofilaria.* The lesion presents as a single (rarely multiple) coin lesion; the incidence is higher in the southeastern United States. There is a necrotizing granuloma with a fibrous wall and a necrotic center. Eosinophils may be prominent. Sectioning of the nodule may reveal the degenerate worm fragments within a necrotic pulmonary artery in the center.

References

Dail DH, Hammer SP (eds). Pulmonary Pathology. New York, Springer-Verlag, 1988.

Thurlbeck WM (ed). Pathology of the Lung. New York, Thieme, 1988.

■ *Toxoplasma gondii* Pneumonia (Figs. 5-121 to 5-123)

T. gondii rarely involves the lungs, and most affected patients are immunosuppressed. Although an interstitial pneumonia with scattered *Toxoplasma* cysts may occur, the most characteristic lesions are necrotizing nodules, usually microscopic, with central coagulative necrosis, containing tachyzoites, with the typical cysts seen in the surrounding tissue.

References

Dail DH, Hammer SP (eds). Pulmonary Pathology. New York, Springer-Verlag, 1988.

Figures 5-121, 5-122, 5-123. Pulmonary toxoplasmosis in a heart transplant patient. Biopsy material showed multiple microscopic nodular foci of coagulative necrosis. Careful evaluation in the necrotic foci revealed occasional *toxoplasma* cysts as well as free organisms (tachyzoites) from recently ruptured cysts (Fig. 5-122). A Wright-Giemsa stained touch imprint from the specimen also showed the organisms (Fig. 5-123).

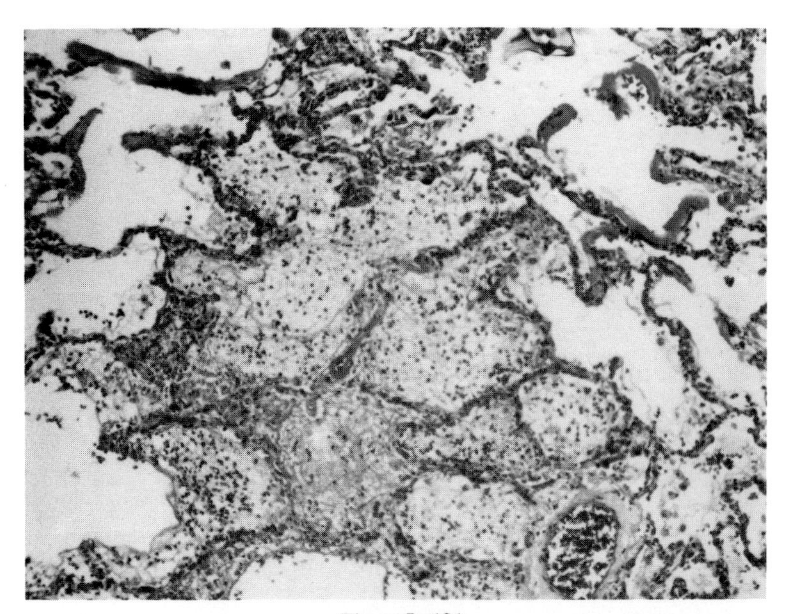

Figure 5-121.

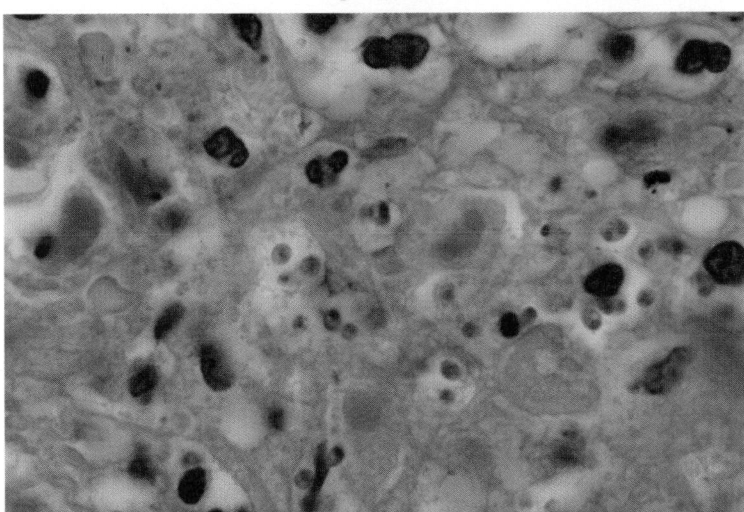

Figure 5-122.

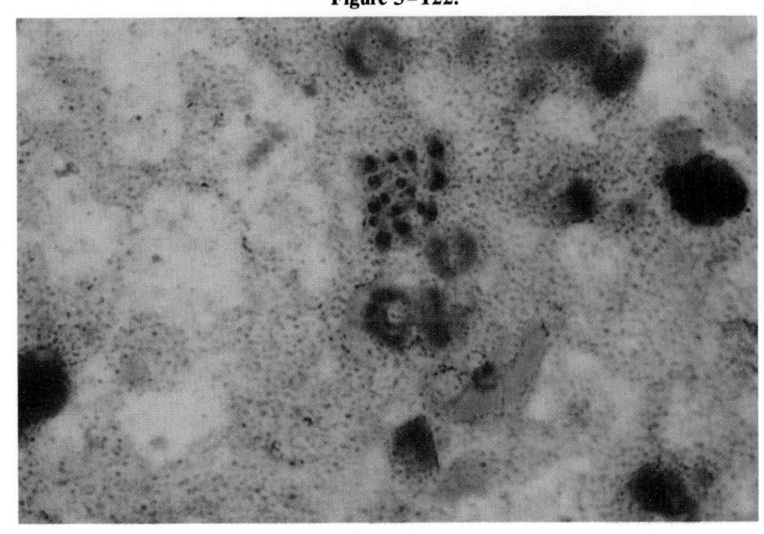

Figure 5-123.

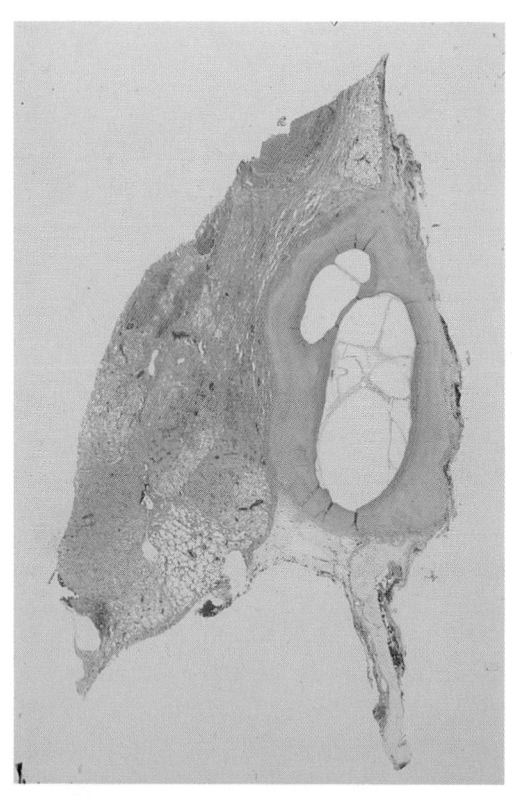

Figure 5-124.

■ Echinococcal Cyst of the Lung (Figs. 5-124 to 1-126)

Pulmonary cysts may be caused by *Echinococcus granulosus* or *Echinococcus multilocularis. E. granulosus* is a parasite in sheep and dogs, and *E. multilocularis* affects wildlife, with foxes being the definitive host. The infective organisms are passed in the animal feces.

Histologically, the echinococcal cyst usually appears as a unilocular cyst showing the characteristic wall with the typical germinal layer and the acellular laminated membrane. The surrounding lung may show an infiltrate rich in eosinophils that mimics eosinophilic pneumonia. Rupture of the cysts into airways or secondary infection may occur. Diagnosis is based on the demonstration of parasitic structures, usually hooklets, or on the characteristic appearance of the cyst wall.

References

Dail DH, Hammer SP (eds). Pulmonary Pathology. New York, Springer-Verlag, 1988.

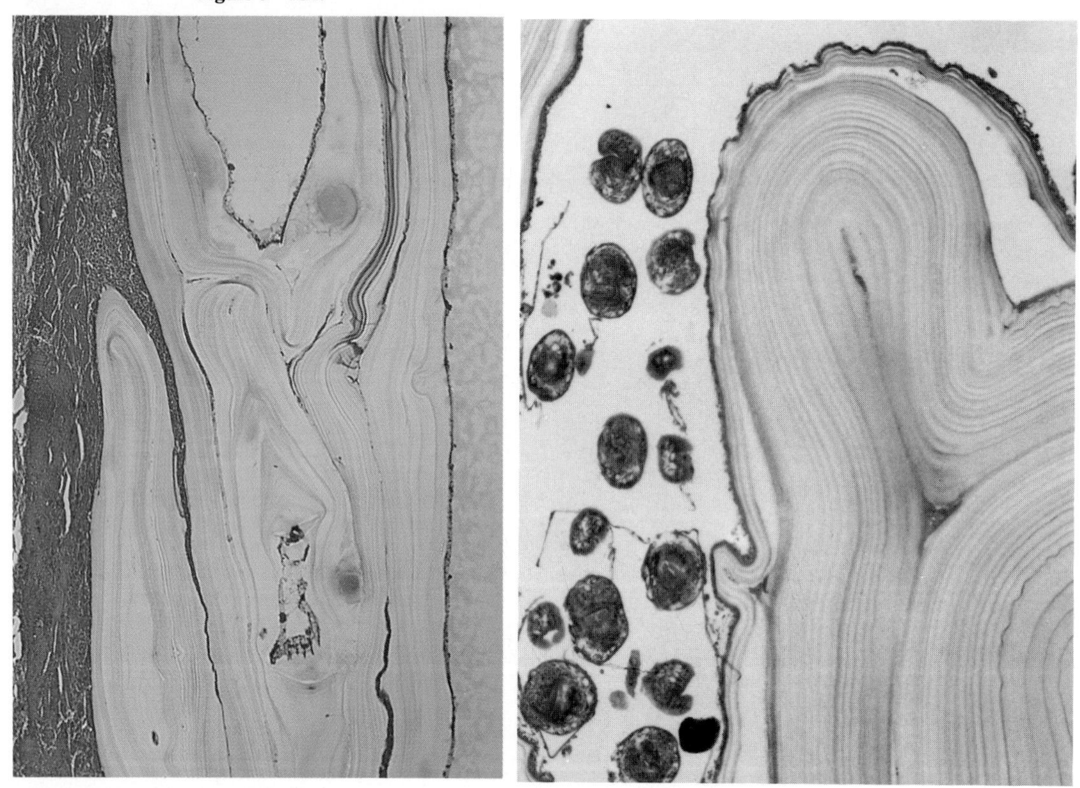

Figure 5-125. **Figure 5-126.**

Figures 5-124, 5-125, 5-126. Echinococcal cyst of the lung. There is a septated cyst with a thick, fibrous wall. Detail of the cyst wall shows the typical laminar appearance of *Echinococcus granulosus* as well as numerous scolices (Fig. 5-126).

CHAPTER 6

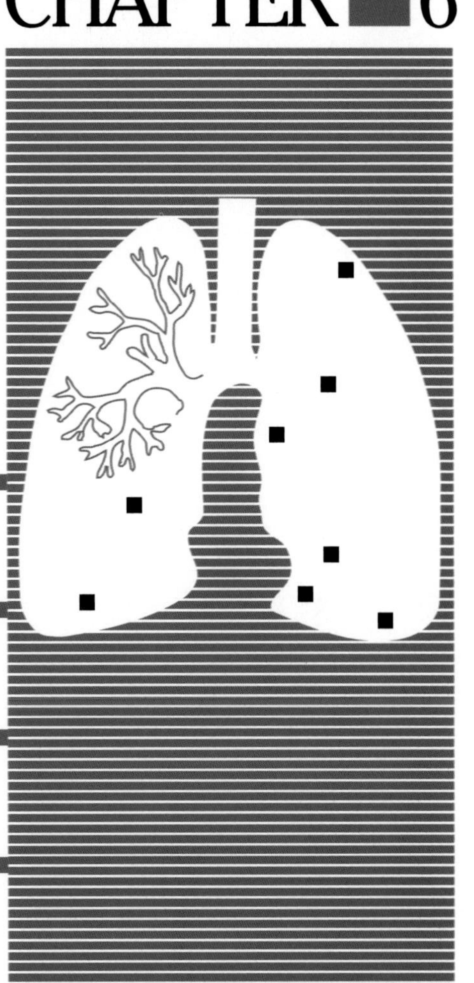

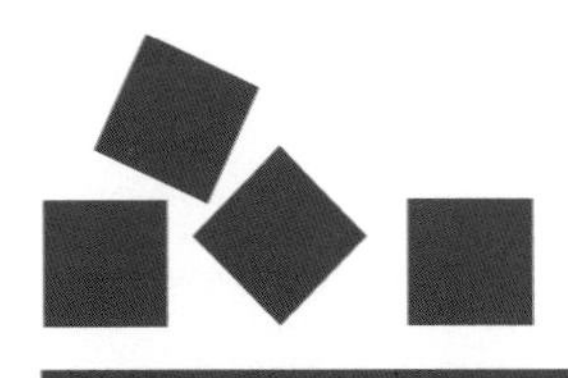

AIRWAY AND OBSTRUCTIVE DISEASES

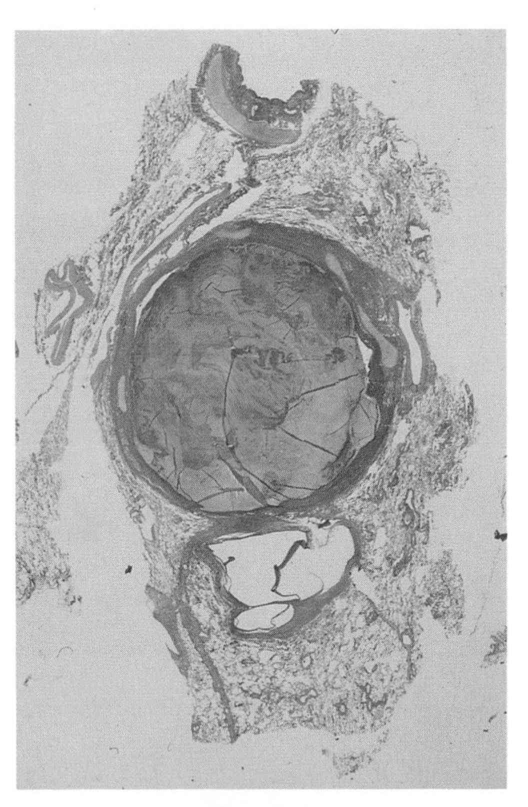

Figure 6-1.

■ Mucoid Impaction (Figs. 6-1 to 6-3)

This condition is characterized by impacted mucus in a medium-sized airway that usually presents as a persistent radiographic infiltrate, often occurring in a patient with a history of asthma. Resected specimens show a dense mucous plug; more distal parenchyma may show distal bronchocentric granulomatosis, eosinophilic pneumonia, or both. Histologically, the mucous plug should be evaluated for fragments of fungal hyphae, *which may take some time to find;* the mucus typically has a lamellar character, with layers of neutrophils, eosinophils, flocculent granular eosinophilic debris, and Charcot-Leyden crystals (so-called allergic mucin). The differential diagnosis includes impacted mucus distal to an obstructing lesion in the airway.

References

Dail DH, Hammer SP (eds). Pulmonary Pathology. New York, Springer-Verlag, 1988.

Katzenstein ALA, Askin FB. Surgical Pathology of Non-Neoplastic Lung Disease, 2nd ed. Philadelphia, WB Saunders Co, 1990.

Thurlbeck WM (ed). Pathology of the Lung. New York, Thieme, 1988.

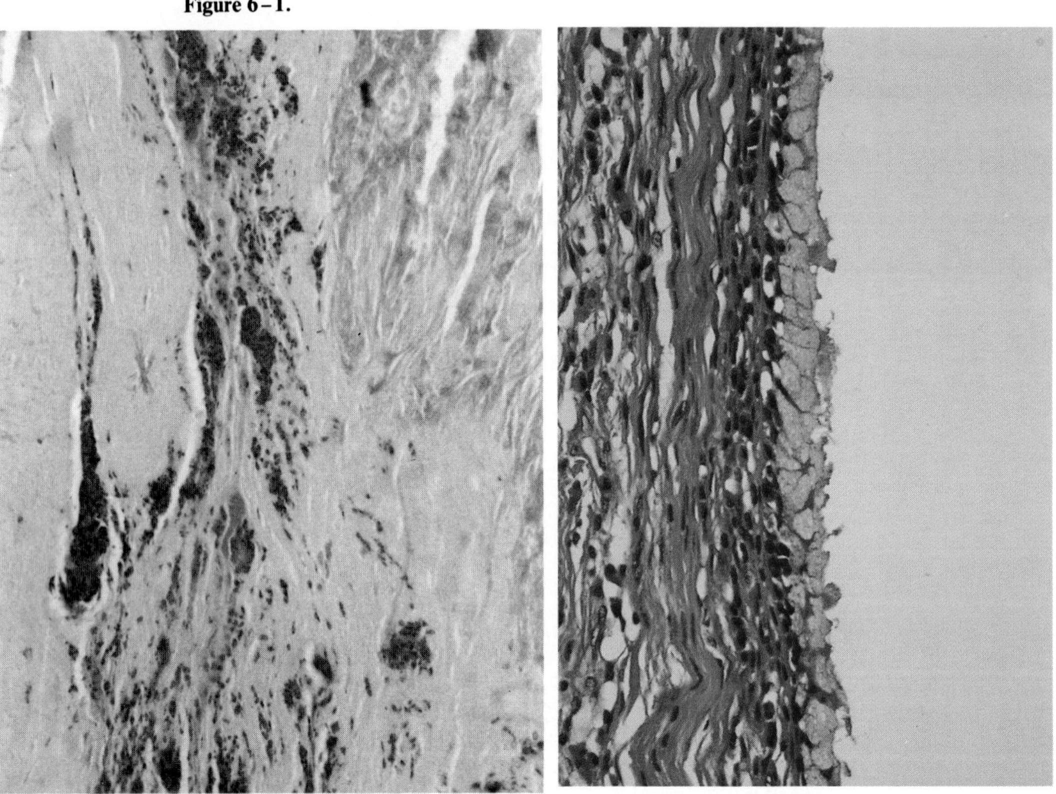

Figure 6-2. Figure 6-3.

Figures 6-1, 6-2, 6-3. Mucoid impaction. There is a medium-sized bronchus that contains a large mucous plug. The mucus is layered with eosinophilic and basophilic zones; within the layers, large numbers of eosinophils and eosinophilic breakdown debris are often discernible. In such cases, silver stains should be performed and evaluated for the presence of fragmented *Aspergillus* hyphae. The mucosa is often composed entirely of goblet cells (Fig. 6-3).

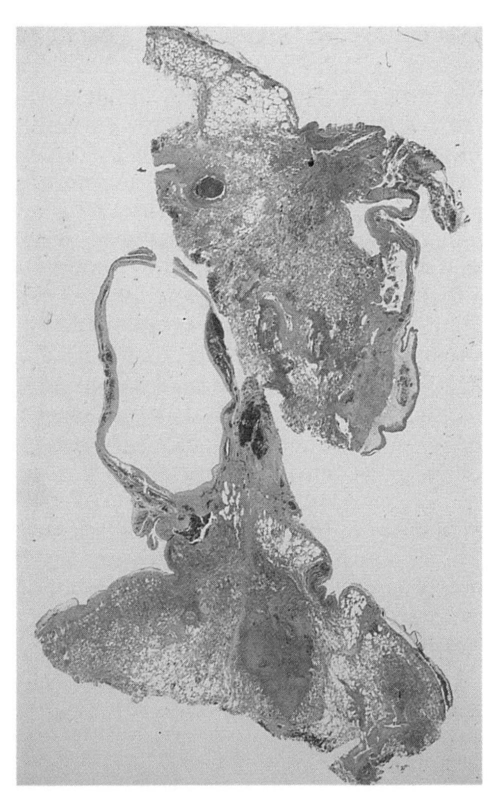
Figure 6–4.

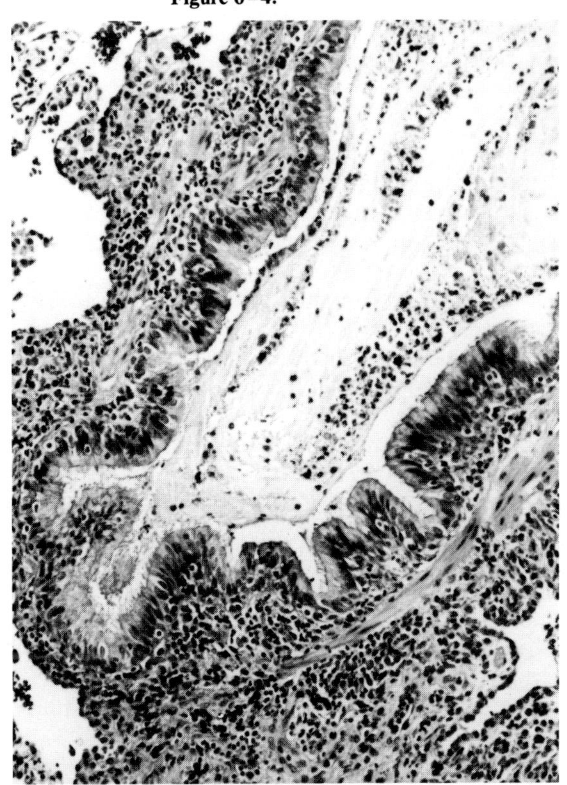
Figure 6–5.

Figures 6–4, 6–5. Cystic fibrosis. A patient underwent lobectomy for recurrent pneumothoraces, which were related to subpleural blebs. The underlying parenchyma shows acute and chronic cellular bronchiolitis with zones of organization and scarring. The bronchioles contain a purulent exudate and show bronchiolectasis.

■ Cystic Fibrosis (Figs. 6–4 and 6–5)

Specimens from patients with cystic fibrosis are seen only occasionally by the surgical pathologist. Severe localized bronchiectasis may sometimes lead to a surgical resection, or excision of blebs may be performed in patients who have had recurrent pneumothoraces.

Histologic changes in cystic fibrosis include bronchiectasis and in bronchiolectasis with secondary inflammatory changes in the parenchyma consisting of bronchopneumonia, sometimes with organization and scarring. Typically, the airways are filled with dense purulent mucus, which frequently contains large numbers of neutrophils and bacterial colonies (often *Pseudomonas*).

If large airways are included in the pathologic specimen, one should examine the submucosal glands for the typical small concretions of impacted mucus with the acini. Mesothelial cells on the visceral pleural surface may show cuboidal change.

References

Dail DH, Hammer SP (eds). Pulmonary Pathology. New York, Springer-Verlag, 1988.
Thurlbeck WM (ed). Pathology of the Lung. New York, Thieme, 1988.

■ Fume and Smoke Inhalation (See Fig. 6–27)

A large number of fumes, and also fire smoke, may be associated with acute pulmonary injury. Silo-filler's disease represents one of the better known examples. In general, there is a known history of exposure, although clinical signs and symptoms do not always develop immediately. Biopsies are rarely performed in the acute state, although occasionally they are performed after some weeks to assess the degree of damage and histologic changes.

Acutely, there is necrosis and acute inflammation of the airways, with edema and diffuse alveolar damage (DAD) involving the alveolar parenchyma. The lesion may heal entirely or may leave a residue of fibrosis, usually manifesting as airflow obstruction as the result of injury and scarring to the small airways. As such, the healed phase falls into the generic group of small airway injury (see 211).

References

Churg A, Green FHY. Pathology of Occupational Lung Disease. New York, Igaku-Shoin Medical Publishers, 1988.
Dail DH, Hammer SP (eds). Pulmonary Pathology. New York, Springer-Verlag, 1988.
Thurlbeck WM (ed). Pathology of the Lung. New York, Thieme, 1988.

■ Bronchiectasis and Localized Chronic Bronchitis or Bronchiolitis with or without Abscess Formation (See Figs. 3–4 to 3–6)

These are localized infiltrates on the chest radiograph. Radiographic features of bronchiectasis may be present.

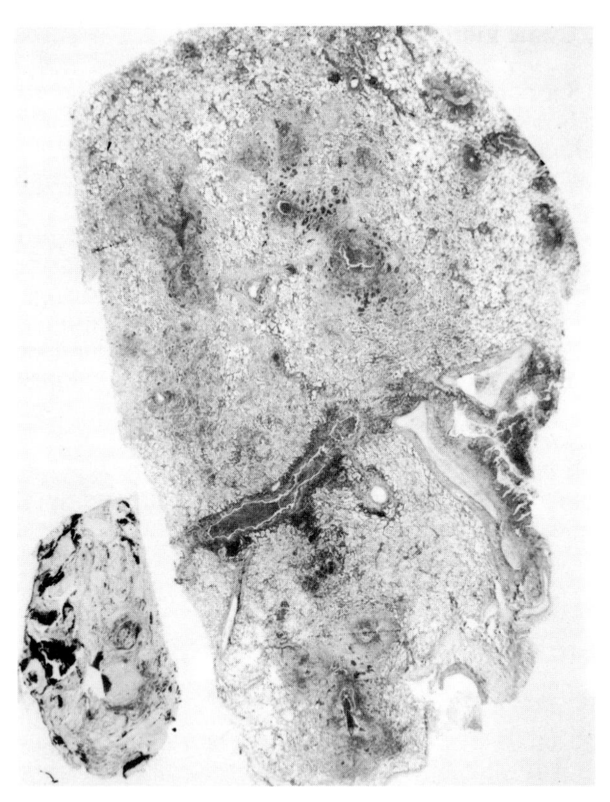

Figure 6–6.

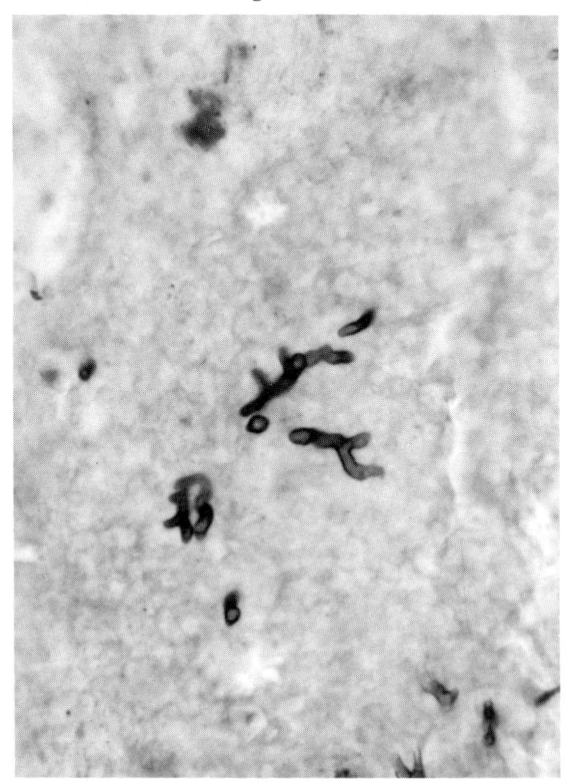

Figure 6–7.

Figures 6–6, 6–7. Bronchocentric granulomatosis (BCG). BCG begins as an acute and chronic inflammatory lesion of the small airways, and this can be best appreciated on gross inspection of the slide or scanning microscopy. The airway lesions are often of different ages, and it may take some time to find the classic bronchocentric granuloma. A section of the associated mucoid impaction is represented by the smaller piece of tissue (Fig. 6–6). Within the mucus, fragments of *Aspergillus* hyphae were found (Fig. 6–7).

There is nonspecific acute and chronic inflammation with scarring and airway ectasia. In the case of bronchiectasis, a number of subtypes have been described, and gross evaluation of the specimen is very important.

Histologically, scarred and chronically inflamed airways are the major finding. Gross features are important in recognizing bronchiectasis; microscopy is generally quite nonspecific except for bronchocentricity of the mixed acute and chronic inflammatory process with airway epithelial ulceration and metaplasia. A few nonnecrotizing granulomas may be present in the wall of the airway or surrounding lung tissue, and a distal obstructive and/or organizing pneumonia is common. Squamous metaplasia may be marked and sufficiently pseudoepitheliomatous to raise the possibility of carcinoma; markedly atypical cells may be seen in cytologic specimens.

Note: In cases of localized bronchiectasis or chronic bronchitis, careful gross examination should exclude the possibility of a proximal obstructing lesion, although this has often been done clinically with bronchoscopy prior to any resection.

References

Dail DH, Hammer SP (eds). Pulmonary Pathology. New York, Springer-Verlag, 1988.

Thurlbeck WM (ed). Pathology of the Lung. New York, Thieme, 1988.

■ Bronchocentric Granulomatosis (Figs. 6–6 to 6–13)

Bronchocentric granulomatosis (BCG) is a necrotizing bronchocentric process in which the airways show acute and chronic inflammation and destruction of the bronchiolar wall, which is replaced by a rim of palisaded histiocytes surrounding a central plug of necrotic tissue, often necrotic eosinophils.

Clinically, a mass or localized infiltrate is apparent in a patient with a history of asthma and in the setting of allergic bronchopulmonary aspergillosis. Cases occurring in nonasthmatics are occasionally recognized, and multifocality is seen rarely.

Bronchiolocentric necrosis and wall destruction are the major features. In the early lesions, acute inflammation and early epithelial necrosis are seen, whereas in late full-blown lesions the bronchiolar wall is replaced by palisaded histiocytes and there is a central core of eosinophilic and/or neutrophilic debris. Associated findings include obstructive pneumonia, eosinophilic pneumonia, organizing pneumonia, scattered granulomas in the parenchyma, and proximal mucoid impaction. If a mucous plug is identified, a silver stain should be performed to look for fragments of *Aspergillus,* the causative allergen in many cases.

Note: Bronchocentric granulomatosis is a diagnosis of exclusion of infection; therefore, cultures and special stains should be performed in all cases. This is especially true of BCG in nonasthmatics, in whom the central core of the granuloma often contains neutrophils. BCG-like reactions have been observed in patients with a variety of granulomatous infections, and chronic bronchocentric

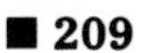

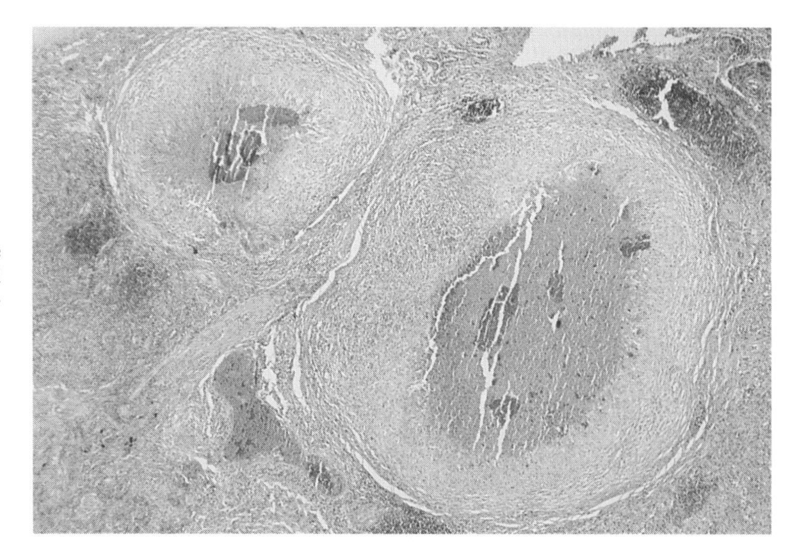

Figure 6-8. Bronchocentric granulomatosis (BCG). The typical well-developed granulomas of BCG have a central plug of necrotic material and a thick, rounded rim of palisaded histiocytes.

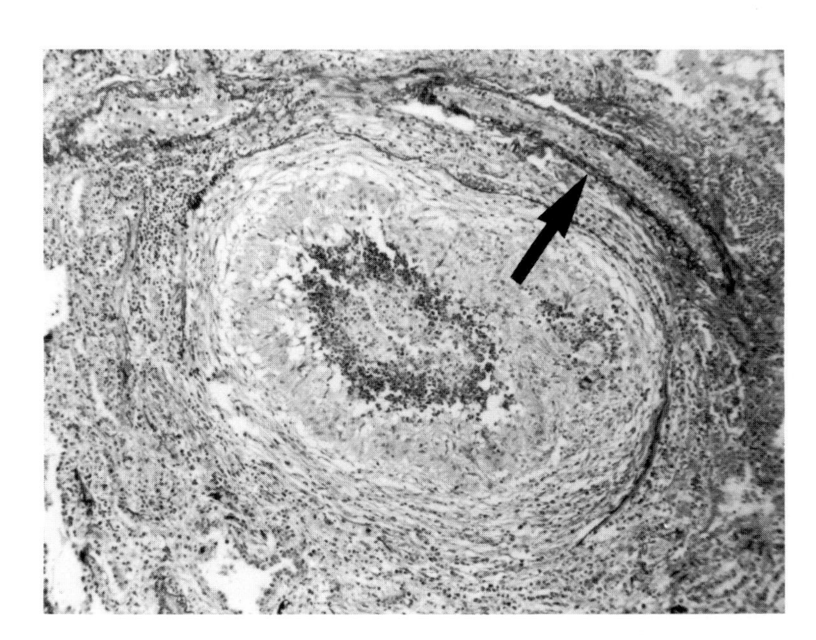

Figure 6-9. Bronchocentric granulomatosis (BCG). This section is stained for elastic tissue and shows a pulmonary artery (arrow) adjacent to a necrotizing granuloma centered on a bronchiole with necrosis and a thick cuff of palisaded histiocytes. There is partial destruction of the elastica of the airway.

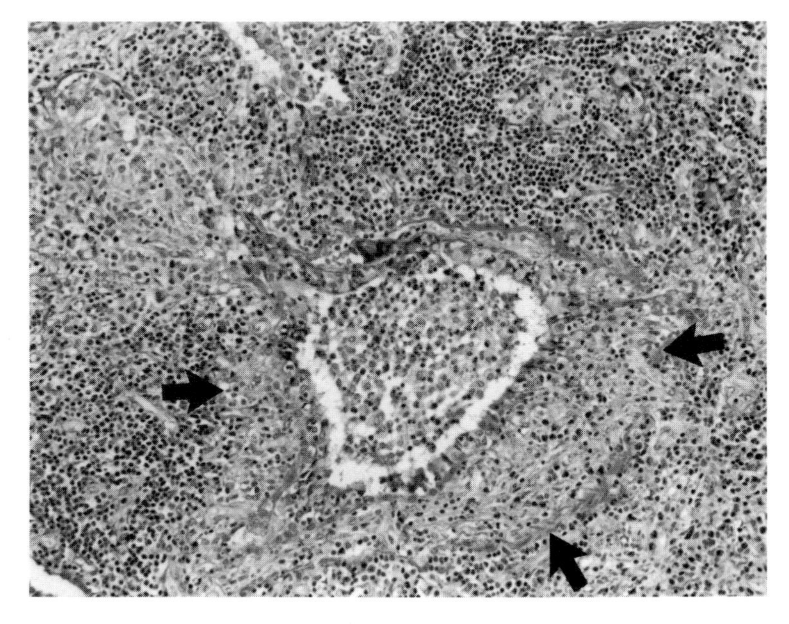

Figure 6-10. Bronchocentric granulomatosis (BCG). Another focus from the case illustrated in Figure 6-9 shows an earlier lesion with inflammation centered on bronchioles and an acute and chronic bronchiolitis with focal histiocytic infiltrate. Partial replacement of the airway wall by histiocytes can be seen (arrows).

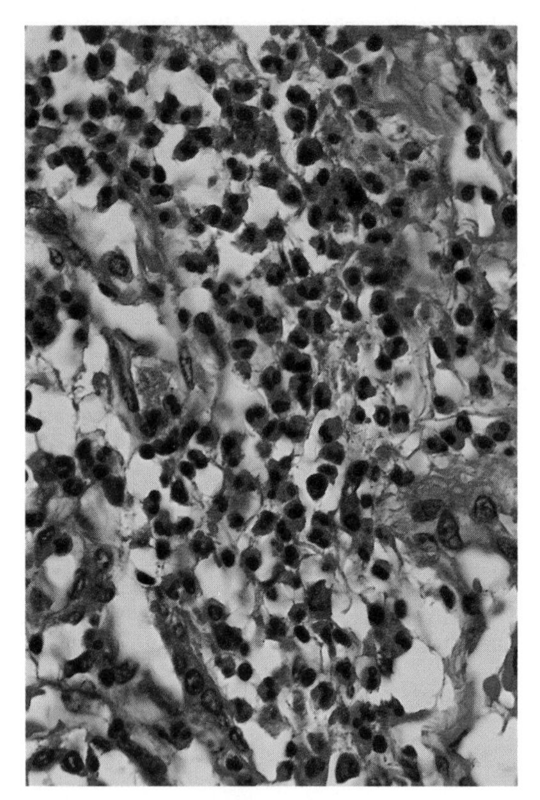

Figure 6–11.

fungal infections in transplant patients have been termed bronchocentric mycosis (Fig. 6–13).

References

Dail DH, Hammer SP (eds). Pulmonary Pathology. New York, Springer-Verlag, 1988.

Katzenstein ALA, Askin FB. Surgical Pathology of Non-Neoplastic Lung Disease, 2nd ed. Philadelphia, WB Saunders Co., 1990.

Katzenstein ALA, Liebow AA, Friedman PJ. Bronchocentric granulomatosis, mucoid impaction, and hypersensitivity reaction to fungi. Am Rev Respir Dis 141:497–537, 1975.

Myers JL. Bronchocentric granulomatosis. Disease or diagnosis (editorial)? Chest 96:3–4, 1989.

Myers JL, Katzenstein ALA. Granulomatous infection mimicking bronchocentric granulomatosis. Am J Surg Pathol 10:317–322, 1986.

Tazelaar HD, Baird AM, Mill M, et al. Bronchocentric mycosis occurring in transplant recipients. Chest 96:92–95, 1989.

Thurlbeck WM (ed). Pathology of the Lung. New York, Thieme, 1988.

■ Allergic Bronchopulmonary Aspergillosis (See Figs. 6–9 to 6–12)

Allergic bronchopulmonary aspergillosis is a clinical syndrome of asthma and recurrent pulmonary infiltrates

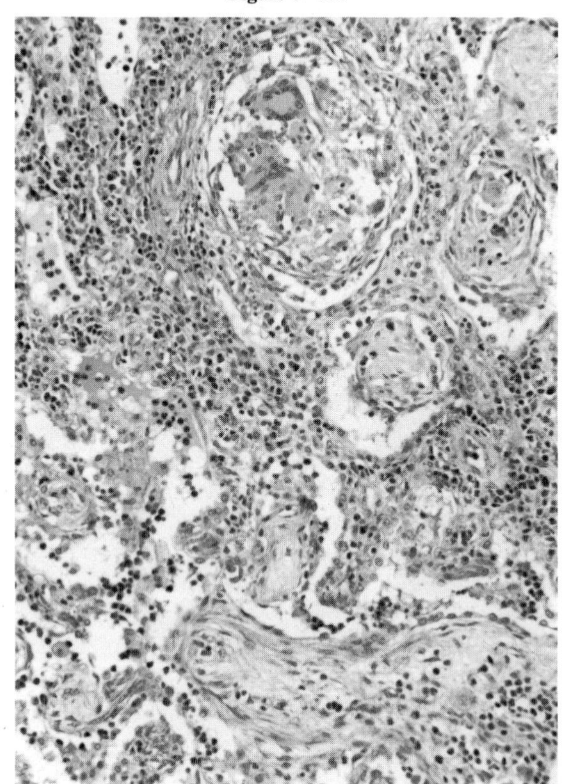

Figure 6–12.

Figures 6–11, 6–12. Bronchocentric granulomatosis (BCG). Alveolar parenchyma from the case illustrated in Figures 6–9 and 6–10 showed the pattern of eosinophilic pneumonia, granulomatous inflammation, and obstructive pneumonia. Adjacent to the granuloma, tufts of organization can be seen both within the alveoli and the alveolar ducts, indicative of the associated organizing pneumonia.

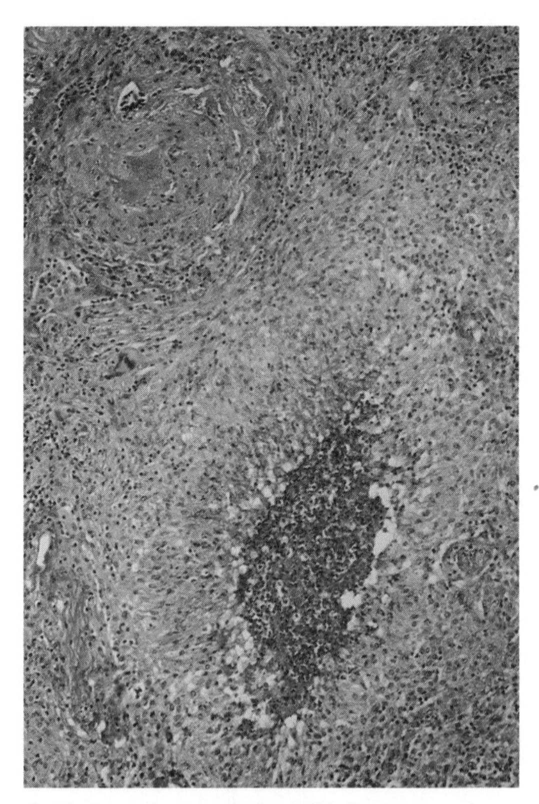

Figure 6–13. A reaction identical to BCG distal to a carcinoma of the lung. No infection could be identified, and there was no history of asthma.

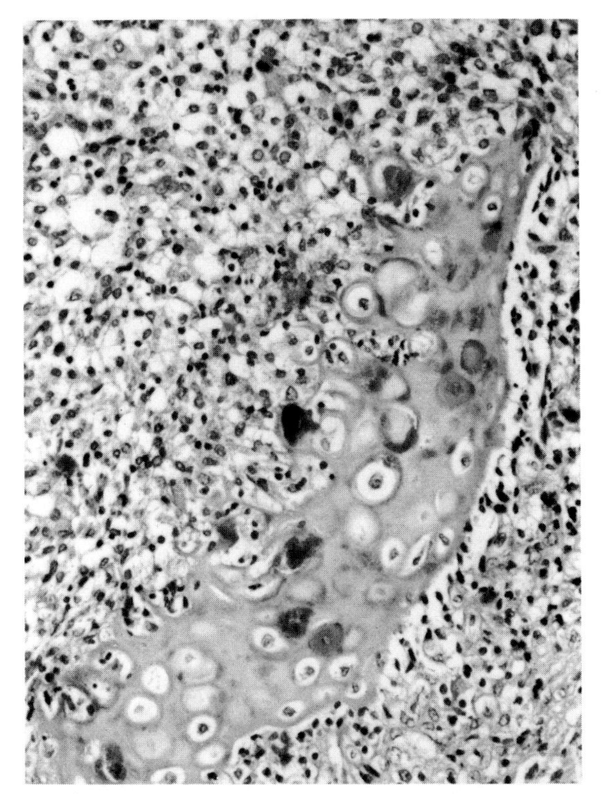

Figure 6-14. Relapsing polychondritis. This patient had recurrent episodes of pneumonia on the basis of airway obstruction secondary to large airway collapse. The cartilaginous plates of the bronchi were being destroyed by an acute and chronic inflammatory process. An appearance very similar to this may be seen with Wegener's granulomatosis.

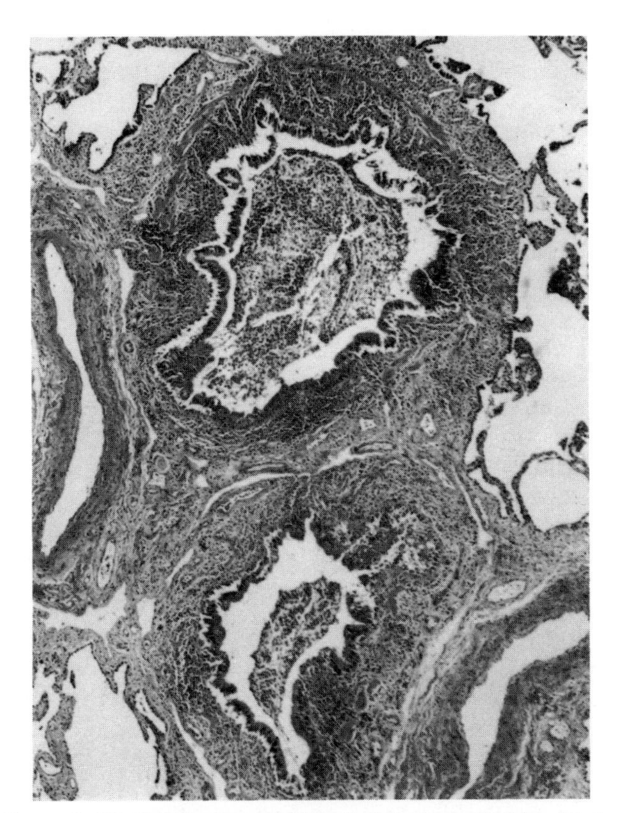

Figure 6-15. Cellular bronchiolitis. Cellular bronchiolitis with luminal acute inflammatory exudate and mural chronic inflammation. (From a case of *Mycoplasma pneumoniae* pneumonia.)

caused by sensitivity to *Aspergillus.* It is more common in England.

The histologic changes, which usually overlap one another, include those of asthma, cellular bronchiolitis, mucoid impaction, bronchocentric granulomatosis, obstructive pneumonia, and eosinophilic pneumonia alone or in combination.

References

Bosken CH, Myers JL, Greenberger PA, Katzenstein ALA. Pathologic features of allergic bronchopulmonary aspergillosis. Am J Surg Pathol 12:216-222, 1988.

Dail DH, Hammer SP (eds). Pulmonary Pathology. New York, Springer-Verlag, 1988.

Thurlbeck WM (ed). Pathology of the Lung. New York, Thieme, 1988.

■ Relapsing Polychondritis (Fig. 6-14)

Relapsing polychondritis is an inflammatory condition affecting cartilage at many sites. The large airway cartilagenous plates are often involved, but biopsy is rarely performed.

There is perichondral inflammation associated with chondromalacia and destruction. This leads to airflow obstruction. The distal alveolar parenchyma may show changes of obstruction and recurrent infection. Some cases are associated with vasculitis, including Wegener's granulomatosis.

References

Dail DH, Hammer SP (eds). Pulmonary Pathology. New York, Springer-Verlag, 1988.

■ Small Airways Injury and Inflammatory Disorders of Small Airways (Figs. 6-15 to 6-27, See Figs. 6-32 to 6-46)

Pathologic changes in the small airways, including inflammation and scarring, are associated with a large number of diseases, and the changes are generally nonspecific. Nevertheless, there are cases in which the salient findings appear (either clinically or pathologically) to be limited to the small airways. A number of labels for these cases have appeared in the literature, including small airways disease, acute and/or chronic bronchiolitis, bronchiolitis obliterans, cryptogenic obliterative bronchiolitis, bronchiolitis in adults (adult bronchiolitis), and others. The literature concerning these conditions is very confusing because terms (such as bronchiolitis obliterans) are used in a clinical sense in some studies and in a histologic or physiologic sense in others; consequently, comparison of series is difficult. To make the situation even more complicated, lesions that show pathologic changes in the small airways morphologically are not always associated with evidence of airways disease clinically or physiologically. Respiratory bronchiolitis-associated interstitial lung disease and bronchiolitis obliterans organizing pneumonia (BOOP) (pp. 253, 255) are examples.

We have chosen the generic term small airways injury to refer to pathologic changes in the small airways, whether they be inflammatory, fibrotic, or both. We have then attempted to define pathologic subgroups

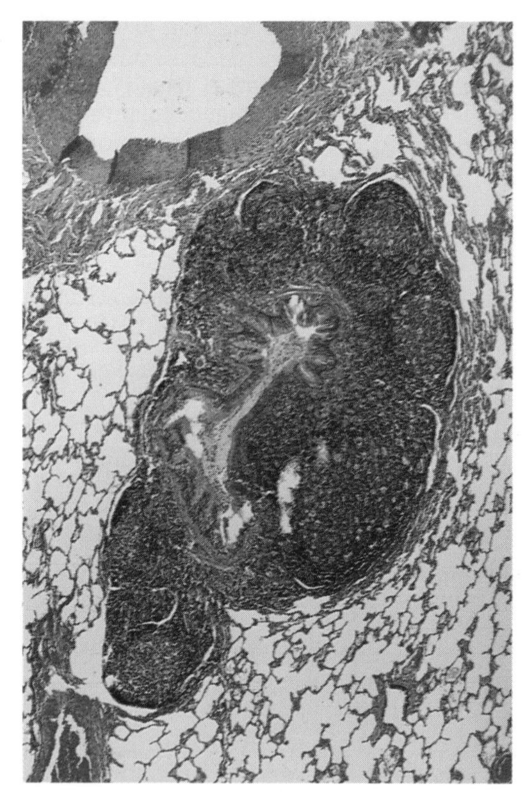

Figure 6–16.

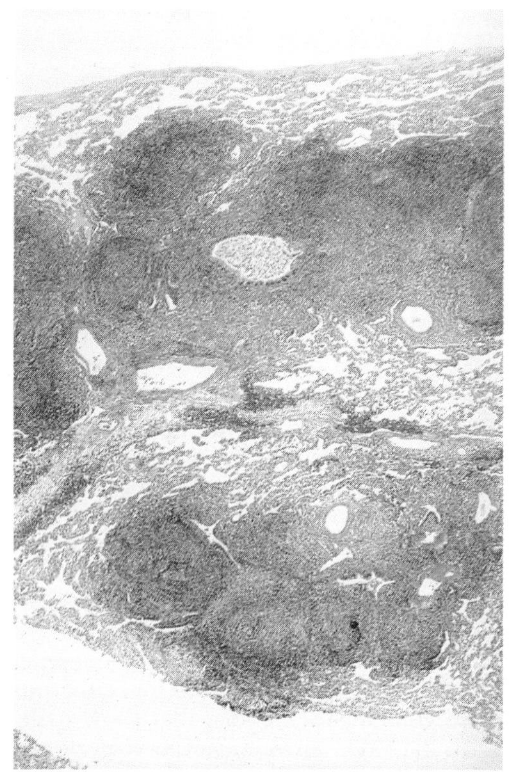

Figure 6–17.

Figures 6–16, 6–17. Follicular bronchiolitis. Examples of follicular bronchiolitis from a case of asthma (Fig. 6–16) and a case of immunodeficiency in a child with peribronchiolar lymphoid hyperplasia (Fig. 6–17). Although "follicular bronchiolitis" is descriptively appropriate, cases such as this have also been termed "diffuse lymphoid hyperplasia of the lung" and "lymphoid interstitial pneumonitis."

among cases of small airways injury that can be identified morphologically. Finally, clinical lesions that show the pathologic changes are discussed. Thus, we have attempted to start from a morphologic foundation and work toward clinical lesions.

Because changes in the small airways occur in many common conditions, such as chronic bronchitis, clinicopathologic correlation is necessary before suggesting that small airways injury is the primary pathologic process.

Small airways injury can usually be included in one of the following groups based on microscopic evaluation:

- Cellular bronchiolitis
- Proliferative bronchiolitis obliterans (i.e., Cases of bronchiolitis obliterans with intralumenal polyps of proliferating granulation tissue)
- Constrictive bronchiolitis (to include cases of bronchiolitis obliterans with concentrically scarred or stenotic airways as well as those entirely destroyed and replaced by scar tissue.

Note that *bronchiolitis obliterans as traditionally defined includes the latter two histologic groups.*

Cellular Bronchiolitis (Figs. 6–15 to 6–17)

Acute or chronic inflammation involves small airways sometimes with mural or peribronchiolar fibrosis. Purulent exudate in the lumen may be present. When germinal centers are present, follicular bronchiolitis is an appropriately descriptive term.

Cellular bronchiolitis is quite nonspecific and common. It is seen alone in such conditions as viral infections, hypersensitivity pneumonitis, chronic bronchitis, or cystic fibrosis. It may be associated with proliferative bronchiolitis obliterans or constrictive bronchiolitis. Respiratory bronchiolitis is a common reaction to cigarette smoking and is discussed in Chapter 7 (p. 253).

Proliferative Bronchiolitis Obliterans (Figs. 6–18 and 6–19)

Proliferative granulation tissue polyps fill the lumens of terminal and respiratory bronchioles and, in appropriately oriented sections, can be seen to extend into alveolar ducts and sometimes distal airspaces (in which case the term organizing pneumonia has been used). Other descriptive terms for proliferative bronchiolitis obliterans include early, intraluminal, polypoid, or unorganized bronchiolitis obliterans, and BOOP pattern. In most cases, this reaction is most extensive in alveolar ducts, but it may be restricted to membranous bronchioles, in which case it is more often associated with clinical evidence of obstruction. When organizing pneumonia is present, a variable alveolar wall infiltrate of chronic inflammatory cells is frequent, as is obstructive pneumonia with foamy macrophages in the airspaces. When organizing pneumonia accompanies proliferative bronchiolitis obliterans, clinical evidence of restrictive lung disease or mixed obstruction and restriction is common. *Proliferative bronchiolitis obliterans is an ex-*

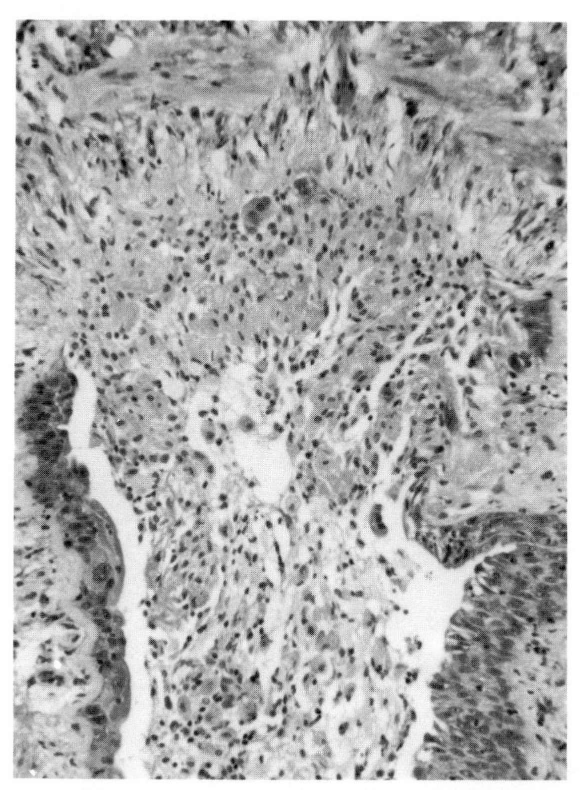

Figure 6–18. Proliferative bronchiolitis obliterans. Proliferative bronchiolitis obliterans with focal ulceration and loss of the bronchiolar epithelium with replacement by an organizing exudate. (From a case of progressive bronchiolitis obliterans with physiologic obstruction following bone marrow transplantation.)

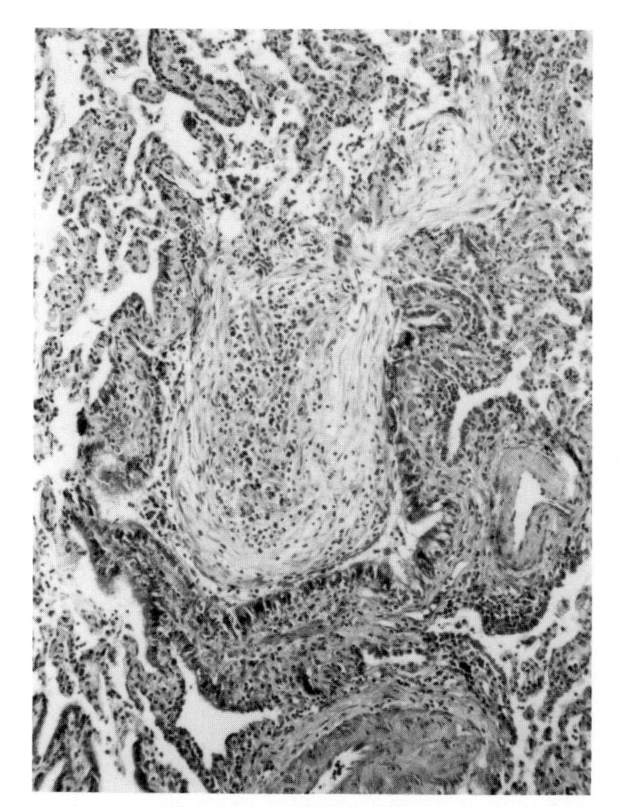

Figure 6–19. Proliferative bronchiolitis obliterans. A large granulation tissue polyp filling a terminal bronchiole at the juncture with a respiratory bronchiole is shown. (From a case of extrinsic allergic alveolitis.)

tremely common reparative reaction, is seen in many conditions, and is most commonly associated with a lesion interpreted clinically as a pneumonitis rather than an airways disease.

Lesions associated with proliferative bronchiolitis obliterans (which often have associated organizing pneumonia and hence resemble BOOP) include the following categories, most of which are discussed in other sections:

Organizing diffuse alveolar damage (organizing adult respiratory distress syndrome [ARDS])
Organizing infections
- Viral
- Mycoplasmal
- Bacterial
- Fungal
- *Pneumocystis*
- Distal to obstruction
- Associated with chronic bronchitis, bronchiectasis, cystic fibrosis, and so forth

Organizing aspiration pneumonia
Fume and toxic exposure
Collagen vascular diseases (especially rheumatoid arthritis)
Extrinsic allergic alveolitis
Eosinophilic pneumonia
Drug reactions
Bone marrow and heart–lung transplantation
Bronchiolitis obliterans organizing pneumonia (BOOP)
As a focal reaction (focal organizing pneumonia) or associated with another lesion (e.g., tumors, abscesses, Wegener's granulomatosis)

Constrictive Bronchiolitis (Figs. 6–20 to 6–27)

Constrictive bronchiolitis displays one or more of the following: (1) complete fibrous obliteration of small airways (bronchiolitis obliterans), (2) stenosis of small airways due to concentric or eccentric mural fibrosis or submucosal granulation tissue formation, (3) irregular smooth muscle hypertrophy, (4) dilatation of small airways with mucostasis, and (5) metaplastic epithelium growing onto surrounding alveolar spaces along peribronchiolar scars. Other descriptive terms for constrictive bronchiolitis include late, mural, fibrotic, cicatricial, and organized bronchiolitis obliterans.

Constrictive bronchiolitis may follow identifiable proliferative bronchiolitis obliterans, but most cases of proliferative bronchiolitis obliterans resolve entirely and do not result in constrictive bronchiolitis. In the transplantation setting proliferative bronchiolitis obliterans may be seen in association with constrictive bronchiolitis. Generally, however, when constrictive bronchiolitis is seen histologically, a concurrent proliferative bronchiolitis obliterans is lacking.

Constrictive bronchiolitis includes many cases clinically called bronchiolitis obliterans (with airflow obstruction). Since these cases show a broad spectrum of changes in the small airways with only a minority of airways showing frank occlusion (i.e., bronchiolitis obliterans), the term constrictive bronchiolitis was chosen to encompass the spectrum.

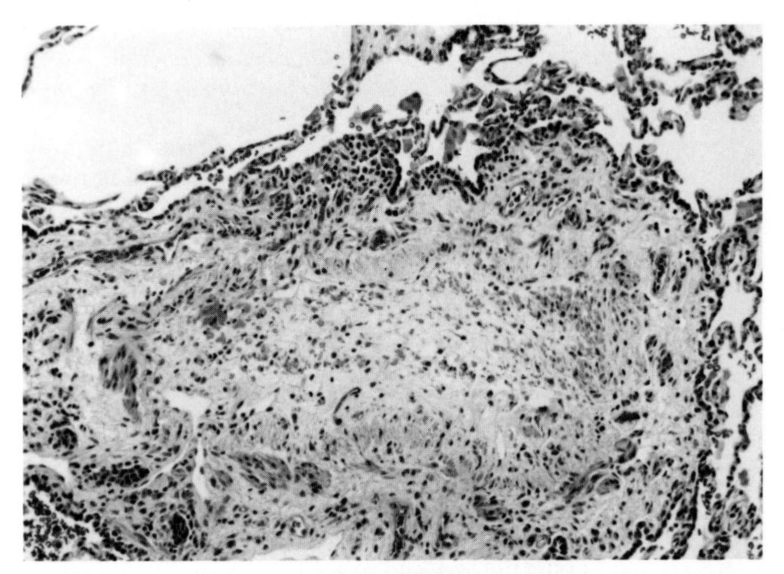

Figure 6-20.

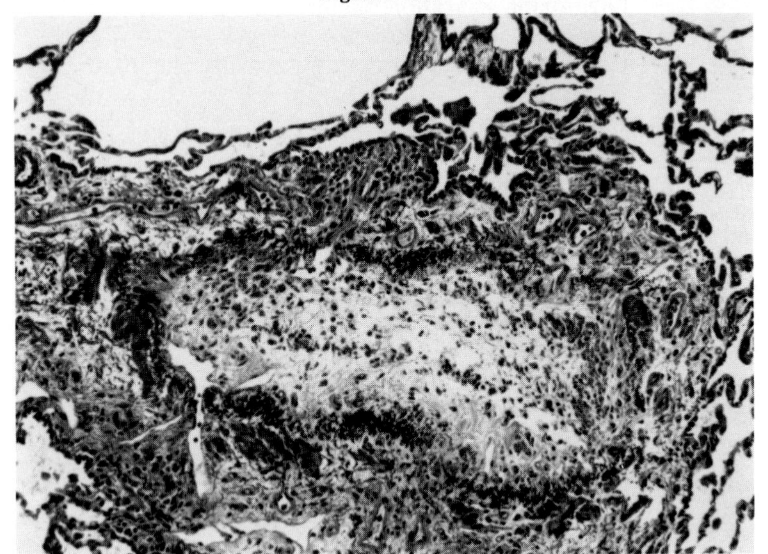

Figure 6-21.

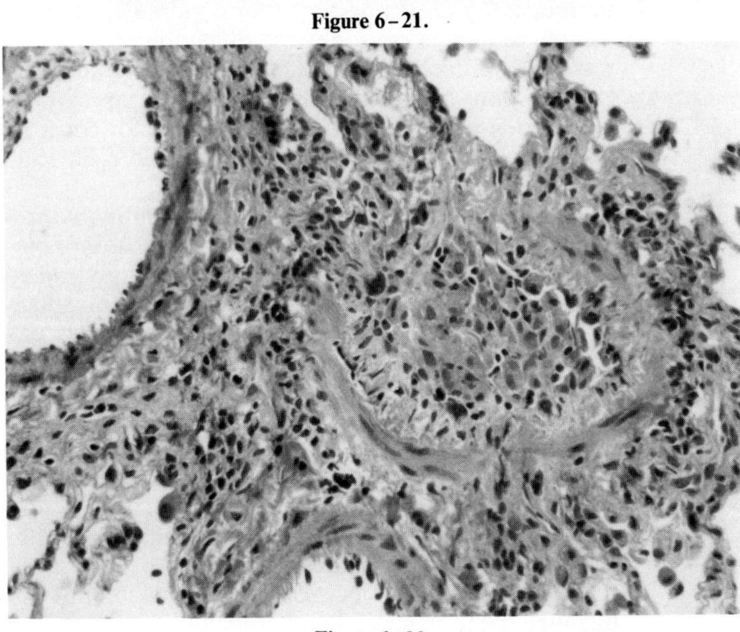

Figure 6-22.

Figures 6-20, 6-21, 6-22. *See legend on opposite page.*

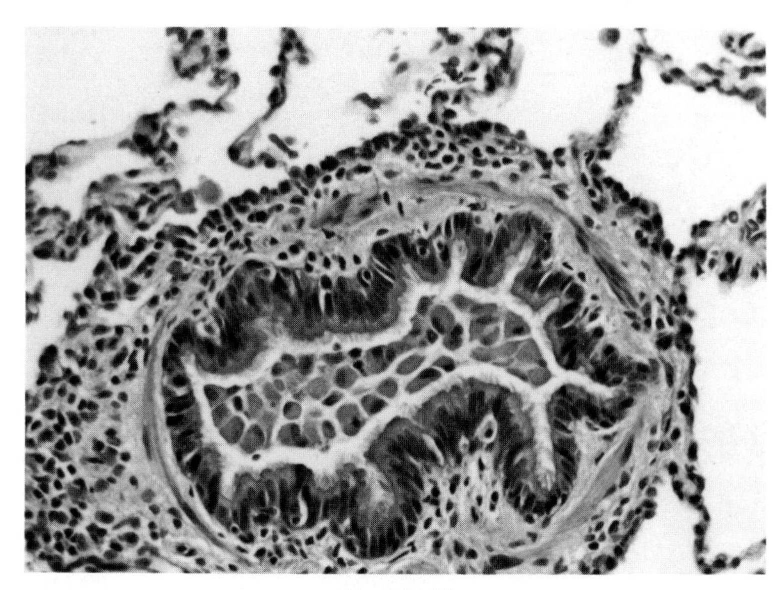

Figure 6-23.

Figures 6-20, 6-21, 6-22, 6-23, 6-24, 6-25. Constrictive bronchiolitis following adenovirus pneumonia in a young girl. The entire spectrum of lesions that may be seen is illustrated, including the following: (1) complete occlusion of small airways with the original bronchiolar wall highlighted by elastic tissue stain (Figs. 6-20, 6-21); (2) decrease in luminal size (Fig. 6-22), accumulation of mucin, macrophages, or both within the lumen (Figs. 6-22, 6-23); (3) bronchiolar dilatation, with stasis of mucus (Fig. 6-24); and (4) peribronchiolar inflammation (Fig. 6-25).

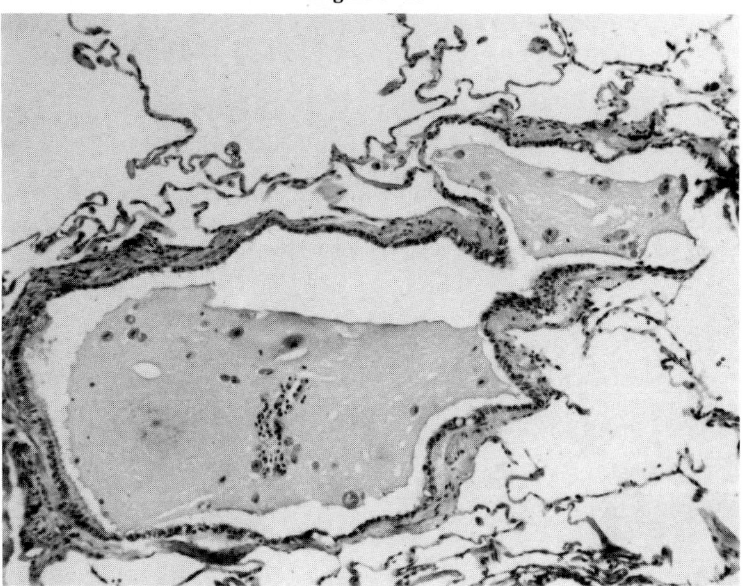

Figure 6-24.

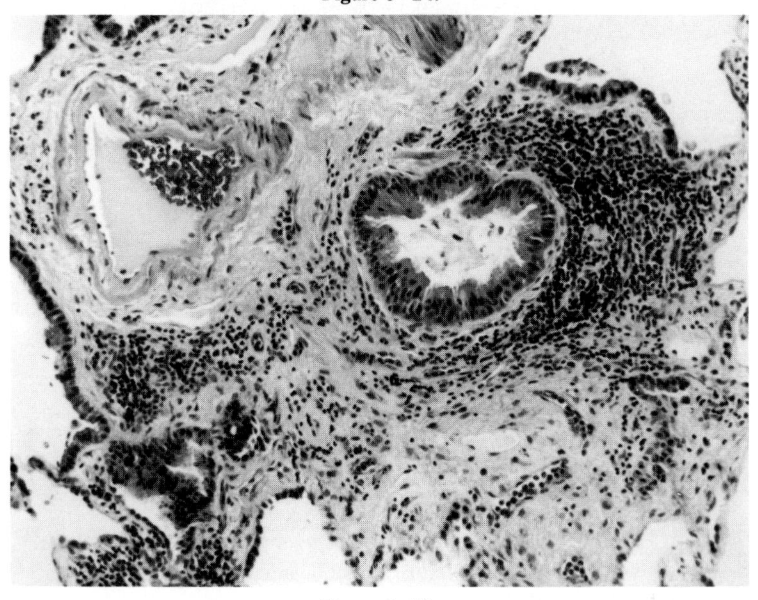

Figure 6-25.

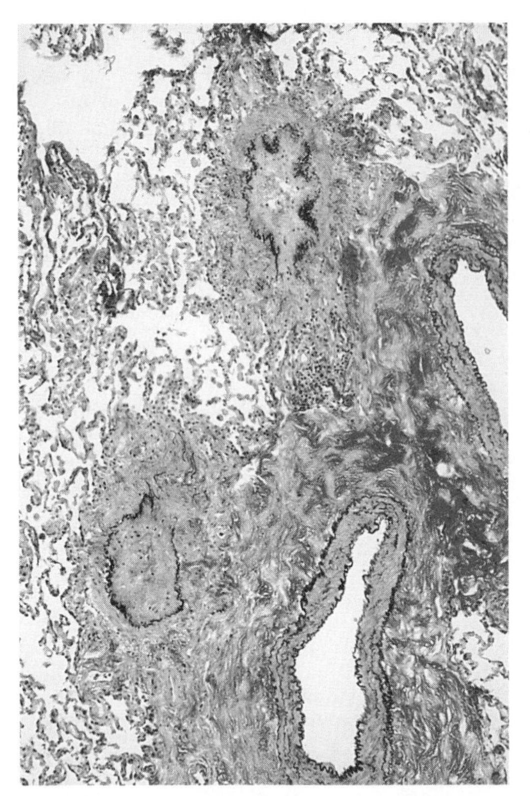

Figure 6–26. Constrictive bronchiolitis with complete occlusion of small airways (highlighted by elastic stain) following documented *Mycoplasma pneumoniae* infection in a young boy with severe airflow obstruction.

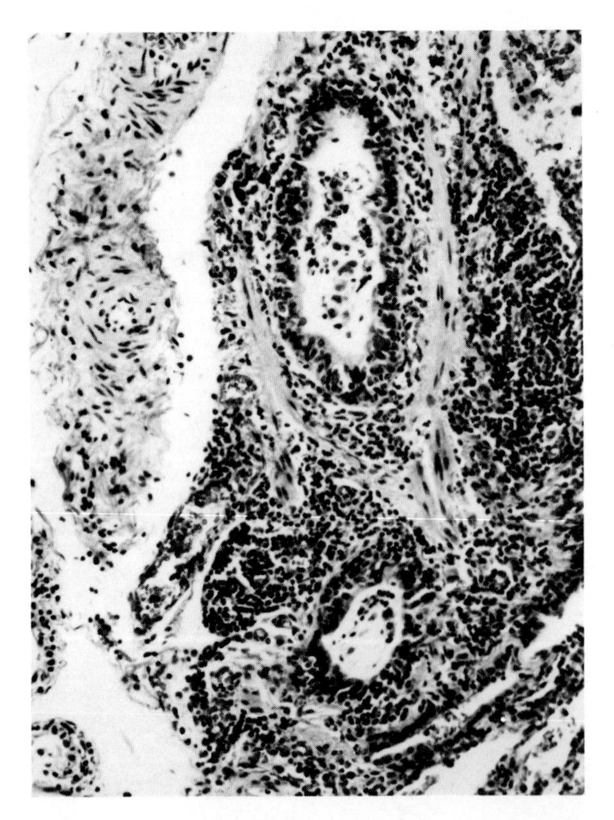

Figure 6–27. Constrictive bronchiolitis with chronic cellular bronchiolitis and decrease in lumen size associated with thickening of the bronchiolar wall. (From a case of smoke inhalation bronchiolitis obliterans associated with obstructive pulmonary functions.)

Constrictive bronchiolitis can be seen in the following settings:

Healed infections (especially viral, mycoplasma)
Chronic bronchitis, cystic fibrosis, chronic asthma, bronchiectasis
Healed toxic and fume exposure
Collagen vascular disease (especially rheumatoid arthritis)
Bone marrow and heart–lung transplantations
Drug reactions (e.g., penicillamine)
Healed DAD (healed ARDS, and neonatal hyaline membrane disease/bronchopulmonary dysplasia)
Chronic allergic alveolitis
Diffuse panbronchiolitis
Idiopathic conditions (see below)

Once constrictive bronchiolitis is present, the abnormal airways are apparently prone to recurring infection and inflammation, starting a vicious circle that leads to further damage.

Among many of the conditions associated with changes in the airways, assessment of the pathologic features in the various anatomic compartments may be useful, as illustrated in Table 6–1.

References

Colby TV, Churg A. Patterns of pulmonary fibrosis. Part 2. Pathol Annu 21:277–310, 1986.

Colby TV, Myers JL. The clinical and histologic spectrum of bronchiolitis obliterans including bronchiolitis obliterans organizing pneumonia (BOOP). Sem Resp Med. In press.

Guerry-Force ML, Muller NL, Wright JL, et al. A comparison of bronchiolitis obliterans organizing pneumonia, usual interstitial pneumonia, and small airways disease. Am Rev Respir Dis 135:705–712, 1987.

Kitaichi M. Pathology of diffuse panbronchiolitis from the viewpoint of differential diagnosis. *In* Grassi C, Rizzato G, Pozzi E (eds). Sarcoidosis. Amsterdam, Elsevier Scientific 1988, pp 741–746.

Macklem PT, Thurlbeck WM, Fraser RG. Chronic obstructive disease of small airways. Ann Intern Med 74:167–177, 1971.

Table 6-1
PATHOLOGIC FEATURES OF AIRWAYS INJURY IN SELECTED CONDITIONS

	Anatomic Compartment				
Condition	***Bronchus***	***Membranous Bronchiole***	***Respiratory Bronchiole***	***Alveolar Duct***	***Alveolus***
Chronic Bronchitis	Increase of glands and goblet cells	Increase of goblet cells with mucin stasis Mural inflammation	Mucostasis	Mucostasis	Mucostasis
Bronchiectasis	Dilatation with inflammation and hypervascularization Denudation of epithelial layer		Rare interstitial accumulation of foamy cells	Rare interstitial accumulation of foamy cells	Rare interstitial accumulation of foamy cells
Cystic Fibrosis	Eosinophilic muco-stasis Dilatation with mural hypervascularization and luminal acute inflammation Denudation of epithe-lial layer	Mild mural inflammation			
Mycoplasma Pneumonia		Reparative epithelial metaplasia Mural inflammation Organizing exudates in airspaces	Organizing exudates in airspaces	Organizing exudates in airspaces	Organizing exudates in airspaces
Extrinsic Allergic Alveolitis		Mural inflammation	Granulation tissue in airspaces Cellular interstitial infiltrates and sarcoid-like granulomas	Granulation tissue in airspaces Cellular interstitial infiltrates and sarcoid-like granulomas	Granulation tissue in airspaces Cellular interstitial infiltrates and sarcoid-like granulomas
BOOP			Granulation tissue in airspaces Mural inflammation	Granulation tissue in airspaces Cellular interstitial infiltrates	Granulation tissue in airspaces Cellular interstitial infiltrates
Cryptogenic Obliterative Bronchiolitis (see text)	Mild mural inflamma-tion	Granulation tissue formation in lumen, variable acute inflamma-tion Muscular hyper-trophy, chronic inflammation and subepithelial fibrosis			
Follicular Bronchitis and Bronchiolitis	Germinal centers and lymphoid fol-licles in and around the wall	Germinal centers and lymphoid fol-licles in and around the wall			
Diffuse Panbronchiolitis	Chronic mural inflammation Dilatation in late stage	Chronic mural inflammation Dilatation in late stage	Mural and luminal inflammation with foamy histiocytes in the wall	Interstitial accumulation of foamy cells	Interstitial accumulation of foamy cells

Modified from Kitaichi M. Pathology of diffuse panbronchiolitis from the viewpoint of differential diagnosis. *In* Grassi C, Rizzato G, Pozzi E. (eds). Sarcoidosis. Amsterdam, Elsevier Scientific, 1988, pp 741–746.
Abbreviation: BOOP, bronchiolitis obliterans organizing pneumonia.

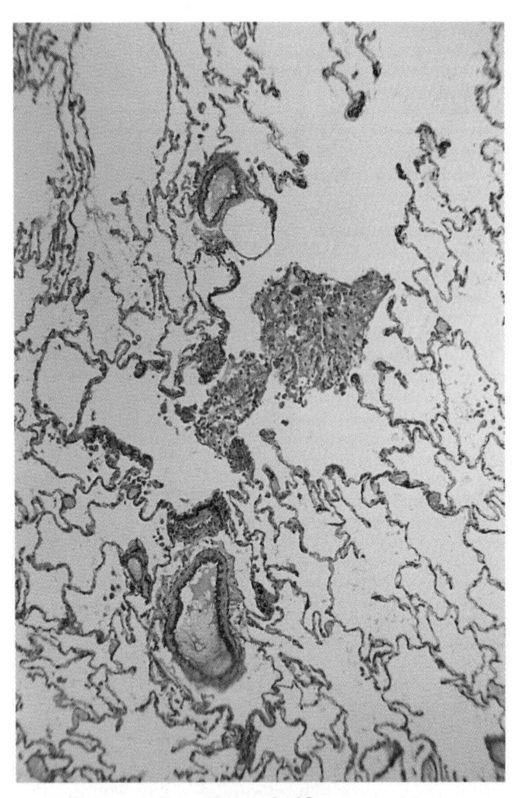

Figure 6–28.

■ Asthma (Figs. 6–28 to 6–31)

Asthma is rarely the reason for performing a lung biopsy. Pathologic changes seen may be the result of the asthma itself, a condition associated with asthma, or the asthma may be an incidental finding to some other unrelated process.

The histologic appearance is variable; it may be entirely normal there may be cellular bronchiolitis with eosinophils and/or a few lymphocytes; a constrictive bronchiolitis with peribronchiolar scarring (probably due to healed microscopic pneumonias) may be seen; or basement membrane thickening, smooth muscle hypertrophy, and goblet cell metaplasia may be found.

Classic changes of status asthmaticus with mucous plugs involving nearly all the small airways is unusual in biopsy specimens.

Some conditions associated with asthma that may lead to the need for biopsy include eosinophilic pneumonia, Churg-Strauss syndrome, unclassified allergic reactions, and allergic bronchopulmonary aspergillosis.

Note: Asthmatics cough up mucous plugs, which may be sent to the surgical pathology laboratory for testing. These should be examined histologically for the presence of fungi, particularly if there is a clinical suspicion of allergic bronchopulmonary aspergillosis.

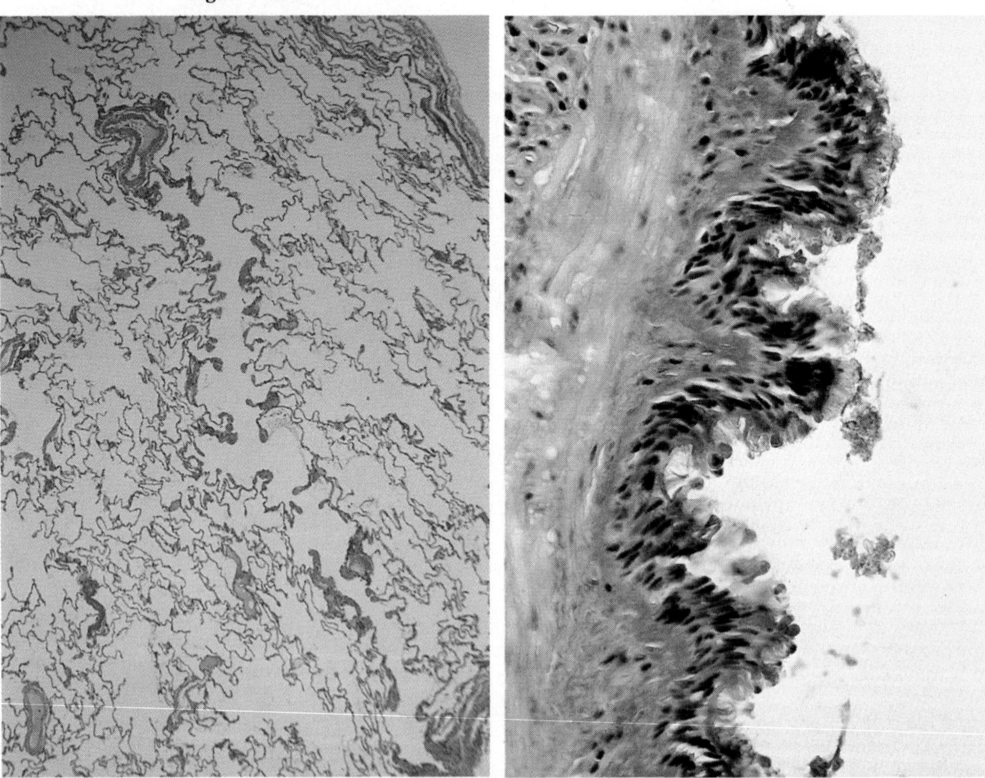

Figure 6–29. Figure 6–30.

Figures 6–28, 6–29, 6–30. Asthma. In patients with asthma, there may be no pathologic changes whatsoever identified on a lung biopsy specimen, especially when the biopsy is performed for some other process. Frequently, however, mild nonspecific changes can be appreciated as shown, including mucostasis in small airways, slight thickening in the walls of small airways, goblet cell metaplasia (stained green), and prominent basement membranes in the mucosa.

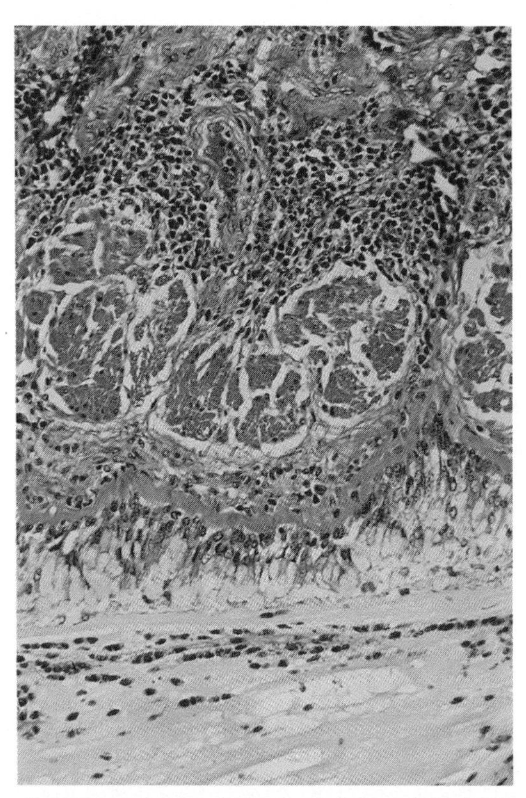

Figure 6-31. Fatal asthma. This photomicrograph depicts luminal plugs of mucus containing eosinophils, marked goblet cell metaplasia of the bronchiolar epithelium, thickening of the basement membrane, marked smooth muscle hypertrophy, and mural inflammatory infiltrate rich in eosinophils.

References

Dail DH, Hammer SP (eds). Pulmonary Pathology. New York, Springer-Verlag, 1988.
Thurlbeck WM (ed). Pathology of the Lung. New York, Thieme, 1988.

■ Idiopathic Small Airways Injury and Inflammatory Disease (Figs. 6-32 to 6-46)

There are conditions with pathologic changes in the small airways without recognizable cause, usually associated with clinical evidence of airflow obstruction. Some cases are diagnosed by clinical findings, others by the surgical pathologist. Two broad groups emerge:

- Idiopathic small airways inflammatory disease with cellular bronchiolitis
- Idiopathic small airways injury with constrictive bronchiolitis

Idiopathic Small Airways Inflammatory Disease with Cellular Bronchiolitis (Acute and Chronic Bronchiolitis)

In this group, cellular infiltrates along bronchioles are apparent, often acute and chronic or chronic alone. The changes may be superimposed on changes of constrictive bronchiolitis. Foci of proliferative bronchiolitis obliterans and organizing pneumonia may also be seen. Acute inflammation may represent secondary infection of anatomically abnormal airways, leading to a vicious

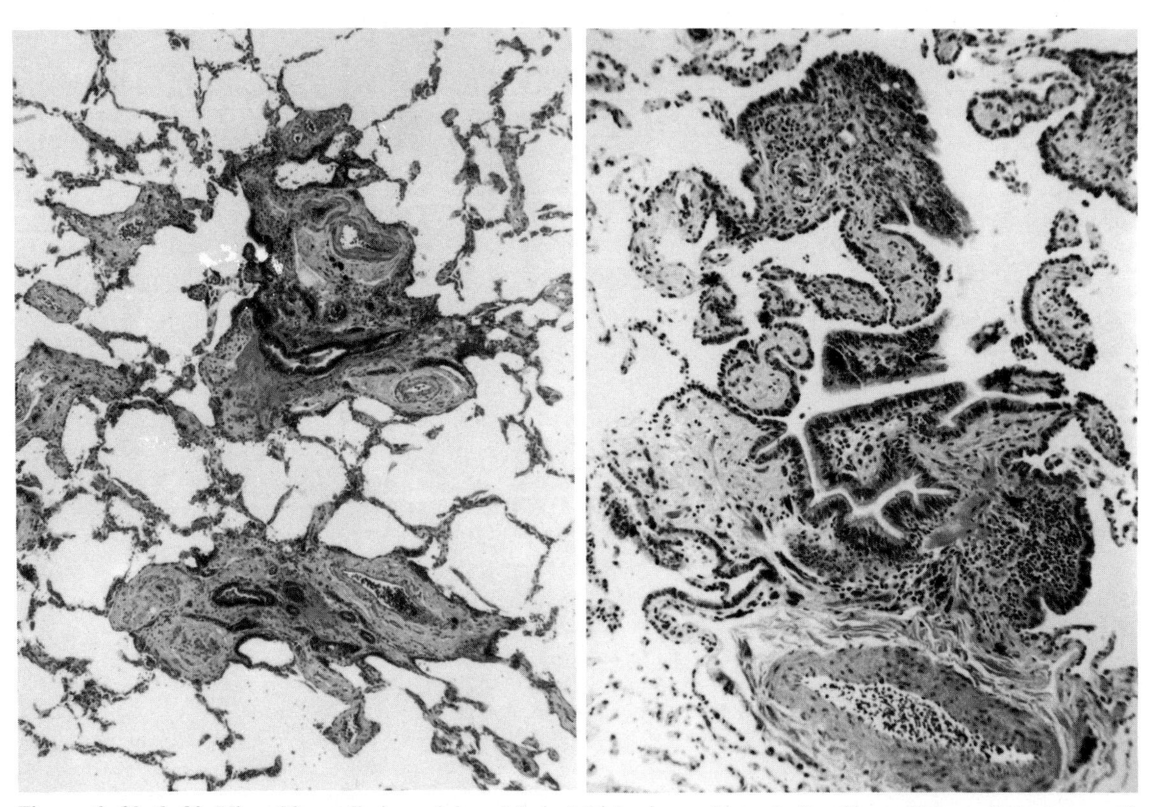

Figures 6-32, 6-33. Idiopathic small airway injury. Marked thickening and irregularity of bronchiolar walls is shown with extension of metaplastic bronchiolar epithelium into surrounding airspaces (lambertosis).

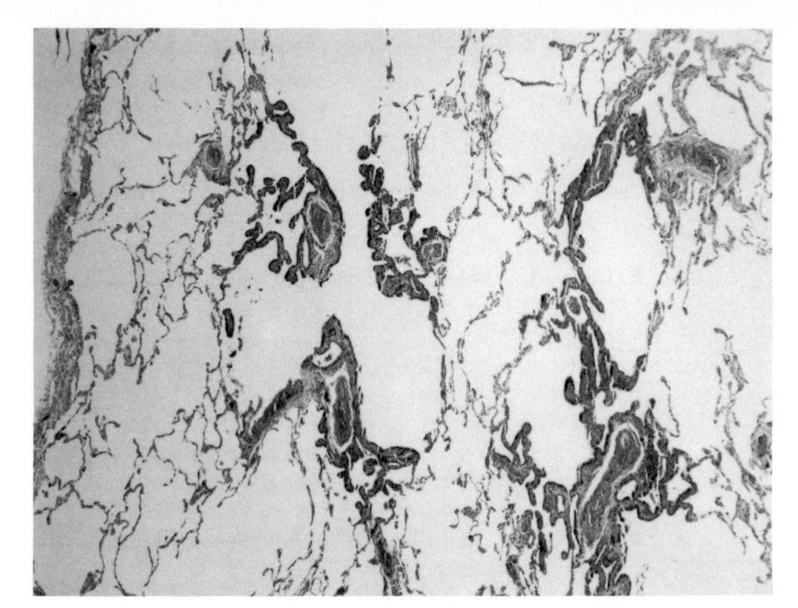

Figure 6–34. Idiopathic small airways injury (constrictive bronchiolitis) manifesting as bronchiolar dilatation and mural thickening with irregular and distorted lumens and extension of metaplastic bronchiolar epithelium into surrounding airspaces.

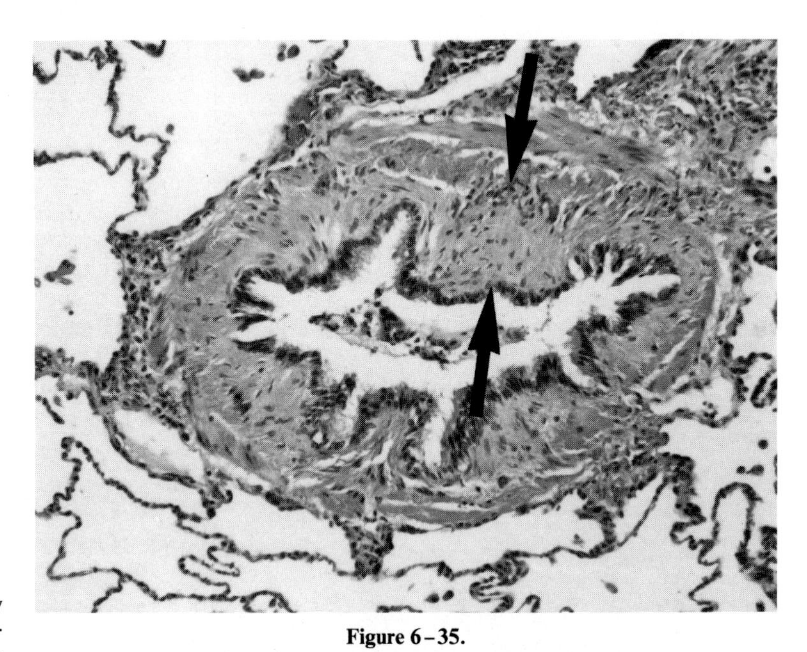

Figure 6–35.

Figures 6–35, 6–36. Idiopathic small airways injury (constrictive bronchiolitis) illustrating very subtle submucosal thickening (arrows); however, severe airway obstruction was present clinically. A similar finding from another case is highlighted with an elastic tissue stain (Fig. 6–36).

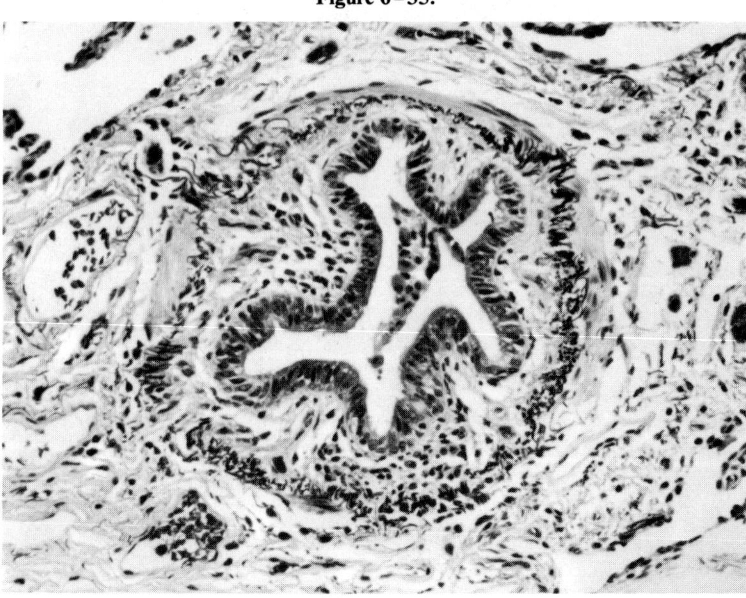

Figure 6–36.

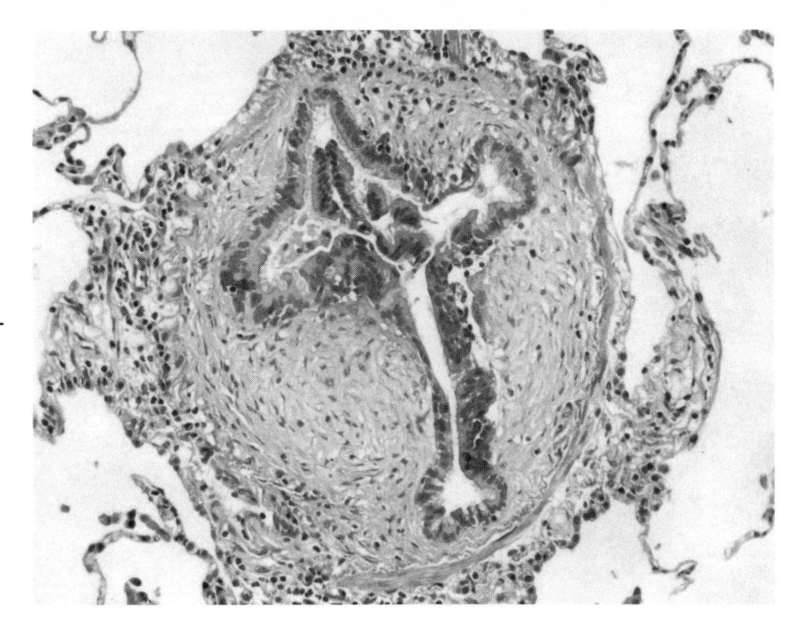

Figures 6-37. Idiopathic small airways injury (constrictive bronchiolitis) with marked submucosal scarring.

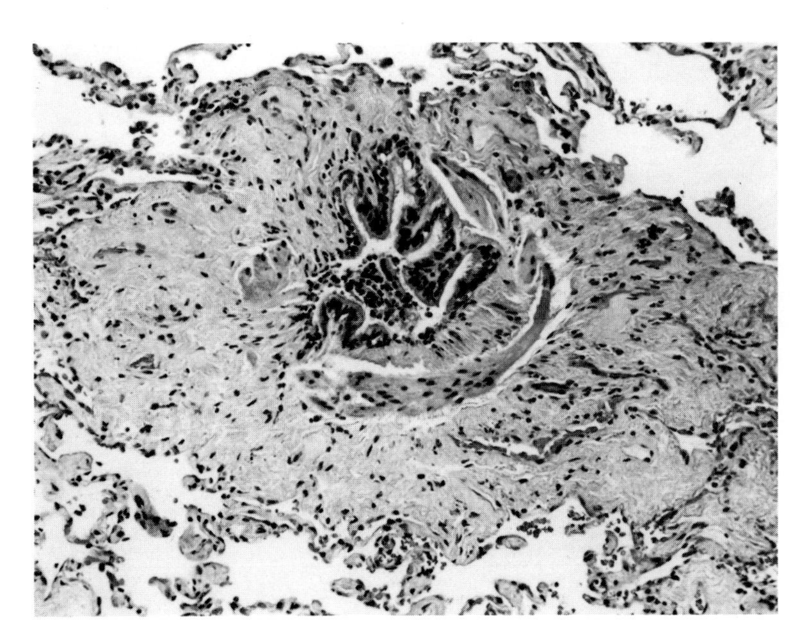

Figure 6-38. Idiopathic small airways injury (constrictive bronchiolitis) with adventitial scarring of the airway outside the smooth muscle layer.

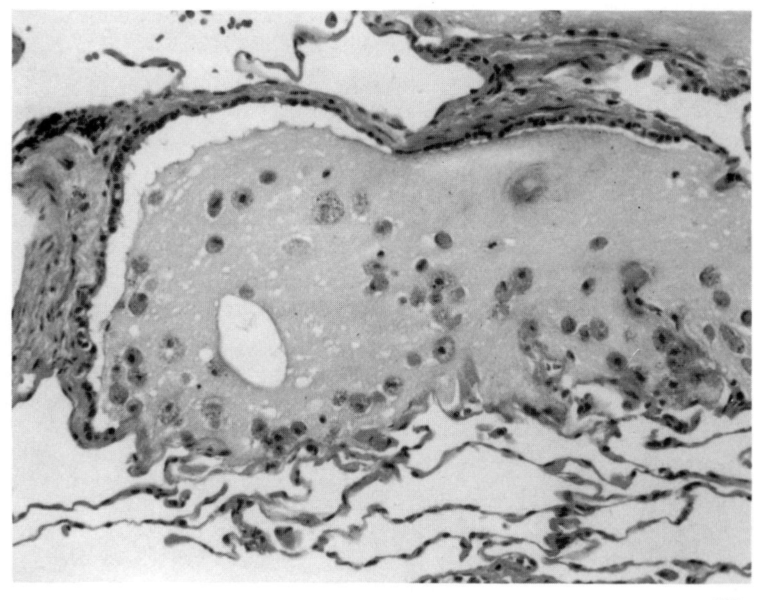

Figure 6-39. Idiopathic small airways injury (constrictive bronchiolitis) with bronchiolar dilatation and mucus stasis, which suggests a lack of air flow through the airway.

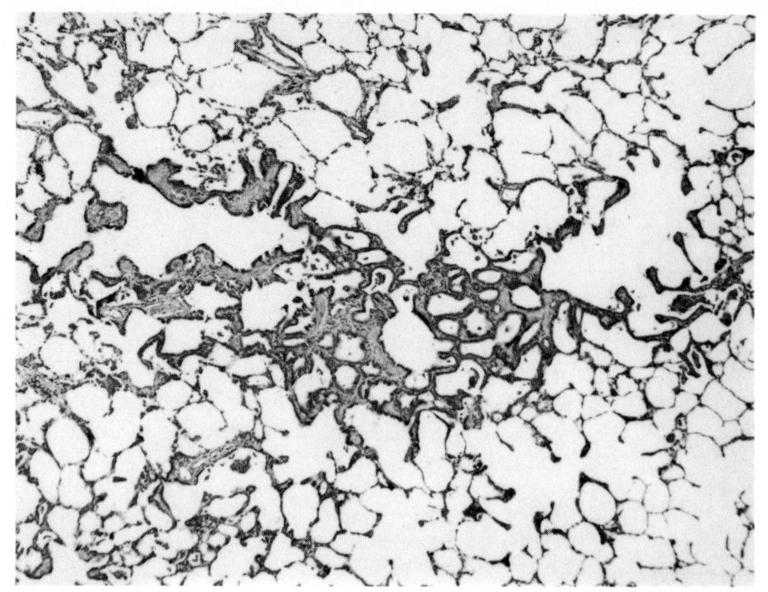

Figure 6-40.

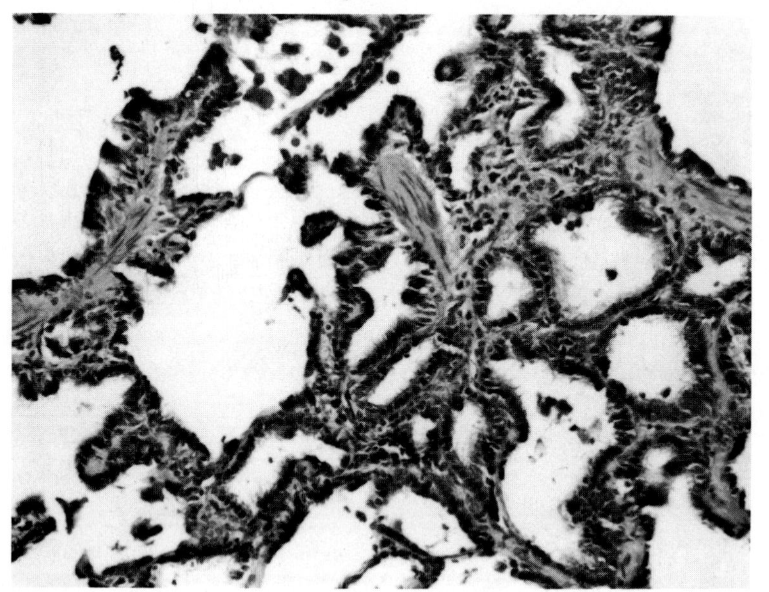

Figure 6-41.

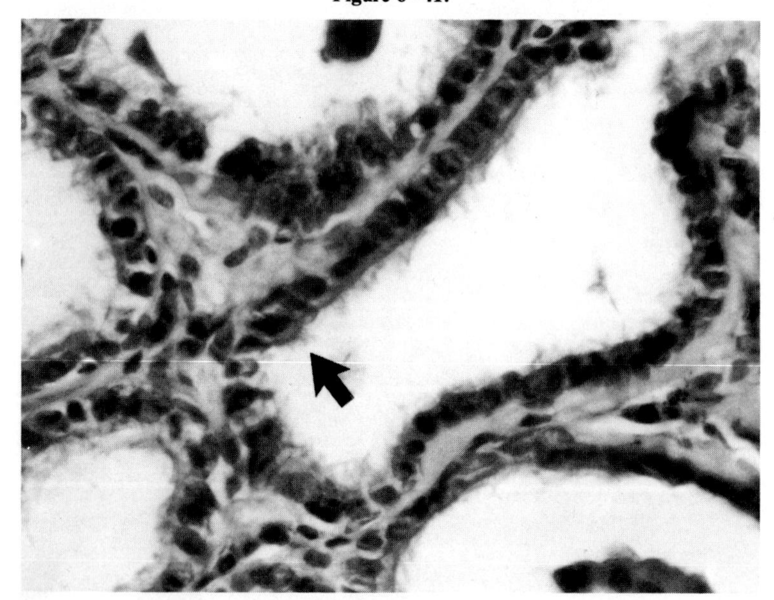

Figure 6-42.

Figures 6-40, 6-41, 6-42. Idiopathic small airways injury with prominent lambertosis. The airway architecture is mildly distorted, and the pattern suggests a chronic interstitial pneumonia or even a bronchioloalveolar carcinoma; however, the lesion can be traced to distorted and scarred airways. In such cases, metaplastic epithelium may extend a considerable distance beyond the airway itself. In this case, ciliated cells were prominent in the metaplastic epithelium (arrow).

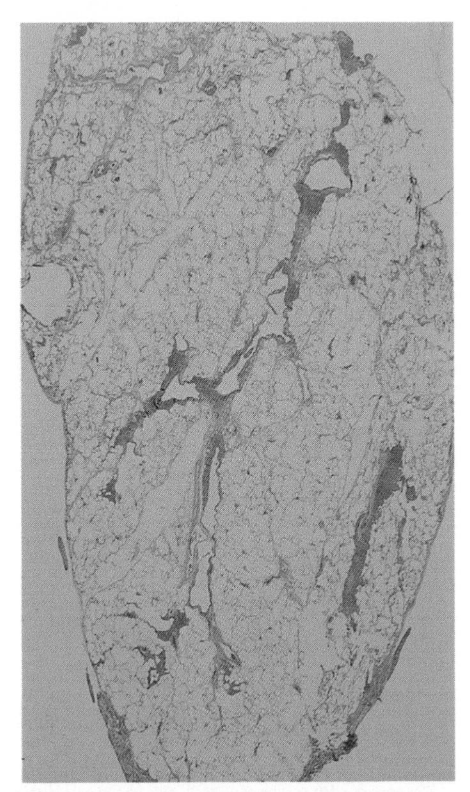

Figure 6-43. Idiopathic small airway injury (chronic cellular bronchiolitis) with chronic inflammatory infiltrates around small airways.

circle of infection and repair with scarring. These cases often feature reticulonodular infiltrates on chest radiograph in addition to physiologic evidence of airflow obstruction.

Idiopathic Small Airways Injury with Constrictive Bronchiolitis (Including Cryptogenic Obliterative Bronchiolitis)

All that is visible is the residue or prior bronchiolar injury without any clue as to its cause. There may be total obliteration of airways; more frequently, however, one sees concentric stenosis, decrease in airway size, mucostasis, bronchiolar dilatation, evidence of obstruction in the distal parenchyma, and sometimes mild histologic emphysema. Cases are often misdiagnosed as normal or as interstitial pneumonia if scarring is recognized. Nevertheless, low-power evaluation is invaluable in recognizing the bronchiolocentricity of the process. The findings in this condition *may be extremely subtle,* and careful evaluation of the small airways should always be performed with biopsy specimens that appear normal at first glance. Trichrome and elastic tissue stains may aid interpretation. These cases are usually associated with a normal or hyperinflated lung on chest radiographs and, less frequently, interstitial infiltrates. Physiologic obstruction is often marked.

There is a poorly understood subset of cases that show prominent peribronchiolar scarring and bronchiolar metaplasia and the other changes of constrictive bronchiolitis (Figs. 6-40 to 6-42). The lesions are best appreciated at scanning power microscopy, which highlights the distribution. An associated cellular bronchiolitis may be present, as may focal honeycombing. This last feature may result in a diagnosis of interstitial fibrosis if the bronchiolocentric distribution in other foci is not appreciated. These cases are occasionally associated with interstitial infiltrates on chest radiographs and physiologic restriction. Because of all these features, this is the least understood of the patterns of small airways injury. Chronic extrinsic allergic alveolitis and probably some healed viral infections may result in this pattern, and should be considered in differential diagnosis.

References

Colby TV, Myers JL. The clinical and histologic spectrum of bronchiolitis obliterans including bronchiolitis obliterans organizing pneumonia (BOOP). Sem Resp Med. In press.

Guerry-Force ML, Muller NL, Wright JL, et al. A comparison of bronchiolitis obliterans organizing pneumonia, usual interstitial pneumonia, and small airways disease. Am Rev Respir Dis 135:705-712, 1987.

Kindt GC, Weiland JE, Davis WB, et al. Bronchiolitis in adults. Am Rev Respir Dis 140:483-492, 1989.

Macklem PT, Thurlbeck WM, Fraser RG. Chronic obstructive disease of small airways. Ann Intern Med 74:167-177, 1971.

Turton CW, Williams G, Green M. Cryptogenic obliterative bronchiolitis in adults. Thorax 36:805-810, 1981.

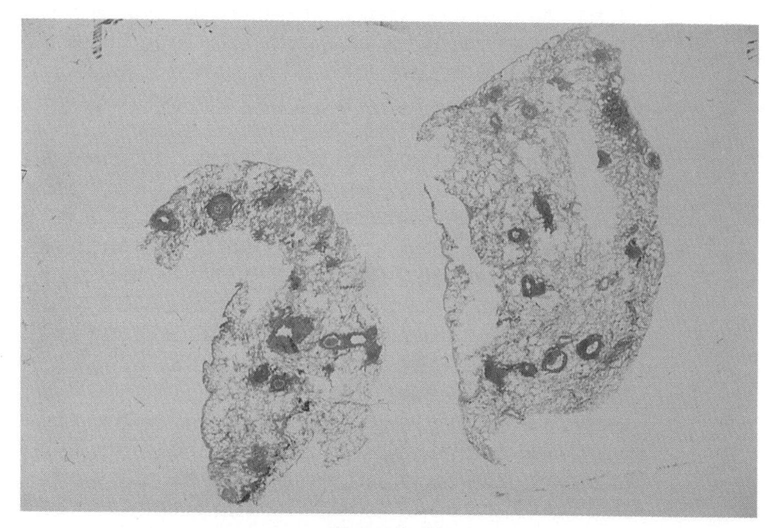

Figure 6–44.

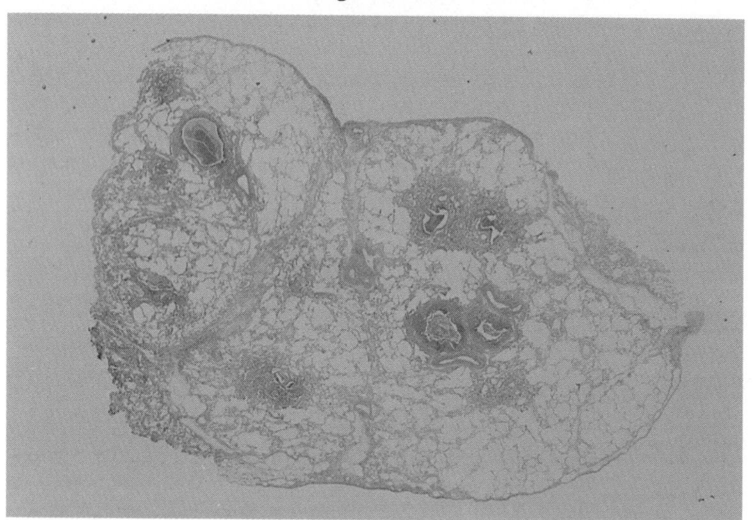

Figure 6–45.

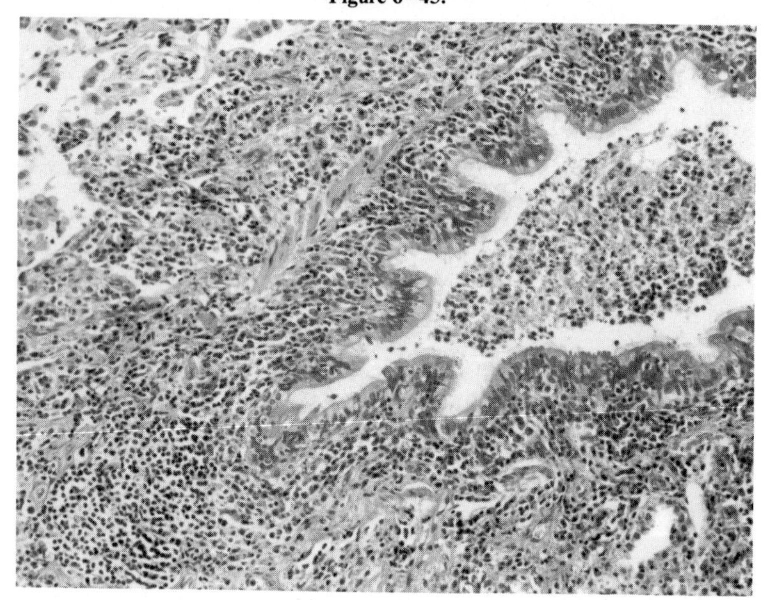

Figure 6–46.

Figures 6–44, 6–45, 6–46. Two cases of idiopathic small airway injury associated with acute and chronic cellular bronchiolitis. The lesions are centered on small airways and consist of an acute inflammatory exudate in the lumen and chronic inflammation in the wall. The cause was not identified in either case, although one was steroid-responsive for several years. Obstructive lung disease and reticulonodular infiltrates on chest radiographs were found in both patients.

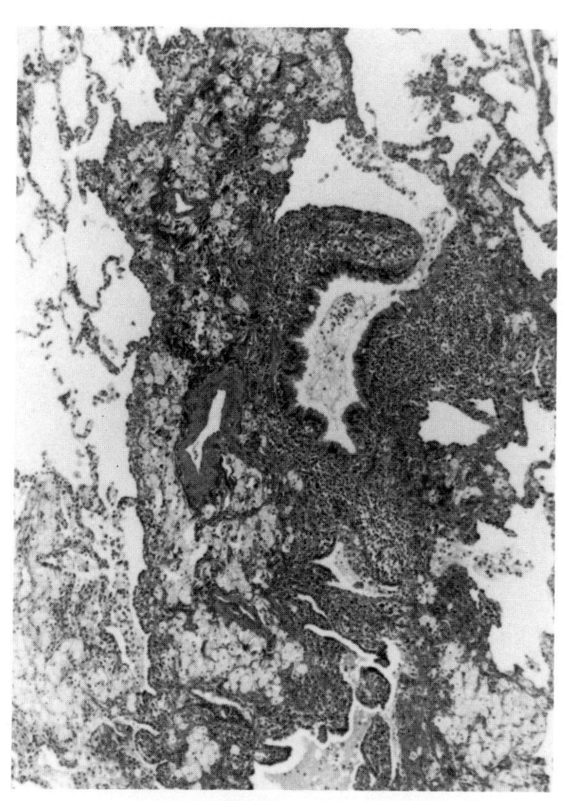

Figure 6-47.

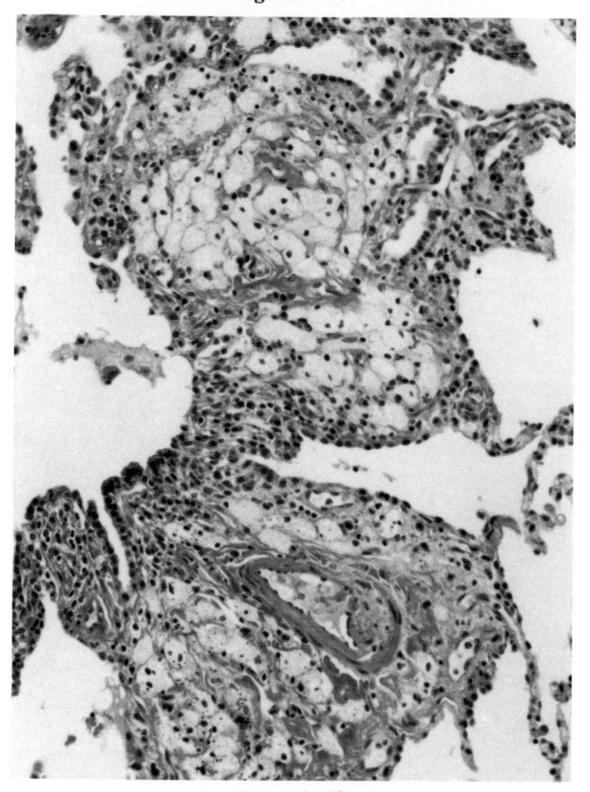

Figure 6-48.

Figures 6-47, 6-48. Diffuse panbronchiolitis. Cellular bronchiolitis is characterized by marked chronic inflammation and thickening around small airways (predominantly respiratory bronchioles) with accumulation of foamy histiocytes, most of which are interstitial.

■ **Diffuse Panbronchiolitis** (Figs. 6-47 and 6-48)

Diffuse panbronchiolitis was described in Japan and appears to be almost entirely restricted to individuals of Japanese heritage. Patients experience cough, dyspnea, and increased sputum production, and the chest radiograph shows small nodular shadows associated with hyperinflation. Obstruction and hypoxemia are seen on pulmonary function tests. Often, there is a history of chronic sinusitis.

Pathologically, inflammation is most marked in the respiratory bronchioles with a cellular bronchiolitis and prominent interstitial and airspace accumulations of foam cells. The foam cells are the most striking feature. Secondary bronchiolectasis and infection with *Pseudomonas* develop.

Because diffuse panbronchiolitis rarely, if ever, occurs in non-Japanese, it has taken some time for this condition to be accepted in the United States. It is, however, a distinct clinicopathologic entity that has been well characterized in Japan, and it is distinct from chronic bronchitis and emphysema, bronchiectasis, cystic fibrosis, and disorders of cilia.

A histologic lesion similar to diffuse panbronchiolitis has been described in patients with chronic ulcerative colitis.

References

Desai SJ, Gephardt GN, Stoller JK. Diffuse panbronchiolitis preceding ulcerative colitis. Chest 45:1342-1344, 1989.

Homma H, Yamanaka A, Tanimoto S, Tamera M, Chijimatsu Y, Kira S, Izumi T. Diffuse panbronchiolitis. Chest 83:63-69, 1983.

Kitaichi M. Pathology of diffuse panbronchiolitis from the viewpoint of differential diagnosis. *In* Grassi C, Rizzato G, Pozzi E (eds). Sarcoidosis. Amsterdam, Elsevier Scientific 1988, pp 741-746.

■ **Ciliary Disorders (Immotile Cilia Syndrome)**

Patients with ultrastructurally abnormal cilia may have recurrent pneumonias, and bronchiectasis may develop. Some patients have Kartagener's syndrome with situs inversus, chronic sinusitis, and bronchiectasis.

Histologically, there are manifestations of recurrent infections with acute and chronic cellular bronchiolitis with or without proliferative bronchiolitis obliterans and organizing pneumonia. Follicular bronchiolitis may be seen and bronchiectasis ultimately develops.

Ultrastructural abnormalities include an absence of dynein arms, abnormalities of radial spokes, and combinations thereof. These changes are thought to lead to abnormal transport of mucus, resulting in recurrent infections.

Because a small number of cilia may be abnormal in normal individuals, *considerable experience is required in interpreting ultrastructural changes.*

A biopsy specimen taken from the nasal tissue or another site in the respiratory tract can be routinely prepared for electron microscopy for study of the cilia. Also, a wet mount scraping of cells on a glass slide can be used, and with the condenser lowered, the beating cilia can be seen.

References

Eliasson R, Mossberg B, Camner P, Afzelius B. The immotile cilia syndrome. N Engl J Med 297:1-6, 1977.
Rutland J, Cole PJ. Noninvasive sampling of normal cilia for measurement of beat frequency and study of ultrastructure. Lancet 2:564-565, 1980.

■ **Mineral Dust Airways Disease** (Figs. 7-112 to 7-114)

Inhalation of rock dusts may lead to their deposition along small airways associated with pigmentation, scarring, and minimal inflammation in their walls. Respiratory bronchioles are particularly affected, and the term "mineral dust-induced airways disease" has been suggested. Asbestos airways disease is well recognized as a morphologic lesion, but whether it represents early asbestosis or is a separate lesion from asbestosis is debated. In some patients with asbestos airways disease, there is indeed airflow obstruction.

References

Churg A, Green FHY. Pathology of Occupational Lung Disease. New York, Igaku-Shoin Medical Publishers, 1988.
Churg A, Wright JL. Small airways disease and mineral dust exposure. Part 2. Pathol Annu 18:233-251, 1983.
Wright JL, Churg A. Morphology of small-airway lesions in patients with asbestosis exposure. Hum Pathol 15:68-74, 1984.

CHAPTER 7

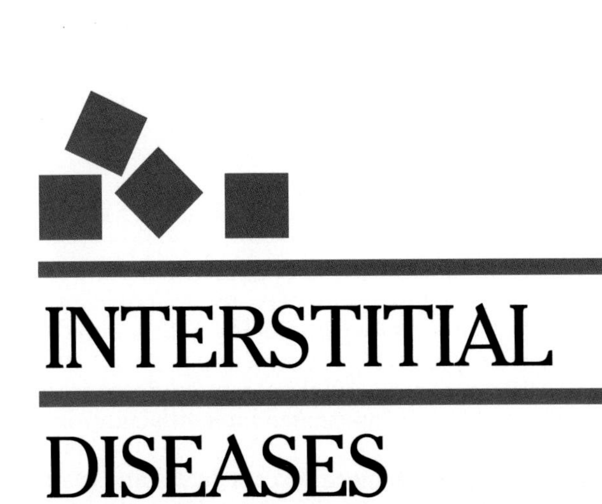

INTERSTITIAL DISEASES

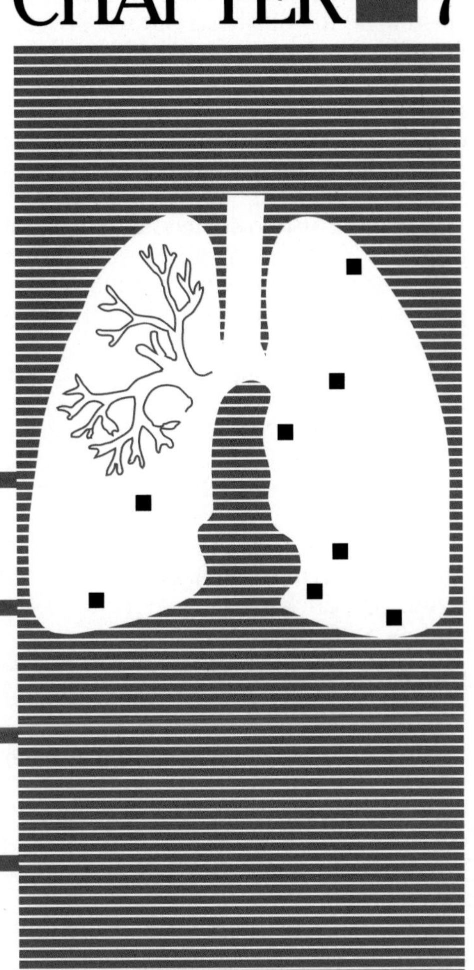

■ General Approach to Interstitial Lung Disease

Interstitial lung diseases are commonly a problem for the surgical pathologist. Nowhere else in lung pathology is clinicopathologic correlation more important. In fact, the differential diagnosis can usually be narrowed considerably just by knowing the history. Some useful considerations and questions one should ask oneself include:

1. Is infection reasonably excluded? (Never forget *Pneumocystis.*)
2. Do the histologic findings fit with the clinical findings?
3. Can a specific clinicopathologic diagnosis be suggested, if not diagnosed (versus giving a purely descriptive diagnosis)?
4. Are the histologic findings worse than the history suggests? or vice versa (i.e., sampling error)?
5. Are incidental changes (e.g., pleural, smoking-related, old scar, or granuloma) present?
6. Are transbronchial biopsy findings being overinterpreted?
7. Is the "fibrosis" that is present of the organizing pneumonia type? The interstitial type? Does it appear recent (in which case it may be reversible) or old and heavily collagenized?
8. How much irreversible, old interstitial scarring and honeycombing are present? How cellular is the process?

Among chronic interstitial pneumonias, the pathology report should include (1) an assessment of the degree of architectural loss by *interstitial* scarring and honeycombing and (2) the degree and type of inflammation present because both may impact on prognosis and therapy.

It is useful to divide interstitial lung diseases into acute or chronic categories and to attempt to determine whether or not the patient is immunosuppressed, although this may not always be possible. In general, acute interstitial lung disease shows relatively little overlap with chronic interstitial lung disease, and previous concepts suggesting that chronic interstitial pneumonias evolved from diffuse alveolar damage (DAD) are probably erroneous. Our approach has been to keep these two groups of interstitial lung diseases separate. The classic categorization of chronic interstitial pneumonias of Liebow is shown:

- Usual interstitial pneumonia (UIP)
- Desquamative interstitial pneumonia (DIP)
- Lymphocytic (lymphoid) interstitial pneumonia (LIP)
- Giant cell interstitial pneumonia (GIP)
- Bronchiolitis obliterans with organizing interstitial pneumonia or organizing diffuse alveolar damage (BIP)

A current interpretation of this classification follows:

- UIP and DIP equate with idiopathic pulmonary fibrosis (IPF), which is a term favored by clinicians. UIP is still often used by pathologists. DIP usually is included as IPF, but DIP is at most one tenth as common as UIP; some cases of DIP can be confused with smoker's bronchiolitis-associated interstitial lung disease.
- LIP is relatively unchanged, except that some cases have been reclassified as diffuse pulmonary lymphomas of small lymphocytes.
- GIP usually signifies hard metal (cobalt) lung disease.
- BIP has been renamed bronchiolitis obliterans organizing pneumonia (BOOP).

UIP, DIP, LIP, and BOOP have all been used to refer both to nonspecific reaction patterns and to specific clinicopathologic lesions, and one should be sure of the context in which the terms are being used.

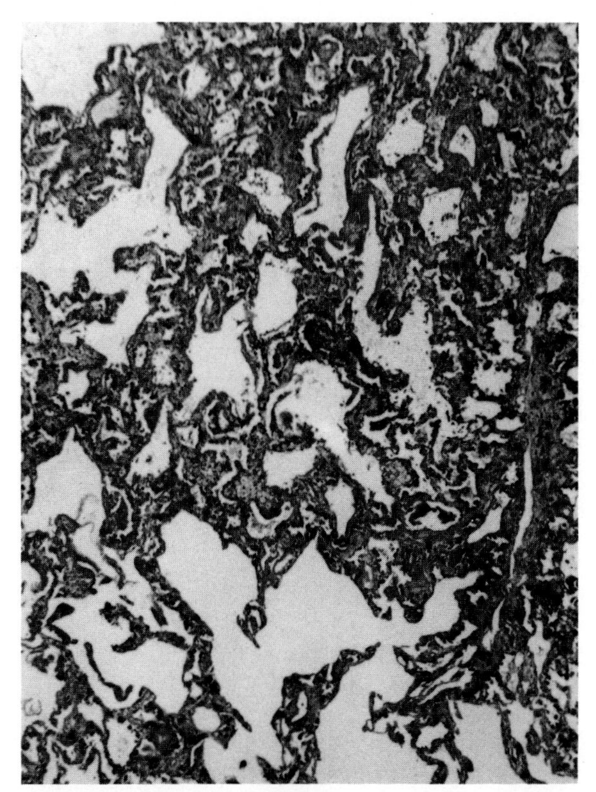

Figure 7 - 1.

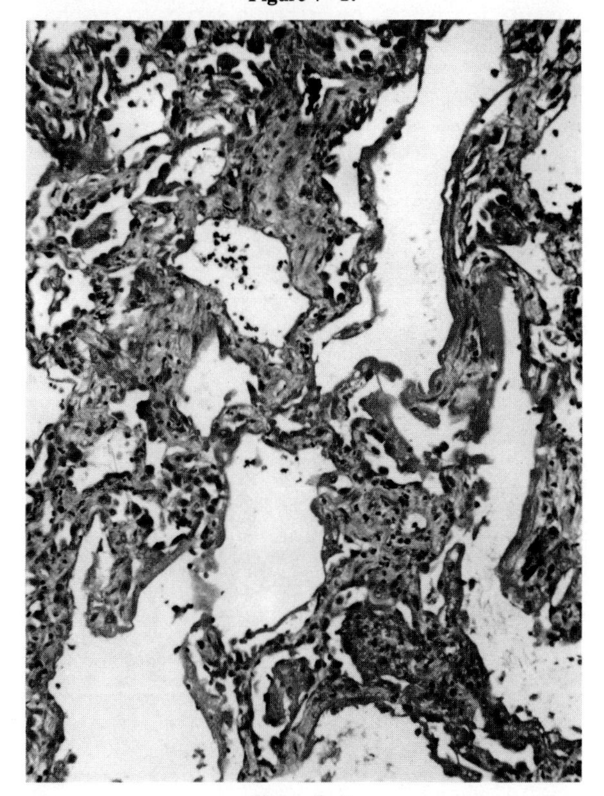

Figure 7 - 2.

Figures 7 - 1, 7 - 2. Diffuse alveolar damage. Hyaline membranes lining airspaces, interstitial edema, and atelectasis are shown. The remnants of atelectatic alveoli are discernible in between the larger airspaces, many of which are dilated alveolar ducts lined by hyaline membranes. (From a case of acute interstitial pneumonia.)

■ Diffuse Alveolar Damage (Figs. 7 - 1 to 7 - 14)

Diffuse alveolar damage is a pattern of diffuse lung injury and repair that is usually associated with acute bilateral interstitial lung disease, clinically labeled adult respiratory distress syndrome (ARDS). Diffuse alveolar damage has many causes and associations; a similar histologic picture affecting immature lungs is seen in neonates with hyaline membrane disease (respiratory distress syndrome of infants). Causes of diffuse alveolar damage include (1) infections, (2) radiation, (3) shock, (4) oxygen toxicity, (5) trauma, (6) sepsis, (7) neurologic disease, (8) drugs (especially chemotherapeutics), (9) acute allergic reactions, (10) noxious gases and chemical lung injury, (11) collagen-vascular diseases, (12) idiopathic (see AIP below), (13) Goodpasture's syndrome, (14) capillaritis, and (15) miscellaneous rare entities.

The histologic appearance is best understood if one separates DAD into injury, repair, and healed or resolved phases, although overlap between these phases exists. In general, the lung is diffusely involved in DAD, although the severity of damage and repair may vary from one field to the next. In early cases, only portions of the lung may be affected (i.e., regional alveolar damage).

Injury Phase: Alveolar and/or interstitial edema with or without alveolar hemorrhage, hyaline membranes (usually arising in alveolar ducts), fibrinous alveolar exudate, mild interstitial mononuclear cell infiltrate, and fibrin microthrombi, rarely with subpleural microinfarcts. A *few* neutrophils may be present in airspaces. Large numbers of neutrophils should suggest bacterial infection or superinfection, which is common in patients who have been on a ventilator or who are terminally ill.

Repair Phase: The repair phase usually shows epithelial metaplasia and regrowth of type II cells over hyaline membranes, and denuded alveolar walls with prominent type II cells, often bizarre in appearance. Fibroblastic proliferation around fragmented hyaline membranes is seen in the edematous interstitium and/or within airspaces in a pattern of organizing pneumonia (i.e., intra-alveolar organization). Immature squamous metaplasia may be prominent in and around bronchioles; it is nonspecific, although characteristic of virally-induced DAD.

Healed Phase: The healed phase may show entirely normal lung tissue or nonspecific changes, including increased alveolar macrophages, nonspecific interstitial and septal scarring, mural scarring in airways, and/or metaplastic epithelium within bronchioles or lining alveolar spaces. In some cases, the appearance of the scarring resembles UIP. Prolonged respiratory or oxygen therapy may result in a cystic and honeycombed appearance, analogous to bronchopulmonary dysplasia in neonates.

Most cases are seen in the injury or early repair phase. The degree of fibroblastic proliferation varies from case to case. In some, it is predominantly interstitial, in others predominantly airspace; or it may be mixed. Airspace organization, field for field, may resemble that seen in bronchiolitis obliterans organizing pneumonia. Airspace organization in the healing phase is eventually

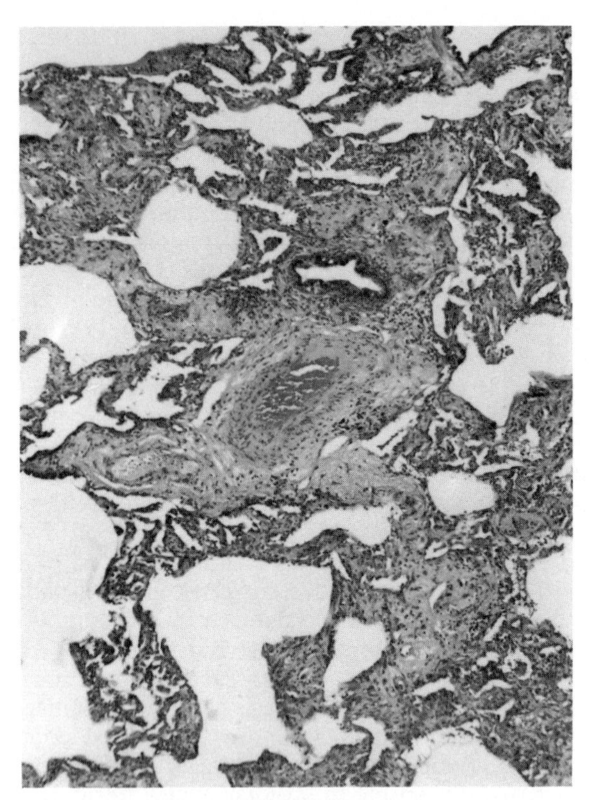

Figure 7–3.

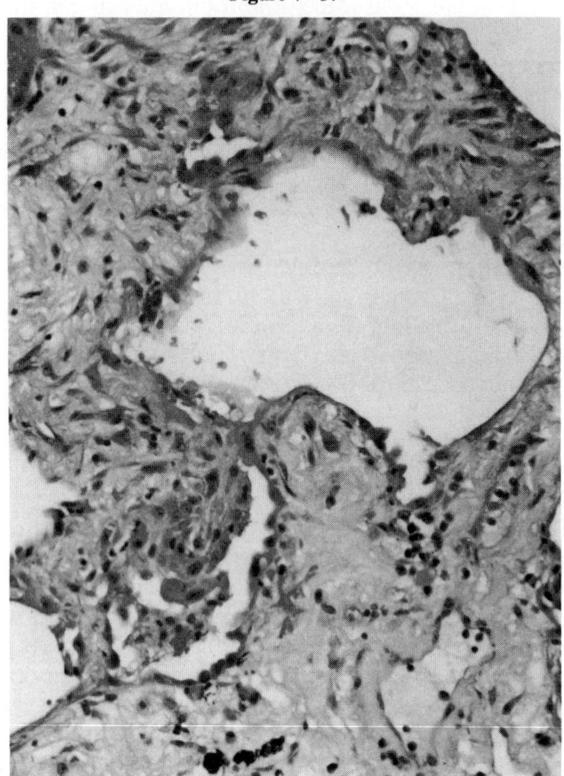

Figure 7–4.

Figures 7–3, 7–4. Diffuse alveolar damage with atelectasis and interstitial edematous thickening. The edematous myxoid interstitium (in conjunction with the history) is a clue to the acuteness of the process. Atelectatic alveoli are apparent. (From a case of acute interstitial pneumonia.)

incorporated into the interstitium with overlying proliferative type II pneumocytes.

References

Churg A, Golden J, Fligiel S, Hogg JC. Bronchopulmonary dysplasia in the adult. Am Rev Respir Dis 127:117–120, 1983.

Flint A, Colby TV. Surgical Pathology of Diffuse Infiltrative Lung Disease. Orlando, Grune & Stratton, Inc, 1987.

Katzenstein ALA, Askin FB. Surgical Pathology of Non-Neoplastic Lung Disease, 2nd ed. Philadelphia, WB Saunders Co, 1990.

Katzenstein ALA, Bloor CM, Liebow AA. Diffuse alveolar damage—the role of oxygen, shock, and related factors. Am J Pathol 85:210–228, 1976.

Pratt PC. Pathology of adult respiratory distress syndrome. *In* Thurlbeck WM, Abell MR (eds). The Lung. Baltimore, Williams & Wilkins, 1978.

Thurlbeck WM (ed). Pathology of the Lung. New York, Thieme, 1988.

Yazdy AM, Tomashefski JF, Yagan R, Kleinerman J. Regional alveolar damage. Am J Clin Pathol 92:10–15, 1989.

■ Acute Interstitial Pneumonia (Figs. 7–1 to 7–14)

Acute interstitial pneumonia (AIP) is synonomous with Hamman-Rich syndrome, acute interstitial pulmonary fibrosis (acute IPF), and accelerated interstitial pneumonia.

Histologically, DAD occurs in previously healthy individuals for which no apparent cause can be found. The term acute interstitial pneumonia serves to emphasize the fulminant clinical features.

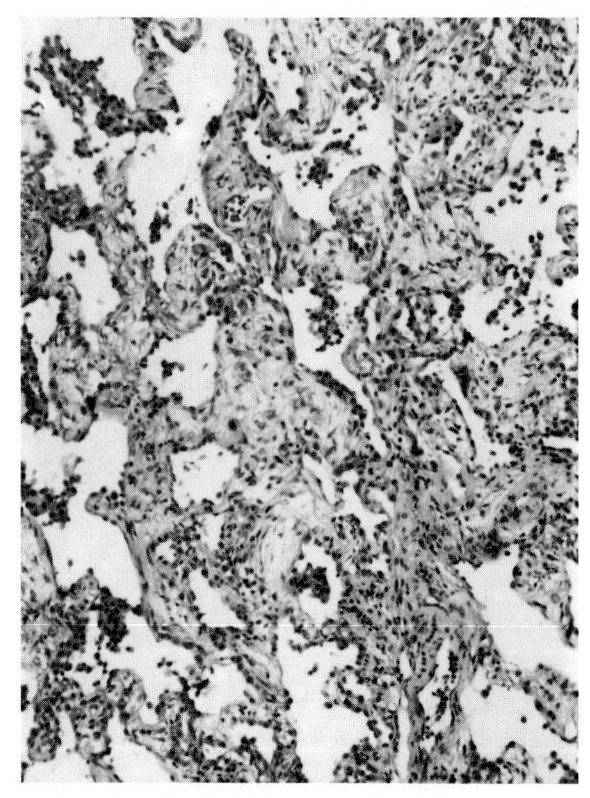

Figure 7–5. Diffuse alveolar damage with prominent interstitial edema and prominent type II cells. (From a case of acute interstitial pneumonia. The patient survived.)

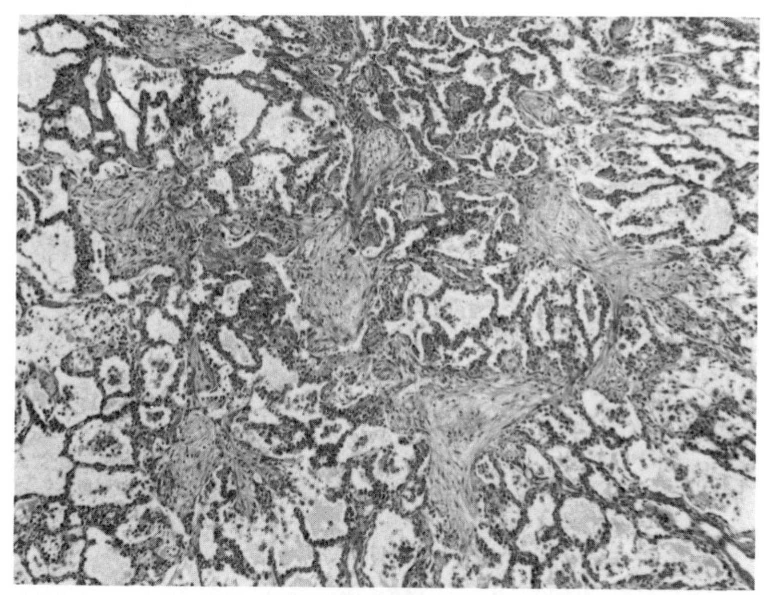

Figure 7–6.

Figures 7–6, 7–7, 7–8. Organizing diffuse alveolar damage. There is an organizing myxomatous connective tissue proliferation in the alveolar ducts. The pattern is indistinguishable from that seen in bronchiolitis obliterans organizing pneumonia (BOOP) and many other reparative processes, and the clinical history is helpful in differential diagnosis. The intervening alveolar walls contain a modest inflammatory infiltrate and are lined by reactive type II cells. In some foci there is edematous myxomatous thickening of alveolar walls. From a case of acute interstitial pneumonia that was fatal over a total course of 4 weeks.

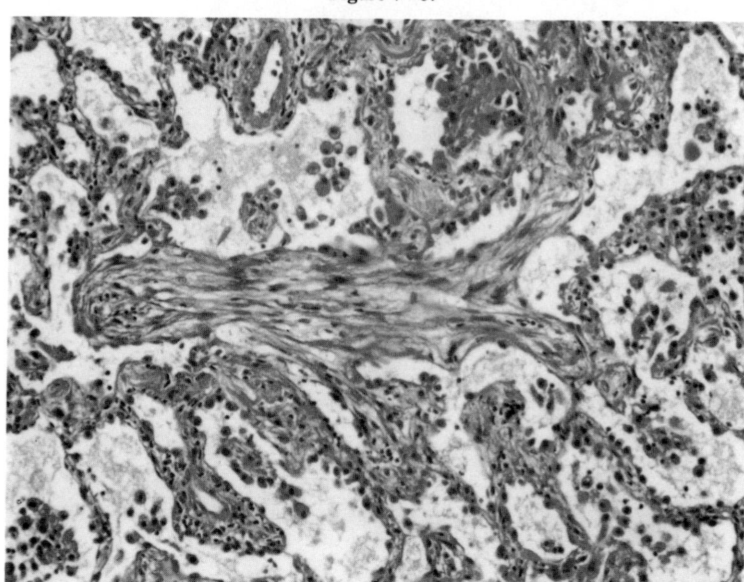

Figure 7–7.

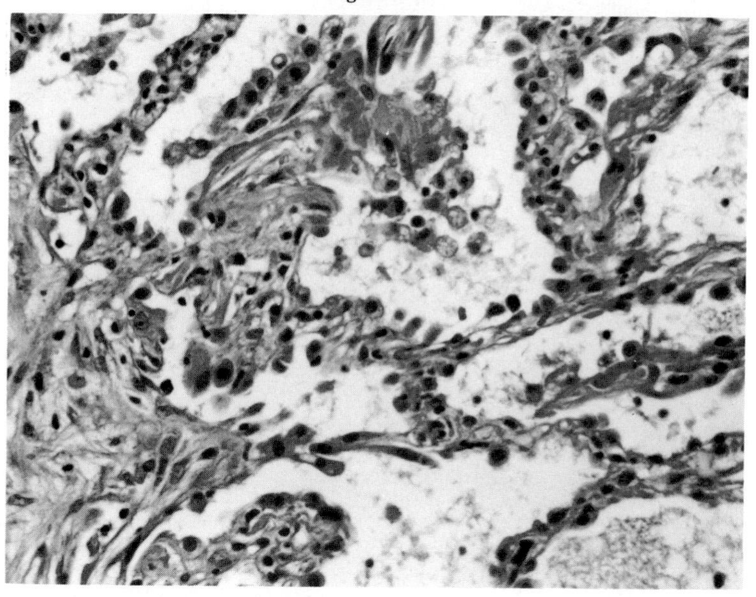

Figure 7–8.

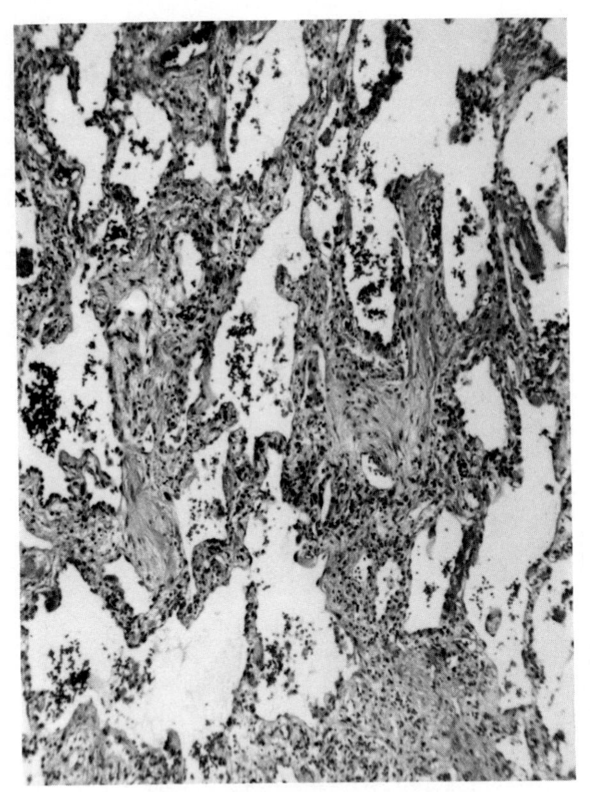

Figure 7-9. Organizing diffuse alveolar damage. This case is at a somewhat later stage than the one illustrated in Figures 7-6 through 7-8. Myxomatous connective tissue is being incorporated into the interstitium with interstitial fibrosis and architectural distortion.

Some patients with subclinical UIP (see below) may present with a fulminant process simulating AIP except for a background of *chronic* scarring and honeycombing that may be recognized grossly, on prior chest radiographs, or microscopically.

References

Ashbaugh DG, Maier RV. Idiopathic pulmonary fibrosis in adult respiratory distress syndrome: diagnosis and treatment. Arch Surg 120:530, 1985.

Hamman L, Rich AR. Fulminating diffuse interstitial fibrosis of the lungs. Trans Am Clin Climatol Assoc 51:154-163, 1935.

Katzenstein ALA, Myers JL, Mazur MT. Acute interstitial pneumonia: a clinicopathologic, ultrastructural, and cell kinetic study. Am J Surg Pathol 10:256-267, 1986.

Olsen J, Colby TV, Elliott CG. Hamman-Rich syndrome revisited. Submitted for publication.

Porte A, Stoeckel ME, Mantz JM, Tempe JD, Jaeger A, Batzenschlager A. Acute interstitial pulmonary fibrosis: comparative light and electron microscopic study of 19 cases. Pathogenic and therapeutic implications. Intensive Care Med 4:181-191, 1978.

Pratt DS, Schwartz MI, May JJ, Dreisin RB. Rapidly fatal pulmonary fibrosis: the accelerated variant of interstitial pneumonitis. Thorax 34:587-593, 1979.

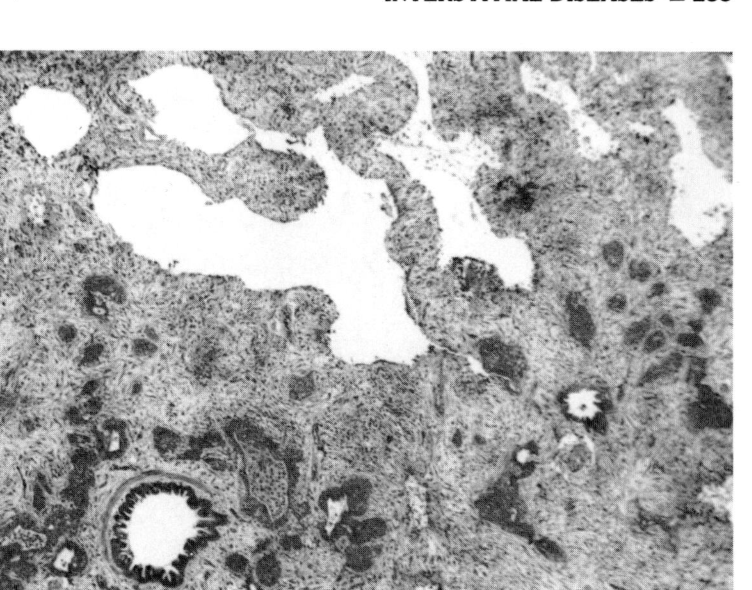

Figure 7–10.

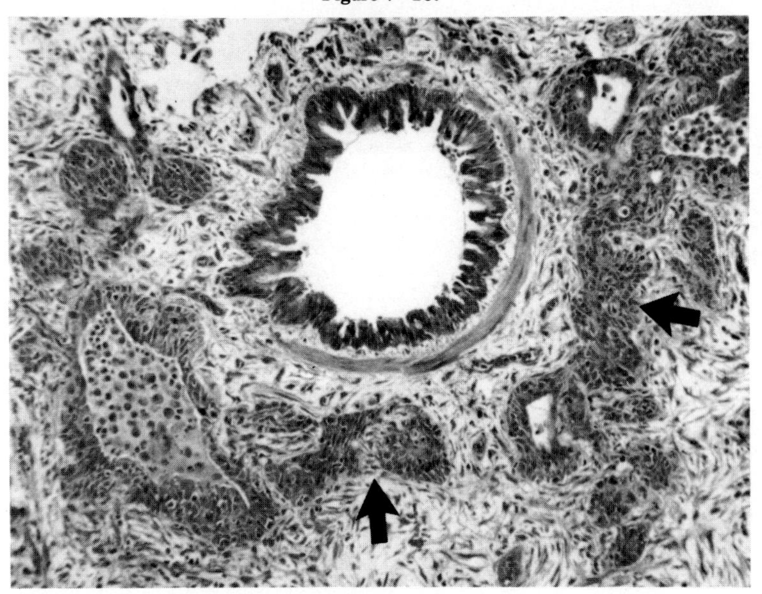

Figure 7–11.

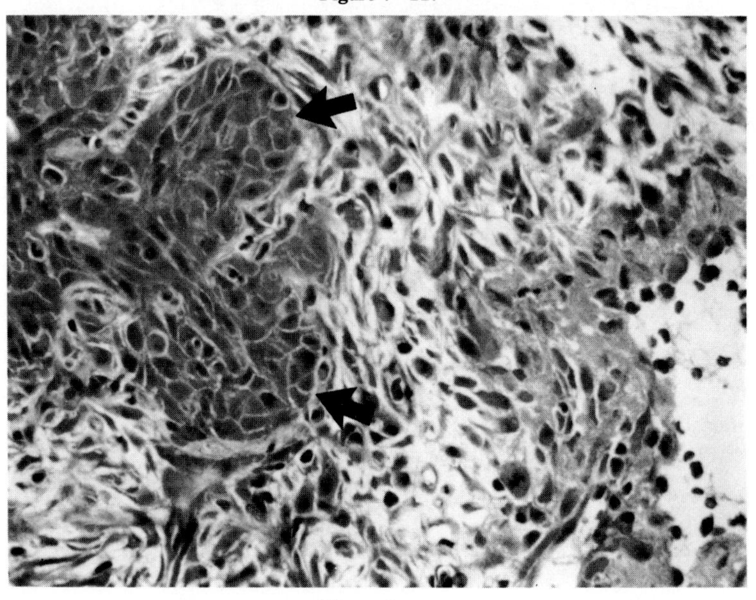

Figure 7–12.

Figures 7–10, 7–11, 7–12. Organizing diffuse alveolar damage. There is dramatic distortion of lung architecture and diffuse thickening by myxomatous connective tissue. Peribronchiolar squamous metaplasia (arrows) is prominent (a common nonspecific finding). (From a case of acute interstitial pneumonia in a 7-year-old boy who survived and recovered and was without clinical evidence of pulmonary disease 1 year after this biopsy procedure was performed.)

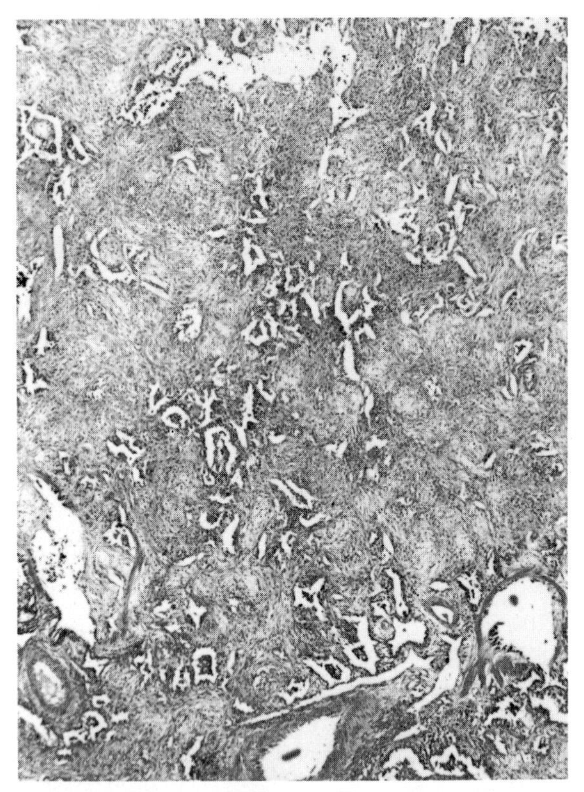

Figure 7–13.

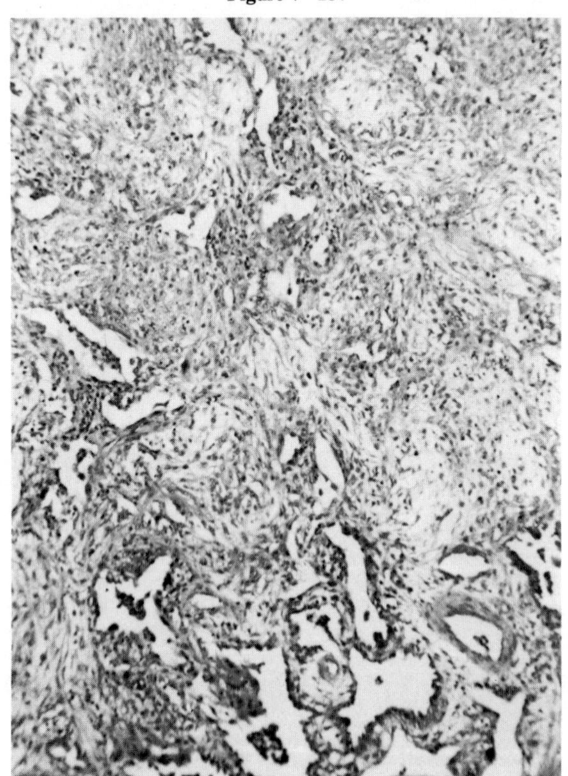

Figure 7–14.

Figures 7–13, 7–14. Organizing diffuse alveolar damage. Architectural distortion from fibroblastic proliferation is evident. (From a case of acute interstitial pneumonia. The patient survived.)

■ Pulmonary Edema (Figs. 7–15 to 7–20)

Pulmonary edema is rarely seen in biopsy material, except in some specimens taken to exclude the possibility of some other lesion, such as an infection.

Histologic findings are not prominent because edema fluid is usually washed out during processing. Septal edema and dilated septal, perivascular, and peribronchial lymphatics can generally be visualized, and sometimes some proteinaceous edema fluid may be appreciated in alveolar spaces. Splaying apart of the connective tissue may erroneously suggest perivascular fibrosis. Margination of neutrophils in vessels may be seen. In a number of chronic interstitial lung diseases, a dense proteinaceous exudate may be apparent in some airspaces ("dense edema"); this is a nonspecific finding. Pulmonary edema is included in the differential diagnosis of the "normal" biopsy specimen. Pulmonary edema is also prominent in the early phases of DAD. Artifactual edema occurs with prolonged surgical clamping prior to the biopsy procedure as a result of vascular and lymphatic occlusion.

References

Thurlbeck WM (ed). Pathology of the Lung. New York, Thieme, 1988.

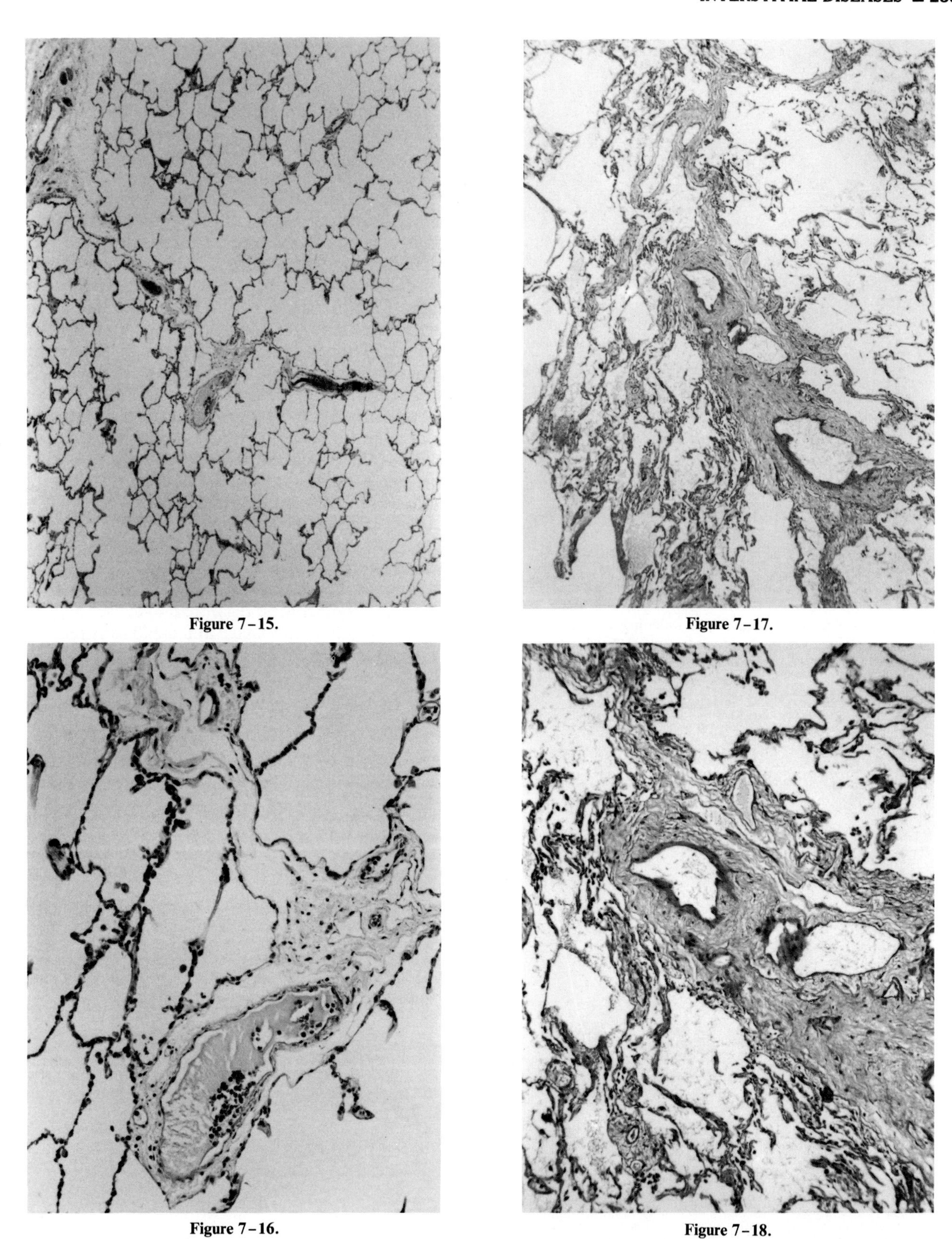

Figure 7–15.

Figure 7–17.

Figure 7–16.

Figure 7–18.

Figures 7–15, 7–16. Pulmonary edema. There is interstitial edema in the septum and dilatation of septal lymphatics. This biopsy specimen was obtained from a patient with systemic lupus erythematosus (SLE) and evidence of heart failure. Despite the presence of immune complexes by immunofluorescence, no pathologic feature other than edema was present and the patient responded to diuresis. (From Colby, TV and Yousem, S: Pulmonary histology for the surgical pathologist. Am J Surg Pathol 12:223–239, 1988. With permission of Raven Press.)

Figures 7–17, 7–18. Pulmonary edema. This biopsy specimen was obtained from a patient with presumed acute interstitial lung disease. The only finding was interstitial and perivascular edema. The appearance might suggest perivascular fibrosis, but the patient responded to diuresis for fluid overload. (With permission of Raven Press.)

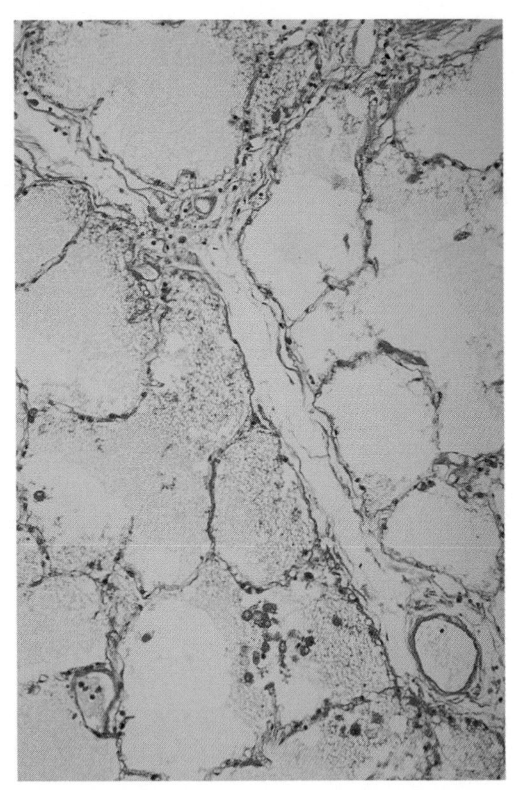

Figure 7-19. Pulmonary edema. Septal widening, dilatation of lymphatics, and a faint eosinophilic proteinaceous material in the alveoli are shown.

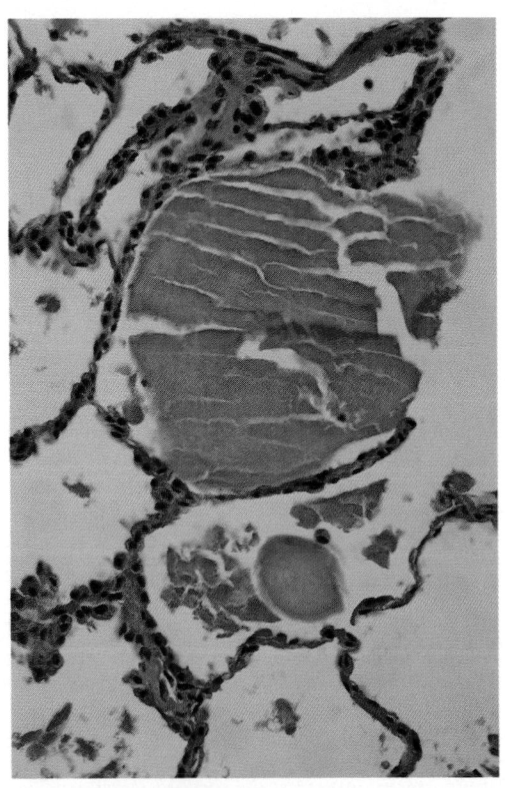

Figure 7-20. "Dense edema." This dense, hard-appearing eosinophilic material within the alveoli is usually seen as an incidental finding. Descriptively termed "dense edema," this change is probably related to chronic alveolar proteinaceous fluid accumulations.

■ **Capillaritis** (Fig. 7-21; see also Figs. 7-24, 7-25, and 8-15 to 8-18)

There is mural inflammation (vasculitis) of the capillaries analogous to leukocytoclastic vasculitis at other sites.

The usual histologic appearance consists of increased interstitial neutrophils in capillary walls without concomitant airspace neutrophils. Capillary wall necrosis, thrombosis, and karyorrhectic debris are observed on occasion. Granulomatous capillaritis with necrosis and giant cell reaction may be observed in Wegener's granulomatosis, although neutrophilic capillaritis is more common. With injury and necrosis of the capillary wall the alveolar spaces become filled with hemorrhage and inflammatory material, and the process resembles an acute hemorrhagic pneumonia.

Capillaritis is nonspecific and may be seen in a number of conditions, including (1) Wegener's granulomatosis and other vasculitides; (2) systemic lupus erythematosus and other collagen vascular diseases; (3) Goodpasture's disease; (4) infections and sepsis; (5) unclassified pulmonary alveolar hemorrhage syndromes, many of which are immune complex mediated; and (6) unclassified reactions.

Capillaritis is a frequent histologic feature in alveolar hemorrhage syndromes, regardless of cause.

Some cases of hemorrhage and capillaritis may never be completely solved, even with extensive clinical evaluations.

References

Mark EJ, Ramirez ME. Pulmonary capillaritis and hemorrhage in patients with systemic vasculitis. Arch Pathol Lab Med 109:413-418, 1985.

Myers J, Katzenstein A. Microangitis in lupus-induced pulmonary hemorrhage. Am J Clin Pathol 85:552-556, 1986.

Myers JL, Katzenstein ALA. Wegener's granulomatosis presenting with massive pulmonary hemorrhage and capillaritis. Am J Surg Pathol 11:895-898, 1987.

Travis WD, Carpenter HA, Lie JT. Diffuse pulmonary hemorrhage: an uncommon manifestation of Wegener's granulomatosis. Am J Surg Pathol 11:702-708, 1987.

Travis WD, Colby TV, Lombard C, Carpenter HA. A clinicopathologic study of 34 cases of diffuse pulmonary hemorrhage with lung biopsy confirmation. Am J Surg Pathol. In press.

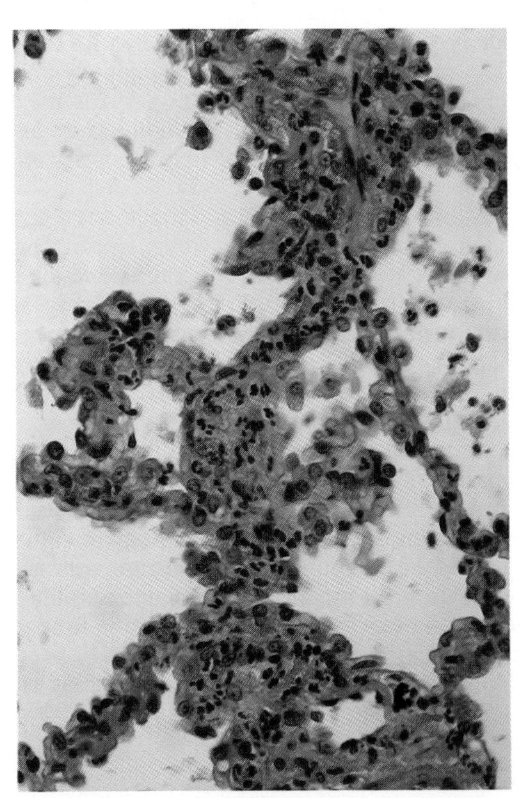

Figure 7-21. Capillaritis. Transbronchial biopsy specimen from a patient with clinical evidence of pulmonary hemorrhage, showing capillaritis with clustering neutrophils in alveolar walls. This finding should evoke a differential diagnosis (see text), although no specific diagnosis was identified in this case, even with subsequent open lung biopsy.

■ Fume and Toxic Exposure (Including Silo-Filler's Disease)

Careful evaluation of the history is important for making the diagnosis. Some fume or toxic exposures may be associated with delayed pulmonary disease manifesting some hours or days after exposure. Offending agents include nitrogen dioxide, sulfur dioxide, ammonia, phosgene, chlorine, metal fumes (cadmium, mercury, zinc), acetaldehyde, acrolein, antimony chloride, beryllium, boranes, cobalts, hydrogen chloride, hydrogen sulfide, hydrogen selenide, methyl bromide, nickel carbonyl, ozone, perchloroethylene, titanium tetrachloride, zirconium chloride.

Inflammation and necrosis in the airways may or may not be evident. The usual histologic findings are those of DAD ("chemical pneumonitis") with an acute bronchiolitis. Late "healed" cases may be histologically normal or may show subtle abnormalities of the small airways and constrictive bronchiolitis. Some cases show prominent desquamative change in the airspaces.

References

Churg A, Green FHY. Pathology of Occupational Lung Disease. New York, Igaku-Shoin Medical Publishers, 1988.

Dail DH, Hammer SP (eds). Pulmonary Pathology. New York, Springer-Verlag, 1988.

Douglas WW, Hopper NGG, Colby TV. Silo-filler's disease. Mayo Clin Proc 64:291-304, 1989.

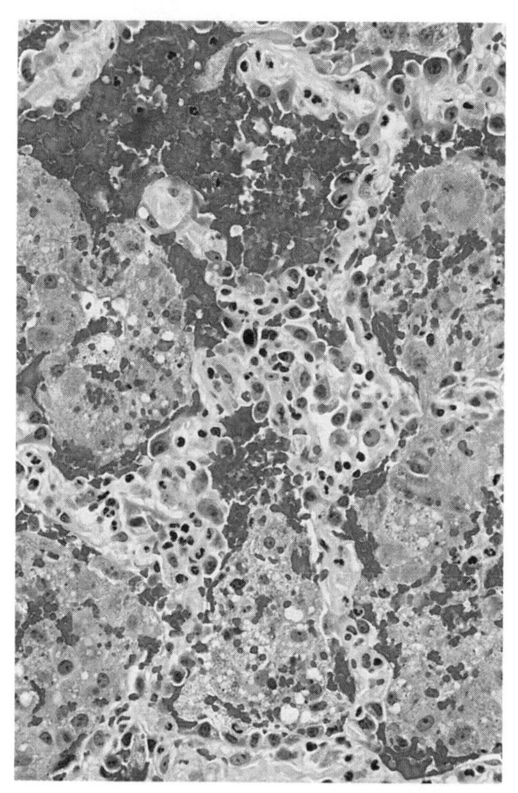

Figure 7-22.

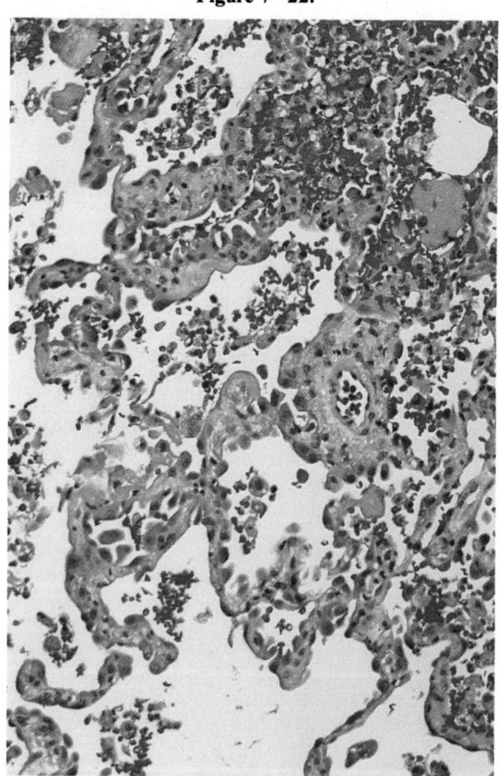

Figure 7-23.

■ Goodpasture's Disease (Figs. 7-22 to 7-25)

There is acute renal and/or pulmonary disease caused by antiglomerular basement membrane antibodies. Pulmonary and renal involvement may be synchronous or dyssynchronous.

Acute and old alveolar hemorrhage with hemosiderin-filled macrophages and fresh hemorrhage are present in the airspaces. Focal organization with granulation tissue, usually in alveolar ducts, may also be present. In some cases, the histologic appearance is that of a hemorrhagic diffuse alveolar damage with hyaline membrane formation and prominent reparative type II cells. Capillaritis may be seen.

The approach for the pathologist in cases of possible Goodpasture's disease includes (1) freezing tissue and performing immunofluorescence for anti-glomerular basement membrane antibody (a negative result does not exclude the diagnosis of Goodpasture's disease), and (2) serologic tests for antiglomerular basement membrane antibodies. Concomitant evaluation for collagen-vascular diseases and vasculitis (especially Wegener's granulomatosis with antineutrophilic cytoplasmic antibody) is appropriate.

References

Dail DH, Hammer SP (eds). Pulmonary Pathology. New York, Springer-Verlag, 1988.

Lombard CM, Colby TV, Elliott CG. Surgical pathology of the lung in anti-basement membrane antibody associated Goodpasture's syndrome. Hum Pathol 20:445-451, 1989.

Thurlbeck WM (ed). Pathology of the Lung. New York, Thieme, 1988.

Figures 7-22, 7-23. Goodpasture's disease. Fresh alveolar hemorrhage and increased macrophages, some of which contain brownish hemosiderin, are apparent. A mild inflammatory infiltrate is present. In other foci, the reactive changes in the alveolar walls (reminiscent of those seen in diffuse alveolar damage) overshadow the alveolar hemorrhage.

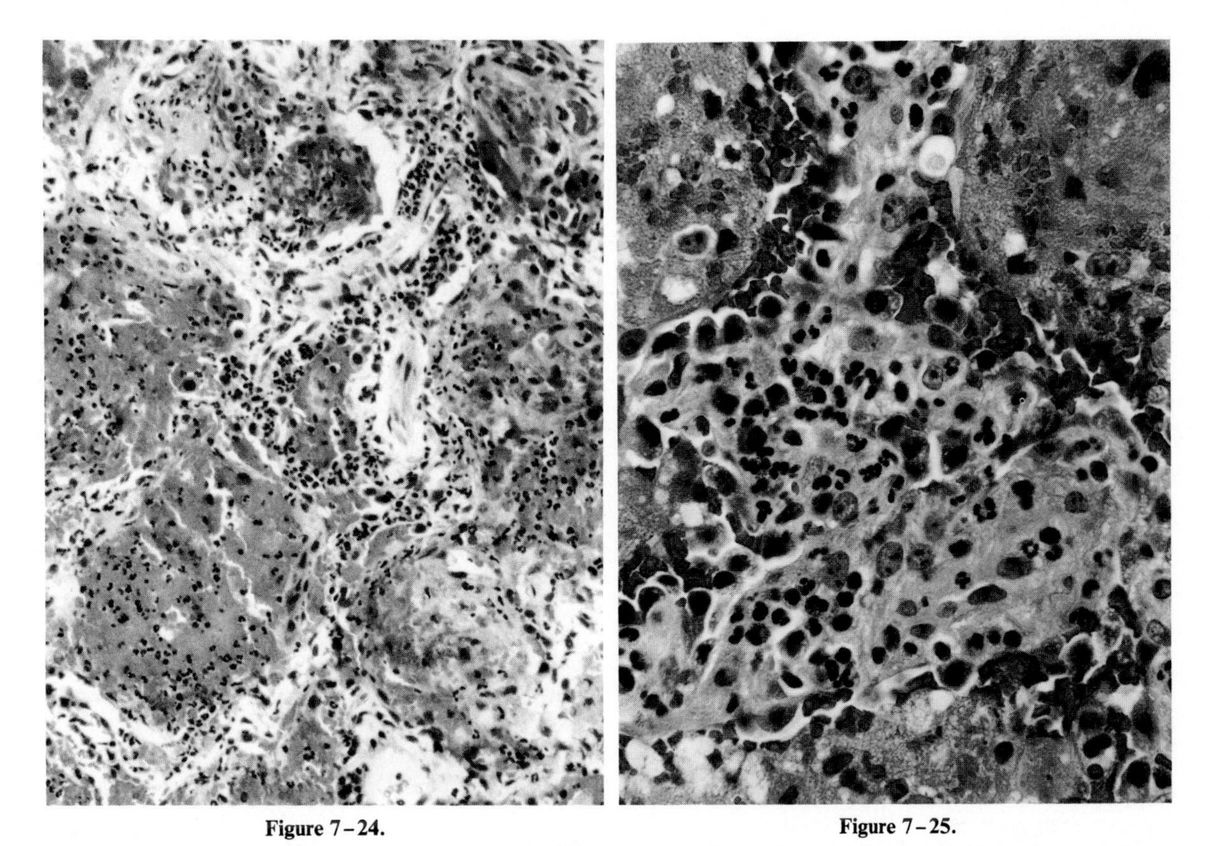

Figure 7-24. **Figure 7-25.**

Figures 7-24, 7-25. Goodpasture's disease. Many cases of Goodpasture's disease show only recent and old alveolar hemorrhage with a few tufts of organization in the airspaces. This case illustrates capillaritis with infiltrates of neutrophils along the capillaries in the alveolar walls. Although some airspace accumulations of neutrophils are present, neutrophils are most marked in the interstitium. Fibrinous exudate, fresh hemorrhage, and refractile hemosiderin can be seen in the alveoli.

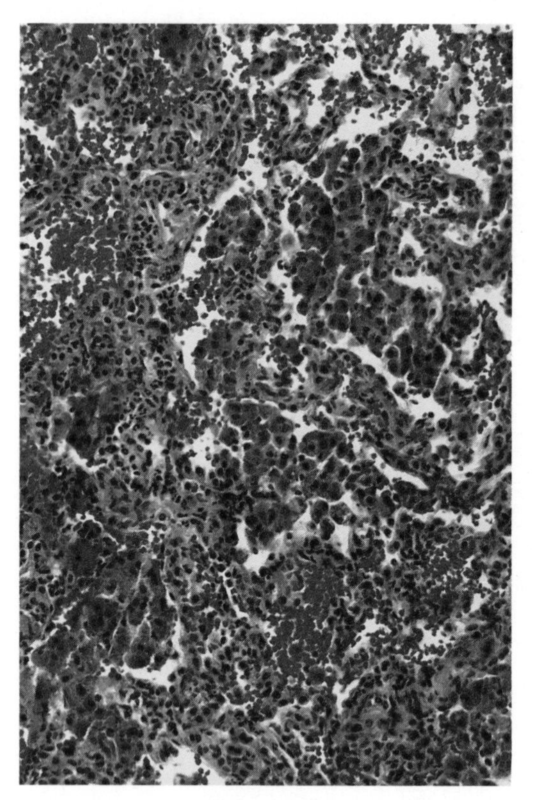

Figure 7–26.

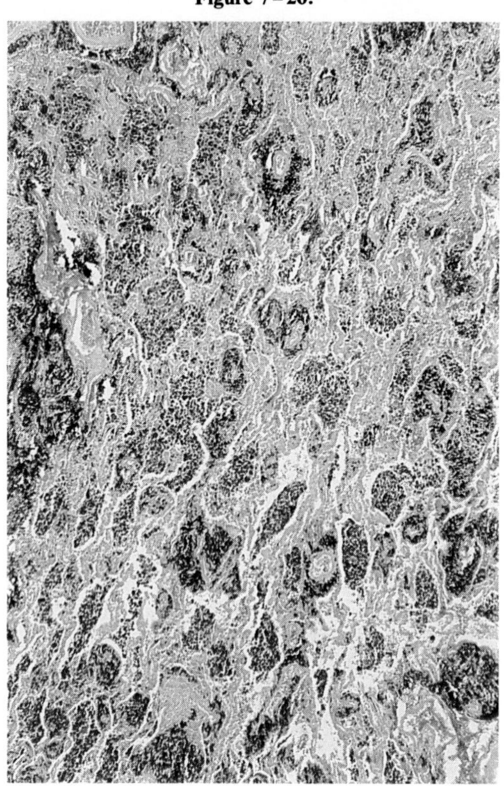

Figure 7–27.

■ Idiopathic Pulmonary Hemosiderosis (Figs. 7–26 to 7–28)

There is chronic recurring pulmonary hemorrhage without evidence of extrapulmonary disease for which no specific cause can be found. Idiopathic pulmonary hemosiderosis (IPH) is a diagnosis of exclusion. It is usually seen in children or young adults with hemoptysis and anemia. In some cases diagnosed as IPH, follow-up results in a different diagnosis. The prognosis is variable; some patients fare poorly over the long term.

Alveolar hemorrhage with prominent hemosiderin-filled macrophages is seen. Slight interstitial thickening and fibrosis may be present with prominent type II alveolar lining cells, especially in chronic cases. These may resemble DIP. Iron and calcium may be seen to encrust elastic fibers. Electron microscopy may show basement membrane reduplication and splitting. Immunofluorescence is negative.

Chronic cigarette smokers commonly show increased numbers of alveolar macrophages, which stain positive with iron stains, and one may consider the possibility of alveolar hemorrhage. In smokers, the iron-positive granules are smaller and finer and are associated with small black flecks of carbonaceous material in the cells. (See Figs. 7–56, 7–57).

References

Dail DH, Hammer SP (eds). Pulmonary Pathology. New York, Springer-Verlag, 1988.

Katzenstein ALA, Askin FB. Surgical Pathology of Non-Neoplastic Lung Disease, 2nd ed. Philadelphia, WB Saunders Co, 1990.

Thurlbeck WM (ed). Pathology of the Lung. New York, Thieme, 1988.

Figures 7–26, 7–27. Idiopathic pulmonary hemosiderosis. Idiopathic pulmonary hemosiderosis in a biopsy specimen from a child with recurrent pulmonary infiltrates and anemia. The histologic features are reminiscent of desquamative interstitial pneumonia, although iron stain shows a large amount of coarse hemosiderin positivity in the macrophages (Fig. 7–27).

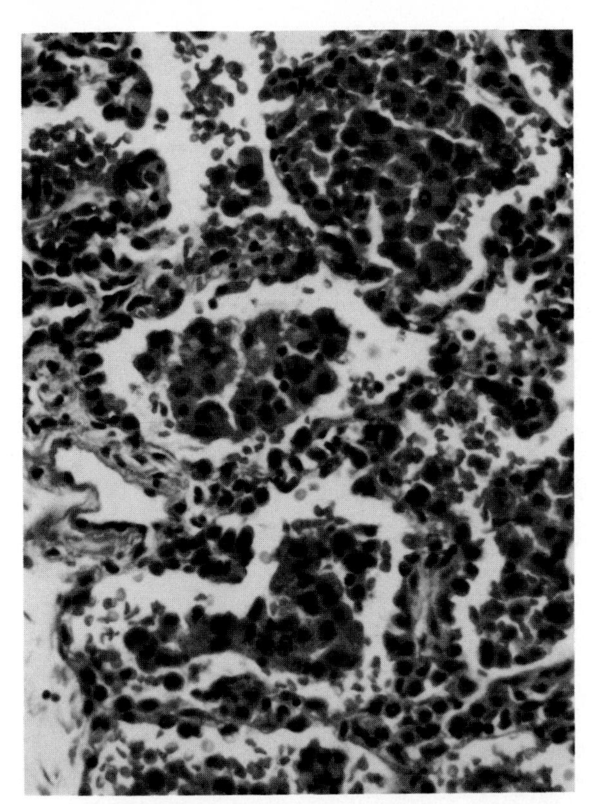

Figure 7–28. Idiopathic pulmonary hemosiderosis. There are large accumulations of macrophages in the airspaces and mild thickening of the alveolar septa with prominent type II cells. The appearance is reminiscent of desquamative interstitial pneumonia. Clinically, however, this specimen was obtained from a child with anemia and interstitial lung disease, and the macrophages contained abundant hemosiderin.

■ Unclassified Pulmonary Hemorrhage Syndromes

An appreciable percentage (up to 25 per cent) of patients who present with specific acute or chronic alveolar hemorrhage cannot be placed into a diagnostic category; however, they may have evidence of multisystem disease, or their condition may be too severe to be considered IPH. Capillaritis may or may not be present. Patients often improve with only steroid therapy. A reasonable approach is as follows: (1) exclude Goodpasture's disease, collagen vascular diseases, Wegener's granulomatosis and other vasculidities as well as vascular malformations, vascular tumors (especially metastatic angiosarcoma) and infections; and (2) adopt a wait-and-see attitude because diagnosis may be forthcoming with follow-up. Traumatic and artifactual hemorrhage from the biopsy procedure should also be excluded.

References

Travis WD, Colby TV, Lombard C, Carpenter HA. A clinicopathologic study of 34 cases of diffuse pulmonary hemorrhage with lung biopsy confirmation. Am J Surg Pathol. In press.

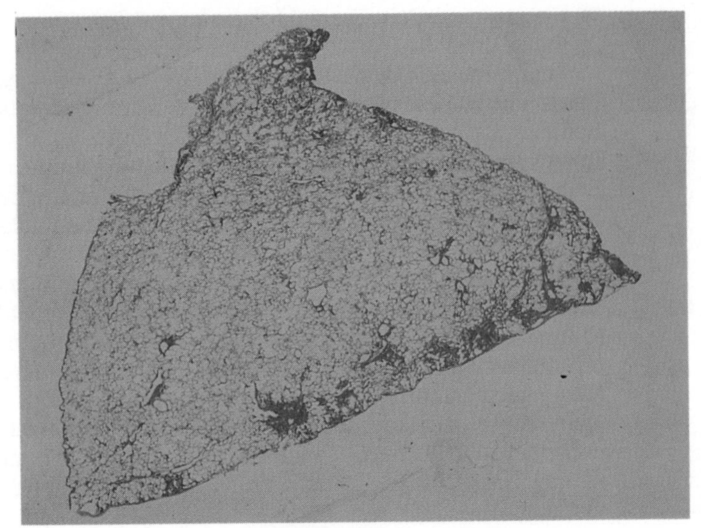

Figure 7-29.

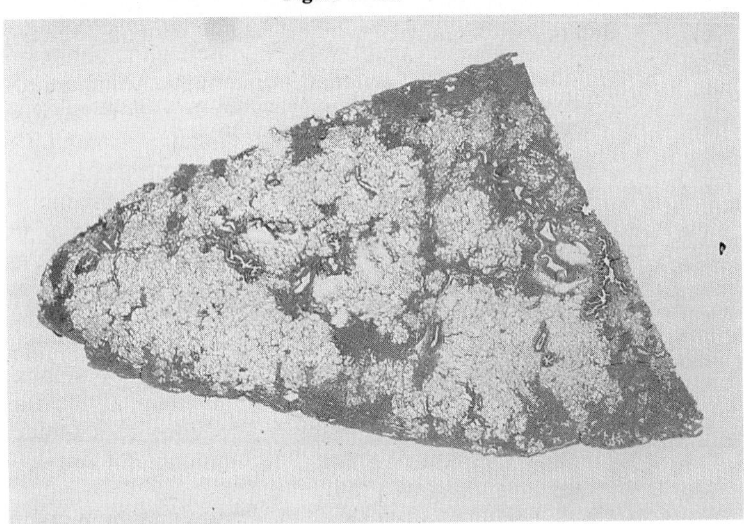

Figure 7-30.

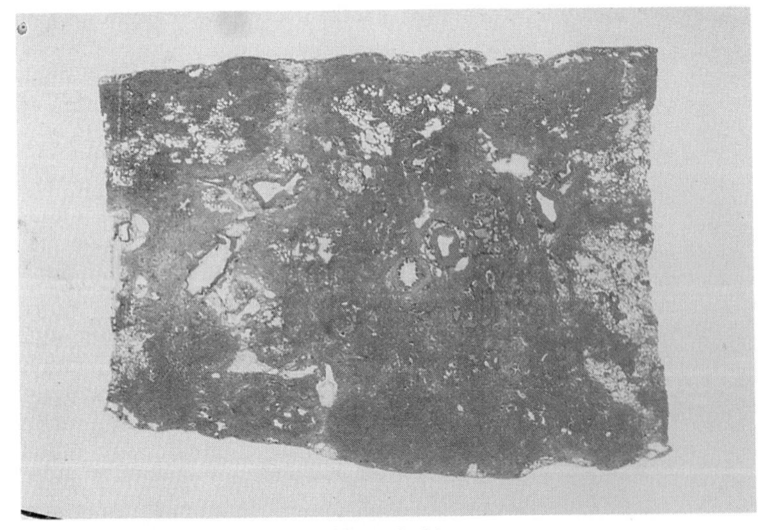

Figure 7-31.

Figures 7-29, 7-30, 7-31. Usual interstitial pneumonia (UIP). This series of illustrations is from biopsy specimens of the upper lobe (Fig. 7-29), middle lobe (Fig. 7-30), and lower lobe (Fig. 7-31), respectively. The figures show the variation in severity that may be seen in UIP. The earliest infiltrates are visible in the upper and middle lobe biopsy specimen in a peripheral acinar distribution and often can be discerned emanating from the septa and the pleura and around bronchovascular structures. Such a peripheral acinar distribution is often apparent in UIP, although there is no discernible distribution in severely affected portions of the lung, as illustrated in the biopsy specimen from the lower lobe.

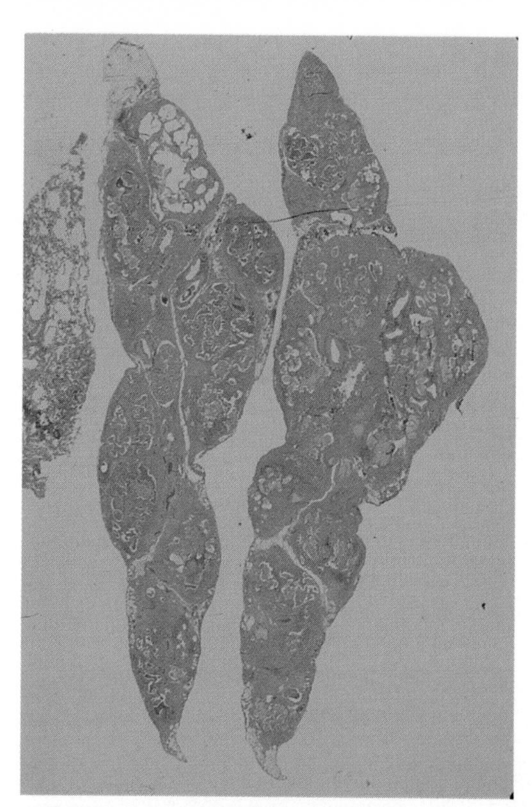

Figure 7–32. Usual interstitial pneumonia (UIP). This is a typical appearance of a biopsy specimen from a patient with UIP. The surgeon has selected a severely affected area that shows, predominantly, honeycombing and septal contraction, thus producing a lobulated appearance that accounts for the knobby pleural surface. In such a case, one should seek out the least affected portions (small area at far left) to determine the pattern of the pathologic process.

■ Usual Interstitial Pneumonia (Figs. 7–29 to 7–42)

Usual interstitial pneumonia is also known as idiopathic pulmonary fibrosis and cryptogenic fibrosing alveolitis, mural type. Bilateral progressive chronic fibrosing interstitial pneumonitis leads to honeycombing.

Histologically, there is a *patchy* interstitial scarring process that often emanates from the subpleural zones and septa or, occasionally, from one edge of an airway, without actually centering on airways. A pattern of *peripheral acinar distribution* can often be identified in the less fibrotic areas. Such a distribution cannot be appreciated in the foci of honeycombing or severely scarred zones. Interstitial widening and fibrosis of alveolar walls are accompanied by honeycombing and smooth muscle metaplasia as parenchyma is destroyed. The degree of inflammation is usually mild (at most moderate) and is composed of lymphocytes and plasma cells. Lymphoid follicles may be present.

In fibrotic regions, increased alveolar macrophages may be present. Pooling of mucin, often with neutrophilic infiltrate, is common in foci of honeycombing. Fibroblastic proliferation with mucopolysaccharide-rich matrix may be prominent in zones of active fibroblastic proliferation; in general, however, the amount of mature scarring (with honeycombing) overshadows the fibroblastic foci. The fibroblastic zones probably represent organization of foci of airspace fibrinous exudate and alveolar wall damage. Such exudative foci are usually focal, few and far between.

In some patients with UIP, a fulminant, and usually fatal, acute DAD superimposed on the UIP develops. Often the acute changes can be distinguished from the background of honeycombing and chronic scarring. This appearance is typical of that found in autopsy specimens from patients with UIP.

The pathology report should include statements as to the degree of irreversible scarring (i.e., interstitial fibrosis and honeycombing) and the degree of inflammation, as these correlate with prognosis.

Note: Extensive fibroblastic proliferation with a small amount of old scarring should lead to consideration of more acute lesions. Marked chronic inflammation, particularly if uniform and diffuse, is unusual in UIP. The presence of granulomas, even a few, should raise the possibility of chronic extrinsic allergic alveolitis. Abundant organizing pneumonia should raise the possibility of BOOP, organizing eosinophilic pneumonia, organizing DAD, or an organizing allergic reaction. Bronchiolocentric scarring suggesting prior airway injury with abundant bronchiolar metaplasia around small airways should raise the possibility of constrictive bronchiolitis. Stellate bronchiolocentric scars are seen in healed eosinophilic granuloma. Marked lymphoid hyperplasia should raise the possibility of collagen vascular disease. UIP rarely occurs in those under the age of 45; this fact is helpful to keep in mind.

Foci resembling UIP are seen in a number of conditions, and an open biopsy specimen, in which a pattern (especially a peripheral acinar pattern) can be appreciated, is usually necessary for the diagnosis. The diagnosis should not be made from a transbronchial biopsy specimen or in the absence of clinical correlation.

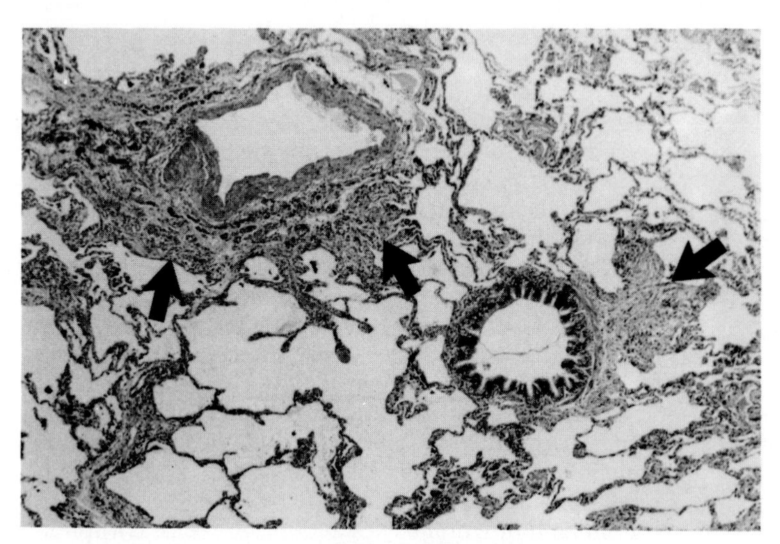

Figure 7–33.

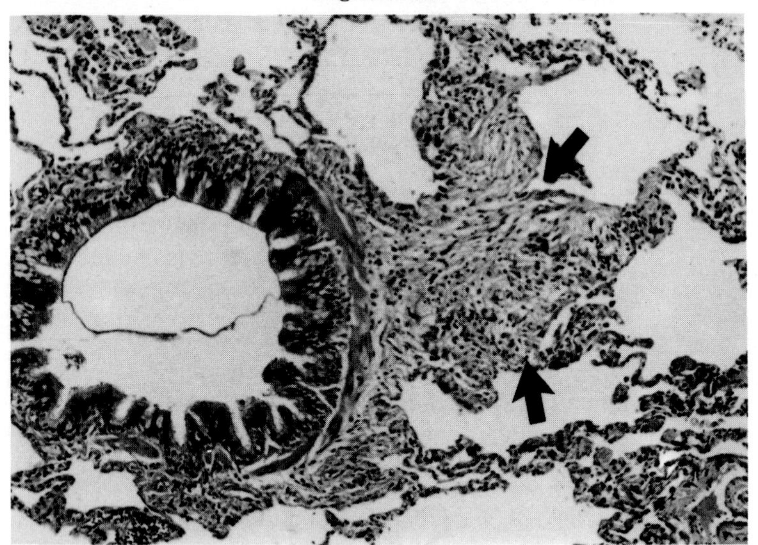

Figure 7–34.

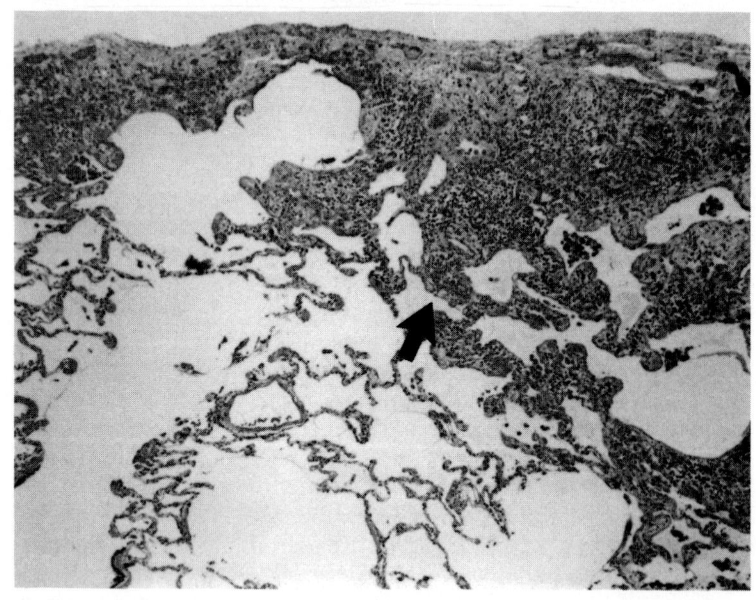

Figure 7–35.

Figures 7–33, 7–34, 7–35. Usual interstitial pneumonia (UIP). Interstitial fibrous thickening emanates from peribronchiolar, perivascular, and subpleural regions (arrows), reflecting a peripheral acinar distribution.

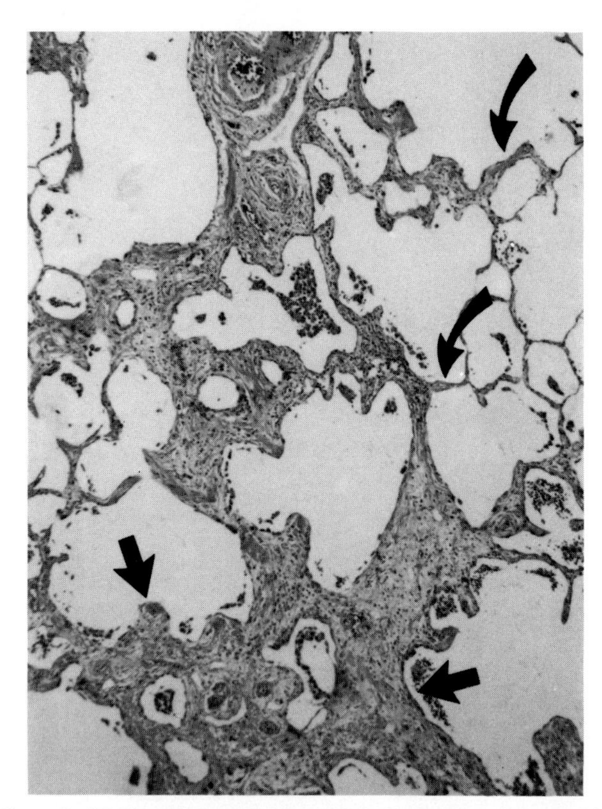

Figure 7-36. Usual interstitial pneumonia (UIP). There is interstitial scarring with no discernible pattern. Micro-honeycombing is present (arrows). Involvement of identifiable alveolar walls (curved arrows) is the earliest lesion seen in this case.

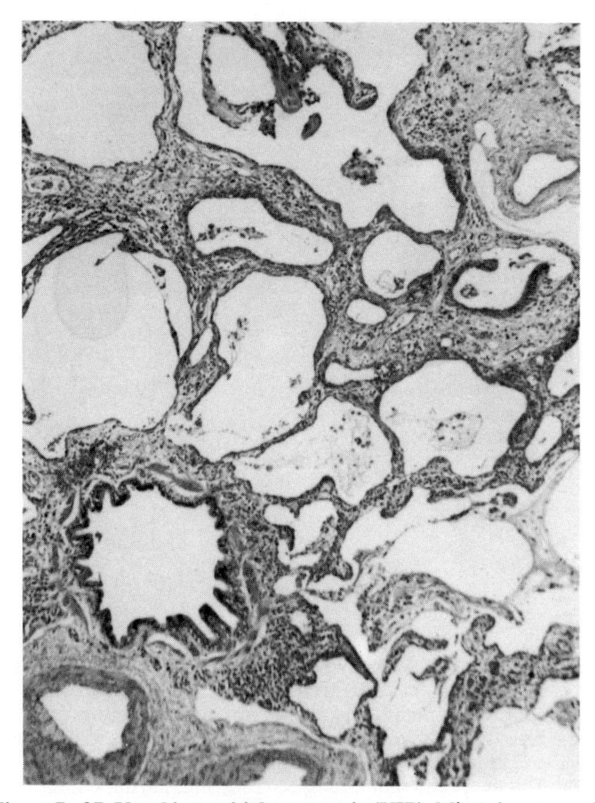

Figure 7-37. Usual interstitial pneumonia (UIP). Micro-honeycombing has occurred. No discernible normal alveoli are present. The bronchiole is unaffected.

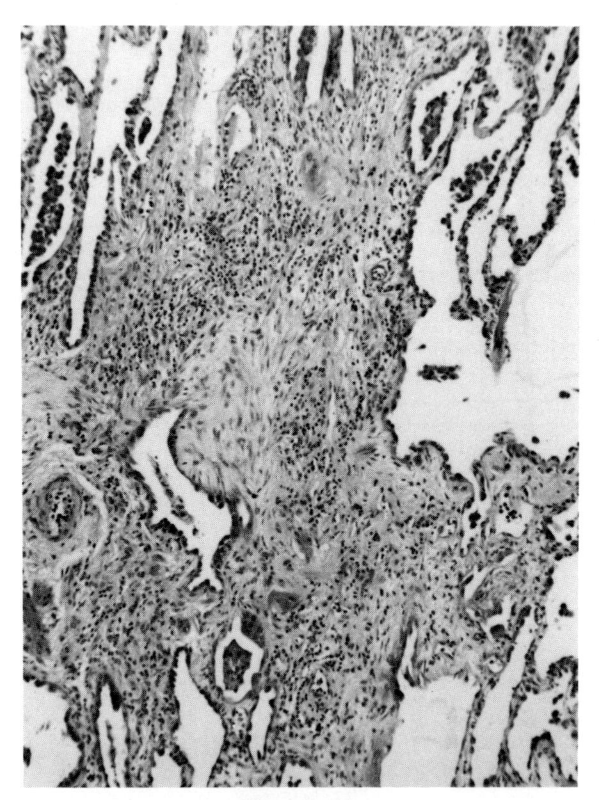

Figure 7-38.

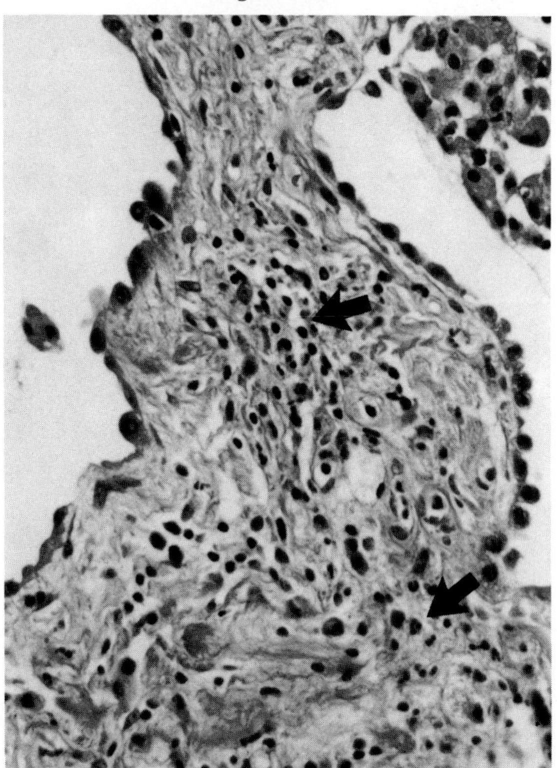

Figure 7-39.

Figures 7-38, 7-39. Usual interstitial pneumonia (UIP). The degree of chronic inflammatory infiltrate is usually sparse to mild and mononuclear in character, although occasionally a few neutrophils (arrows) may be evident. In sites of active interstitial thickening and engulfment of alveolar walls, prominent type II cells are common. A histologic correlate of the neutrophilic alveolitis described in bronchoalveolar lavage specimens from patients with UIP (idiopathic pulmonary fibrosis), is actually uncommon in sites of active interstitial widening identified histologically.

References

Carrington CB, Gaensler EA, Coutu RE, et al. Natural history and treated course of usual and desquamative interstitial pneumonia. N Engl J Med 298:801–810, 1978.
Crystal RG, Bitterman PB, Rennard SI, et al. Interstitial lung diseases of unknown cause. Part I. N Engl J Med 310:154–156, 1984.
Crystal RG, Bitterman PB, Rennard SI, et al. Interstitial lung diseases of unknown causes. Part II. N Engl J Med 310:235–244, 1984.
Dail DH, Hammer SP (eds). Pulmonary Pathology. New York, Springer-Verlag, 1988.
Katzenstein ALA, Askin FB. Surgical Pathology of Non-Neoplastic Lung Disease, 2nd ed. Philadelphia, WB Saunders Co, 1990.
Thurlbeck WM (ed). Pathology of the Lung. New York, Thieme, 1988.

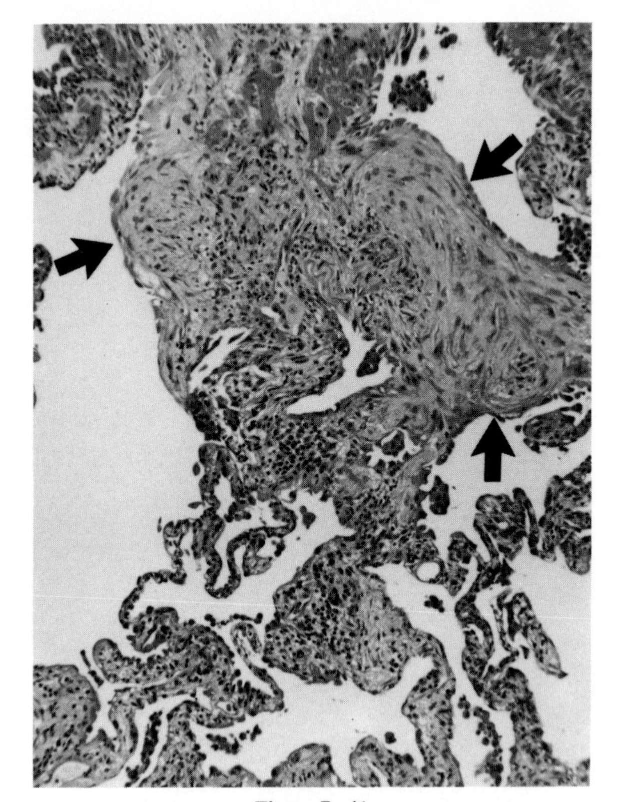

Figure 7–41.

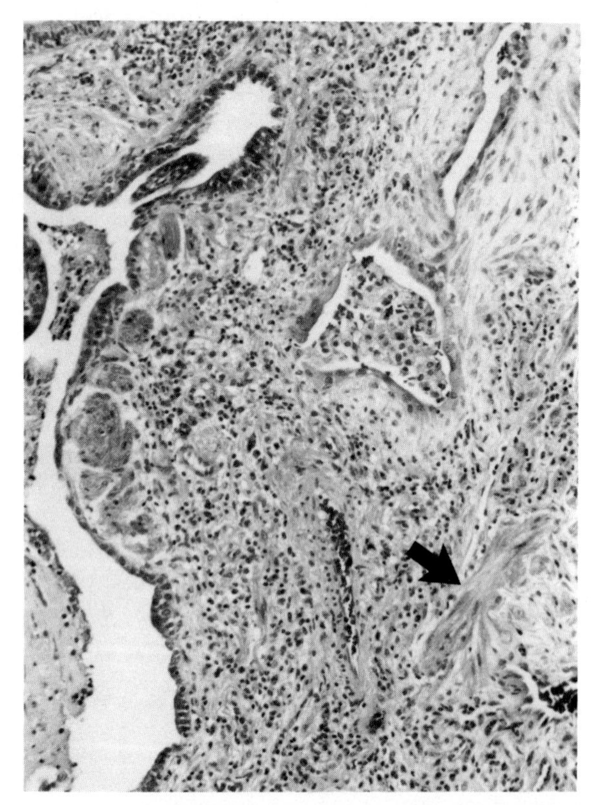

Figure 7–40. Usual interstitial pneumonia (UIP). Zones of marked fibrosis are evident. Alveolar structure is lost, and smooth muscle metaplasia (arrow) is present. The airspaces are lined by a variety of types of metaplastic epithelium. The rounded smooth muscle bundles at the top are probably the remnant of a small airway.

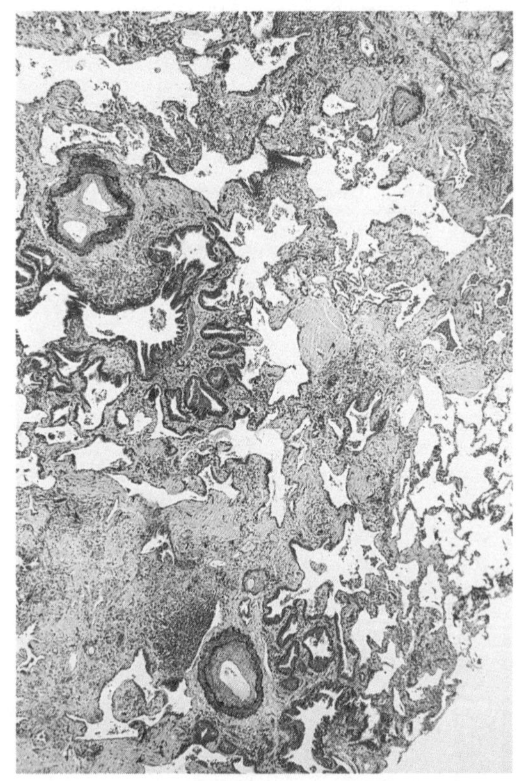

Figure 7–42.

Figures 7–41, 7–42. Usual interstitial pneumonia (UIP). In zones of active destruction of alveoli, myxomatous connective tissue may be present (arrows) and may even be quite prominent, as illustrated by the blue-green staining areas in a pentachrome stain (Fig. 7–42) reflecting the abundant mucopolysaccharide matrix of the young connective tissue. This figure also shows nonspecific myointimal thickening in the vessels.

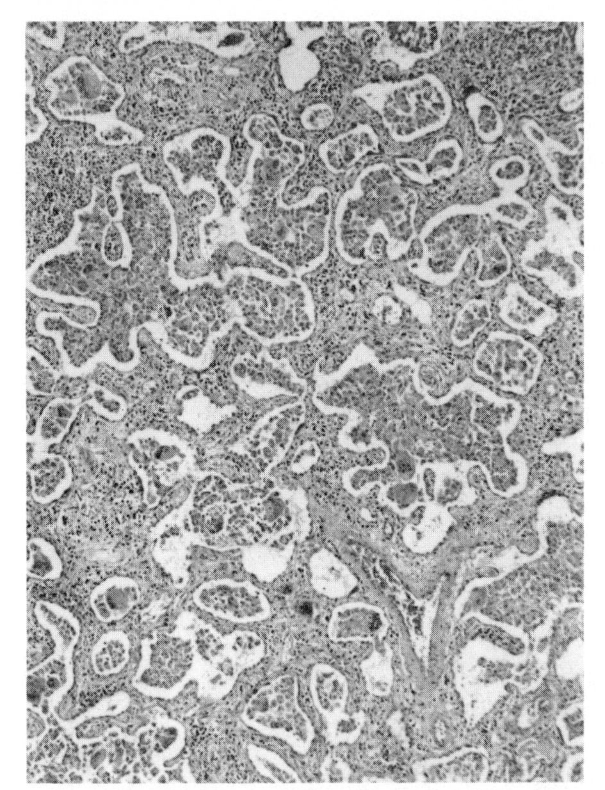

Figure 7–43. Desquamative interstitial pneumonia (DIP). In this classic case of DIP, there is uniform and diffuse interstitial widening with modest interstitial inflammatory infiltrates and uniform filling of airspaces by macrophages, including occasional multinucleated giant cells.

■ Desquamative Interstitial Pneumonia (Figs. 7–43 to 7–47)

DIP is a chronic fibrosing interstitial pneumonia with the potential for honeycombing and progressive pulmonary fibrosis; it is more often steroid responsive than is UIP. Some have considered this an early cellular phase of UIP or the desquamative (exudative) phase of cryptogenic fibrosing alveolitis. DIP is relatively rare, presently less than one tenth as common as UIP.

Generally, DIP is more uniform and diffuse than is UIP, with much more prominent airspace accumulations of macrophages and more uniform interstitial widening with mild fibrosis and mild to moderate chronic inflammatory infiltrate. A few eosinophils and lymphoid aggregates are often part of the infiltrate; the macrophages within airspaces may be positive with iron stains in smokers with DIP. A DIP reaction may be seen with drugs and/or asbestos exposure, as part of eosinophilic pneumonia, and in infections, notably *Pneumocystis.* DIP should be considered a diagnosis of exclusion. The diagnosis should not be made on a transbronchial biopsy.

Note: Pseudo–DIP reactions (see the next section), interstitial pneumonias with large numbers of histiocytes, smoker's bronchiolitis–associated interstitial lung disease, and eosinophilic granuloma should be excluded in considering differential diagnosis.

References

Katzenstein ALA, Askin FB. Surgical Pathology of Non-Neoplastic Lung Disease, 2nd ed. Philadelphia, WB Saunders Co, 1990.

Liebow AA, Steer A, Billingsley JG. Desquamative interstitial pneumonia. Am J Med 39:369–404, 1965.

Patchefsky AS, Israel HL, Hock WS, et al. Desquamative interstitial pneumonia: relationship to interstitial fibrosis. Thorax 28:680–693, 1973.

Thurlbeck WM (ed). Pathology of the Lung. New York, Thieme, 1988.

Tubbs RR, Benjamin SP, Reich NE, et al. Desquamative interstitial pneumonitis: cellular phase of fibrosing alveolitis. Chest 72:159–165, 1977.

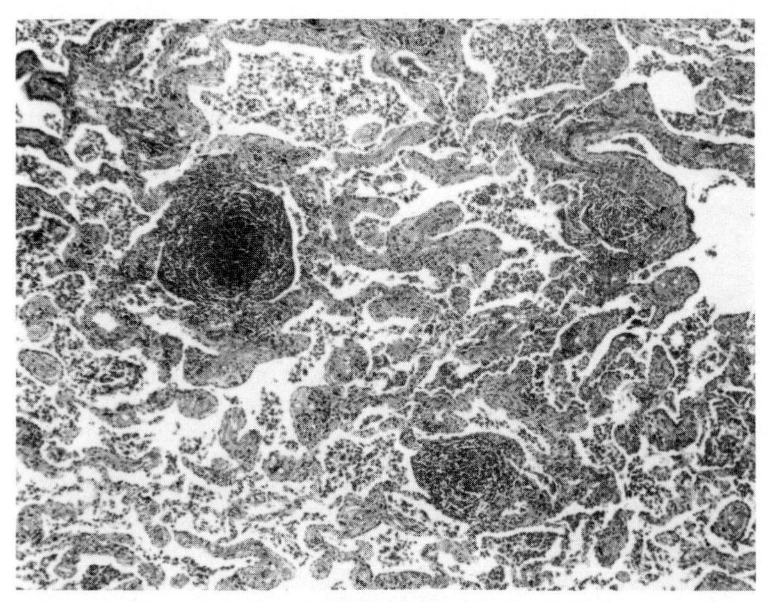

Figure 7–44.

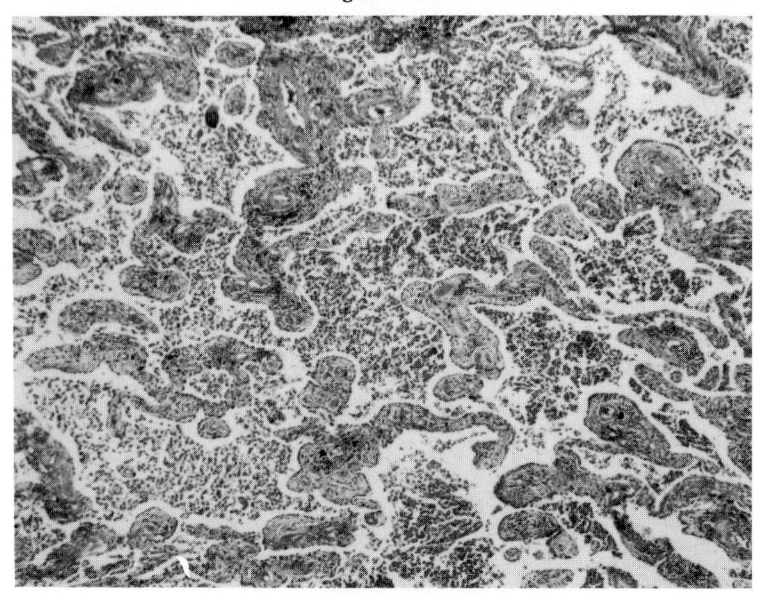

Figure 7–45.

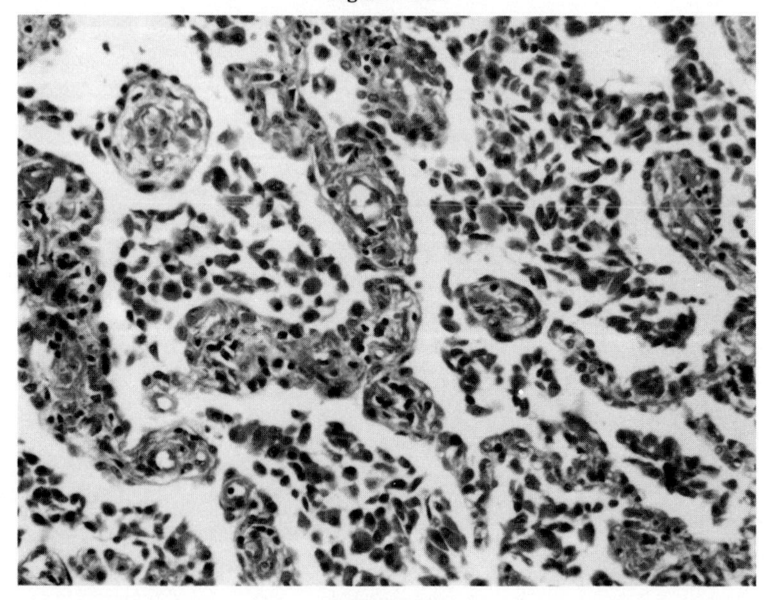

Figure 7–46.

Figures 7–44, 7–45, 7–46. Desquamative interstitial pneumonia (DIP). There is fairly uniform filling of airspaces by macrophages associated with interstitial scarring and modest inflammation. The background architecture in this case suggests emphysema is also present (Fig. 7–45). Occasional lymphoid follicles can be seen.

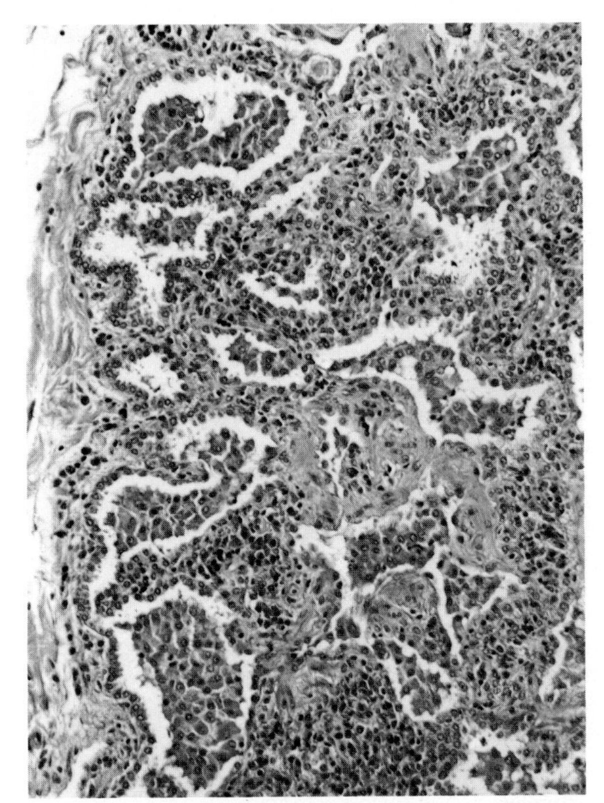

Figure 7-47. Desquamative interstitial pneumonia (DIP). DIP in an 18-year-old boy with shortness of breath and bilateral interstitial infiltrates.

■ Pseudo-Desquamative Interstitial Pneumonia Reactions (Fig. 7-141)

A reaction that mimics desquamative interstitial pneumonia but is caused by another lesion is known as a pseudo-DIP reaction.

A pseudo-DIP reaction may be seen with many lung diseases. Its location is particularly frequent adjacent to the lesions of eosinophilic granuloma. In some foci of UIP, airspace accumulation of macrophages is prominent. Smoker's bronchiolitis-associated interstitial lung disease often mimics DIP.

Because a pseudo-DIP reaction is a very common focal finding with a large number of focal and diffuse lung diseases, a diagnosis of DIP based on transbronchial biopsy is fraught with problems.

References

Bedrossian CWM, Kuhn C, Luna MA, et al. Desquamative interstitial pneumonia-like reaction accompanying pulmonary lesions. Chest 72:166-169, 1977.

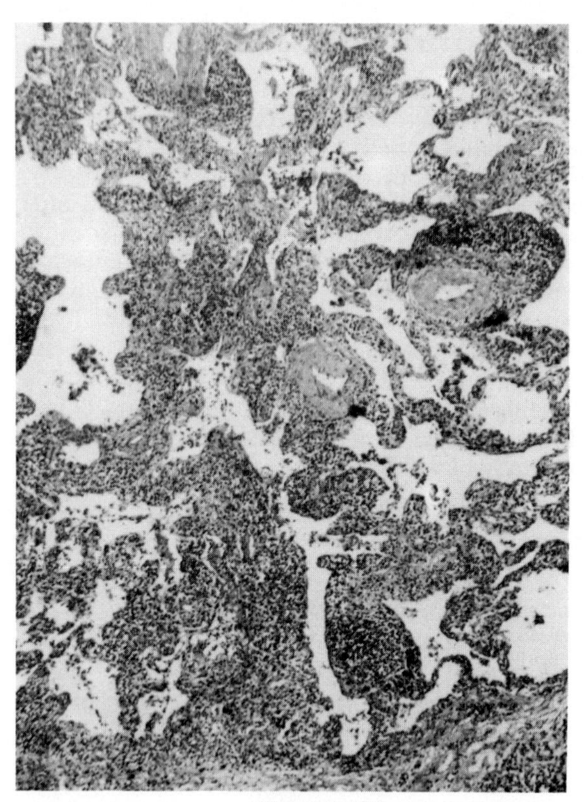

Figure 7–48.

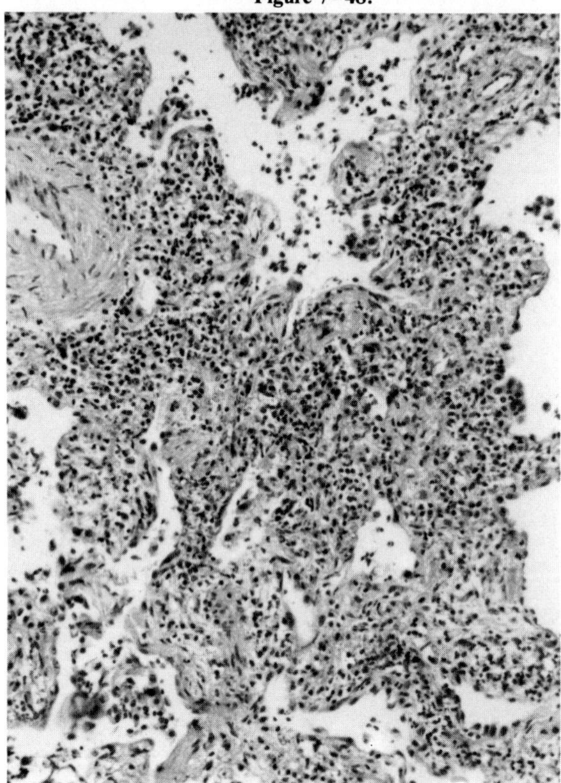

Figure 7–49.

■ Lymphocytic (Lymphoid) Interstitial Pneumonia (Figs. 7–48 to 7–54)

LIP is a bilateral chronic interstitial pneumonia characterized by dense interstitial lymphoid infiltrates. It is associated with collagen-vascular diseases, immunodeficiency states (including acquired immunodeficiency syndrome [AIDS]), and dysgammaglobulinemias.

Dense, diffuse and uniform mixed interstitial infiltrates with lymphocytes, plasma cells, and histiocytes, sometimes forming granulomas, are seen. LIP is polyclonal when studied by immunologic markers, often with significant numbers of T cells. Some cases are characterized by germinal center proliferation along the lymphatic routes around the vessels in the septum and along bronchovascular structures (also called *pulmonary lymphoid hyperplasia)*; a variable degree of scarring and honeycombing may be present.

The diagnosis of lymphocytic interstitial pneumonia should not be made without first considering the following possibilities: (1) well-differentiated lymphocytic and lymphoplasmacytic lymphomas presenting as diffuse lung disease, (2) immunodeficiency states, (3) collagen vascular diseases, and (4) extrinsic allergic alveolitis with marked interstitial infiltrates.

References

Katzenstein ALA, Askin FB. Surgical Pathology of Non-Neoplastic Lung Disease, 2nd ed. Philadelphia, WB Saunders Co, 1990.

Liebow AA, Carrington CB. The interstitial pneumonias. *In* Simon M, Potchen EJ, LeMay M (eds). Frontiers of Pulmonary Radiology. Orlando, Grune & Stratton, 1969, pp 102–141.

Mark EJ. Lung Biopsy Interpretation. Baltimore, Williams & Wilkins, 1984.

Strimlan CV, Rosenow EC, Weiland LH, et al. Lymphocytic interstitial pneumonitis. Ann Intern Med 88:616–621, 1978.

Thurlbeck WM (ed). Pathology of the Lung. New York, Thieme, 1988.

Figures 7–48, 7–49. Lymphocytic interstitial pneumonia (LIP). There is a dense uniform interstitial infiltrate of mononuclear cells. The cells composing the infiltrate in such cases are mixed and include varying numbers of lymphocytes and plasma cells. Occasionally, granulomas are seen in LIP.

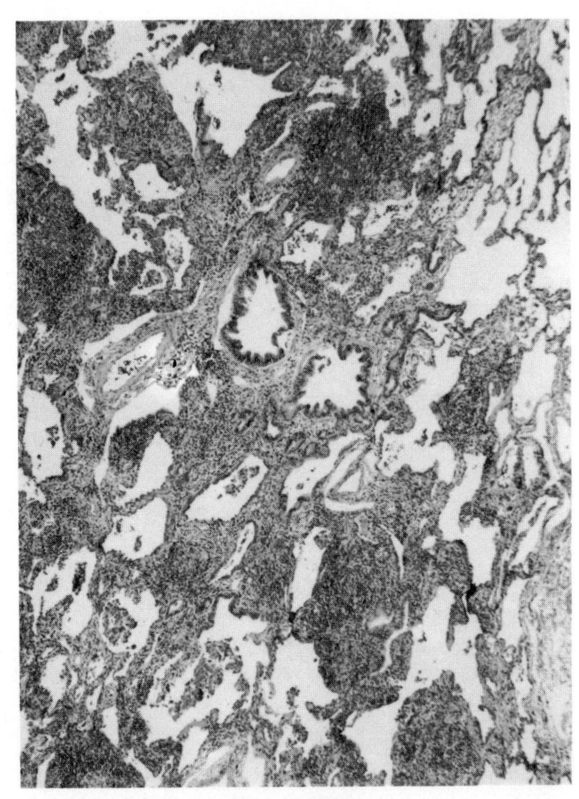

Figure 7–50.

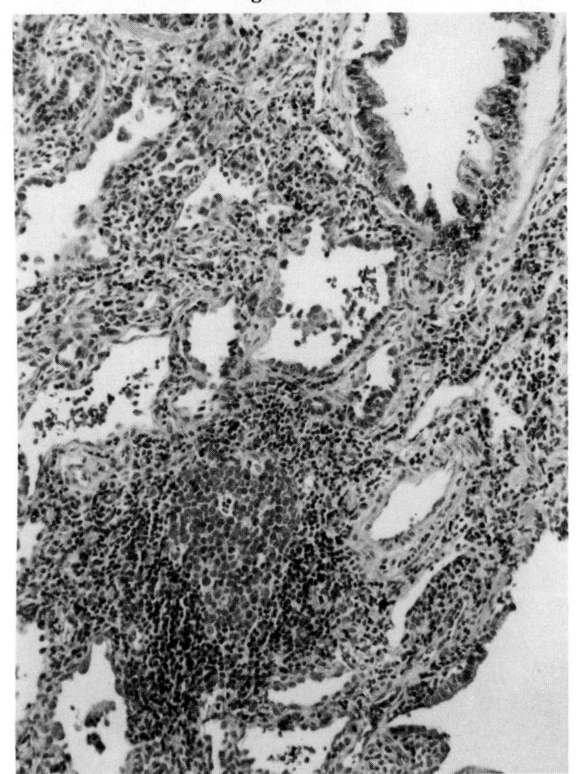

Figure 7–51.

Figures 7–50, 7–51. (LIP). LIP with lymphoid hyperplasia. A marked interstitial infiltrate of mononuclear cells and numerous germinal centers are apparent. There is architectural loss and fibrosis in this case, but the prominent change is lymphoid hyperplasia with lymphoid follicles, most of which contain germinal centers.

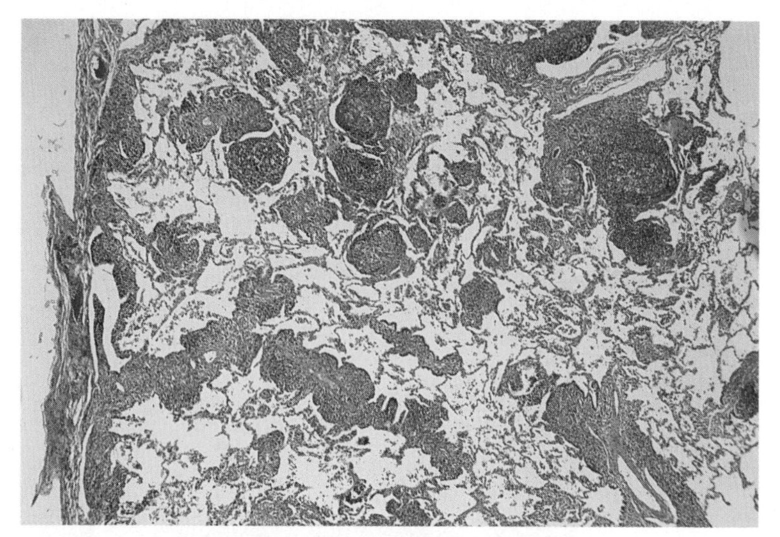

Figure 7–52.

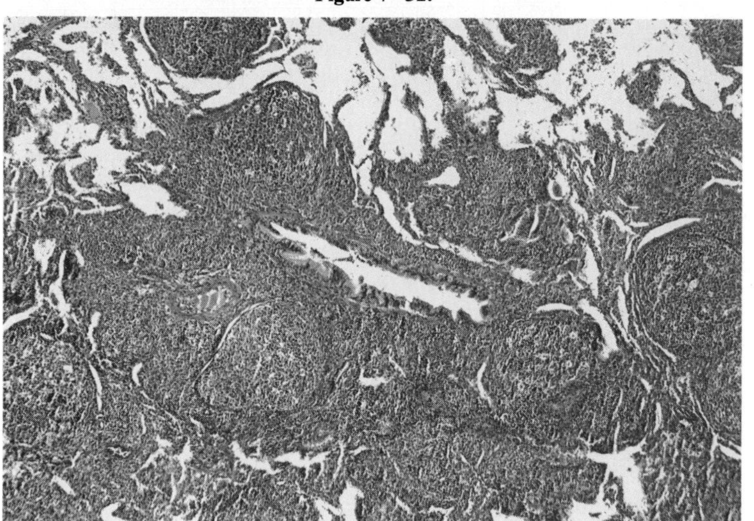

Figure 7–53.

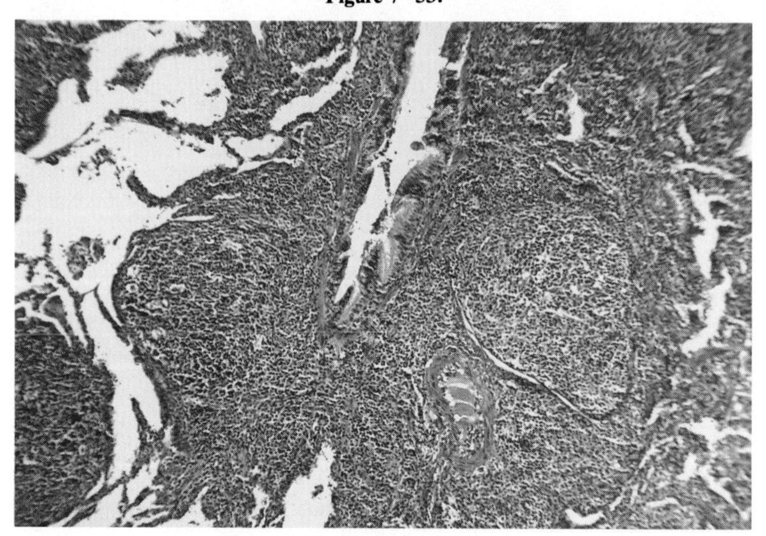

Figure 7–54.

Figures 7–52, 7–53, 7–54. Diffuse lymphoid hyperplasia (lymphocytic interstitial pneumonia [LIP]) in a boy with common variable immunoglobulin deficiency. An open lung biopsy shows diffuse lymphoid hyperplasia with lymphoid follicles around vessels, in the pleura, and along the lung bronchovascular structures. Although, technically, this represents diffuse lymphoid hyperplasia in the lung, it is a pattern that also has commonly been termed lymphocytic or lymphoid interstitial pneumonia.

■ Respiratory (Smoker's) Bronchiolitis–Associated Interstitial Lung Disease (Figs. 7–55 to 7–61)

Mild interstitial lung disease (by clinical, radiographic, and functional parameters) is associated with respiratory (smoker's) bronchiolitis caused by cigarette smoking.

Respiratory (smoker's) bronchiolitis–associated interstitial disease is characterized by mild interstitial infiltrates, fibrosis, and airspace accumulations of macrophages around respiratory bronchioles and alveolar ducts. Macrophages are frequently positive with stains for iron, and they are flecked with dark granules. The pattern is often reminiscent of DIP. As in chronic bronchitis, goblet cell metaplasia, mucous stasis, and bronchiolar metaplasia surround thickened bronchioles.

Respiratory (smoker's) bronchiolitis–associated interstitial disease should be carefully distinguished from DIP and alveolar hemorrhage syndromes. The clinical findings in this condition are rarely those of alveolar hemorrhage. Transbronchial biopsy findings from a smoker showing any of the above histologic findings should be considered nonspecific and non-diagnostic.

References

Bogin RM, Niccoli SA, Waldron JA, et al. Respiratory bronchiolitis: clinical presentation and bronchoalveolar lavage findings. Chest 94:21S, 1988.

Myers JL, Veal CF, Shin MS, Katzenstein ALA. Respiratory bronchiolitis causing interstitial lung disease. Am Rev Respir Dis 135:880–884.

Yousem SA, Colby TV, Gaensler EA. Respiratory bronchiolitis and its relationship to desquamative interstitial pneumonia. Mayo Clin Proc. 64:1373–1380, 1989.

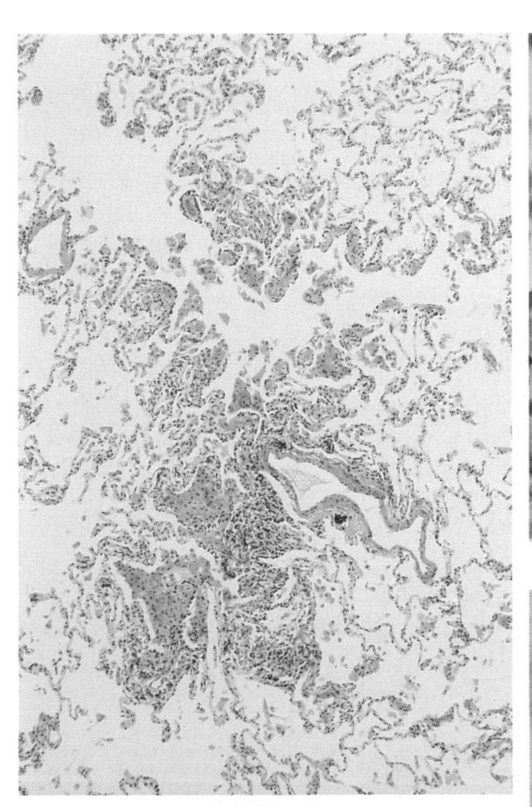

Figure 7–55.

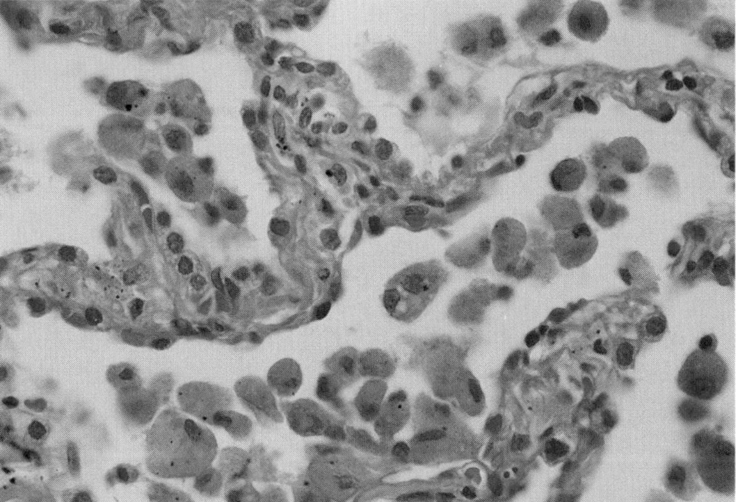

Figure 7–56.

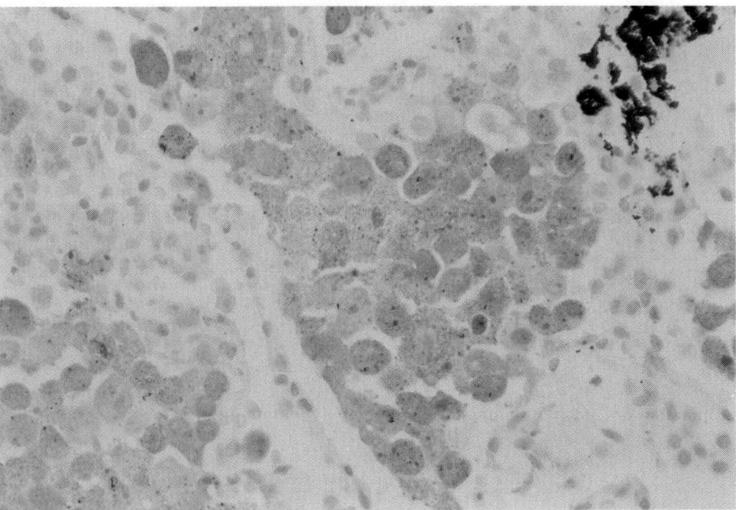

Figure 7–57.

Figures 7–55, 7–56, 7–57. Respiratory bronchiolitis. In respiratory (smoker's) bronchiolitis, there is an accumulation of tan alveolar macrophages, some of which contain flecks of brown or black material in and around a respiratory bronchiole, which shows associated interstitial thickening and modest chronic inflammatory infiltrate. Prussian blue stain shows fine positivity in the smoker's macrophages. This lesion is usually an incidental finding and not associated with a recognizable disease.

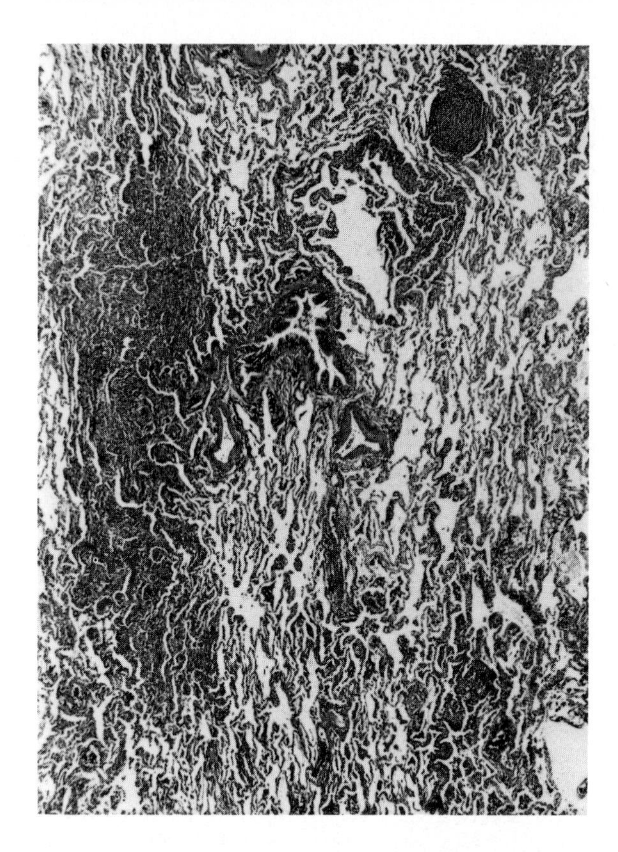

Figure 7–58. Respiratory bronchiolitis-associated interstitial lung disease. In this atelectatic biopsy, one can see accumulations of cells in the airspaces around small bronchioles, and the low-power assessment is critical for their recognition. Signs and symptoms of mild interstitial lung diseae were present, and open lung biopsy was performed for diagnosis. The reaction around the small airways related to smoking (smoker's bronchiolitis) was the only pathologic condition identified.

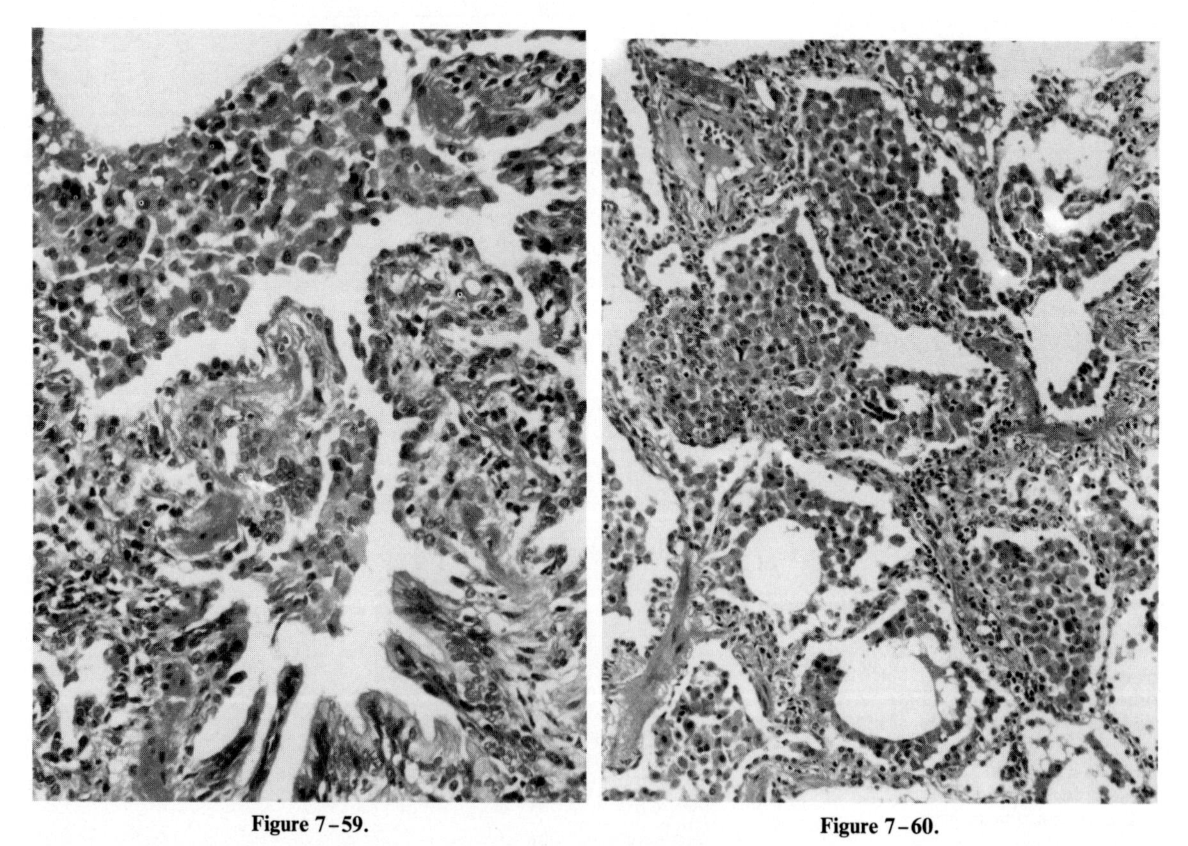

Figure 7–59. **Figure 7–60.**

Figures 7–59, 7–60. Respiratory (smoker's) bronchiolitis-associated interstitial lung disease. There is an accumulation of macrophages in respiratory bronchioles and peribronchiolar alveolar spaces with an appearance indistinguishable from desquamative interstitial pneumonia (DIP).

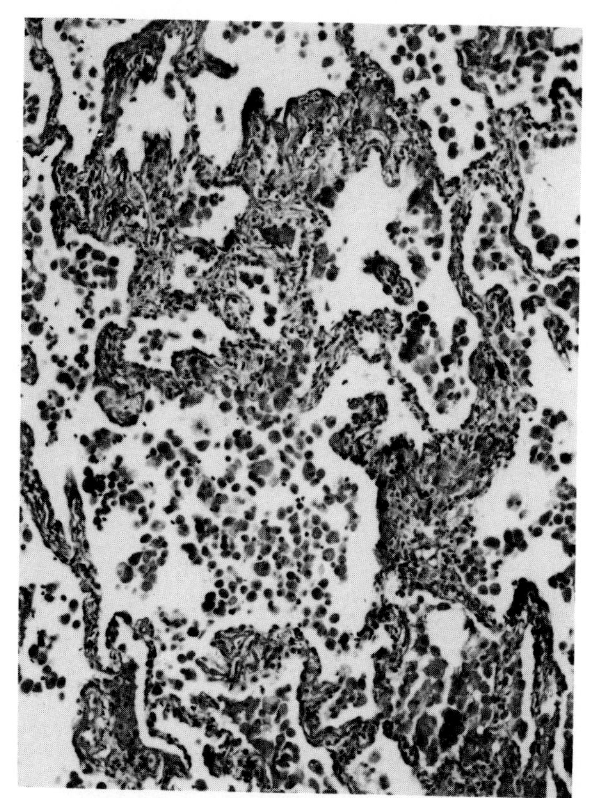

Figure 7–61. Respiratory bronchiolitis-associated interstitial lung disease. Respiratory (smoker's) bronchiolitis-associated interstitial lung disease with airspace accumulations of macrophages and mild interstitial thickening, fibrosis, and chronic inflammatory infiltrate. The thickened alveolar walls are lines by metaplastic type II cells.

■ Bronchiolitis Obliterans Organizing Pneumonia (BOOP) (Figs. 7–62 to 7–73)

Synonyms include cryptogenic organizing pneumonitis, bronchiolitis obliterans, and organizing pneumonia. Because of the connotation often associated with "bronchiolitis obliterans," the term "cryptogenic organizing pneumonitis" is favored because it better reflects the clinical appearance of the disorder, which is that of a pneumonitis rather than of an airway disease.

Most affected individuals are middle-aged adults with an illness that follows some weeks after an upper respiratory infection.

This is a subacute interstitial lung disease characterized by chronic inflammatory interstitial infiltrates associated with patchy bronchiolitis obliterans and organizing pneumonia with granulation tissue filling terminal and/or respiratory bronchioles with extension into distal airspaces. A few eosinophils, changes of obstruction, and cellular bronchiolitis with inflammatory infiltrate in bronchiolar walls may all be present. The presence of granulomas should raise the possibility of an allergic reaction.

Histologic findings of BOOP are nonspecific and may be seen in a number of pulmonary repair reactions: organizing infections, organizing DAD, allergic reactions, drug reactions, collagen-vascular disease, organizing toxic exposures, eosinophilic pneumonia, eosinophilic granuloma, Wegener's granulomatosis, and around other lesions, including abscesses and tumors. *A diagnosis of BOOP is one of exclusion.* Necrosis, microabscesses, marked neutrophilic infiltration, vasculitis, and granulomas contradict the diagnosis.

Some of the conceptual problems that surround the term *BOOP* can be avoided by using the terms *idiopathic BOOP* (for the clinicopathologic lesion described) and *BOOP pattern* (for the nonspecific histologic reaction pattern).

References

Colby TV, Myers JL. The clinical and histologic spectrum of bronchiolitis obliterans including bronchiolitis obliterans organizing pneumonia (BOOP). Sem Resp Med. In press.

Davison AG, Heard BE, McAlister WAC, Turner-Warwick MEH. Cryptogenic organizing pneumonia. Q J Med 52:328–394, 1983.

Epler GR, Colby TV, McLoud TC, et al. Bronchiolitis obliterans organizing pneumonia. N Engl J Med 312:152–158, 1985.

Katzenstein ALA, Myers JL, Prophet WD, et al. Bronchiolitis obliterans and usual interstitial pneumonia. Am J Surg Pathol 10:373–381, 1986.

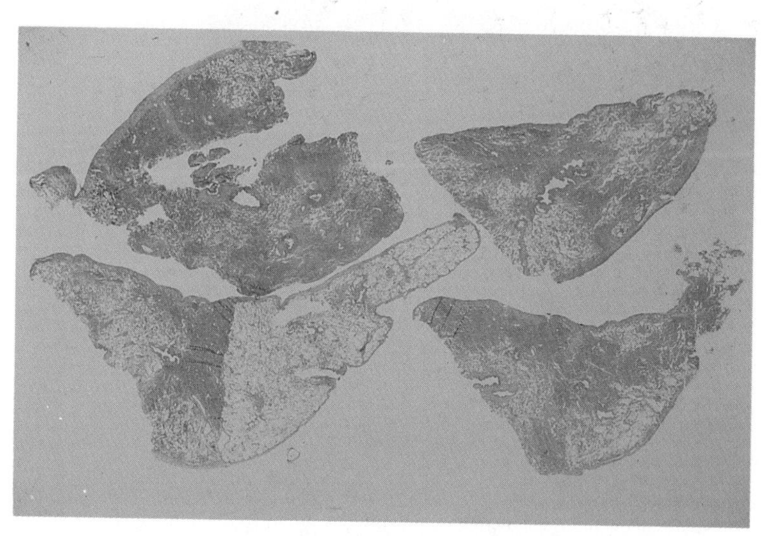

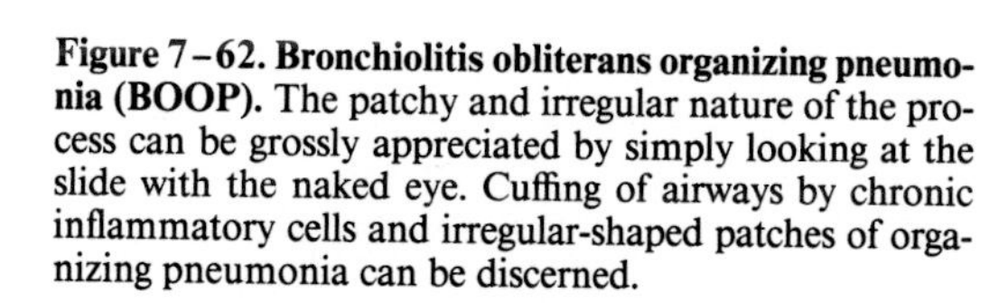

Figure 7–62. Bronchiolitis obliterans organizing pneumonia (BOOP). The patchy and irregular nature of the process can be grossly appreciated by simply looking at the slide with the naked eye. Cuffing of airways by chronic inflammatory cells and irregular-shaped patches of organizing pneumonia can be discerned.

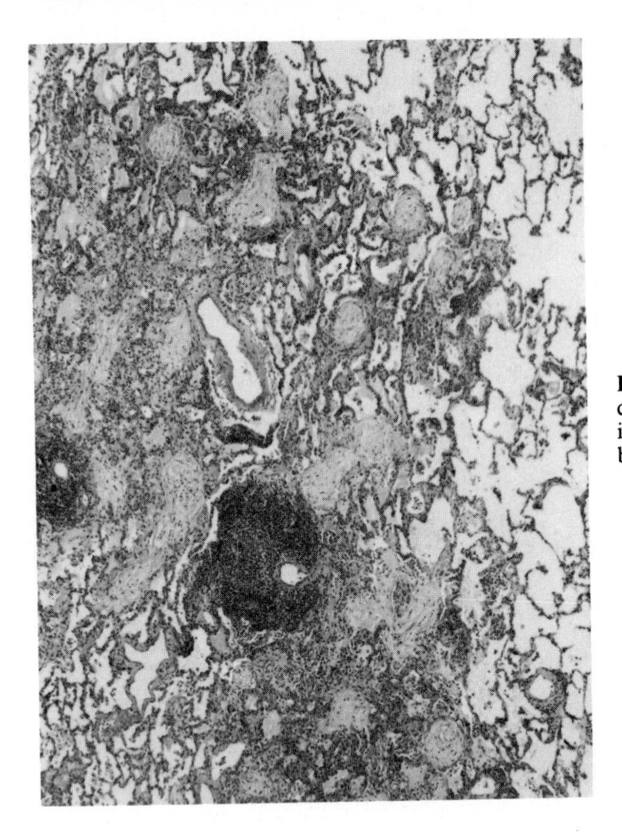

Figure 7-63. Bronchiolitis obliterans organizing pneumonia (BOOP). A discrete patch of organizing pneumonia containing occasional lymphoid follicles is shown. The alveolar walls are mildly inflamed. The evenly spaced, rounded balls of myxomatous connective tissue are characteristic.

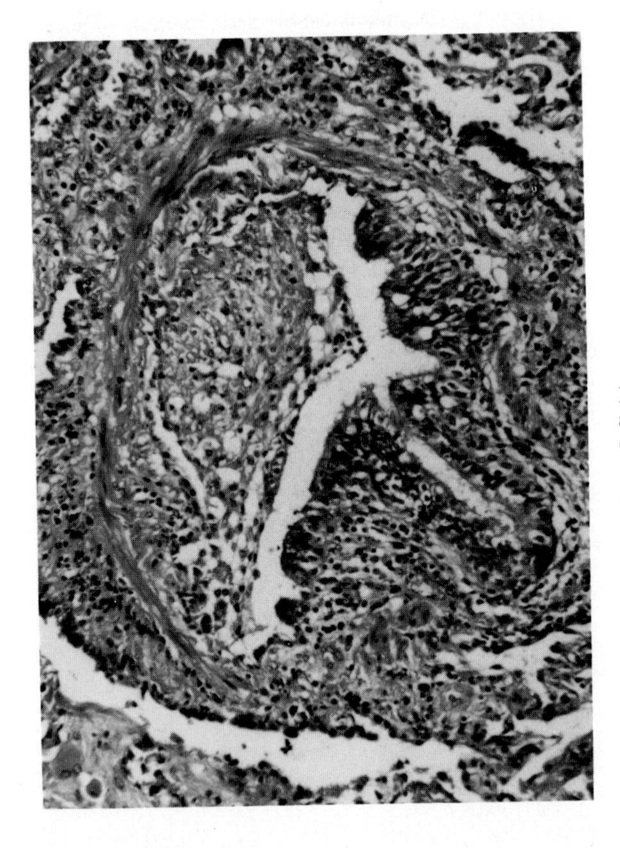

Figure 7-64. Bronchiolitis obliterans organizing pneumonia (BOOP). There is an early proliferation of connective tissue that forms a polyp within the lumen of the small bronchiole (proliferative bronchiolitis obliterans).

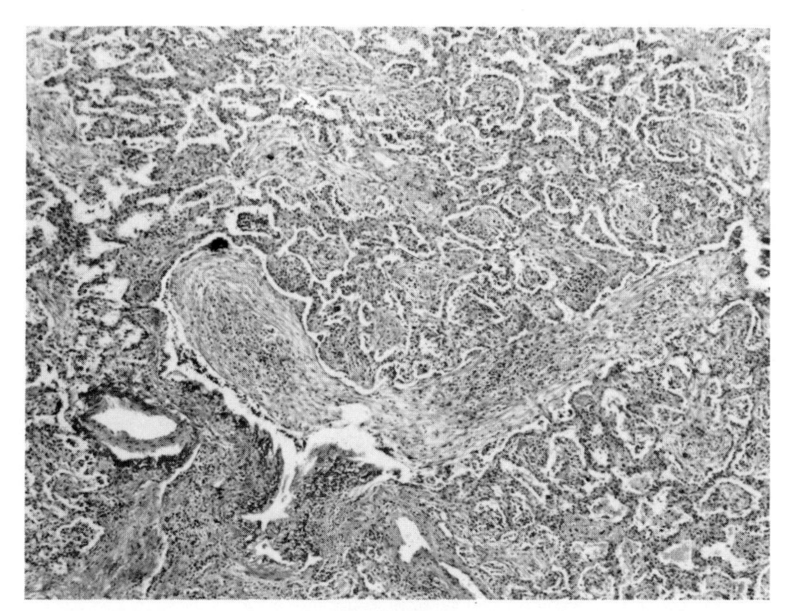

Figure 7-65.

Figures 7-65, 7-66, 7-67. Bronchiolitis obliterans organizing pneumonia (BOOP). BOOP with ramifying masses of myxomatous connective tissue extending from bronchioles along alveolar ducts into alveoli with recognizable alveolar walls. Mild inflammation of the alveolar wall is present.

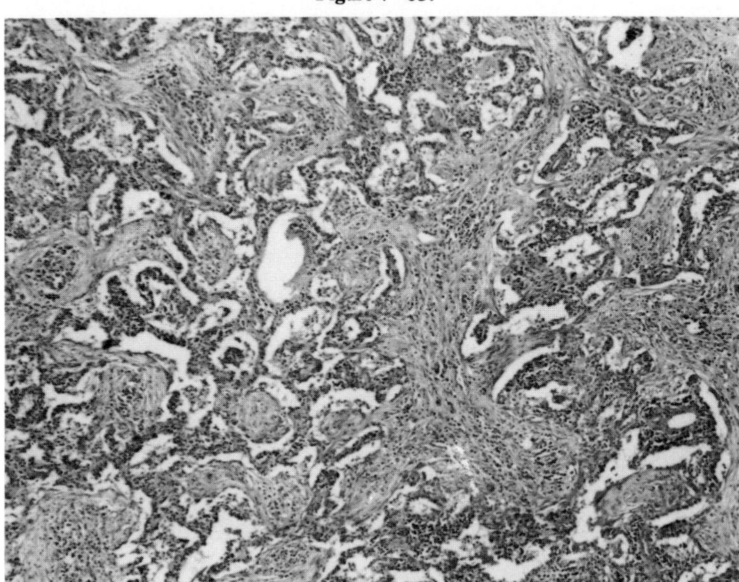

Figure 7-66.

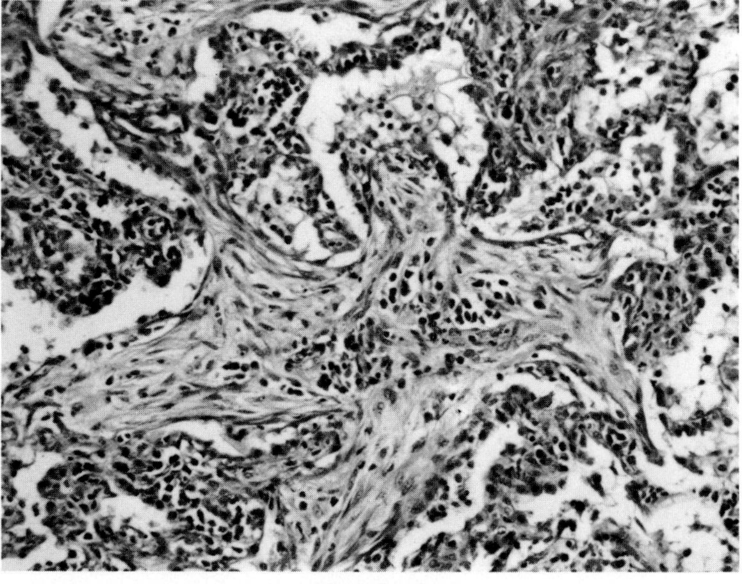

Figure 7-67.

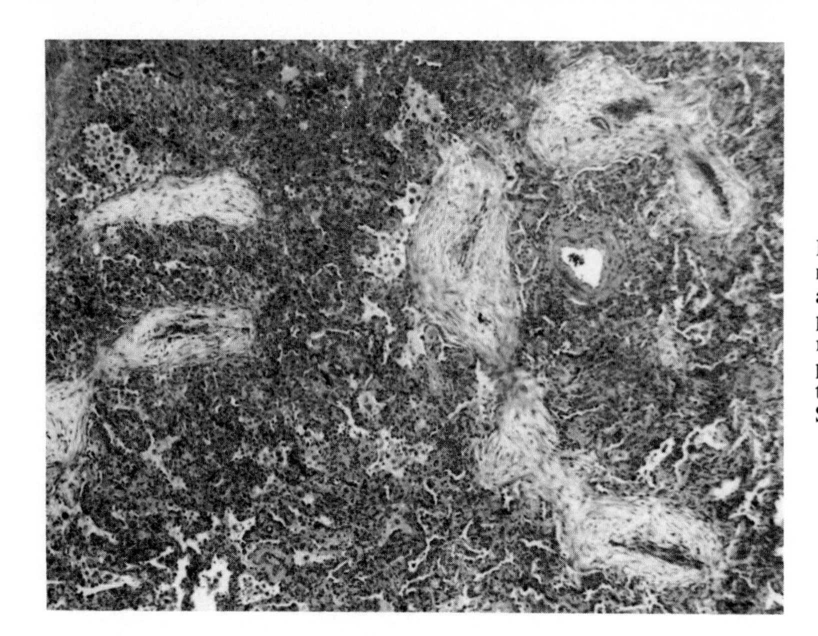

Figure 7–68. Bronchiolitis obliterans organizing pneumonia (BOOP). The biopsy specimen is atelectatic, and the alveolar architecture is difficult to discern. The most prominent features are the evenly spaced, pale masses of myxomatous connective tissue comprising the organizing pneumonia within alveolar ducts. The lesion cleared spontaneously, leaving the patient with entirely normal lungs. Subsequently, cardiac transplant was performed.

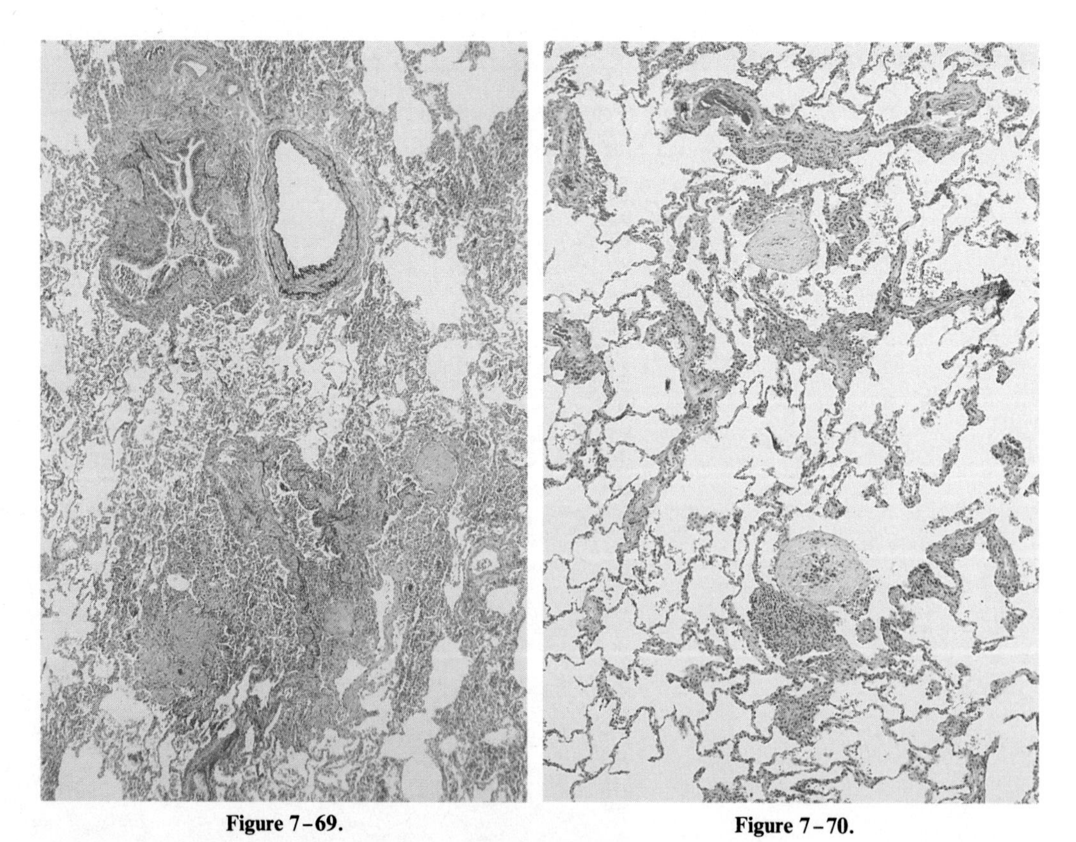

Figure 7–69. **Figure 7–70.**

Figures 7–69, 7–70. Bronchiolitis obliterans organizing pneumonia (BOOP). Pentachrome stain (with alcian green counterstain) from two cases of BOOP shows preservation of architecture and highlights the edematous mucopolysaccharide-rich connective tissue.

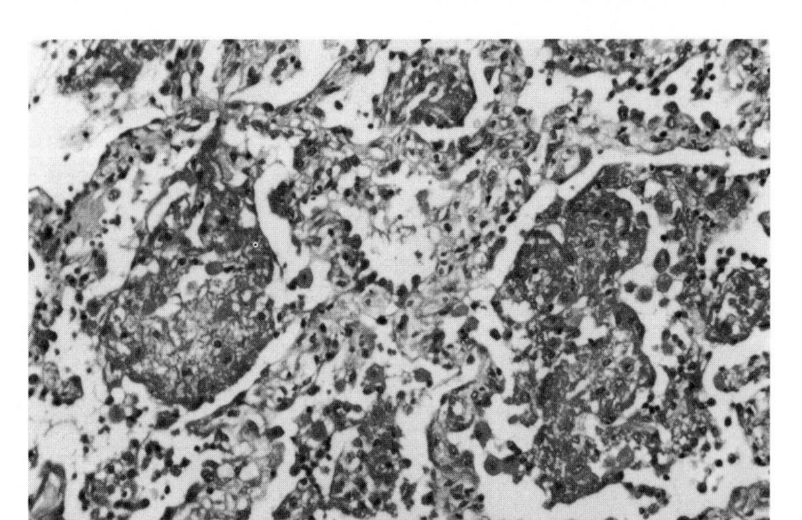

Figure 7-71. Bronchiolitis obliterans organizing pneumonia (BOOP). In relatively early cases, one may see fibrin in airspaces adjacent to the foci of organization.

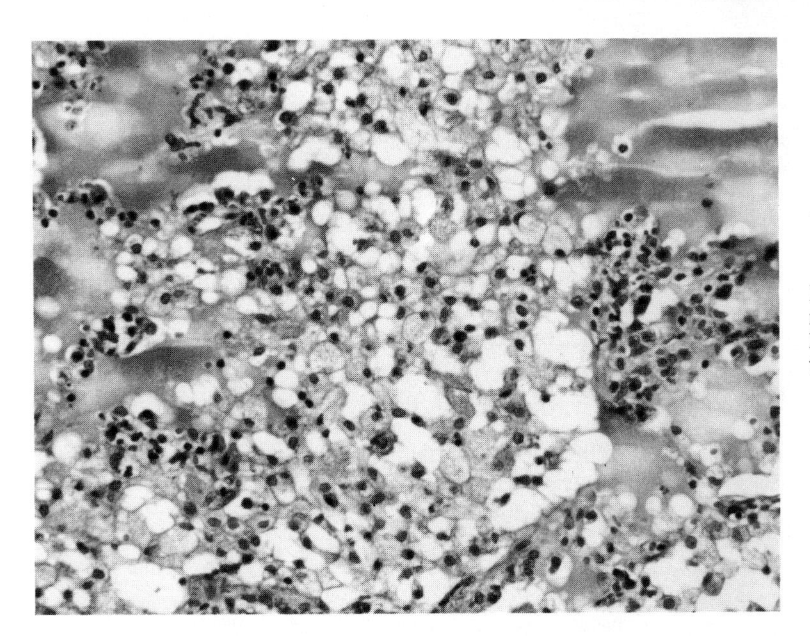

Figure 7-72. Bronchiolitis obliterans organizing pneumonia (BOOP). Evidence of obstruction at the microscopic level in BOOP is often manifested as alveolar accumulations of foamy macrophages.

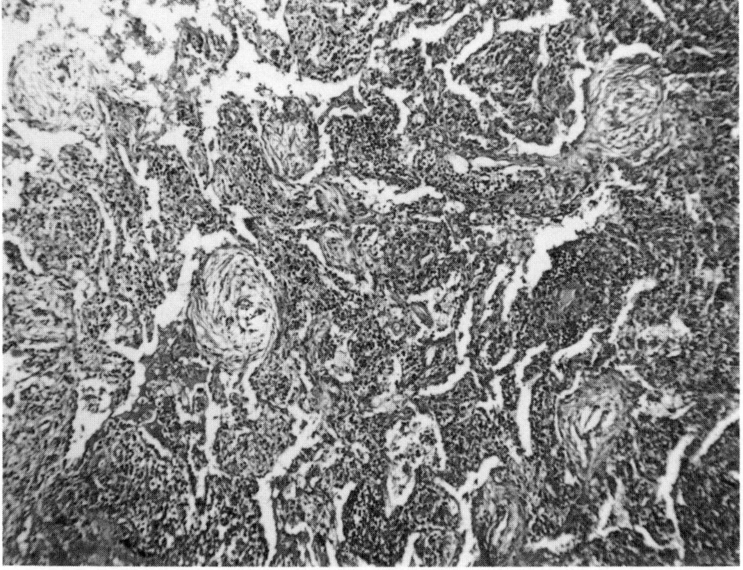

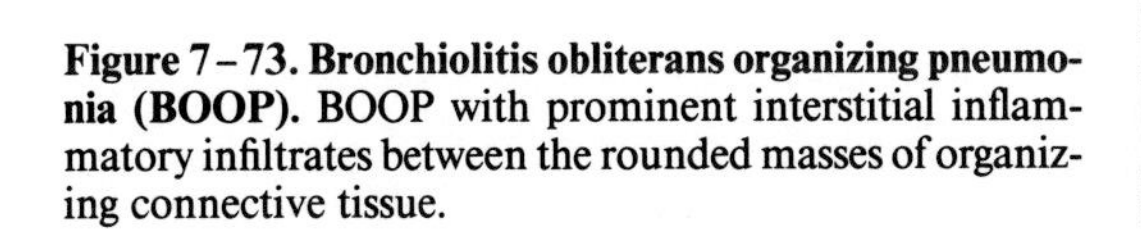

Figure 7-73. Bronchiolitis obliterans organizing pneumonia (BOOP). BOOP with prominent interstitial inflammatory infiltrates between the rounded masses of organizing connective tissue.

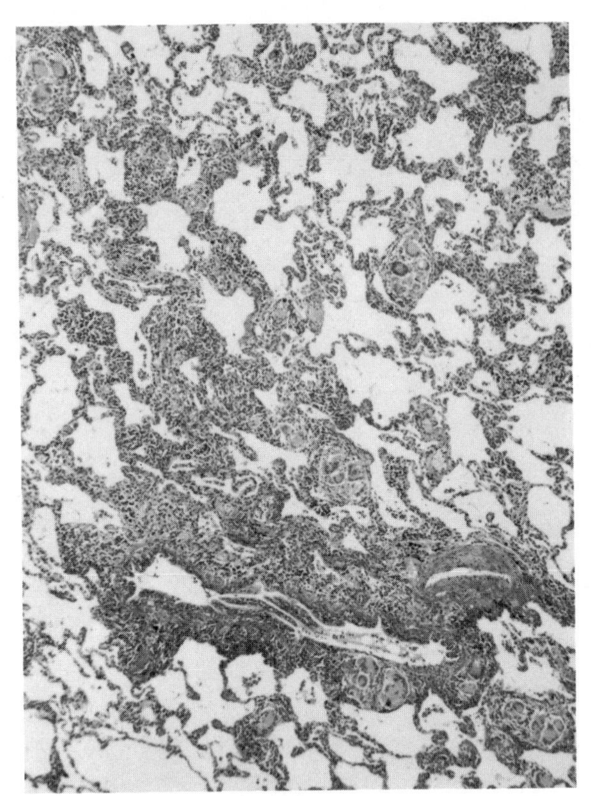

Figure 7–74.

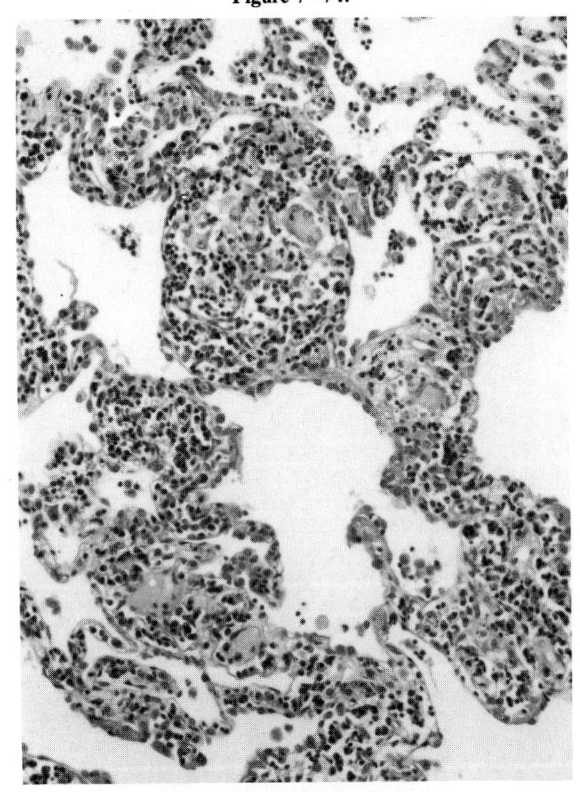

Figure 7–75.

Figures 7–74, 7–75. Extrinsic allergic alveolitis. The classic histologic pattern with peribronchiolar inflammation (cellular bronchiolitis), interstitial inflammation, and scattered small granulomas, which in this case manifest predominantly as clusters of giant cells.

■ Extrinsic Allergic Alveolitis (Hypersensitivity Pneumonitis) (Figs. 7–74 to 7–88)

Extrinsic allergic alveolitis is an acute, subacute, or chronic interstitial pneumonia usually caused by inhalation of organic antigens from a variety of different sources with many colorful names, such as bird fancier's disease, farmer's lung, mushroom picker's disease, and others. The histologic pattern may occasionally be seen with drugs; in some cases, the characteristic histologic appearance cannot be correlated with a definable exposure.

Seventy-five to 80 percent of patients show the histologic triad of cellular bronchiolitis, scattered small interstitial granulomas (sometimes comprising just a few epithelioid cells), and a more diffuse interstitial infiltrate of chronic inflammatory cells. In most cases, pulmonary alveolar architecture is relatively well maintained. Giant cells, either singly or in clusters, often with cholesterol clefts and/or calcifications, are common. Some cases may show change in a BOOP pattern, and distal obstructive pneumonia with airspace accumulations of foamy macrophages. Only in maple bark stripper's disease can the inciting agent *(Cryptostroma corticale)* be seen. In severe acute cases, acute inflammation, hyaline membranes, and/or focal necrosis may be present. In chronic cases, interstitial fibrosis may be present and may be indistinguishable from UIP, although often an airway-centered distribution of the scarring is often apparent.

Granulomas may be few and difficult to find, necessitating considerable search. One may need to lower one's criteria for a granuloma by accepting even small interstitial clusters of epithelioid histiocytes. In any fibrotic lung disease with a few granulomas, the possibility of chronic extrinsic allergic alveolitis should be considered.

When granulomas are numerous, the differential diagnosis includes sarcoid, berylliosis, and infections.

References

Colby TV, Coleman A. Histologic differential diagnosis of extrinsic allergic alveolitis. Prog Surg Pathol 10:11–26, 1989.

Coleman A, Colby TV. Histologic diagnosis of extrinsic allergic alveolitis. Am J Surg Pathol 12:514–518, 1988.

Dail DH, Hammer SP (eds). Pulmonary Pathology. New York, Springer-Verlag, 1988.

Hammar S. Hypersensitivity pneumonitis. Part 1. Pathol Ann 23:195–216, 1988.

Reyes CN, Wenzel FJ, Lawton DR, Emmanuel DA. The pulmonary pathology of farmer's lung disease. Chest 81:142–151, 1982.

Thurlbeck WM (ed). Pathology of the Lung. New York, Thieme, 1988.

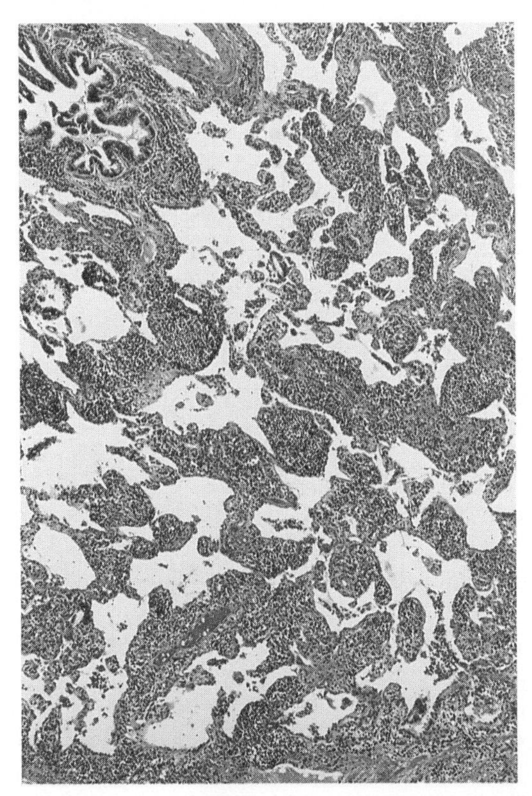

Figure 7-76.

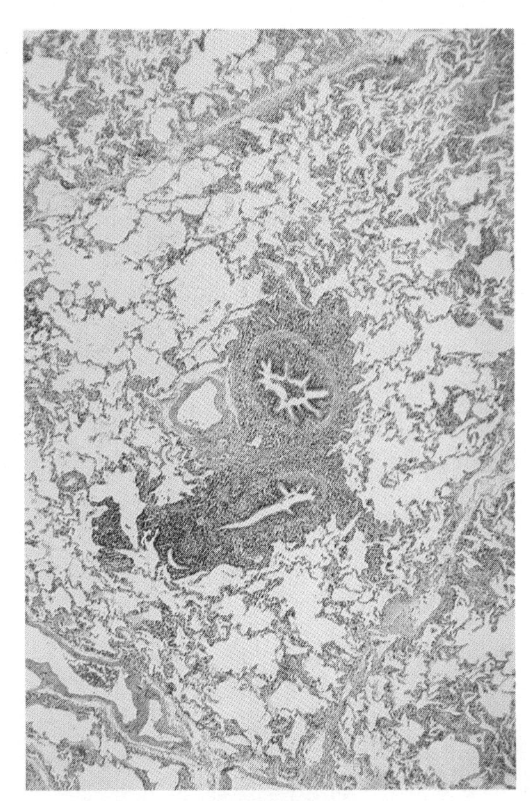

Figure 7-78.

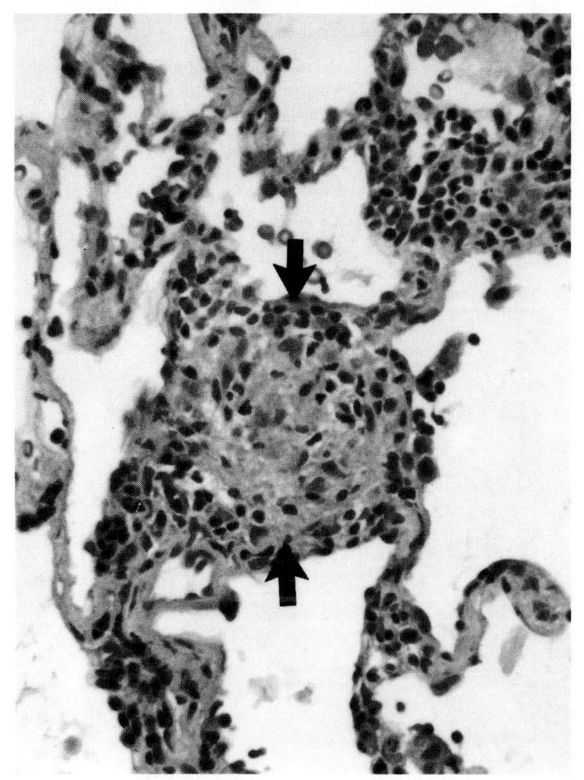

Figure 7-77.

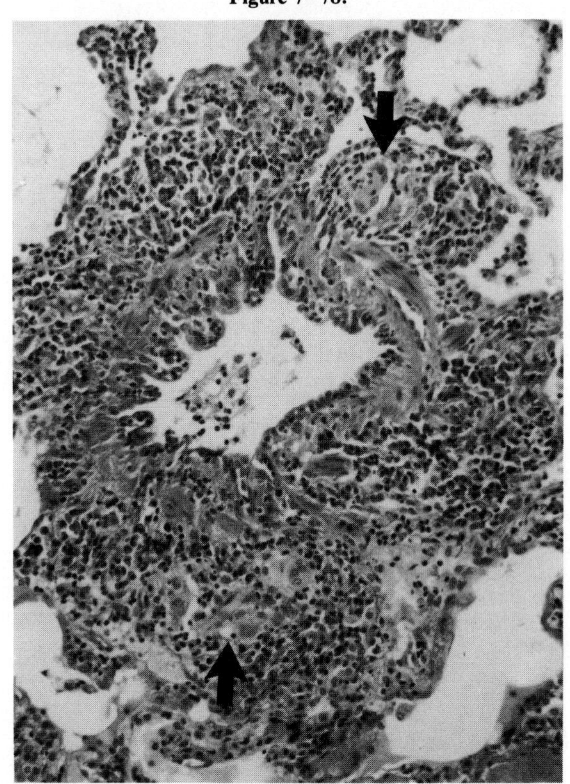

Figure 7-79.

Figures 7-76, 7-77. Extrinsic allergic alveolitis. The interstitial inflammation may be intense enough to suggest a diagnosis of lymphocytic interstitial pneumonia (LIP). The infiltrate is usually rich in plasma cells. The granulomas may manifest as classic sarcoid-like granulomas; clusters of giant cells; small epithelioid granulomas without giant cells; single giant cells, which may have cholesterol clefts; or as tiny accumulations of interstitial epithelioid histiocytes (arrows), which may stretch one's criteria for a granuloma.

Figures 7-78, 7-79. Extrinsic allergic alveolitis. A cellular bronchiolitis is shown, including peribronchiolar accumulations of giant cell (arrows).

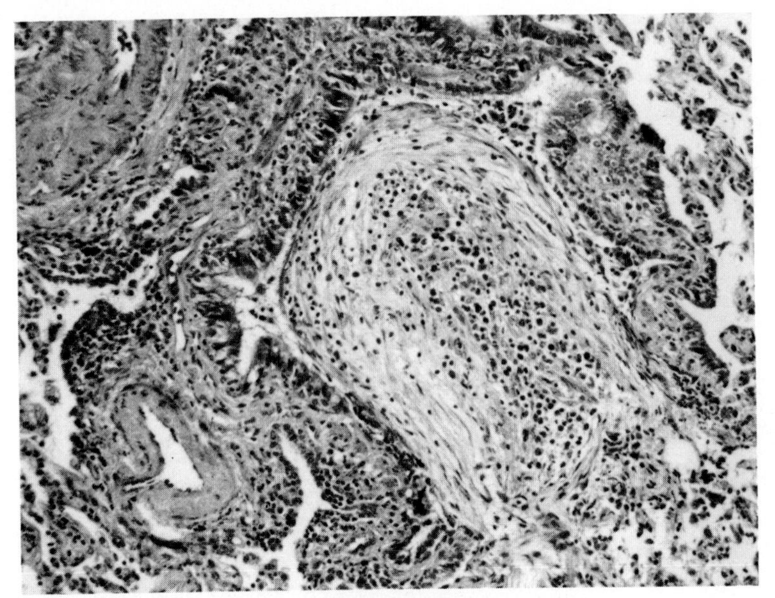

Figure 7-80.

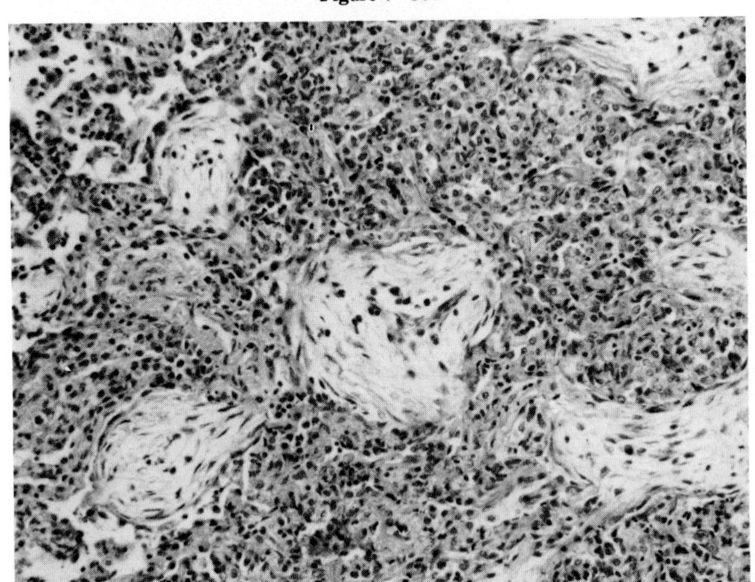

Figure 7-81.

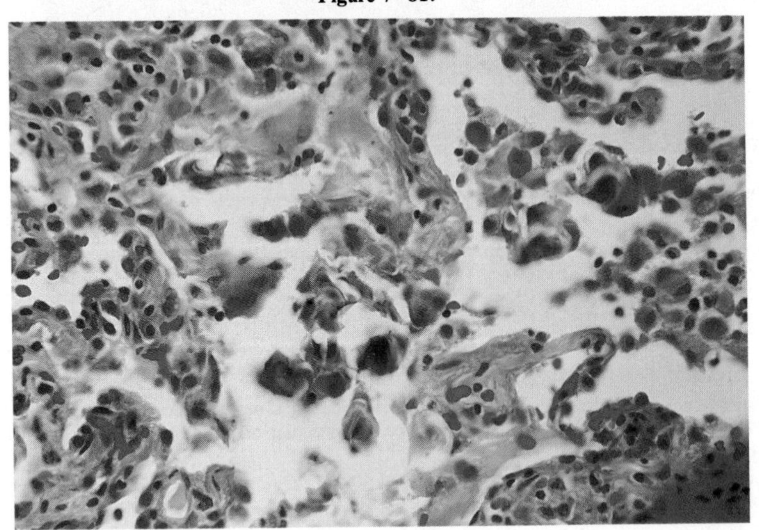

Figure 7-82.

Figures 7-80, 7-81, 7-82. Extrinsic allergic alveolitis. Proliferative bronchiolitis obliterans, organizing pneumonia, and blue bodies may be accompanying features in extrinsic allergic alveolitis.

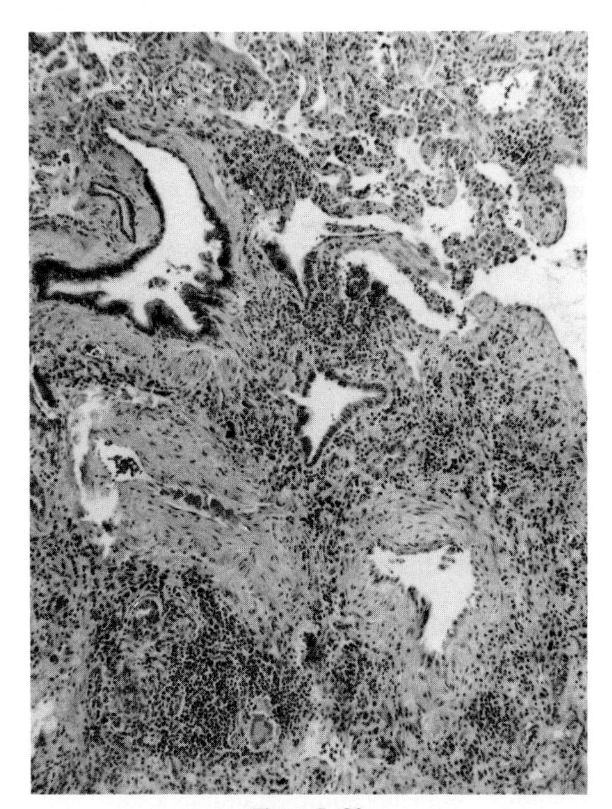

Figure 7-83.

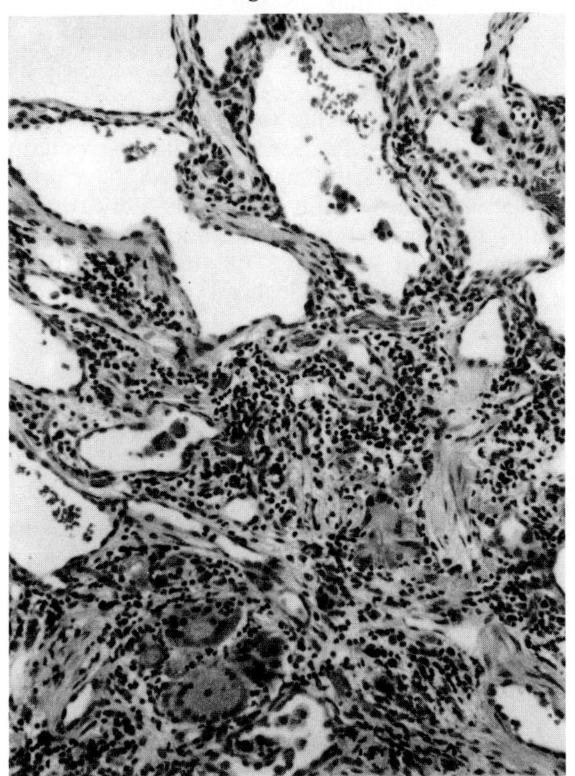

Figure 7-84.

Figures 7-83, 7-84. Chronic extrinsic allergic alveolitis. Interstitial inflammation, scarring, and a few small clusters of giant cells are apparent.

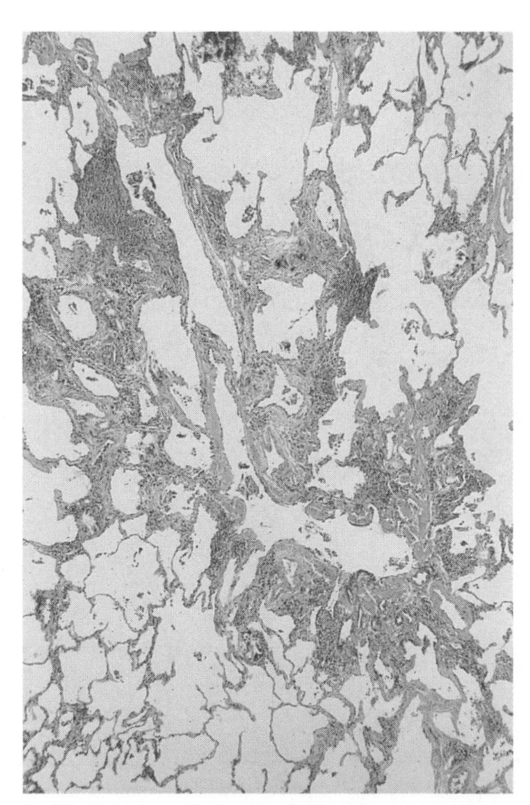

Figure 7-85. Chronic extrinsic allergic alveolitis. The peribronchiolar nature of this inflammatory and fibrosing process is evident.

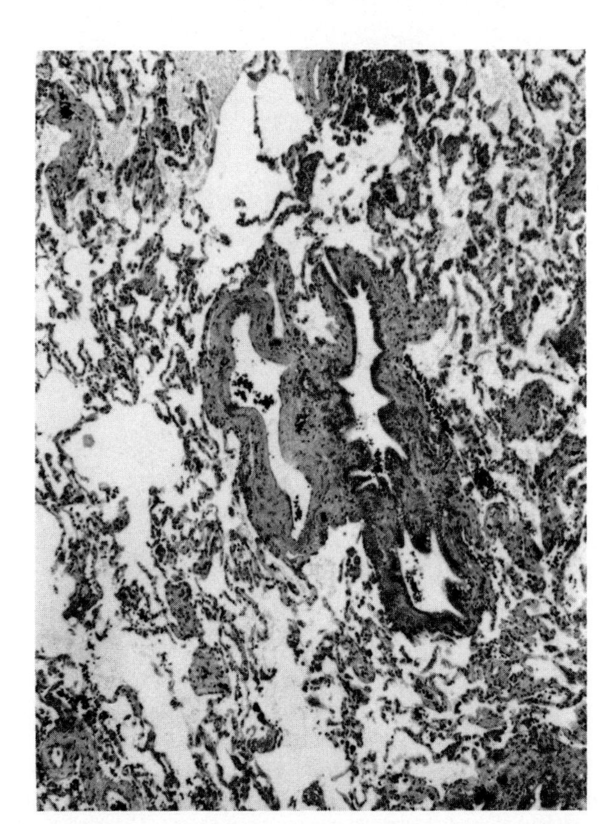

Figure 7-86. Chronic extrinsic allergic alveolitis. Evidence of chronicity is demonstrated by the fibrotic thickening in the bronchiolar wall.

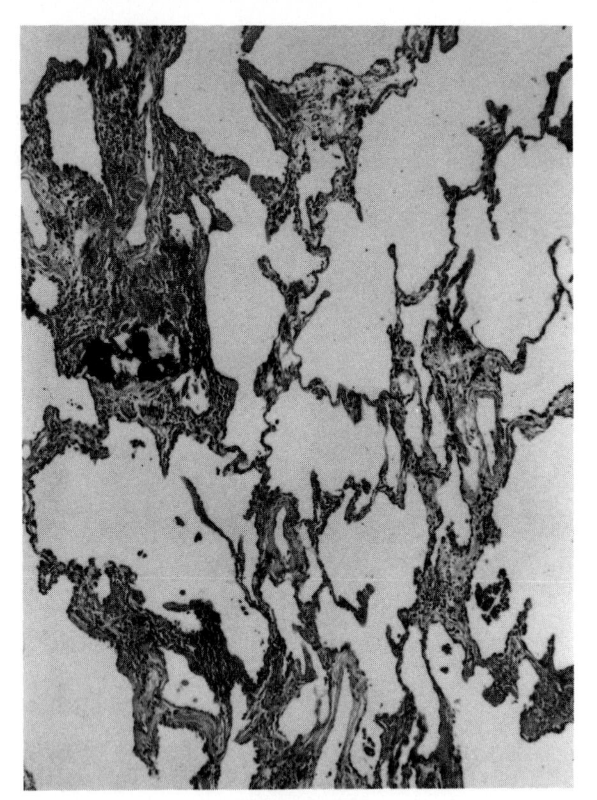

Figure 7-87.

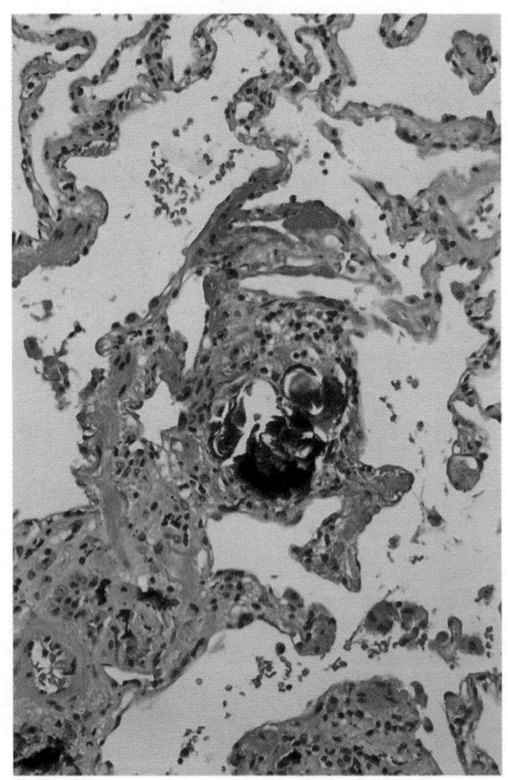

Figure 7-88.

Figures 7-87, 7-88. Chronic extrinsic allergic alveolitis. A pattern reminiscent of usual interstitial pneumonia is shown. The presence of Schaumann's bodies (and granulomas in other fields) was a clue to the cause of the fibrosis in this case. The calcified lamellated Schaumann's bodies, which often show a giant cell reaction around them, are a clue to prior granulomatous inflammation.

■ **Eosinophilic Pneumonia** (Figs. 7-89 to 7-97)

Eosinophilic pneumonia is an acute, subacute, or chronic interstitial lung disease of adults that is typically associated with fever, peripheral blood eosinophilia, and peripheral airspace infiltrates on chest radiograph. Occasional cases feature localized, or even nodular, infiltrates. Fever and/or peripheral blood eosinophilia need not always be present. Although the majority of cases are idiopathic, eosinophilic pneumonia-like reactions may be seen with drugs, parasitic infestations, pulmonary infections (particularly coccidioidomycosis), and vasculitis, especially Wegener's granulomatosis. Eosinophilic pneumonia is a frequent histologic finding in patients with allergic bronchopulmonary aspergillosis.

The histologic pattern includes airspace consolidation by histiocytes and pools of eosinophils with interstitial infiltrates of eosinophils, plasma cells, and lymphocytes. Neutrophils are frequently admixed with eosinophils, and a fibrinous exudate may be prominent. Necrosis of the alveolar exudate with surrounding palisaded histiocytic response (without parenchymal lung necrosis) is typical. Charcot-Leyden crystals, organizing pneumonia, eosinophilic venulitis, bronchiolitis obliterans, scattered granulomas, and obstructive pneumonia all may be found. In patients with allergic bronchopulmonary aspergillosis, bronchocentric granulomatosis, and/or mucoid impaction may be found more proximally. Diagnostic foci of eosinophilic pneumonia are sometimes quite focal, and some cases resemble DIP or organizing pneumonia.

Organizing eosinophilic pneumonia shows some overlap with BOOP; a diagnosis of unclassified pneumonia with features of both may occasionally be appropriate. Patients with systemic hypersensitivity reactions may show histologic features of eosinophilic pneumonia with a prominent venulitis. Differential diagnosis in such cases includes Churg-Strauss syndrome.

References

Carrington CB, Addington WW, Goff AM, Madoff IM, Marks A, Schwaber JR, Gaensler EA. Chronic eosinophilic pneumonia. N Engl J Med 280:787-798, 1969.

Jederlinic PJ, Sicchan L, Gaensler EA. Chronic eosinophilic pneumonia. Medicine 67:154-162, 1988.

Thurlbeck WM (ed). Pathology of the Lung. New York, Thieme, 1988.

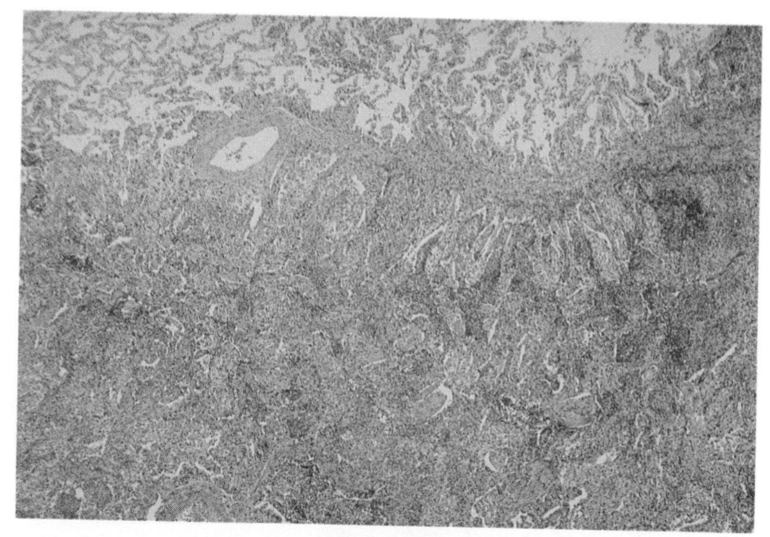

Figure 7–89.

Figures 7–89, 7–90, 7–91, 7–92, 7–93, 7–94. Chronic eosinophilic pneumonia. There is consolidation of airspaces by sheets of histiocytes and accumulations of eosinophils. The eosinophils may occur in sheets or may aggregate to form necrotic eosinophilic microabscesses with surrounding palisaded histiocytic reaction (Fig. 7–93). Eosinophilic and mononuclear cell interstitial infiltrates, as well as an eosinophilic angiitis (Fig. 7–94), are common accompanying features.

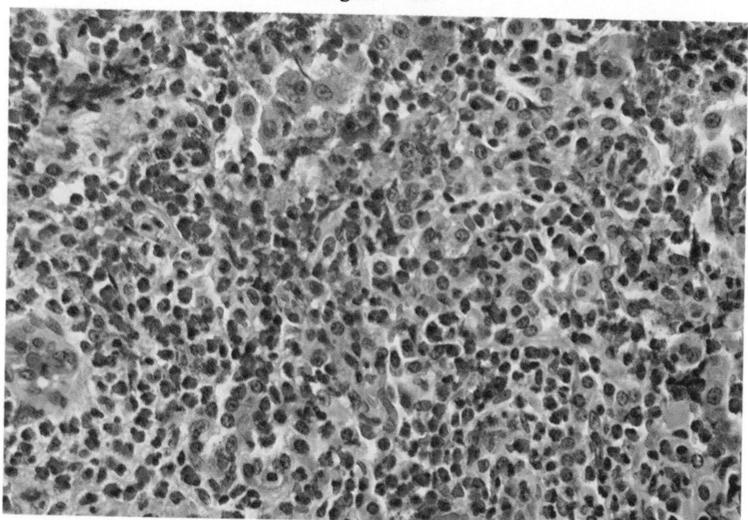

Figure 7–90.

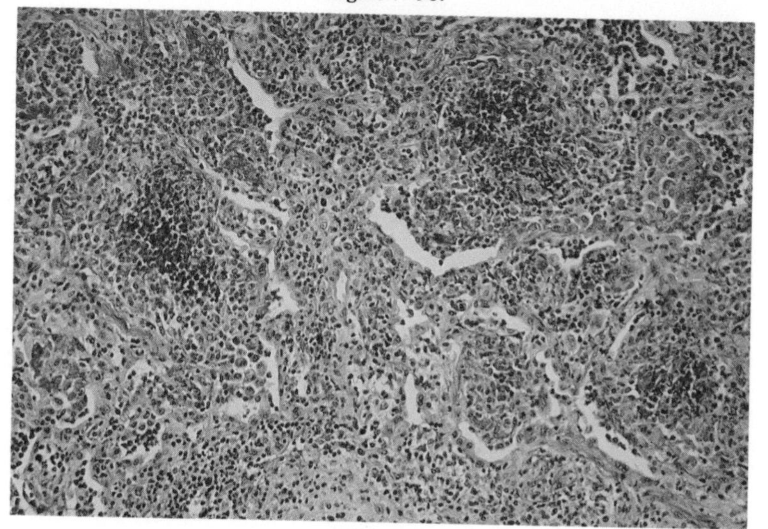

Figure 7–91.

Illustrations continued on following page

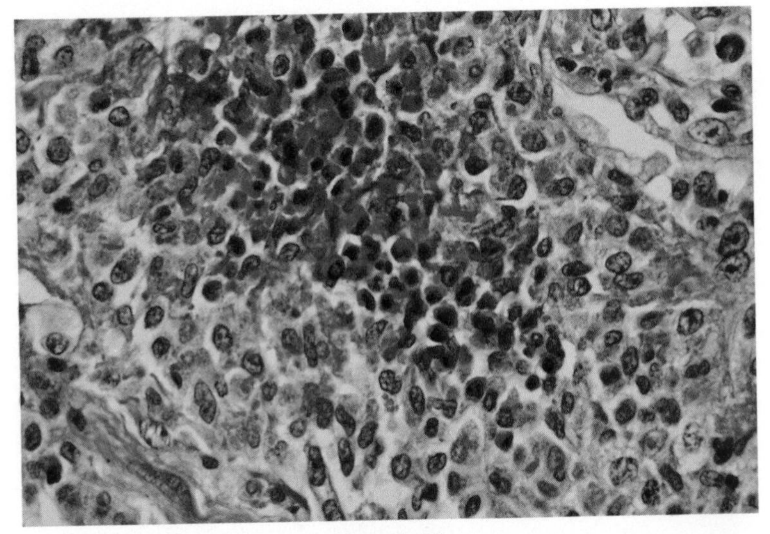

Figure 7–92.

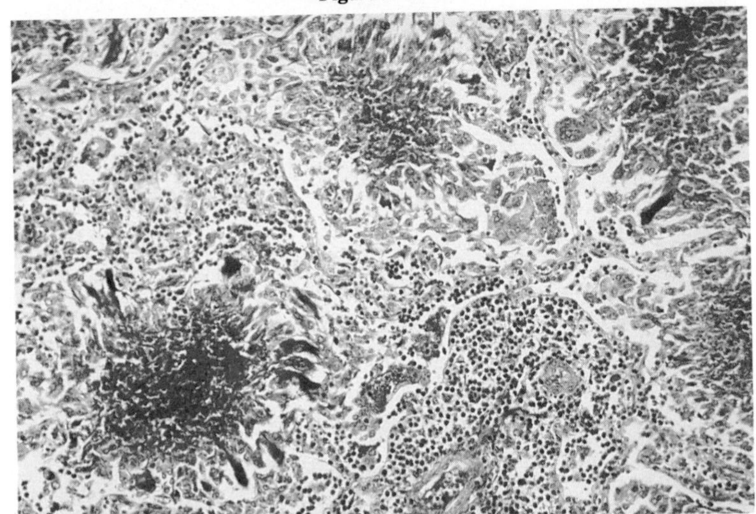

Figure 7–93.

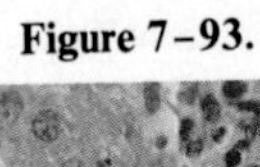

Figures 7–92, 7–93, 7–94 *see legend on previous page*

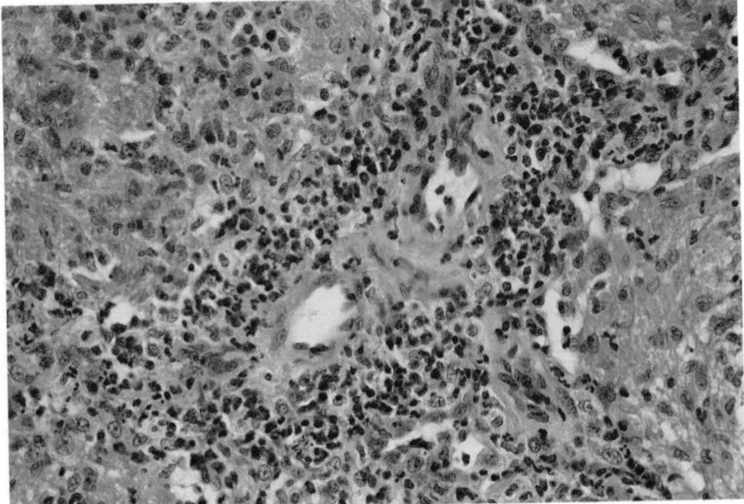

Figure 7–94.

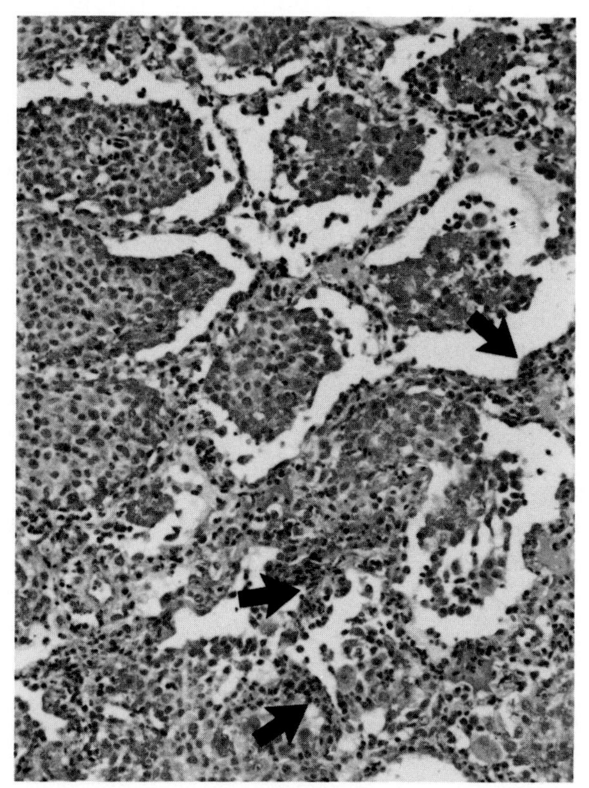

Figure 7-95. Chronic eosinophilic pneumonia. In addition to large numbers of histiocytes and eosinophils in airspaces, some cases are associated with neutrophils (arrows), which may be interstitial or alveolar and appear to correlate with a more acute history.

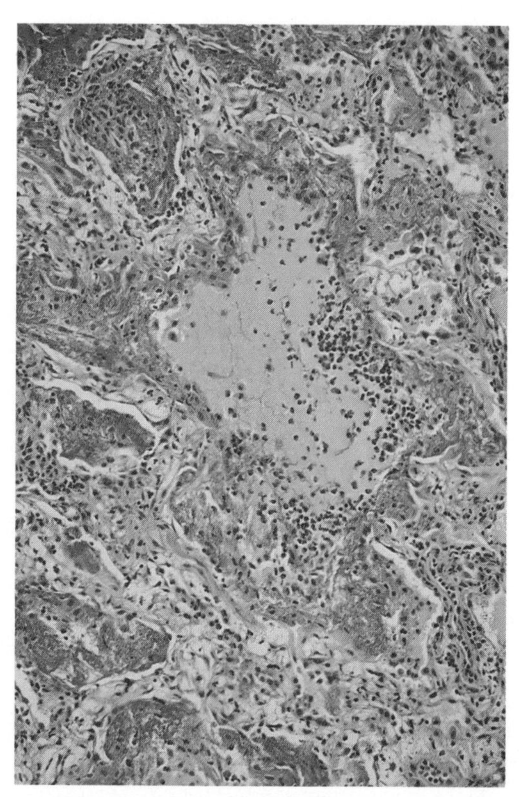

Figure 7-97. Acute eosinophilic pneumonia. Acute eosinophilic pneumonia with accumulations of eosinophils and hyaline membranes in airspaces. Waxing and waning infiltrates associated with peripheral eosinophilia were present. No infection could be identified, and the histologic findings were thought to represent an acute eosinophilic pneumonia.

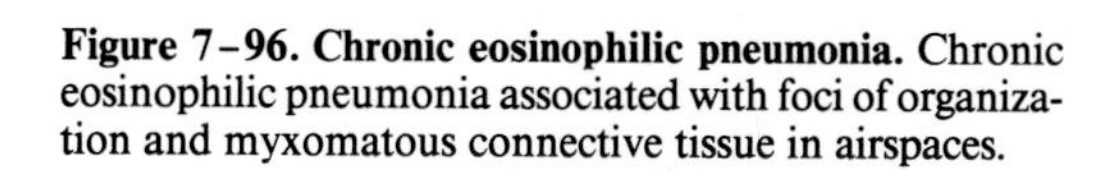

Figure 7-96. Chronic eosinophilic pneumonia. Chronic eosinophilic pneumonia associated with foci of organization and myxomatous connective tissue in airspaces.

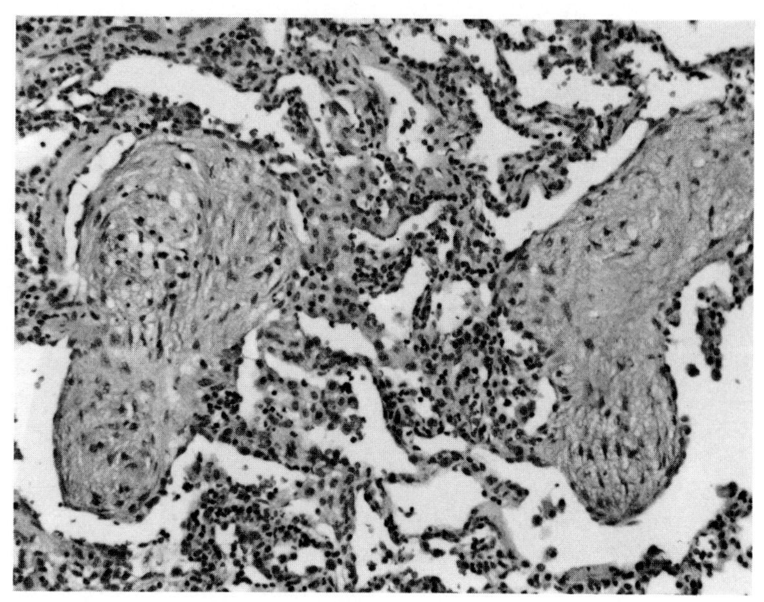

■ Unclassified Interstitial Pneumonias (Figs. 7-98 to 7-106)

Some subacute or chronic interstitial pneumonias cannot be put into any of the well described categories. Examples include BOOP/eosinophilic pneumonia hybrids, cellular interstitial pneumonias without fibrosis or other features to place them into a specific category (a descriptive diagnosis of nonspecific cellular interstitial pneumonia may be appropriate), UIP/BOOP hybrids in which a very active and fibroblastic UIP is difficult to separate from late BOOP with incorporation of the airspace fibroblastic tissue into the interstitium, and BOOP with granulomas versus extrinsic allergic alveolitis with prominent organization. In such cases it is useful to emphasize that the lesion is difficult to classify and to list the clinicopathologic entities to which it comes closest; an example of this is unclassified interstitial pneumonia with features of BOOP versus UIP.

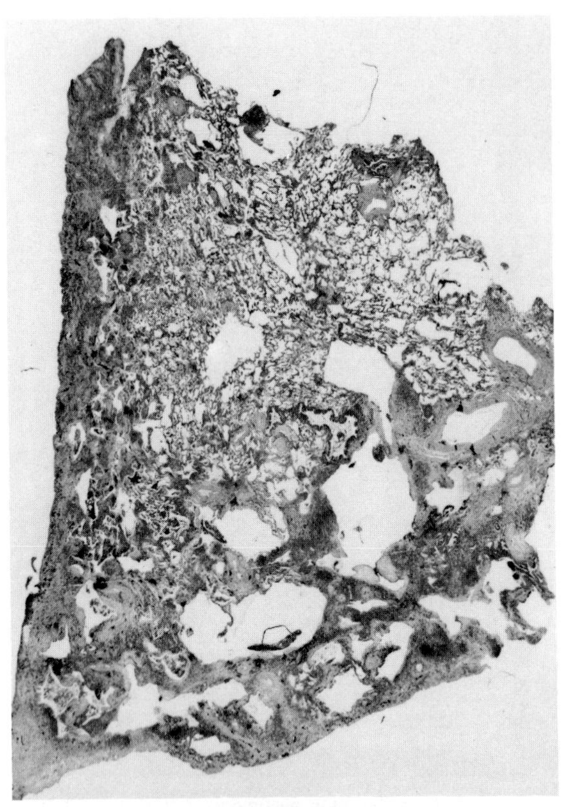

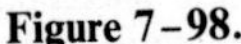

Figure 7-98.

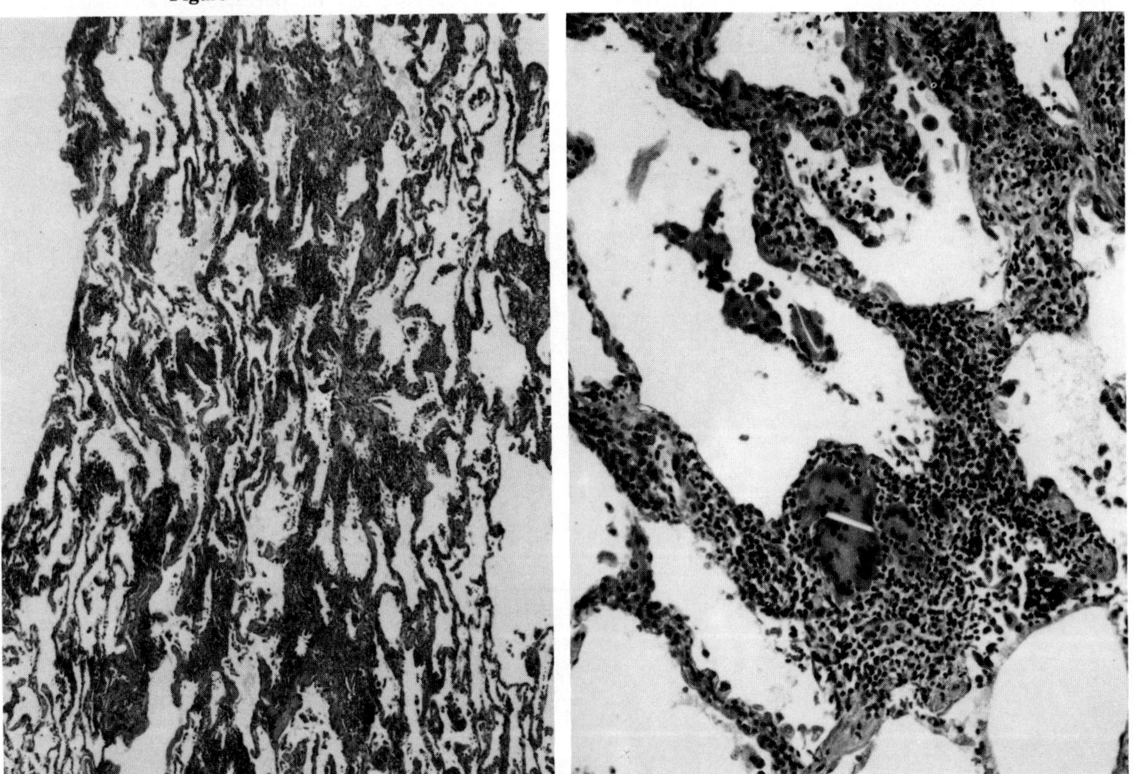

Figure 7-99. **Figure 7-100.**

Figures 7-98, 7-99, 7-100. Unclassified interstitial pneumonia. The low-power appearance is that of a fibrosing interstitial pneumonia with honeycombing that would be most consistent with usual interstitial pneumonia (UIP). A higher-power magnification, however, shows more extensive inflammation than is usually present in UIP as well as occasional clusters of giant cells with cholesterol clefts. The possibility of extrinsic allergic alveolitis was suggested, although no cause was found. The patient did not respond to steroid therapy.

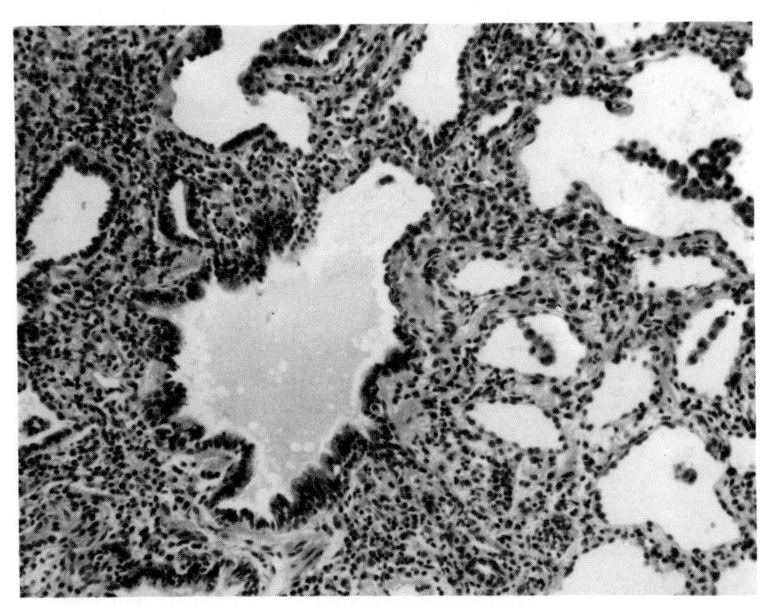

Figure 7-101.

Figures 7-101, 7-102, 7-103. Unclassified interstitial pneumonia (cellular interstitial pneumonia). There is uniform mild to moderate interstitial infiltrate associated with metaplastic type II cells lining the alveolar walls. Relatively little fibrosis is present. This lesion does not fit into any of the well-recognized clinical pathologic groups of interstitial lung disease. A generic designation of cellular interstitial pneumonia is descriptively appropriate, although it does not really help the clinician in classifying the process. This biopsy specimen was obtained from a patient with systemic lupus erythematosus (SLE) with a clinically subacute interstitial pneumonia that responded to steroids.

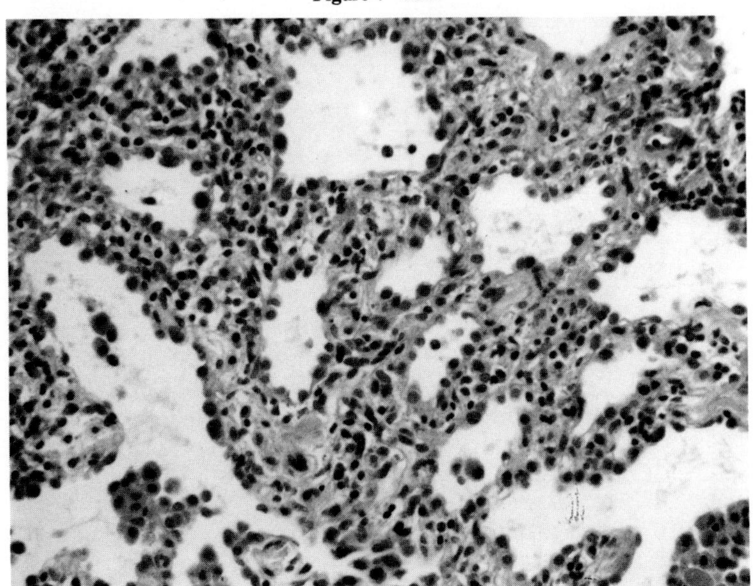

Figure 7-102.

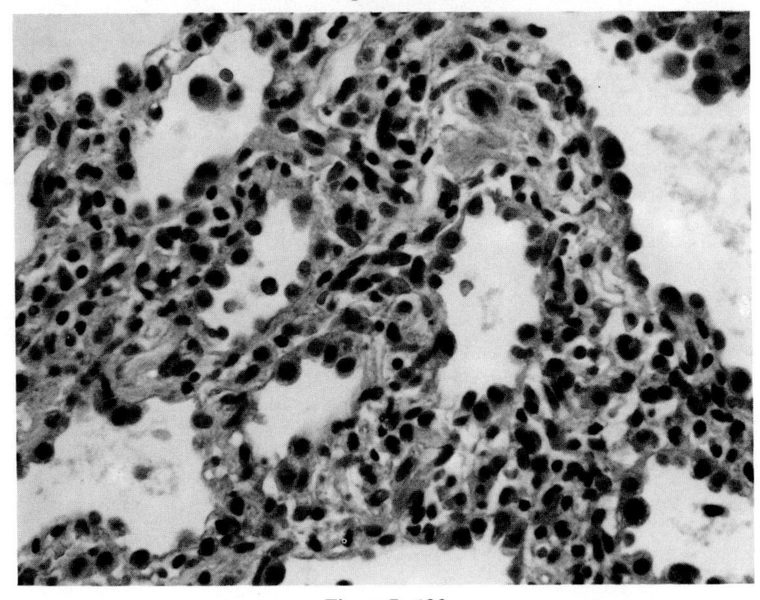

Figure 7-103.

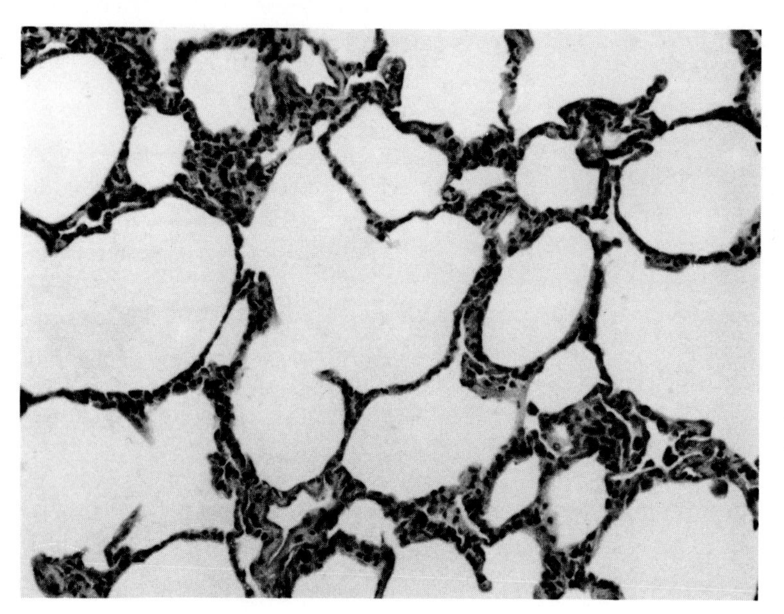

Figure 7-104. Unclassified mild interstitial pneumonia (mild cellular interstitial pneumonia). A young man with mild interstitial lung disease underwent open lung biopsy. The specimen shows preservation of architecture and a mild diffuse infiltrate in the alveolar walls associated with some metaplastic type II cells. No cause could be found, and the patient responded to steroids. Such an appearance could be the residue of a healing viral pneumonia. Nowadays, a case like this should be carefully evaluated for the presence of pneumocystis and other pathogens because of the possibility of human immunodeficiency virus (HIV) infection.

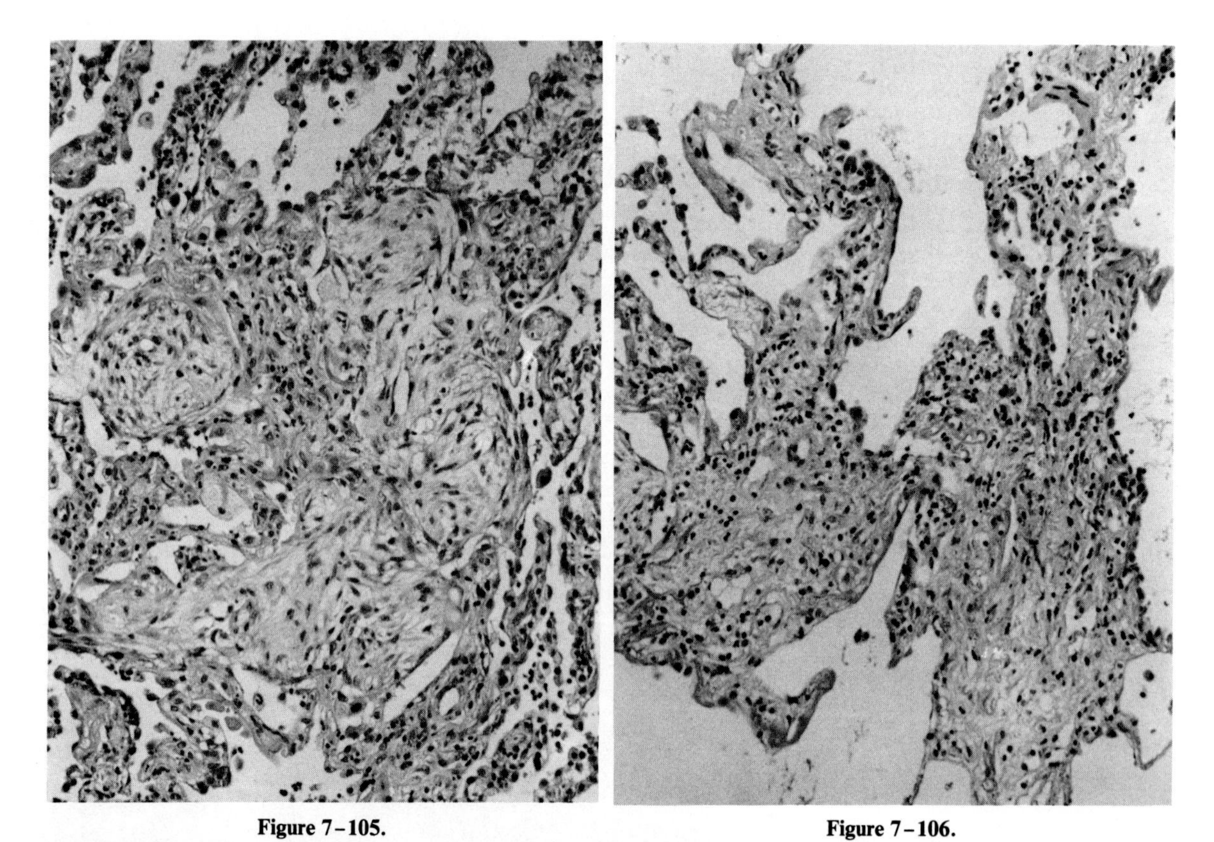

Figure 7-105. **Figure 7-106.**

Figures 7-105, 7-106. Unclassified interstitial pneumonia. Unclassified interstitial pneumonia with some features of bronchiolitis obliterans organizing pneumonia (BOOP) and some features of usual interstitial pneumonia (UIP). In some zones, there was organization within distal airspaces typical of that seen in BOOP (Fig. 7-105), whereas other foci showed interstitial scarring and widening typical of UIP (Fig. 7-106). A designation of unclassified interstitial pneumonia with features of both UIP and BOOP is appropriate, and steroids are probably indicated.

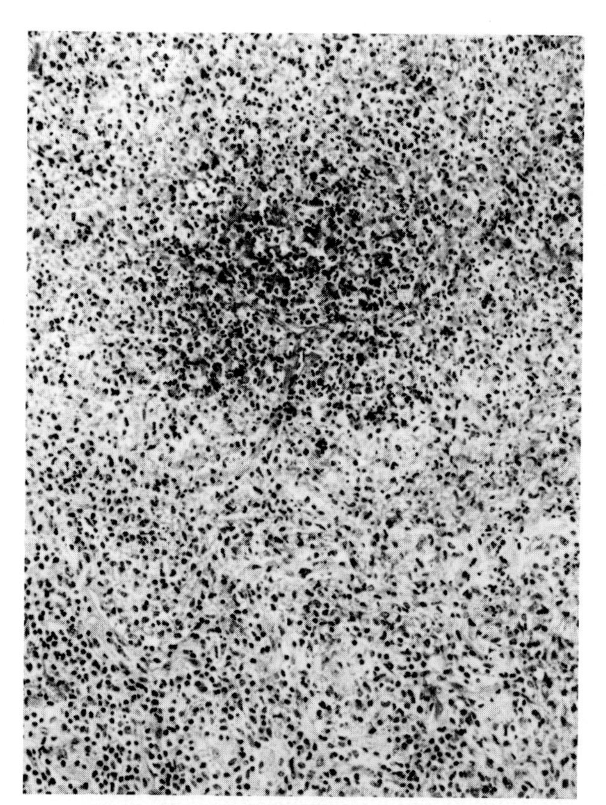

Figure 7–107.

■ Unclassified Allergic Reactions (Figs. 7–107 to 7–109)

Unclassified allergic reaction is a designation that is sometimes useful for cases that cannot be placed into a specific clinicopathologic category but that include one or more of the following: scattered microgranulomas; eosinophilic interstitial or perivascular infiltrates; a suggestive clinical history.

The distinctions in many of these unclassified lesions may be moot because the treatment is usually the same once an infection has been reasonably excluded. Obviously, however, removal of an offending agent, if it can be identified, is most desirable; if extrinsic allergic alveolitis is a consideration, an exposure history should be sought. The key features in terms of prognosis are the degree of architectural destruction by irreversible interstitial fibrosis and honeycombing in contrast to airspace organization and cellular infiltrates, which are potentially reversible, despite the fact that they may be very dramatic in degree.

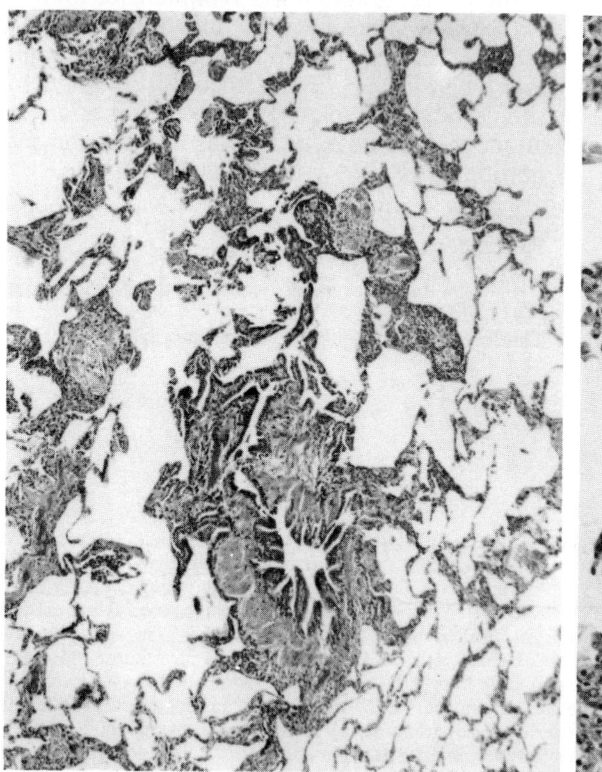

Figure 7–108.

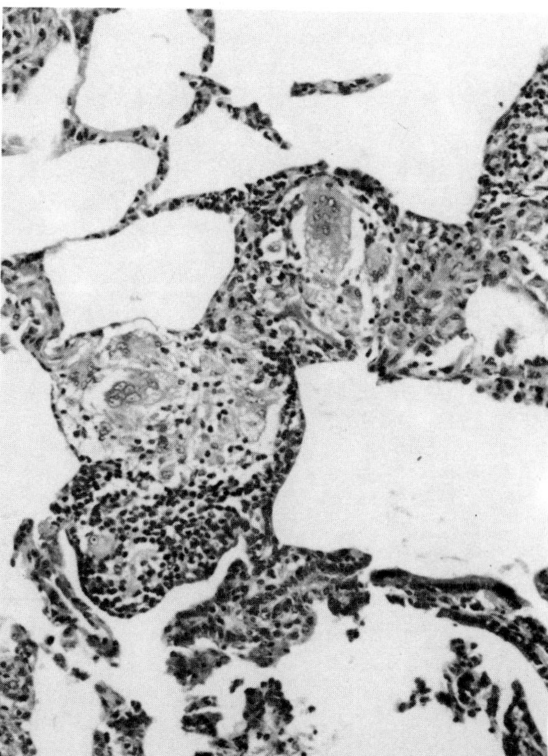

Figure 7–109.

Figures 7–107, 7–108, 7–109. Unclassified allergic reaction. A biopsy specimen obtained from a farmer shows miliary nodules with necrosis and surrounding chronic inflammation (Fig. 7–107). Other fields show peribronchiolar thickening, interstitial infiltrates, and granulomas suggestive of extrinsic allergic alveolitis (Fig. 7–108, 7–109). The presence of necrotic nodules should be considered to be an infection until proven otherwise, although evaluation proved negative in this case, and the patient responded promptly and dramatically to steroids. *In retrospect,* a designation of unclassified allergic reaction appeared appropriate.

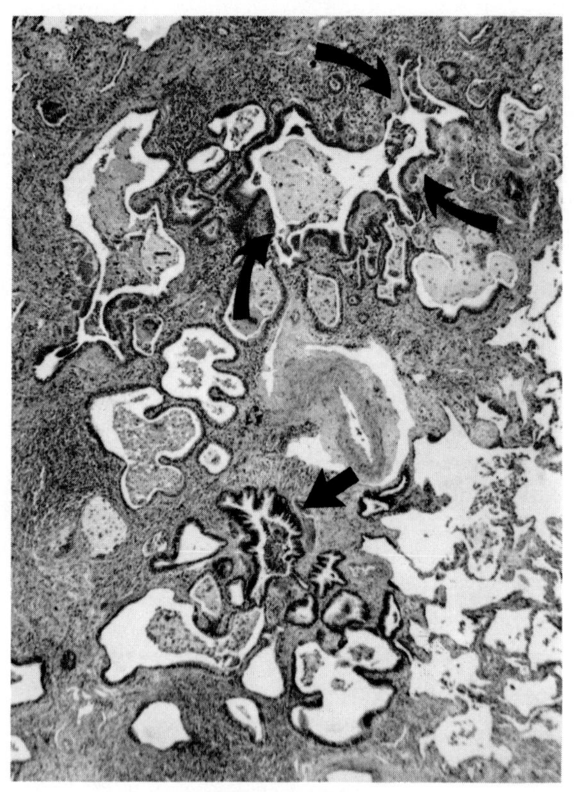

Figure 7-110.

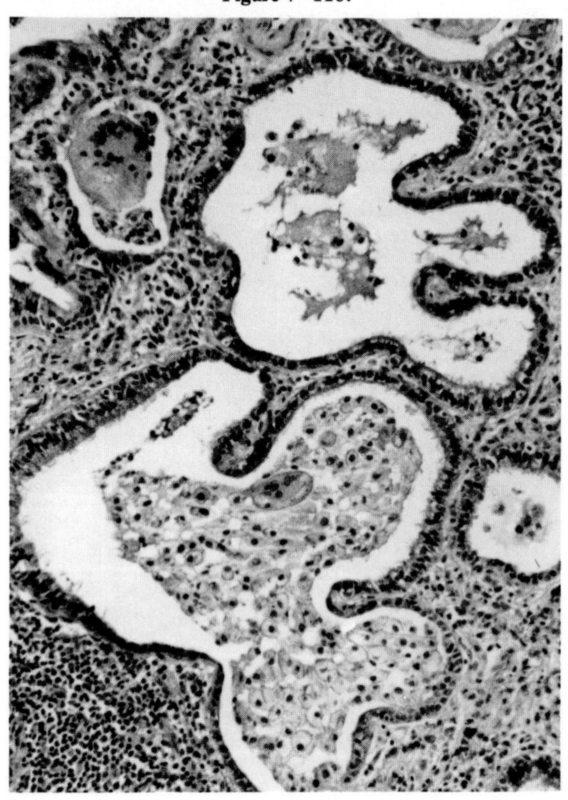

Figure 7-111.

■ Honeycomb Lung (Figs. 7-110, 7-111)

This is a nonspecific endstage appearance of many fibrosing interstitial and/or necrotizing pneumonias represented by functionally useless lung tissue. Some cases can be recognized radiographically.

Macroscopically, the lungs are small and contracted with holes that often contain mucus and that are lined by thick, rigid fibrotic walls. Histologically, there is architectural destruction with interstitial fibrosis and abnormal airspaces lined by metaplastic bronchiolar or type II epithelium. Mucus and neutrophils frequently fill the airspaces as pools. Interstitial changes include fibrosis, chronic inflammation, smooth muscle metaplasia, and sometimes calcification or bone. Vessels often show myointimal thickening. Small saprophytic aspergilliomas are sometimes seen. Microscopic honeycombing may not be appreciated grossly or by chest radiograph. Causes of honeycombing include UIP, DIP, LIP, collagen-vascular diseases, drugs, sarcoidosis, chronic extrinsic allergic alveolitis, organized DAD, eosinophilic granuloma, asbestosis, berylliosis, other pneumoconioses, chronic granulomatous infections, recurrent aspiration, and diffuse low-grade lymphomas. No cause is found in some cases.

An enlarged, hyperinflated lung with fibrosis and honeycombing should raise the possibility of sarcoidosis, eosinophilic granuloma, lymphangioleiomyomatosis (which is technically not honeycombing on histologic grounds because it lacks fibrosis), and an emphysematous lung with superimposed fibrosis. Emphysema alone should be readily distinguishable from honeycombing, although the bullae in bullous emphysema may have fibrotic walls.

References

Heppleston AG. The pathology of honeycomb lung. Thorax 11:77-93, 1956.

Thurlbeck WM (ed). Pathology of the Lung. New York, Thieme, 1988.

Figures 7-110, 7-111. Honeycombing. There is loss of the normal lung architecture and replacement by irregular airspaces lined by metaplastic epithelium and containing accumulations of mucus, macrophages, and other inflammatory cells. Occasional histiocytic giant cells can be seen. The lining epithelium varies from bronchiolar to reactive type II cells. The interstitium in honeycombing is characterized by variable degrees of inflammation, fibrosis, and smooth muscle fibroplasia. Dystrophic ossification may occur. In some foci, honeycombing appears to be the result of bronchiolectasis following the destruction of surrounding alveoli (curved arrows). In others, however, bronchioles (arrow) remain relatively unaffected, and the surrounding alveoli are transformed into the abnormal spaces of honeycombing.

■ Focal Honeycombing

Focal honeycombing is characterized by end-stage inflammatory destruction of lung parenchyma that is localized. Some might prefer the term focal scar or healed pneumonia.

Histologically, there is architecturally abnormal lung tissue with fibrosis and abnormal airspaces lined by metaplastic epithelium and frequently containing inflammatory debris and/or mucin. The walls may contain acute or chronic inflammation, fibrosis, smooth muscle metaplasia, and even metaplastic bone. Thickened vessels with or without intimal thickening occur in such foci.

The differential diagnosis of focal honeycombing includes bronchioloalveolar carcinoma. Features that favor diagnosis of focal honeycombing include marked inflammation, variation in epithelial cell types, marked architectural derangement and thickening of the interstitium, and lack of cytologic features of malignancy.

References

Thurlbeck WM (ed). Pathology of the Lung. New York, Thieme, 1988.

■ Interstitial Pneumonias in Children (Fig. 7–47)

As in adults, a large number of conditions cause interstitial lung disease in children. Many of these are the same lesions as those seen in adults. A lesion resembling DIP occurs, but the possibility that this is a nonspecific reaction pattern to some other process, particularly an infection, should be kept in mind. UIP, as seen in adults, probably does not occur in children. Many cases of idiopathic chronic interstitial pneumonia in children are probably the residue of a prior (usually viral) infection, a conclusion supported in some cases by the history or the histologic appearance with bronchiolocentric scarring and inflammation.

References

Tal A, Maor E, Bar-Ziv J, Gorodischer R. Fatal desquamative interstitial pneumonia in three infant siblings. J Pediatr 104:873–876, 1984.

■ Asbestosis (Figs. 7–112 to 7–117)

Pulmonary parenchymal fibrosis due to asbestos exposure may be subclinical (histologic asbestosis), or associated with overt clinical, radiographic, and functional findings of restrictive lung disease (classic asbestosis).

In many cases, progressive interstitial fibrosis appears to start around small airways and alveolar ducts and to involve more and more interstitium, ultimately resulting in honeycombing. Pleural and subpleural fibrosis may be marked and may sometimes be the main finding. Histiocytes filled with hemosiderin and a giant cell reaction (but without granulomas) may be present. Some cases are reminiscent of DIP. Light microscopic diagnosis depends on identification of asbestos bodies associated with the interstitial fibrosis. Asbestos bodies are beaded, ferruginous bodies with a thin, translucent core that represents the actual mineral fiber. Asbestos bodies are often found in clusters in airspaces or in the interstitium, especially around scarred airways. Nonspecific increases in hemosiderin and anthracotic pigment are common in the lung with increased asbestos bodies and are of the first clues to search for asbestos bodies.

The diagnosis of asbestosis is based on the presence of asbestos bodies (at least one) *and* fibrosis. Fibrosis alone is quite nonspecific. The presence of asbestos bodies alone is indicative only of exposure, and in the absence of fibrosis a diagnosis of asbestosis is not warranted. Practically speaking, the diagnosis rarely rests on the presence of only one asbestos body because others can usually be found. Quantitation of asbestos bodies and fibers requires special techniques and careful standardization. A minimum of 3 to 5 gm of tissue (inflated wet weight) is recommended. Formalin-fixed tissue is sufficient.

Asbestos airways changes must be distinguished from respiratory (smoker's) bronchiolitis, a task that may not always be possible in asbestos-exposed individuals who also smoke.

References

Churg A, Green FHY. Pathology of Occupational Lung Disease. New York, Igaku-Shoin Medical Publishers, 1988.
Craighead JE, Abraham JL, Churg A, et al. The pathology of asbestos-associated diseases of the lungs and pleural cavities: diagnostic criteria and proposed grading schema. Arch Pathol Lab Med 106:544–596,1982.
Dail DH, Hammer SP (eds). Pulmonary Pathology. New York, Springer-Verlag, 1988.
Thurlbeck WM (ed). Pathology of the Lung. New York, Thieme, 1988.

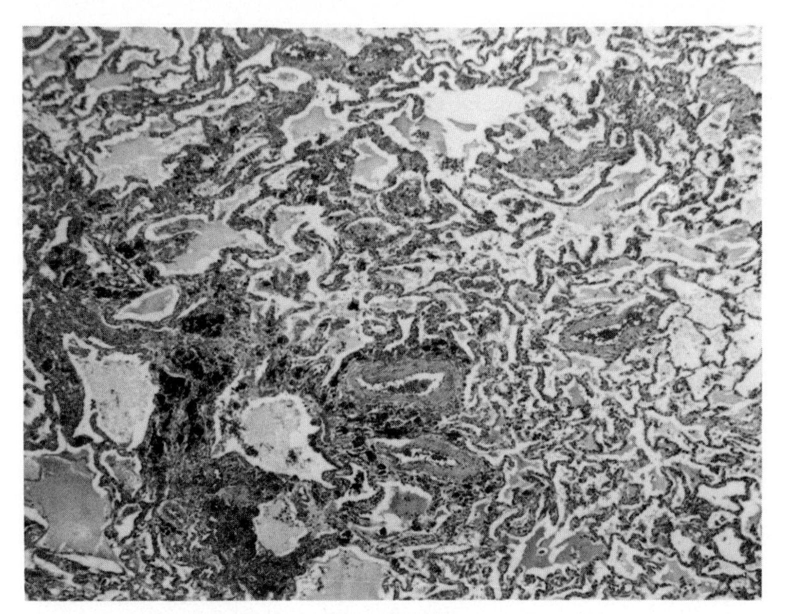

Figure 7-112.

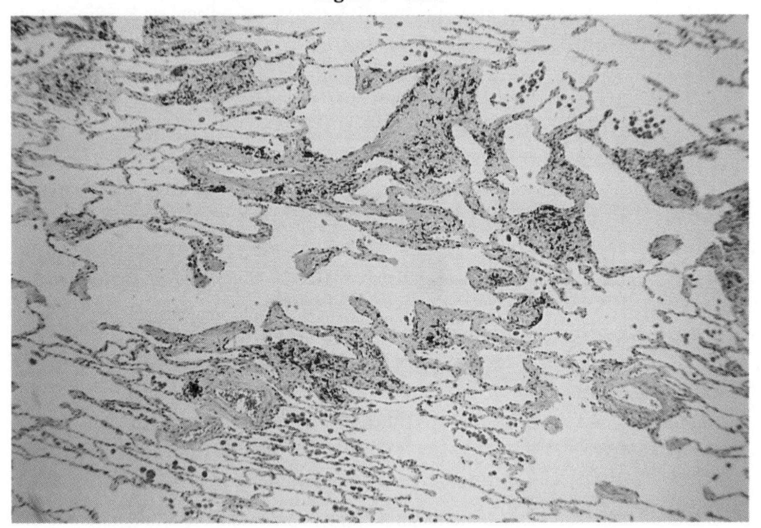

Figure 7-113.

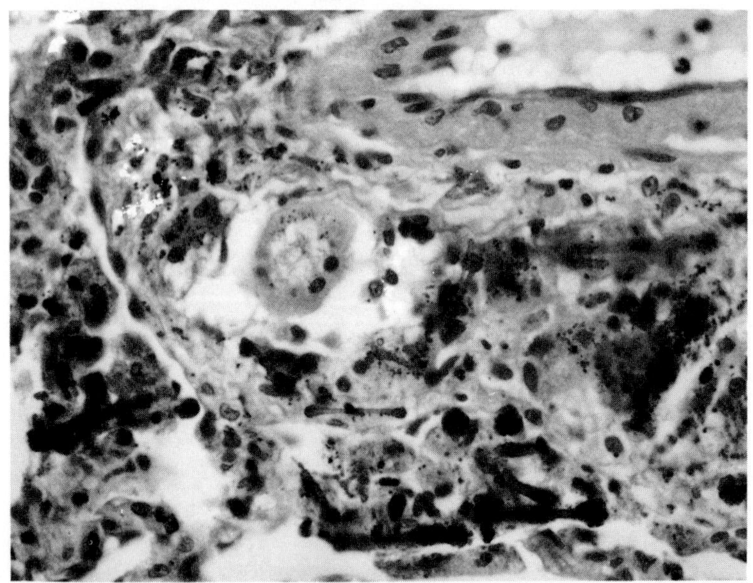

Figure 7-114.

Figures 7-112, 7-113, 7-114. Mild asbestosis. Mural thickening and pigment deposition around small bronchioles, with extension around the alveolar ducts associated with mild interstitial thickening and scarring. In and around the small airway, clusters of asbestos bodies were found (Fig. 7-114).

Figure 7–115. Asbestosis. A giant cell reaction to asbestos bodies is not uncommon; however, a sarcoid-like granulomatous reaction does not occur. Numerous hemosiderin-filled macrophages are common in patients with significant numbers of asbestos bodies.

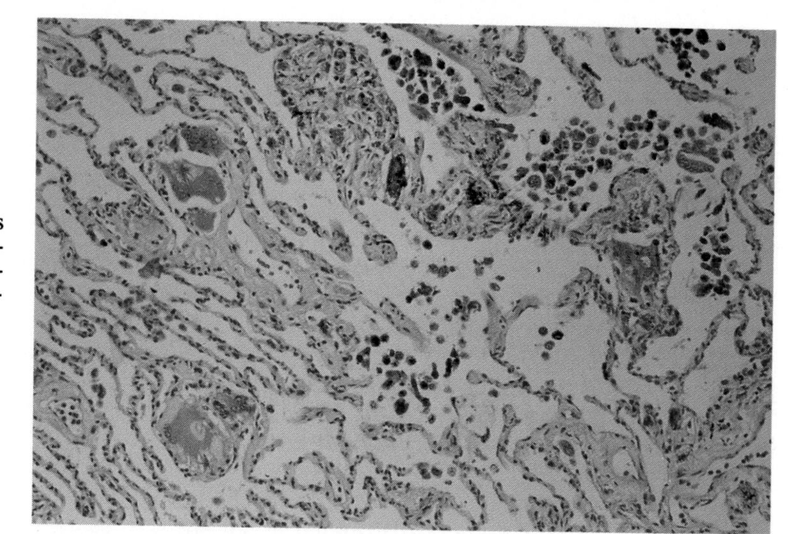

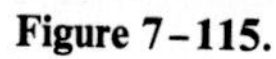

Figure 7–115.

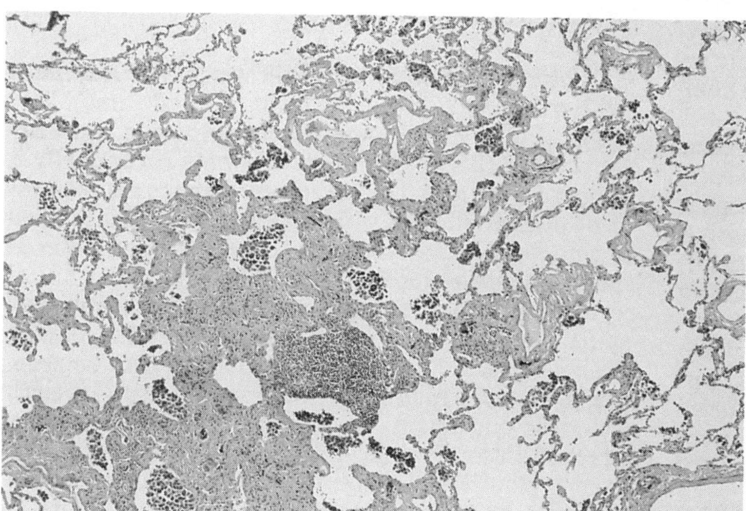

Figure 7–116.

Figure 7–116. Asbestosis. More advanced asbestosis with prominent interstitial scarring. Numerous hemosiderin-filled macrophages can be seen in the airspaces around the fibrosis.

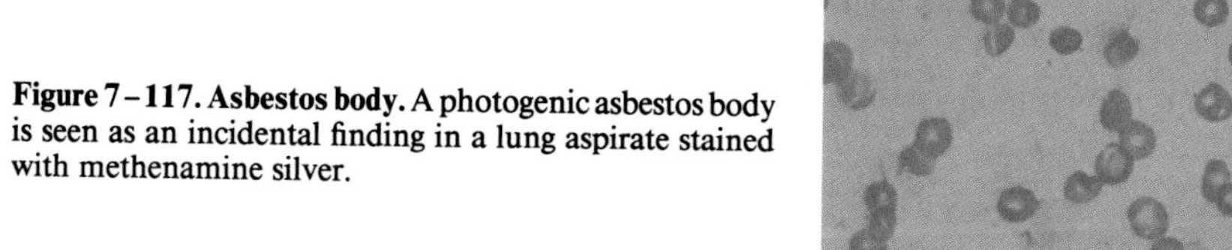

Figure 7–117. Asbestos body. A photogenic asbestos body is seen as an incidental finding in a lung aspirate stained with methenamine silver.

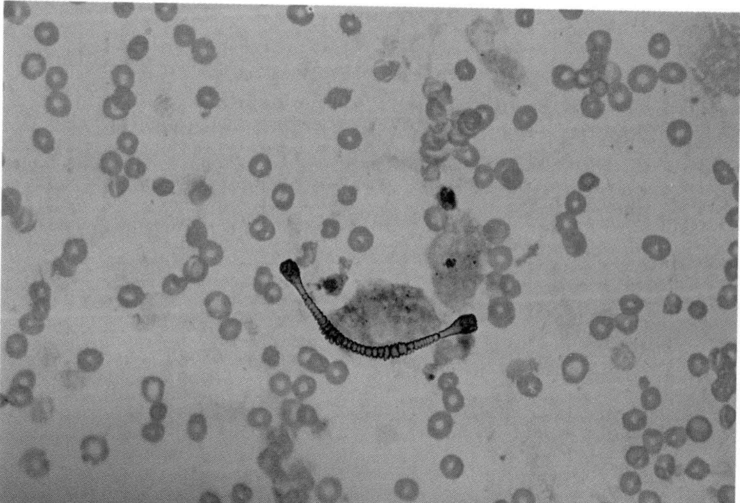

Figure 7–117.

■ Silicosis

Silicosis is a pneumoconiosis caused by exposure to silica, usually resulting in discrete parenchymal fibrotic nodules and interstitial histiocytic infiltrates and rarely other patterns.

Acute, accelerated, and chronic (classic) forms of silicosis are recognized.

In acute silicosis, there is an alveolar proteinosis-like reaction in the airspaces associated with abundant silica particles that are birefringent. This form is rarely seen.

In accelerated silicosis, there are usually signs and symptoms of interstitial lung disease associated histologically with dense aggregates of dust-filled histiocytes along lymphatic routes with or without early fibrous nodule formation.

The chronic form consists of scattered, relatively acellular, whorled, fibrous nodules distributed along lymphatic routes with normal intervening lung parenchyma. A variable amount of anthracotic pigment may be present. In progressive massive fibrosis, there are aggregates of confluent nodules of sufficient size to compromise lung function. Diffuse interstitial fibrosis with or without honeycombing is an uncommon but recognized pattern of silicosis. Silica is recognized as *weakly* birefringent needle-like particles only a few microns in size in contrast to silicates, which tend to be larger, somewhat more irregular in shape, and much more brightly birefringent. Silica is slightly less birefringent than the endogenous collagen fibers in the lung.

Chronic silicosis usually takes many years to develop. There are characteristic radiographic findings, and biopsy is rarely ever performed for diagnosis. Accelerated silicosis usually occurs with heavier exposure over a shorter period of time and a transbronchial or open lung biopsy diagnosis is occasionally made.

Chronic silicotic nodules should be distinguished from old healed granulomas. Granulomas have a granular necrotic center, and silicotic nodules have a whorled collagenous center, although degenerative changes may be present. Dystrophic calcification may occur in both. The presence of a single or a few silicotic nodules in histologic material (especially in hilar nodes) should *not* lead to a diagnosis of silicosis without clinical correlation. Likewise, the presence of birefringent material in the lung, especially along bronchovascular bundles or in the pleura and in association with anthracosis, in the absence of other changes of silicosis should not lead to a diagnosis of silicosis.

Some early silicotic nodules lack much anthracosis and are so cellular that they mimic an inflammatory pseudotumor or a low-grade sarcoma.

References

Churg A, Green FHY. Pathology of Occupational Lung Disease. New York, Igaku-Shoin Medical Publishers, 1988.

Craighead JE, Kleinerman J, Abraham JL, et al. Diseases associated with exposure to silica and nonfibrous silicate minerals. Arch Pathol Lab Med 112:673–720, 1988.

Dail DH, Hammer SP (eds). Pulmonary Pathology. New York, Springer-Verlag, 1988.

Thurlbeck WM (ed). Pathology of the Lung. New York, Thieme, 1988.

■ Non-asbestos Silicates

A number of non-asbestos silicates may be associated with pulmonary disease. These include talc, mica, kaolinate, Fuller's earth, and others. Exposure is usually obvious in the work history, and only occasionally is biopsy performed. The pathologic features are reminiscent of early silicosis with large numbers of dust-filled macrophages along lymphatic routes without the fibrous nodules that develop in silicosis. The infiltrates of histiocytes may be sufficient to cause clinical findings of interstitial lung disease. With massive exposures, massive scarring and diffuse interstitial fibrosis may be seen. Large amounts of brightly birefringent material is characteristic, and a giant cell and sometimes granulomatous reaction occurs, particularly with talc and mica. The lucent, platelike, birefingert particles of talc may be encrusted with hemosiderin, representing a cause of ferruginous bodies.

Many of the non-asbestos silicates have variable amounts of silica mixed with them, resulting in a mixed-dust pneumoconiosis (see below).

References

Churg A, Green FHY. Pathology of Occupational Lung Disease. New York, Igaku-Shoin Medical Publishers, 1988.

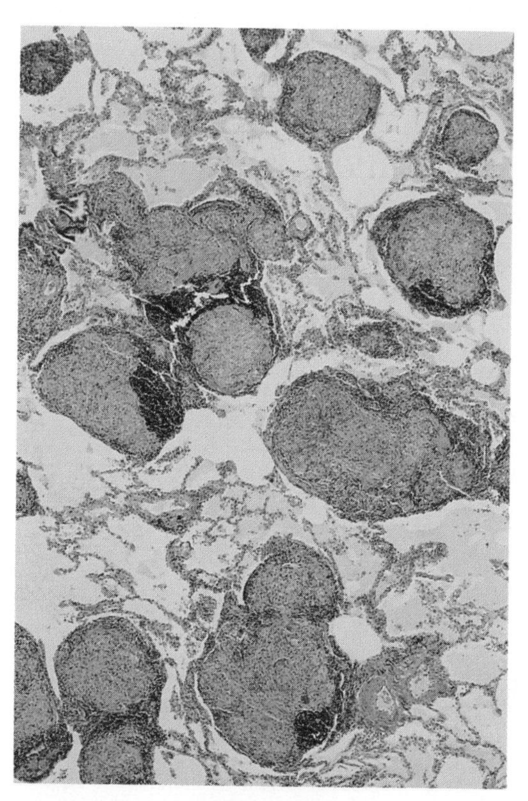

Figure 7-118.

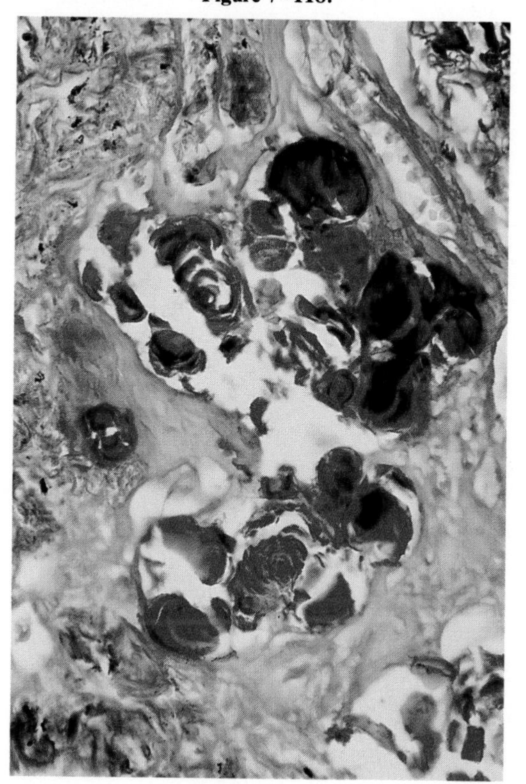

Figure 7-119.

■ Berylliosis (Figs. 7-118, 7-119)

Berylliosis is an acute or chronic lung disease caused by exposure to beryllium or its salts. The acute form follows a massive exposure, usually accidental. The chronic form is a hypersensitivity reaction, which may take decades to develop, underscoring the need for a careful occupational history.

The acute form of berylliosis is histologically identical to that of DAD, and the diagnosis depends on history, tissue analysis or both. The chronic form may be virtually identical to sarcoidosis, with confluent granulomas following lymphatic routes, or may resemble usual interstitial pneumonia with interstitial fibrosis with variable nongranulomatous chronic inflammatory infiltrate. Overlap between the two forms does occur, and honeycombing develops over time.

The diagnosis of berylliosis usually requires a constellation of findings, including occupational exposure; histologic changes consistent with berylliosis, especially granulomatous inflammation; clinical findings consistent with berylliosis; evidence of immunologic reactivity to beryllium; and when possible, documentation of beryllium in tissues. At least 1-7 gm of tissue is needed for analysis.

References

Churg A, Green FHY. Pathology of Occupational Lung Disease. New York, Igaku-Shoin Medical Publishers, 1988.

Dail DH, Hammer SP (eds). Pulmonary Pathology. New York, Springer-Verlag, 1988.

Freiman DG, Hardy HL. Beryllium disease: the relation of pulmonary pathology to clinical course and prognosis based on a study of 130 cases from the U.S. Beryllium Case Registry. Hum Pathol 1:25-44, 1970.

Thurlbeck WM (ed). Pathology of the Lung. New York, Thieme, 1988.

Figures 7-118, 7-119. Berylliosis. A biopsy specimen obtained two decades prior to death for interstitial lung disease shows coalescing non-necrotizing granulomas indistinguishable from those seen in sarcoidosis (Fig. 7-118). At the time of autopsy, granulomas were absent and only extensive fibrosis and honeycombing were found. Within the fibrous tissue, large accumulations of Schaumann's bodies, attesting to the prior granulomatous inflammation, were present (Fig. 7-119).

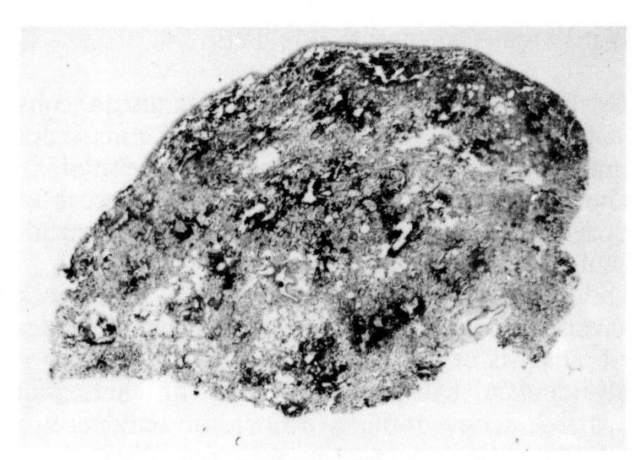

Figure 7–120.

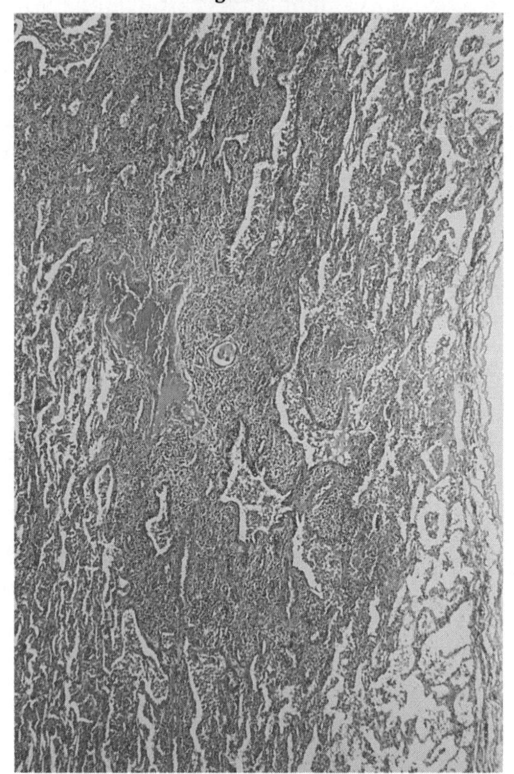

Figure 7–121.

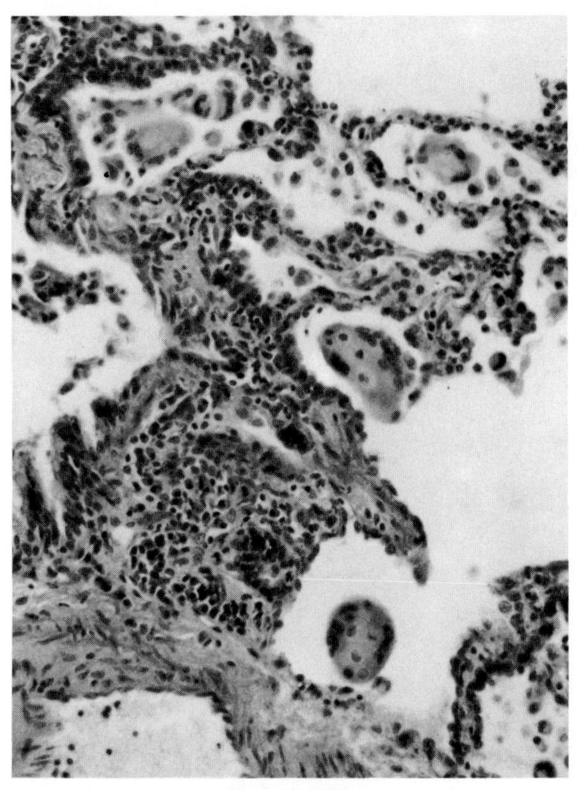

Figure 7–122.

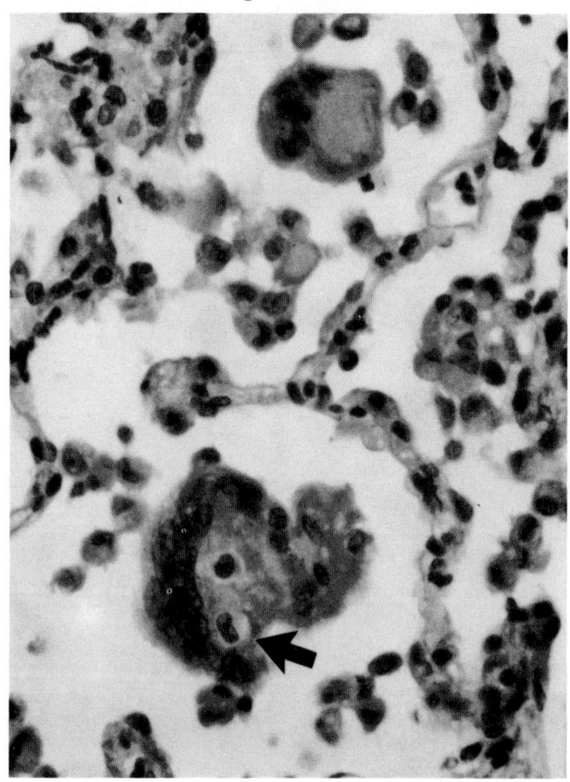

Figure 7–123.

Figures 7–120, 7–121, 7–122, 7–123. Giant cell interstitial pneumonia caused by hard metal pneumoconiosis. Inflammation and scarring are centered on small airways (Figs. 7–120, 7–121). The airways themselves are dilated and many contain mucus. The interstitial infiltrate is moderate to severe and is associated with accumulations of distinctive multinucleated giant cells in the adjacent airspaces. The giant cells show intact macrophages in their cytoplasm (arrow).

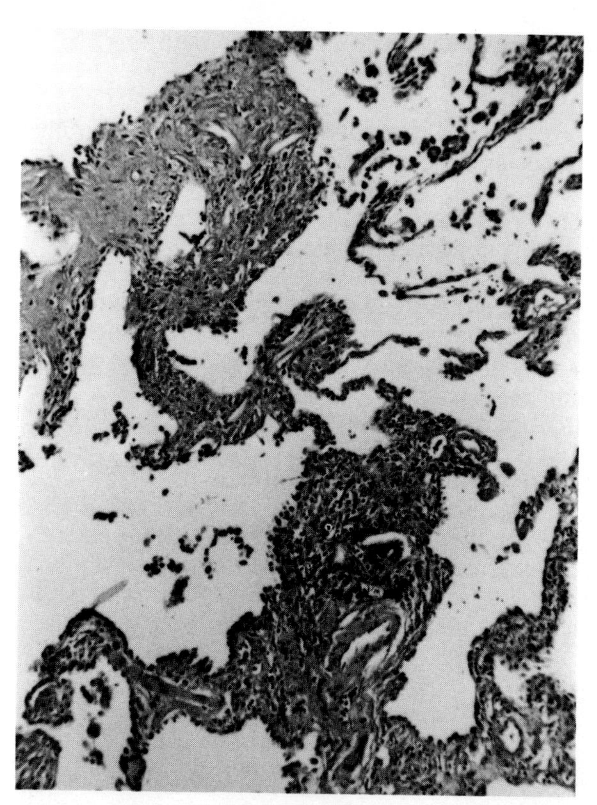

Figure 7–124.

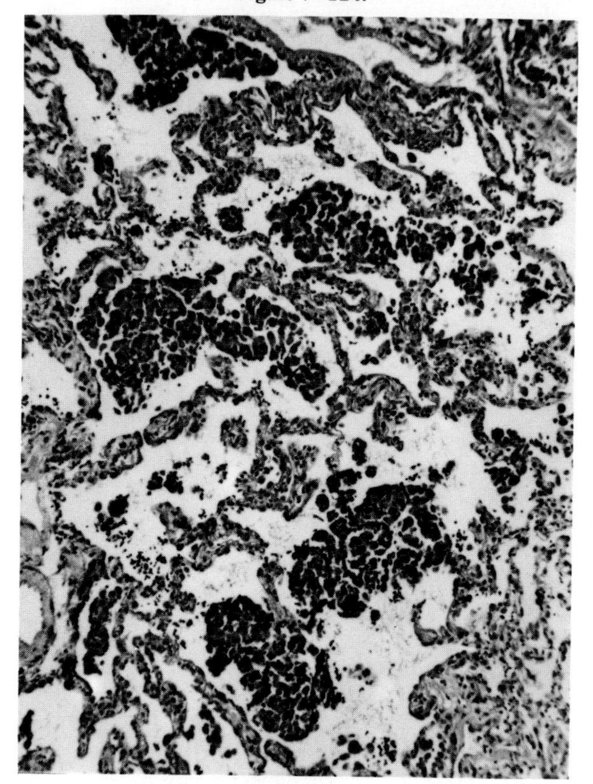

Figure 7–125.

■ Hard Metal Pneumoconiosis (Figs. 7–120 to 7–127)

This pneumoconiosis is caused by exposure to hard metals containing cobalt. Clinical symptoms include asthma or those of a chronic interstitial pneumonia.

The interstitial lung disease typically shows the following pattern of giant cell interstitial pneumonia: bronchiolocentric fibrosing interstitial pneumonia with bronchiolar and peribronchiolar fibrosis and increased macrophages in the airspaces associated with numerous giant cells, which may appear cannibalistic of other histiocytes. Less specific patterns resemble UIP or DIP with or without honeycombing, and diagnosis depends on tissue analysis and occupational history. Tissue from a paraffin block is sufficient for microprobe analysis. Cobalt may not be found because it is soluble, but other hard metals, usually tungsten, serve as a marker of exposure. In cases with only cobalt exposure (such as in diamond polishers), analysis may not be helpful. The classic histologic appearance of GIP should be considered hard metal pneumoconiosis until proven otherwise.

References

Austenfeld J, Colby TV. Hard metal asthma and interstitial lung disease. J Respir Dis 10:65–75, 1989.

Balmes JR. Respiratory effects of hard-metal dust exposure. State Art Rev Occup Med 2:327–344, 1987.

Churg A, Green FHY. Pathology of Occupational Lung Disease. New York, Igaku-Shoin Medical Publishers, 1988.

Ohori NP, Scuirba F, Owens G, Yousem SA. Giant cell pneumonia and hard metal pneumoconiosis. Am J Surg Pathol 13:581–587, 1989.

Figures 7–124, 7–125. Hard metal pneumoconiosis with fields resembling usual interstitial pneumonia (UIP) and desquamative interstitial pneumonia (DIP), respectively.

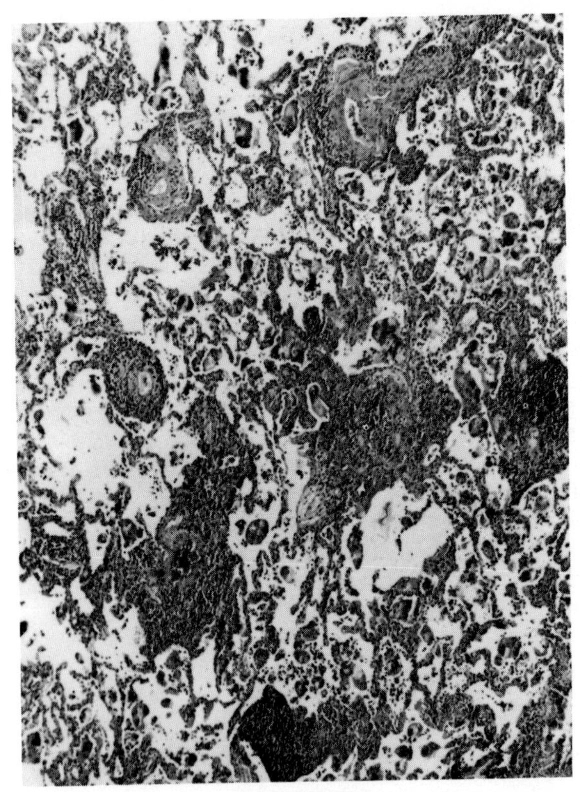

Figure 7-126.

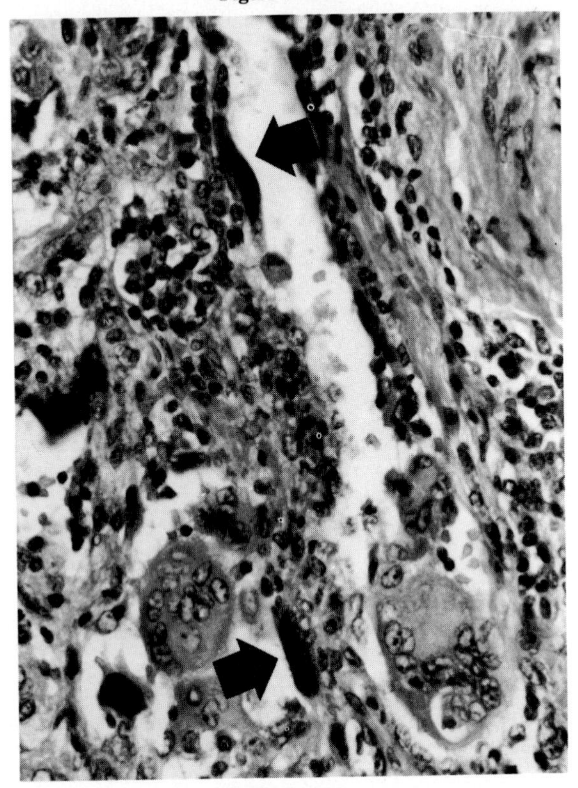

Figure 7-127.

Figures 7-126, 7-127. Giant cell interstitial pneumonia. Giant cell interstitial pneumonia not associated with hard metal exposure. There is patchy interstitial infiltrate associated with accumulations of giant cells, some of which show cannibalism. Multinucleated alveolar lining cells were also present (arrows). The patient was a housewife with no known history of exposure, and analysis failed to show any tungsten. Because an unclassified connective tissue disorder was present, the interstitial pneumonia was ascribed to that.

■ Intravenous Talcosis (Talc Granulomatosis) (Figs. 7-128, 7-129)

Intravenous (IV) talcosis results when talc and other fillers used for drugs intended for oral ingestion are deposited in the lung as a result of intravenous injection. The term IV talcosis is often used to distinguish this condition from inhalation talcosis.

Birefringent gray-white particulate material, ranging from a few microns to 20 or 30 μm in size is distributed along the pulmonary vasculature, usually along small vessels. There is characteristically a giant cell and/or granulomatous reaction.

A small amount of fibrosis may be present, and rarely, massive fibrosis is the result. Changes of pulmonary hypertension may be a concomitant finding.

IV-drug abusers are prone to a variety of pulmonary diseases (including those associated with AIDS), and one must be careful to assess whether IV talcosis is an incidental finding or whether some other problem is the explanation of the clinical problem.

References

Churg A, Green FHY. Pathology of Occupational Lung Disease. New York, Igaku-Shoin Medical Publishers, 1988.

Dail DH, Hammer SP (eds). Pulmonary Pathology. New York, Springer-Verlag, 1988.

Siegel H. Human pulmonary pathology associated with narcotic and other addictive drugs. Hum Pathol 3:55-66, 1972.

Thurlbeck WM (ed). Pathology of the Lung. New York, Thieme, 1988.

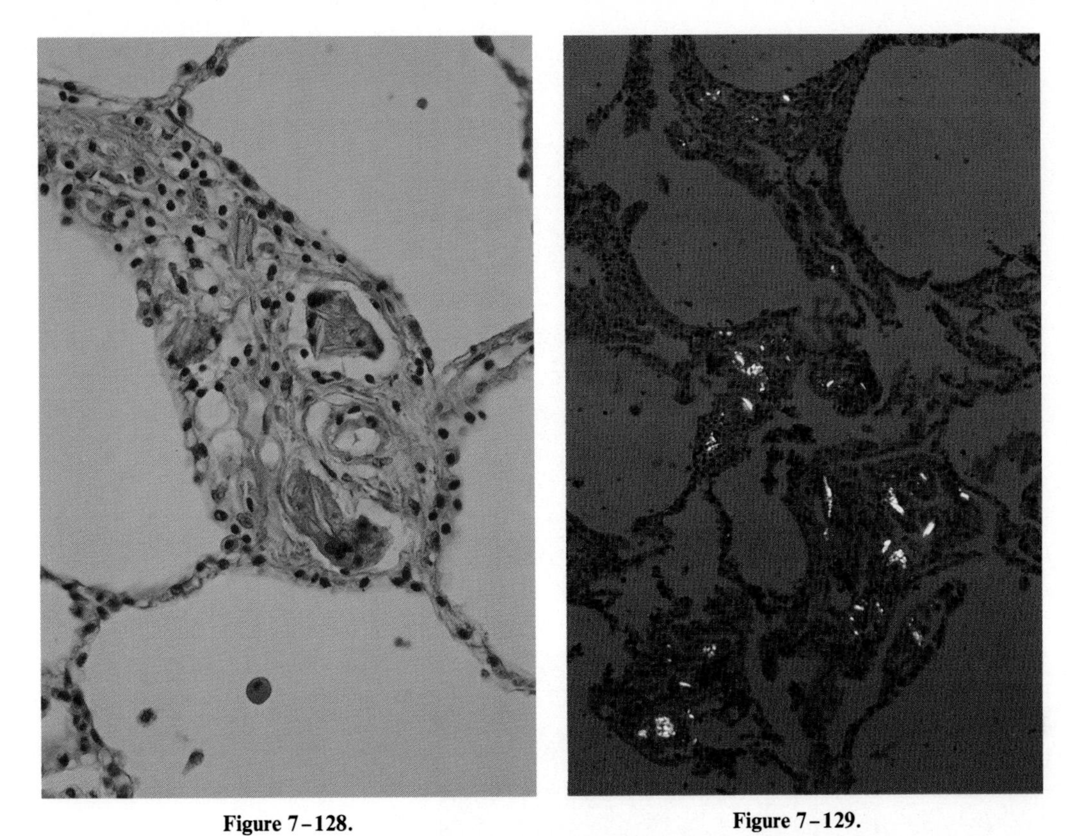

Figure 7-128. **Figure 7-129.**

Figures 7-128, 7-129. Intravenous talcosis (intravenous drug abuse). Interstitial widening and inflammation are restricted to the perivascular zones. Partial polarization reveals abundant birefringent material around the giant cells and granulomatous reaction. The talc can be appreciated without polarization as grayish material in giant cells.

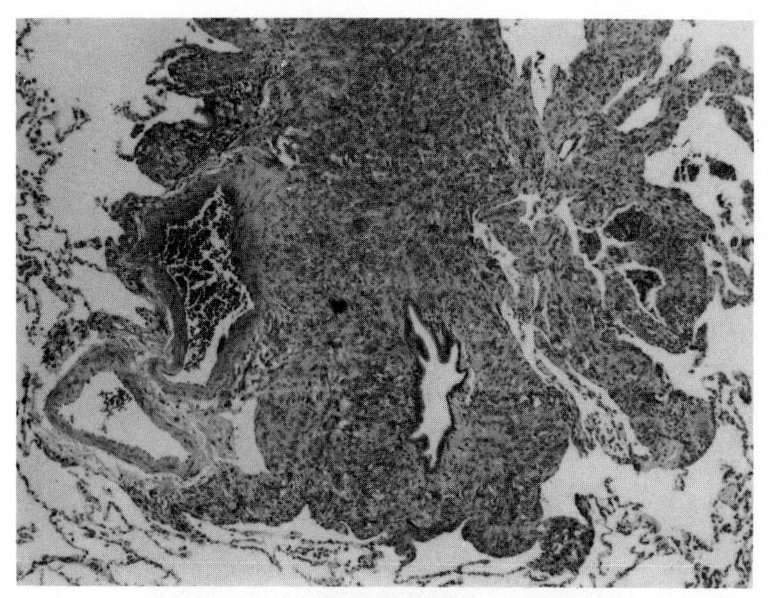

Figure 7–130.

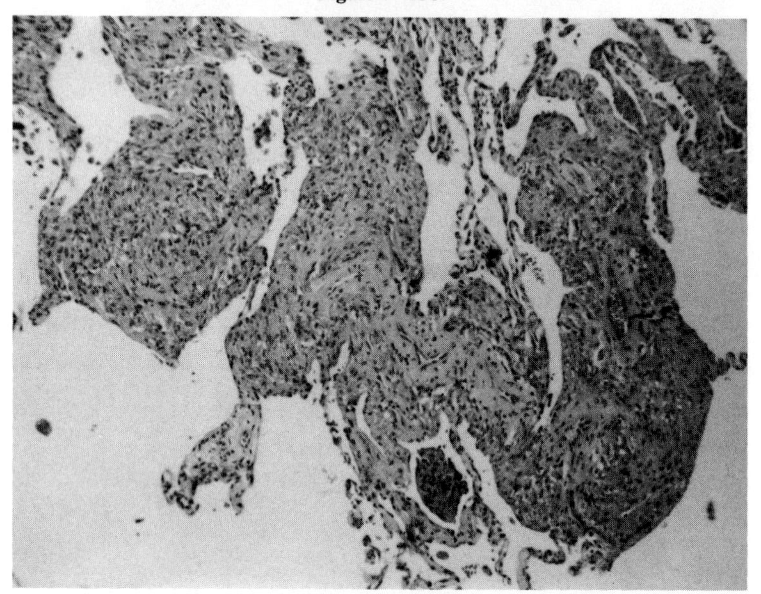

Figure 7–131.

Figures 7–130, 7–131, 7–132. Mixed-dust pneumoconiosis. A predominant pattern of early silicosis is shown. There are peribronchiolar and perivascular infiltrates of histiocytes that contain numerous small flecks of material. Within some of the clusters, early fibrotic silicotic nodule formation is apparent (Fig. 7–132).

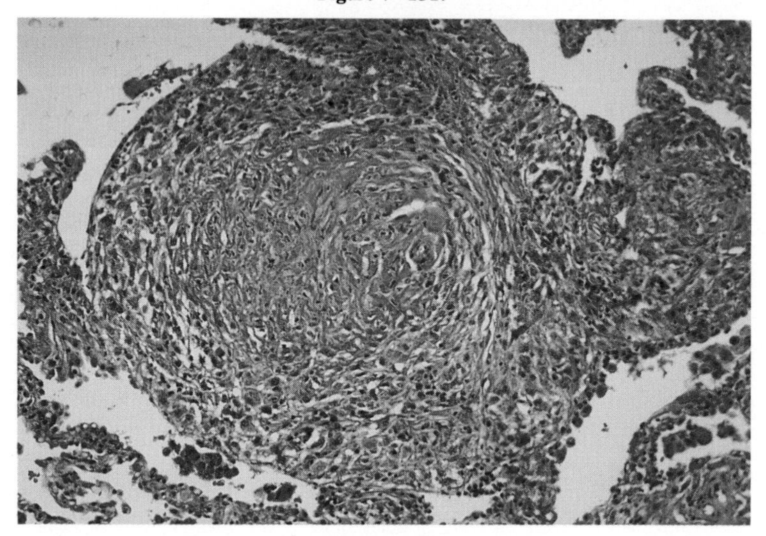

Figure 7–132.

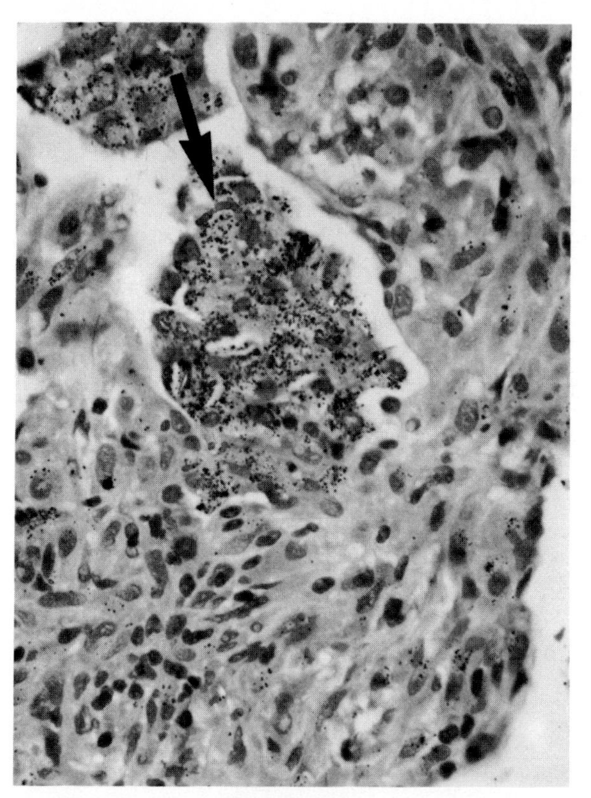

Figure 7-133.

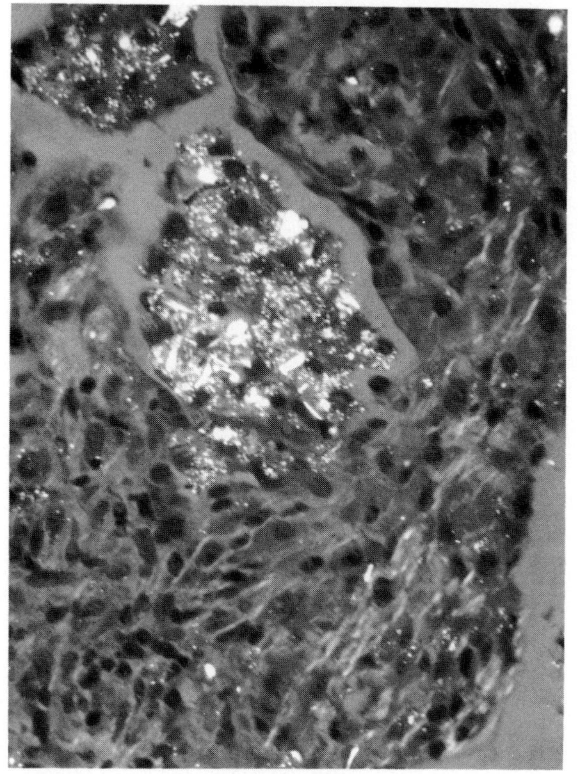

Figure 7-134.

■ Mixed-Dust Pneumoconiosis (Figs. 7-130 to 7-134)

Lung disease caused by a mixture of dusts is relatively common. Anthracosilicosis is such an example. Non-asbestos silicates commonly are contaminated with silica, resulting in a mixed silica/silicate pneumoconiosis. Nodular fibrosis in such cases is probably caused by the silica. Nevertheless, histiocyte infiltrates by themselves, if massive enough, may be associated with clinical findings of interstitial lung disease.

References

Churg A, Green FHY. Pathology of Occupational Lung Disease. New York, Igaku-Shoin Medical Publishers, 1988.

Figures 7-133, 7-134. Mixed-dust pneumoconiosis. The same case illustrated in Figures 7-130 to 7-132 reveals interstitial and airspace accumulations of macrophages with particulate material including an occasional asbestos body (arrow). Polarization of this field shows a large amount of birefringent material. The brightly birefringent large particles represent silicates, and the smaller, more weakly birefringent particles are silica. This case, then, is a mixed-dust pneumoconiosis with evidence of asbestos exposure, silica exposure, silicate exposure, and anthracosis. The basic pattern is that of silicosis with early nodule formation.

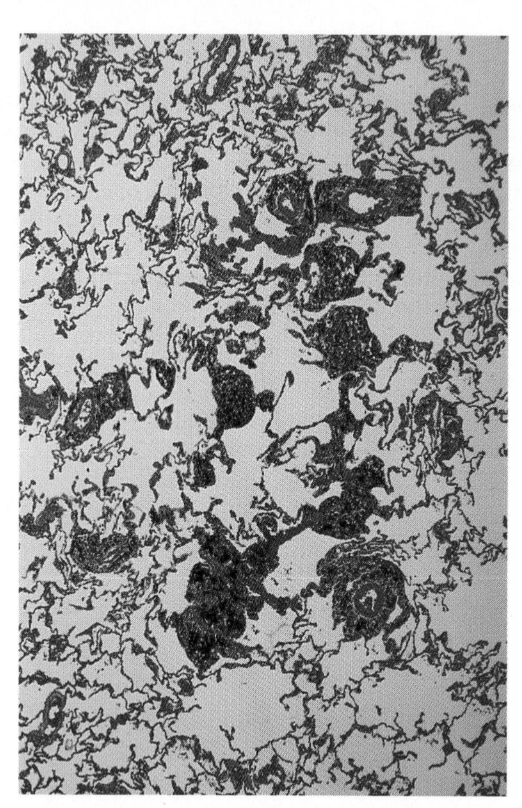

Figure 7–135. Anthracosis. Anthracosis in a coal miner. There is a dust macule caused by accumulations of macrophages containing anthracotic pigment around the respiratory bronchioles.

■ Other Pneumoconioses

Many other dusts may be associated with lung disease, but biopsy is performed only rarely. In most of these cases, there is obvious exposure history and the diagnosis is based on clinical grounds. Anthracosis is common in coal miners (coal workers' pneumoconiosis), and lesser degrees are seen in cigarette smokers and urban dwellers (Fig. 7–135).

References

Churg A, Green FHY. Pathology of Occupational Lung Disease. New York, Igaku-Shoin Medical Publishers, 1988.

Dail DH, Hammer SP (eds). Pulmonary Pathology. New York, Springer-Verlag, 1988.

Thurlbeck WM (ed). Pathology of the Lung. New York, Thieme, 1988.

■ Eosinophilic Granuloma (Langerhans Cell Granulomatosis, Pulmonary Histiocytosis X)
(Figs. 7–136 to 7–146)

This is a chronic interstitial pneumonia caused by a proliferation of Langerhans cells associated with fibrosis and other inflammatory cells in a nodular distribution in the lung. Chest radiograph shows bilateral nodular or reticulonodular infiltrates that often show an upper-lobe predilection. The vast majority of adults with pulmonary eosinophilic granuloma are smokers in the third to fifth decades of life. The female-to-male ratio is 2:1. Patients with this disorder may present with constitutional symptoms, signs and symptoms of interstitial lung disease, pneumothorax, or an abnormal radiograph without symptomatology. The disease is analogous to sarcoid; there is an active phase, following which an inactive healed phase occurs without significant functional deficits in the majority of patients. Some cases are identified by routine radiographic evaluation, making it likely that many cases never come to clinical attention.

Early cellular lesions are peribronchiolar or centered on alveolar ducts. These progress to fibrotic scars with a distribution difficult to discern. Cellular lesions have a proliferation of Langerhans cells and a variable number of eosinophils and other inflammatory cells. Central scarring develops, and there are pigmented macrophages (smoker's macrophages) caught up in the fibrosis with a surrounding pseudo–DIP reaction. As the scar enlarges, the active cellular zones are at the periphery. Holes may develop in the center, and microscopic emphysema—a form of peri-cicatrical emphysema—may be seen in the lung parenchyma surrounding the nodules. In the majority of cases, the lesions burn out and leave scattered fibrous scars with intervening normal or emphysematous tissue. A minority of cases are progressive and lead to death with fibrotic but hyperinflated rather than shrunken lungs.

The classic lesion of eosinophilic granuloma is a stellate or somewhat rounded, discrete interstitial fibrous nodule with a cellular periphery in which the Langerhans cells can be identified. Open lung biopsy usually shows multiple nodules at different stages of histologic evolution: some active and cellular, some old and fibrotic.

Langerhans cells are positive with the following stains: S100, OKT6, and HLA–DR. These stains may be useful in enhancing the presence of Langerhans cells.

The key to the diagnosis is the low-power recognition of scattered nodules centered on airways. Because the nodules are scattered, there is the potential for sampling error. A pseudo–DIP reaction is frequent around the lesions of the eosinophilic granuloma. UIP is also in the differential diagnosis, but UIP is rarely associated with such discrete fibrous nodules. The eosinophils are rarely so prominent or pooled within airspaces as to make eosinophilic pneumonia a serious consideration. Pneumothorax-induced eosinophilic pleuritis may occasionally mimic a lesion of the eosinophilic granuloma; lesions of eosinophilic granuloma should be sought in the deeper parenchyma.

References

Colby TV, Lombard C. Histiocytosis X presenting in the lung. Hum Pathol 14:847–856, 1983.
Dail DH, Hammer SP (eds). Pulmonary Pathology. New York, Springer-Verlag, 1988.
Katzenstein ALA, Askin FB. Surgical Pathology of Non-Neoplastic Lung Disease, 2nd ed. Philadelphia, WB Saunders Co, 1990.
Thurlbeck WM (ed). Pathology of the Lung. New York, Thieme, 1988.

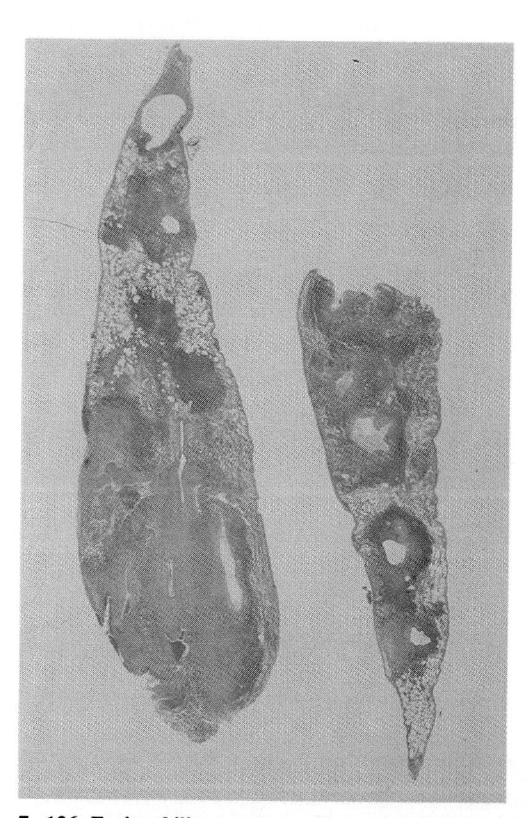

Figure 7–136. Eosinophilic granuloma. The nodules of eosinophilic granuloma are often best appreciated using the naked eye to examine the slide. Typically, the nodules are discrete and vary in cellularity and size. Some of them contain holes.

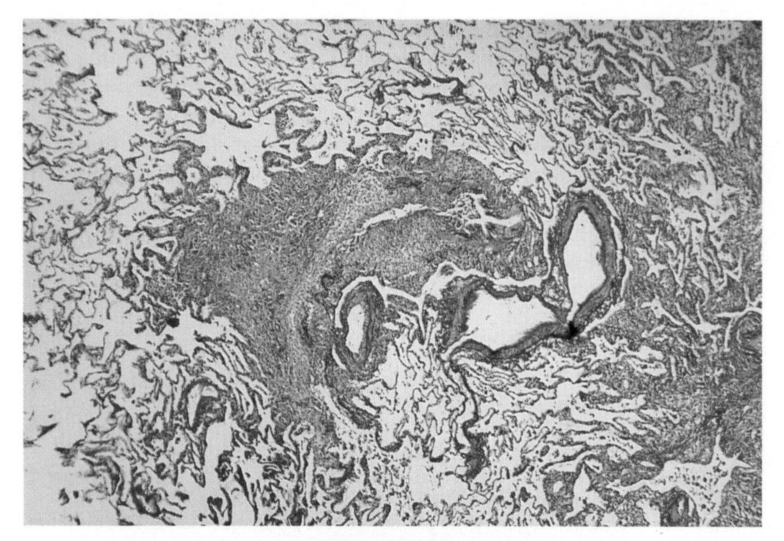

Figure 7–137.

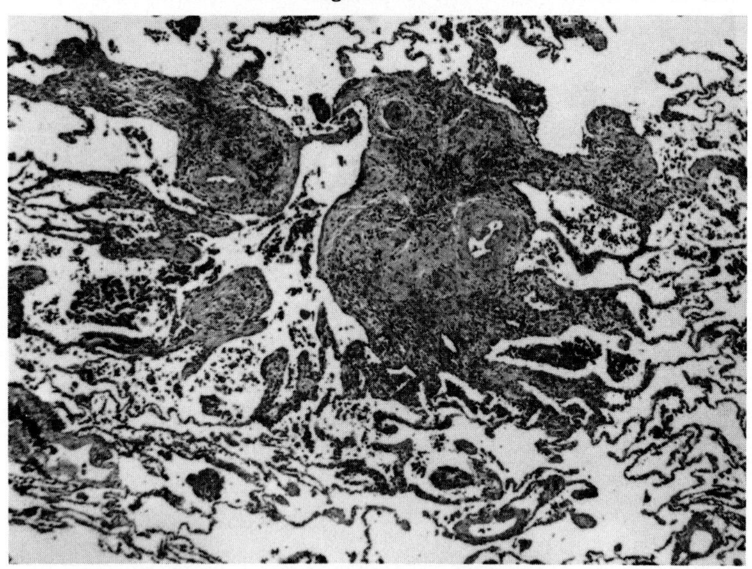

Figure 7–138.

Figures 7–137, 7–138, 7–139. Eosinophilic granuloma. The earliest lesions of eosinophilic granuloma are proliferations of Langerhans cells in the walls of small airways. As the lesions expand, they become stellate, and their bronchiolocentric location may be difficult to identify. They then look simply like an interstitial infiltrate. These three figures all illustrate bronchiolocentricity.

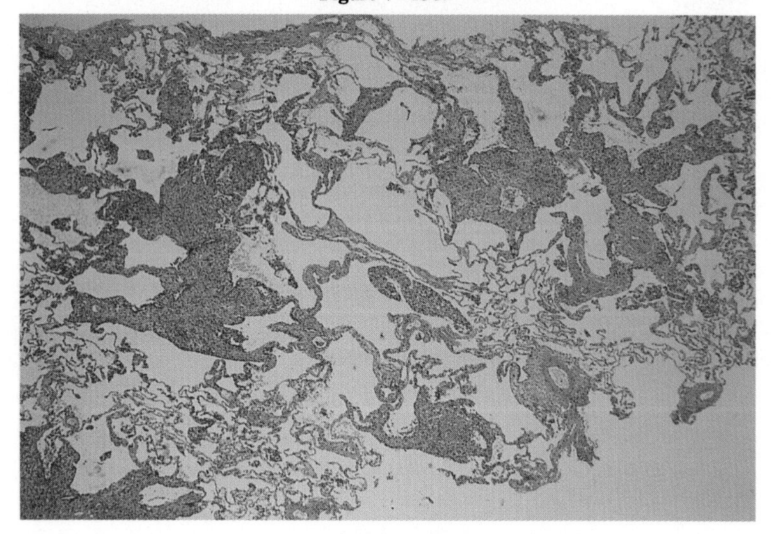

Figure 7–139.

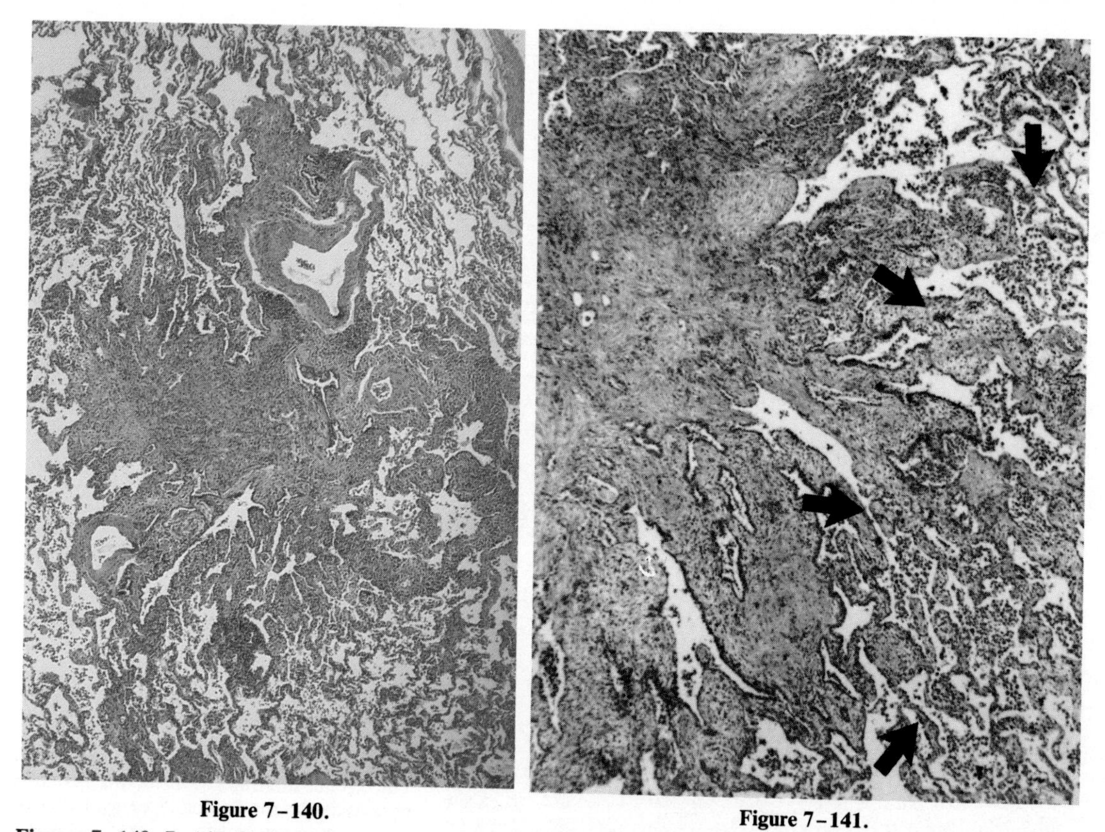

Figure 7-140. **Figure 7-141.**

Figures 7-140, 7-141. Eosinophilic granuloma. The classic lesion of eosinophilic granuloma is a stellate interstitial nodule with central fibrosis and peripheral cellularity in which one searches for clusters of Langerhans cells. A pseudo-DIP (pseudo-desquamative interstitial pneumonia) reaction in the airspaces adjacent to these nodules (arrows) is characteristic and may be extensive.

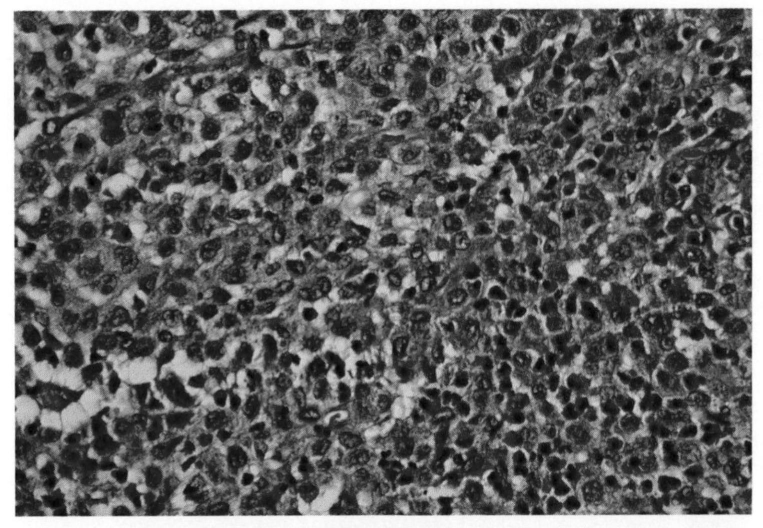

Figure 7-142.

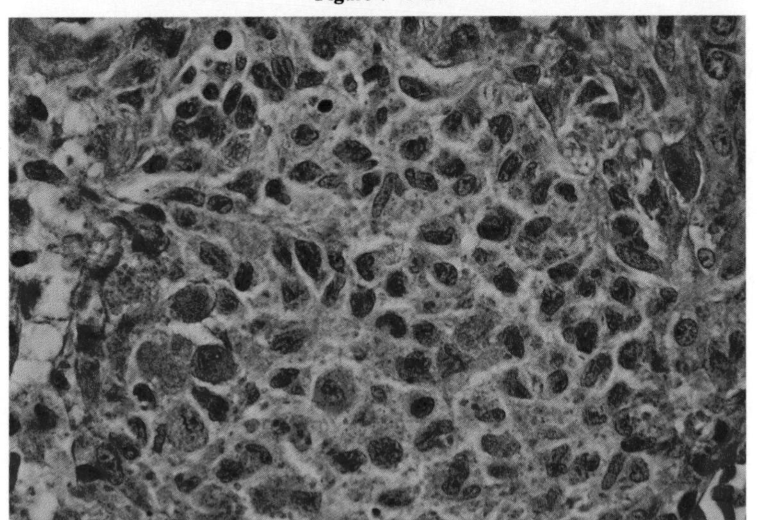

Figure 7-143.

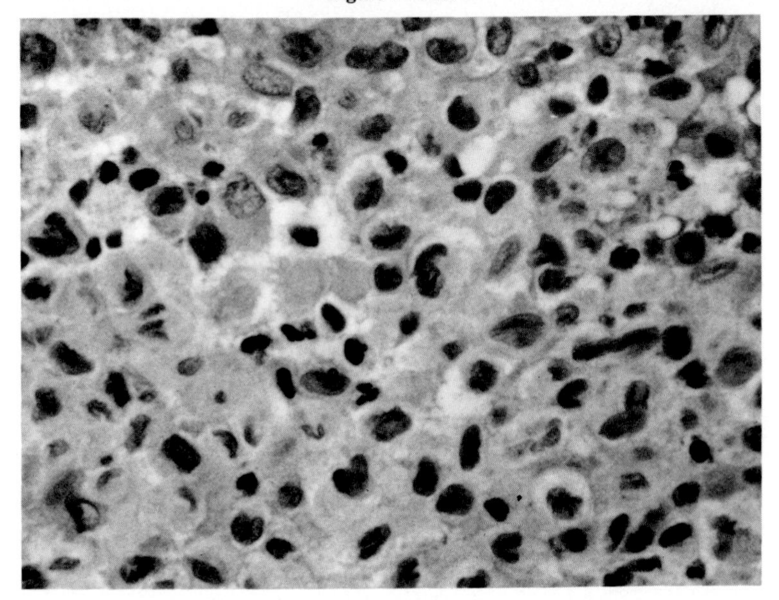

Figure 7-144.

Figures 7-142, 7-143, 7-144. Eosinophilic granuloma. The cellular infiltrates in the nodules are mixed; the diagnosis relies on the finding of Langerhans-type histiocytes with their characteristic nuclear folds and convolutions (Figs. 7-143, 7-144). The amount of eosinophils present ranges from very few to large pools (Fig. 7-142 [See area at lower right]) and even to eosinophil microabscesses. Pigmented alveolar macrophages are often interspersed, and they can be recognized by their tan-brown cytoplasmic pigmentation and prominent cytoplasmic borders (Fig. 7-143).

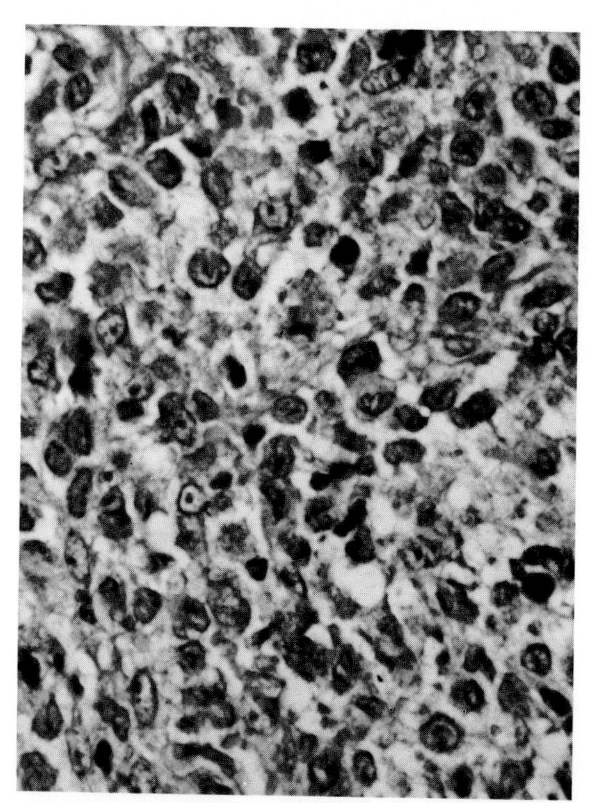

Figure 7-145. Eosinophilic granuloma. In many cases, the nuclear features of the Langerhans cells are somewhat obscured and difficult to appreciate, probably owing to the fixation procedure. They may appear "blown up." In the field illustrated, which consists almost entirely of Langerhans cells, only a few of the cells show the typical nuclear features.

■ Eosinophilic Pleuritis (Figs. 7-147 to 7-149)

In eosinophilic pleuritis, a pleural reaction is induced by the presence of air in the pleural space, usually as a result of pneumothorax. This reaction is limited to the pleura and is associated with sheets of mesothelial cells, macrophages, and numerous eosinophils.

The underlying lung tissue often shows subpleural blebs, and these are thought to be the cause of the pneumothorax. Careful cytologic assessment usually allows one to distinguish mesothelial cells from the Langerhans cells. Eosinophilic pleuritis, of course, can occur in patients with underlying parenchymal disease that has caused pneumothorax, such as eosinophilic granuloma or lymphangioleiomyomatosis.

References

Askin FB, McCann BG, Kuhn C. Reactive eosinophilic pleuritis: a lesion to be distinguished from pulmonary eosinophilic granuloma. Arch Pathol Lab Med 101:187-192, 1977.

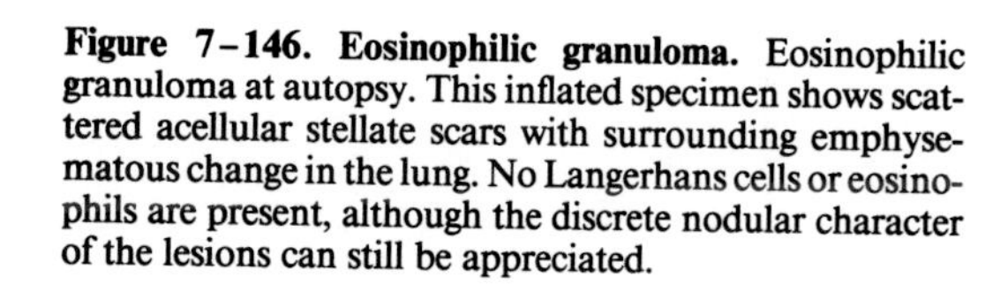

Figure 7-146. Eosinophilic granuloma. Eosinophilic granuloma at autopsy. This inflated specimen shows scattered acellular stellate scars with surrounding emphysematous change in the lung. No Langerhans cells or eosinophils are present, although the discrete nodular character of the lesions can still be appreciated.

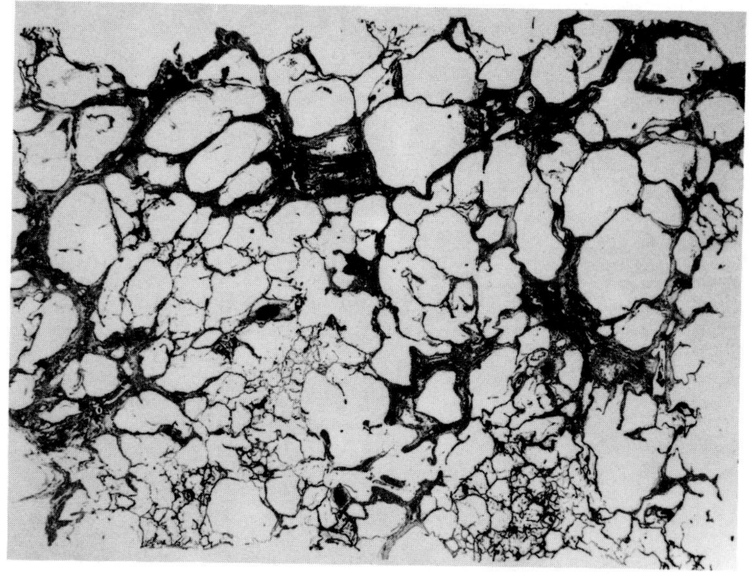

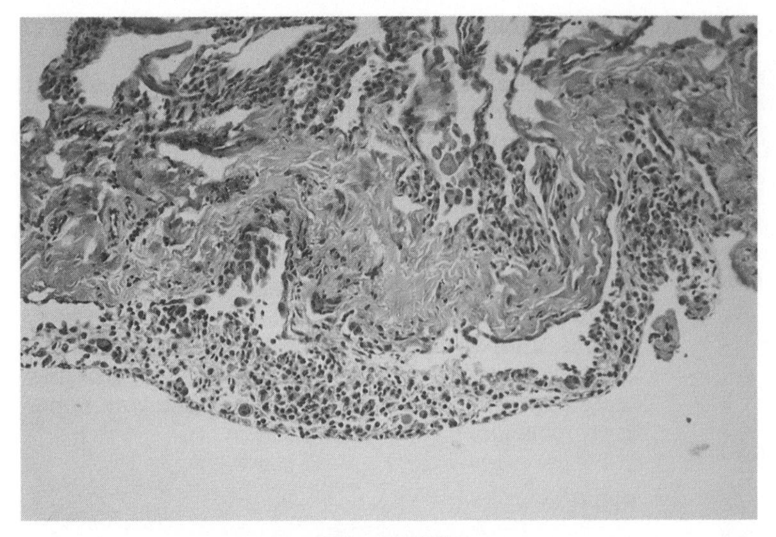

Figure 7-147.

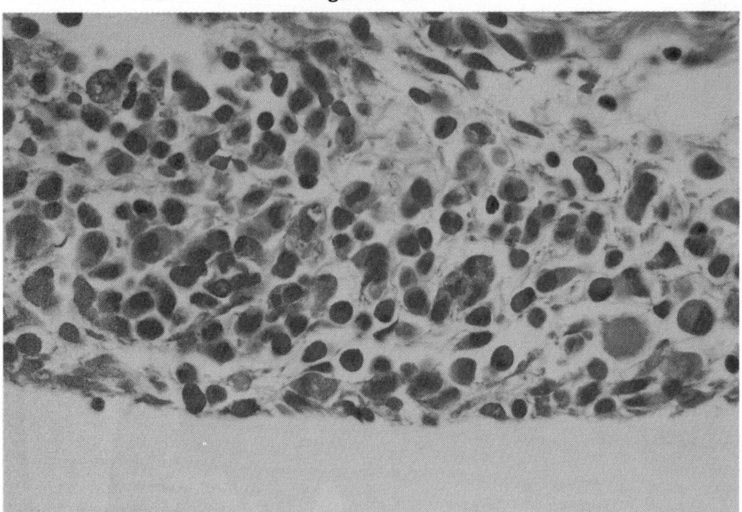

Figure 7-148.

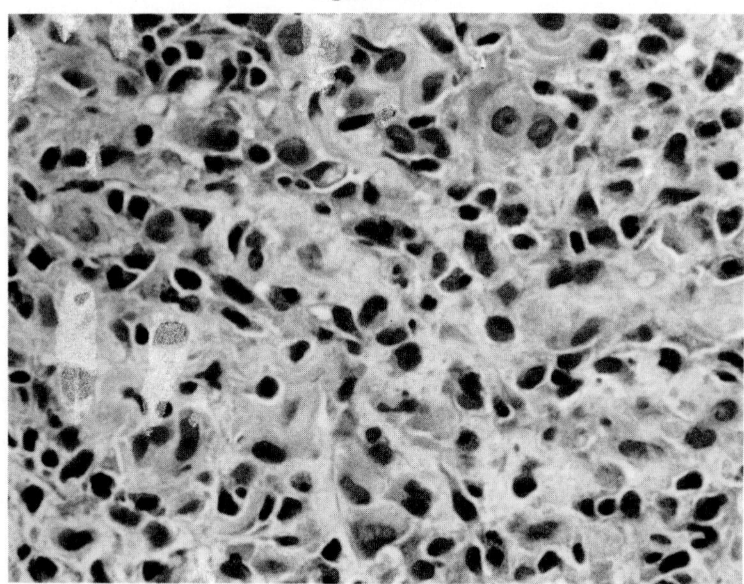

Figure 7-149.

Figures 7-147, 7-148, 7-149. Eosinophilic pleuritis. Eosinophilic pleuritis related to pneumothorax. A cellular proliferation in the pleura is mixed in composition and includes large numbers of eosinophils. Some of the reactive mesothelial cells may have nuclear features suggestive of Langerhans cells. Lesions of eosinophilic granuloma are predominantly intraparenchymal (although the pleura may be affected). One of the specimens (Fig. 7-149) was actually obtained from a patient who had pneumothorax caused by eosinophilic granuloma, the lesions of which were found elsewhere.

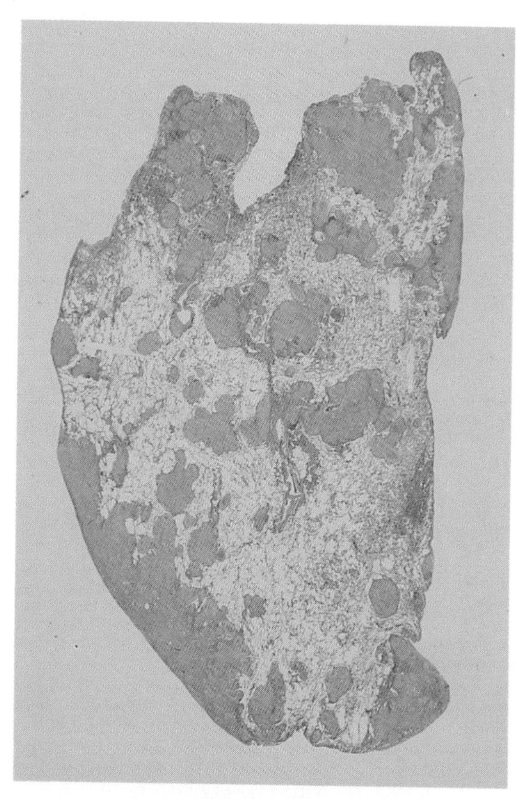

Figure 7-150.

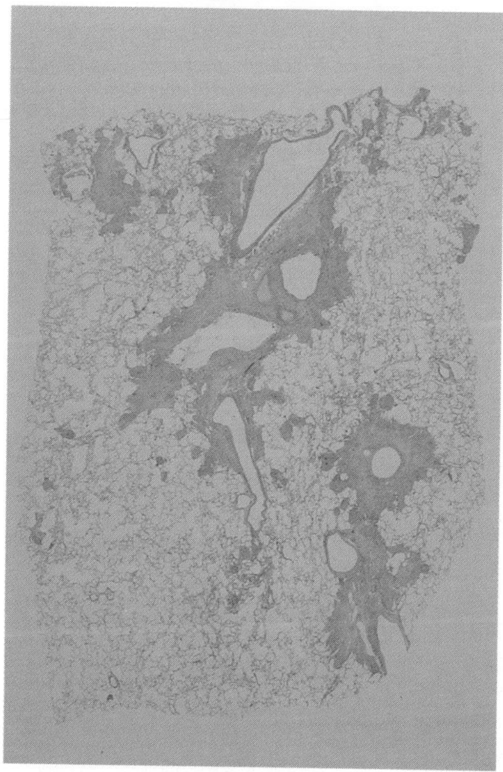

Figure 7-151.

Figures 7-150, 7-151. Sarcoidosis. Sarcoidosis represents an idiopathic granulomatous disease that becomes manifest in the lung as granulomatous inflammation along lymphatic routes. This is shown in an open lung biopsy specimen from a patient with symptoms and a positive chest radiograph (Fig. 7-150) and as an incidental finding at autopsy from a patient who died in a motor vehicle accident (Fig. 7-151).

■ Sarcoidosis (Figs. 7-150 to 7-171)

Sarcoidosis is a systemic granulomatous disease of unknown cause associated with granulomas in a variety of organs. The lung is usually involved even when the chest radiograph is normal. An interstitial reticular or reticulonodular infiltrate with hilar adenopathy is typical and may show an upper-lobe distribution. Some cases feature parenchymal nodules, which may simulate metastatic disease (nodular sarcoid), and in some cases, necrosis may occur in the nodules (necrotizing sarcoid), suggesting an infection.

In *classical sarcoid,* one sees non-necrotizing coalescing granulomas distributed along lymphatic routes in the pleura and septa and along bronchovascular structures. Invasion of vessel walls and intimal granulomas are quite typical but are only rarely associated with necrosis or clinical findings of vascular disease. Granulomas may cause airway obstruction, and obstructive or organizing pneumonia may be seen in otherwise typical sarcoidosis. Sarcoid granulomas tend to form confluent masses, which become quite large in the case of *nodular sarcoid.* A small amount of central fibrinoid degeneration or necrosis is common in classic sarcoid granulomas and should not lead to a diagnosis of necrotizing sarcoid or necrotizing granulomatous inflammation. In most cases, there is an inconspicuous interstitial mononuclear cell infiltrate. In *necrotizing sarcoid,* there is extensive necrosis, sometimes with acute inflammation, and the appearance is more suggestive of an infectious granuloma, which is the main differential diagnosis.

There are a number of unusual patterns, including (1) complete parenchymal consolidation by granulomas, in florid cases of sarcoidosis, (2) pulmonary arterial or venous hypertension caused by vascular involvement (arteriolar and/or venous), (3) massive pleural involvement with effusions, (4) marked cellular interstitial infiltrate associated with the granulomas.

In most cases, sarcoid heals to leave normal or slightly scarred lung with hyalinized lamellar fibrosis with entrapped giant cells and Schaumann's bodies. In a minority of cases, progressive scarring with honeycombing may ensue. Early on in such cases, the fibrosis shows a distribution similar to that of the granulomas (i.e., along lymphatic routes). In healed sarcoid, calcified Schaumann's bodies may remain in the fibrous tissue as a marker of the prior granulomatous inflammation.

Transbronchial biopsy is useful in the diagnosis of sarcoidosis, even in the presence of a normal chest radiograph, because the granulomas are distributed along lymphatic routes and hence are accessible to biopsy through the wall of an airway. Granulomatous lymphadenitis should be distinguished from the histiocytic clusters that are characteristic in normal hilar lymph nodes.

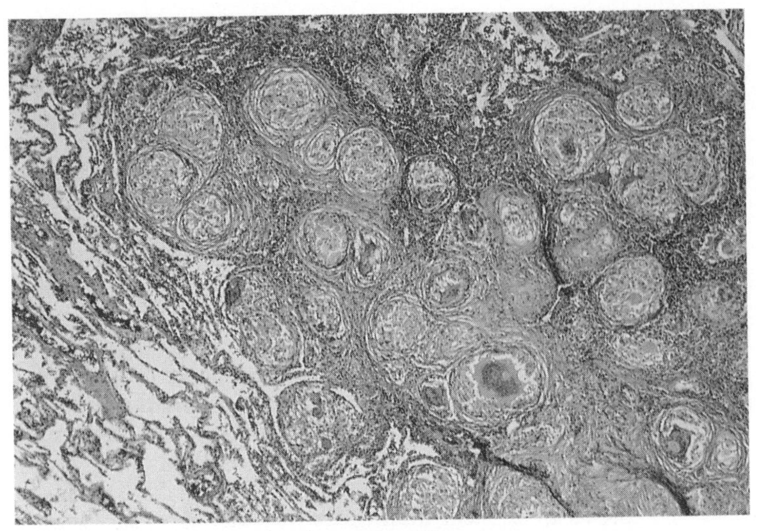

Figure 7-152.

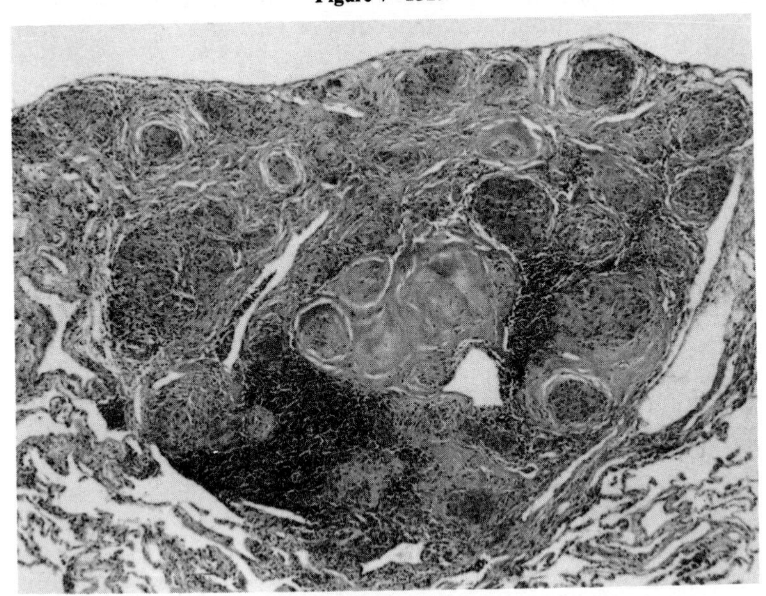

Figure 7-153.

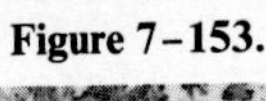

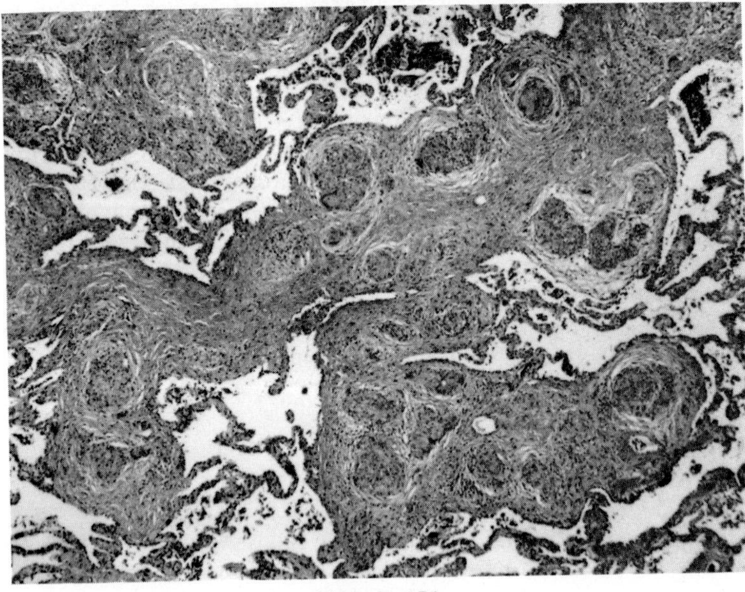

Figure 7-154.

Figures 7-152, 7-153, 7-154. Sarcoidosis. There are confluent nodules of non-necrotizing granulomas associated with a variable degree of inflammation and fibrosis in the pleura (Fig. 7-153) and along the septa and vascular structures (Fig. 7-154).

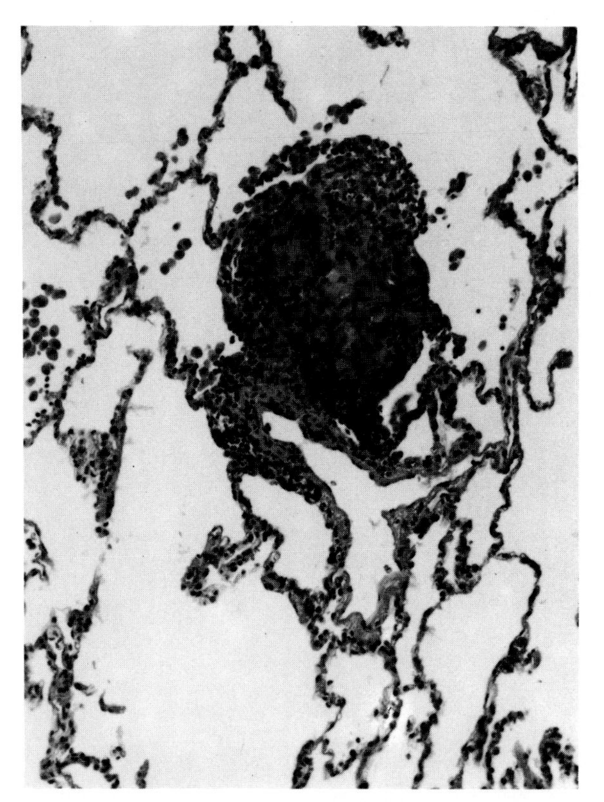

Figure 7–155. Sarcoidosis. An early perivascular granuloma manifests as a loose cluster of epithelioid histiocytes with surrounding lymphocytes.

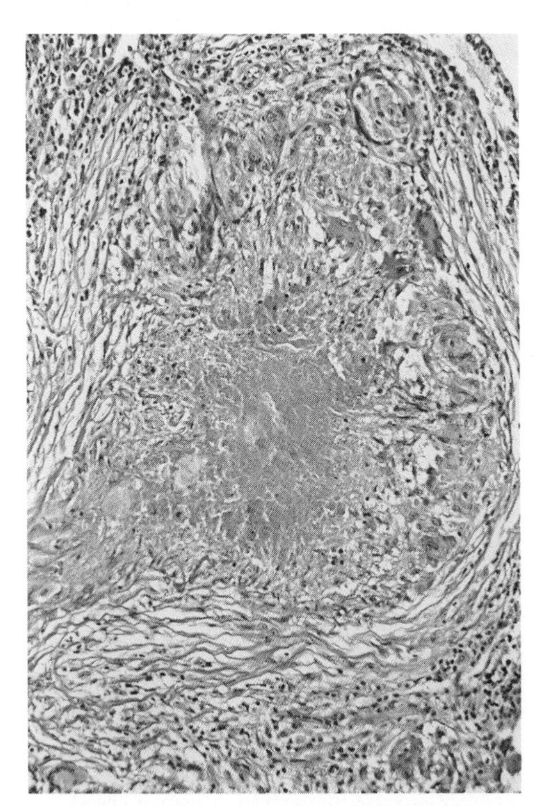

Figure 7–156. Sarcoidosis. A small amount of fibrinoid necrosis in the centers of a few granulomas may be seen in sarcoidosis. In the case illustrated, all cultures and special stains were negative and there was no evidence of infection at 1-year follow-up.

References

Dail DH, Hammer SP (eds). Pulmonary Pathology. New York, Springer-Verlag, 1988.

Flint A, Colby TV. Surgical Pathology of Diffuse Infiltrative Lung Disease. Orlando, Grune & Stratton Co, 1987.

Thurlbeck WM (ed). Pathology of the Lung. New York, Thieme, 1988.

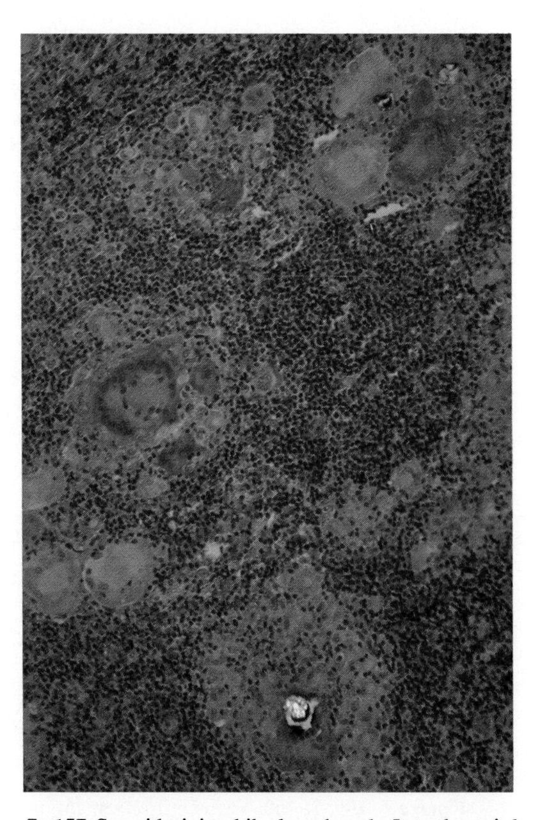

Figure 7–157. Sarcoidosis in a hilar lymph node. Intrathoracic lymphadenopathy is extremely common in sarcoidosis. In this partially polarized biopsy specimen, one can appreciate birefringent calcifications associated with the granulomas. This finding should not be taken as evidence of foreign material.

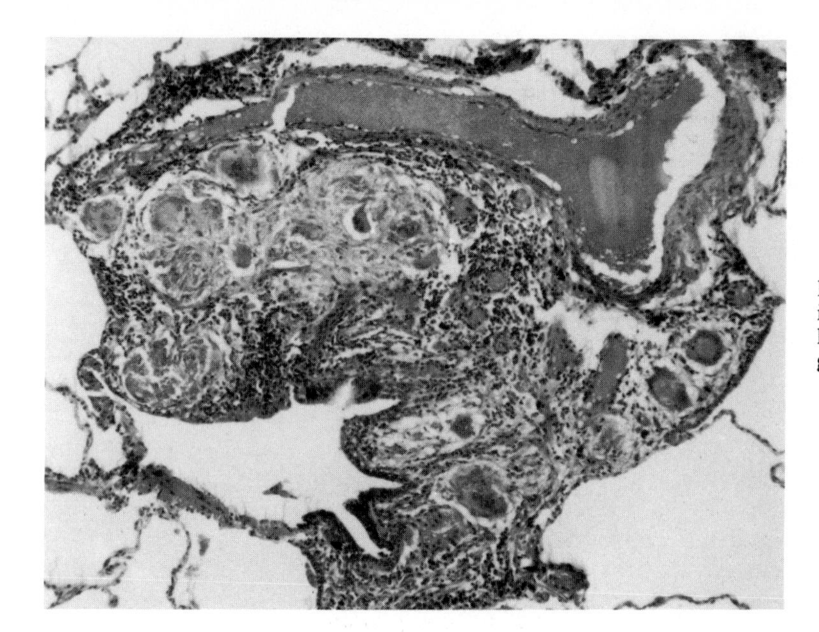

Figure 7–158. Sarcoidosis. Peribronchiolar granuloma in an open lung biopsy specimen from a patient with hilar lymphadenopathy and an otherwise normal chest radiograph.

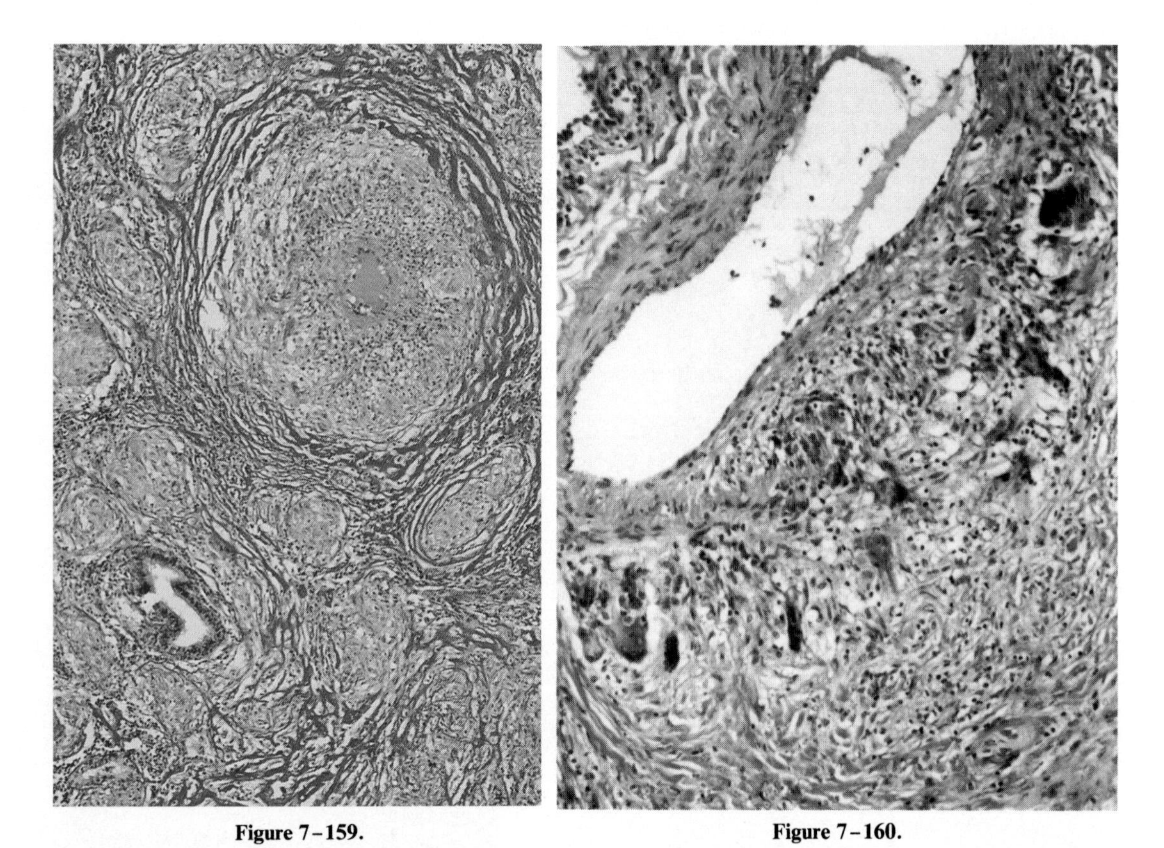

Figure 7–159. **Figure 7–160.**

Figures 7–159, 7–160. Vascular involvement in sarcoidosis. Adventitial, intramural, and even intimal granulomas are extremely common in pulmonary arteries and veins. They may entirely replace the vessel wall with no apparent ill effects clinically. Bright eosinophilic lamellar hyalinized collagen is also a common finding.

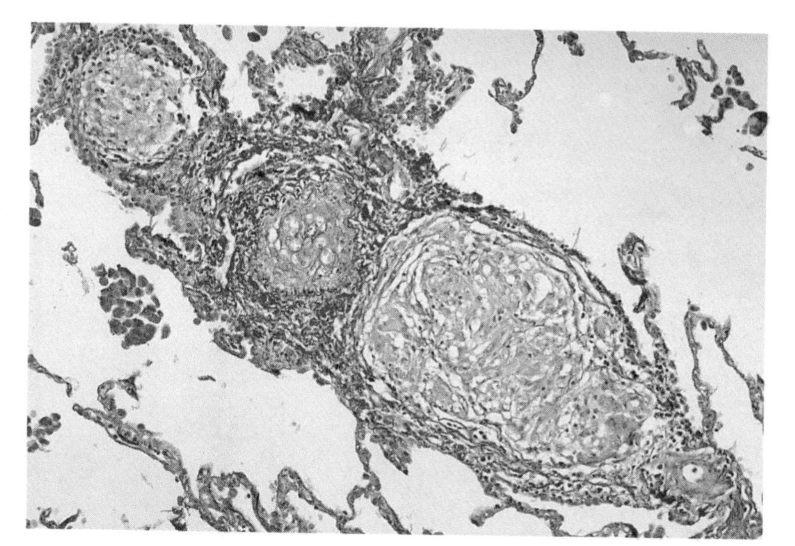

Figure 7-161. Venous occlusion associated with sarcoidosis. Signs and symptoms of pulmonary hypertension were evident, and on the basis of the lung biopsy findings, sarcoidosis with secondary venous obstruction was diagnosed. In the field illustrated, two granulomas can be seen around a small pulmonary vein that is entirely occluded, as highlighted by an elastic tissue stain.

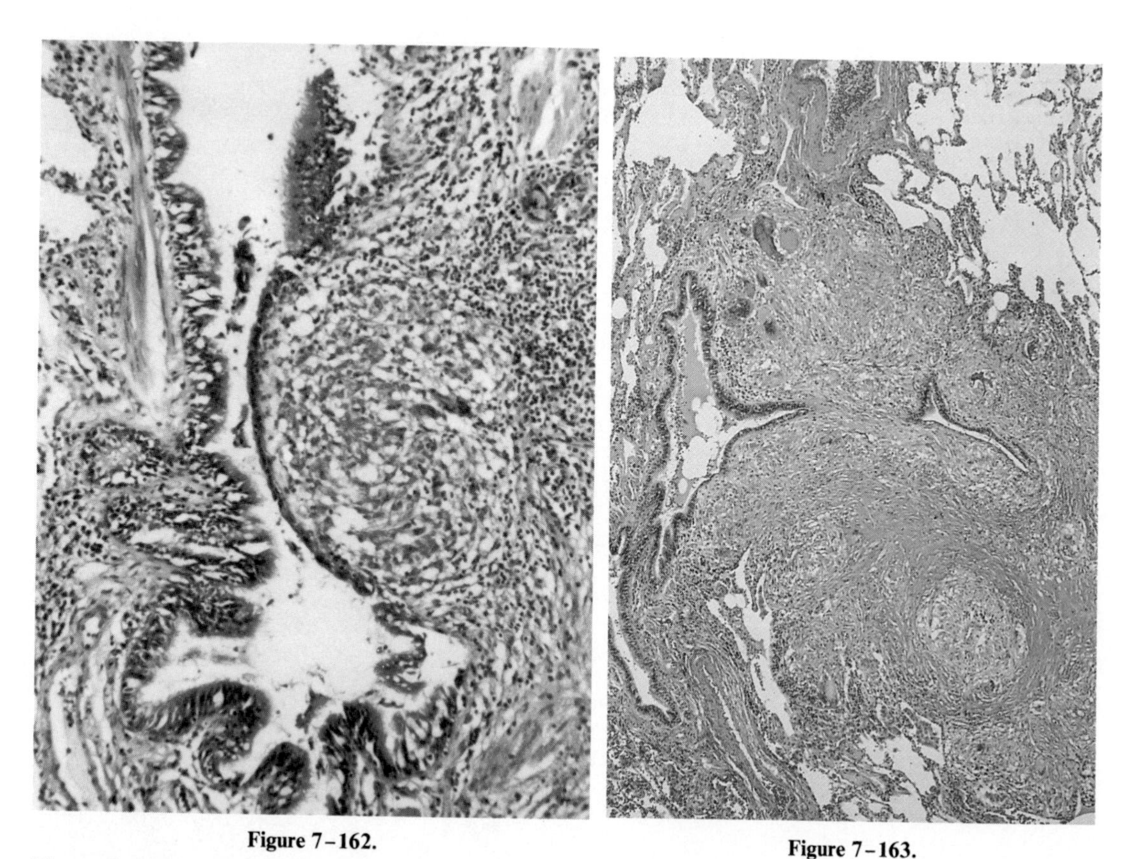

Figure 7-162. **Figure 7-163.**

Figures 7-162, 7-163. Airway involvement in sarcoidosis. Granulomas within the mucosa and wall of small and large airways are common in sarcoidosis and may even be visible bronchoscopically. Only rarely is sarcoidosis associated with clinical evidence of obstruction, but it was in the case illustrated in Figure 7-163, in which luminal narrowing is associated with granulomas.

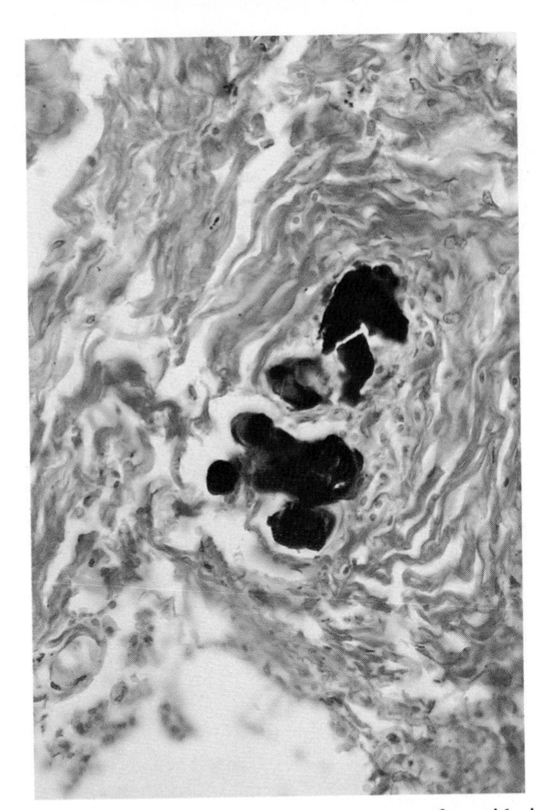

Figure 7–164. Healed sarcoidosis. The granulomas of sarcoidosis may disappear entirely or may leave a residue of scarring behind, which often shows a lymphatic distribution. In some cases, one can find calcified Schaumann's bodies embedded within the fibrous tissue as evidence of the prior granulomatous inflammation.

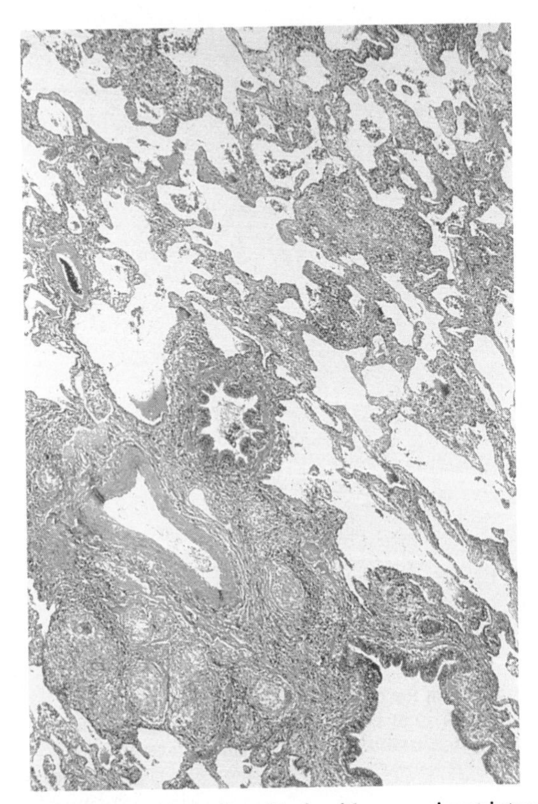

Figure 7–165. Sarcoidosis. Sarcoidosis with a prominent interstitial mononuclear infiltrate. The differential diagnosis in such cases includes berylliosis and extrinsic allergic alveolitis.

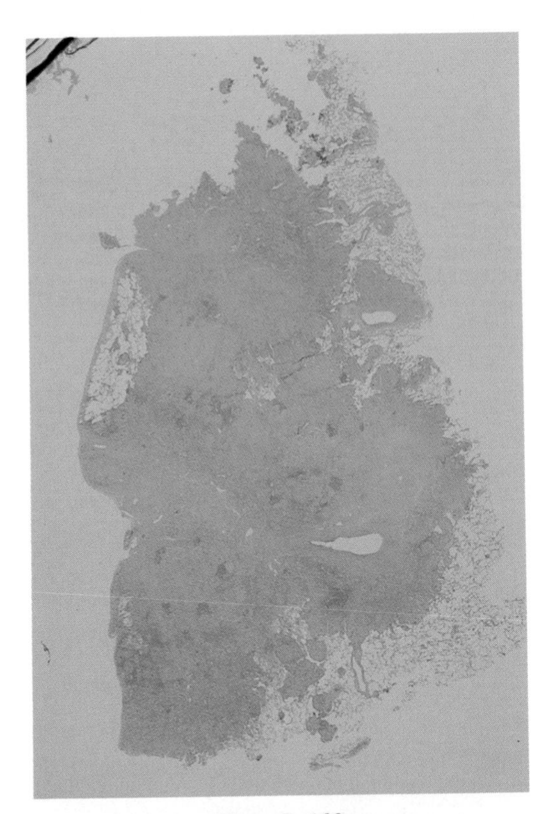

Figure 7–166.

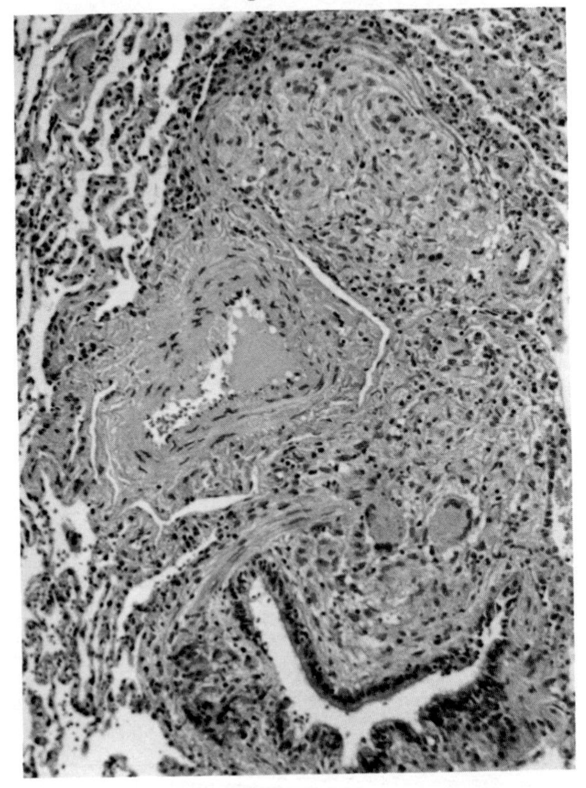

Figure 7–167.

Figures 7–166, 7–167. Nodular sarcoid. Confluent masses of granulomas in sarcoid occasionally coalesce to form nodules several centimeters in size and identifiable on chest radiograph. In this case, the smaller satellite nodules are perivascular in distribution. Away from the large nodules, typical peribronchiolar granulomas of sarcoid could be found (Fig. 7–167).

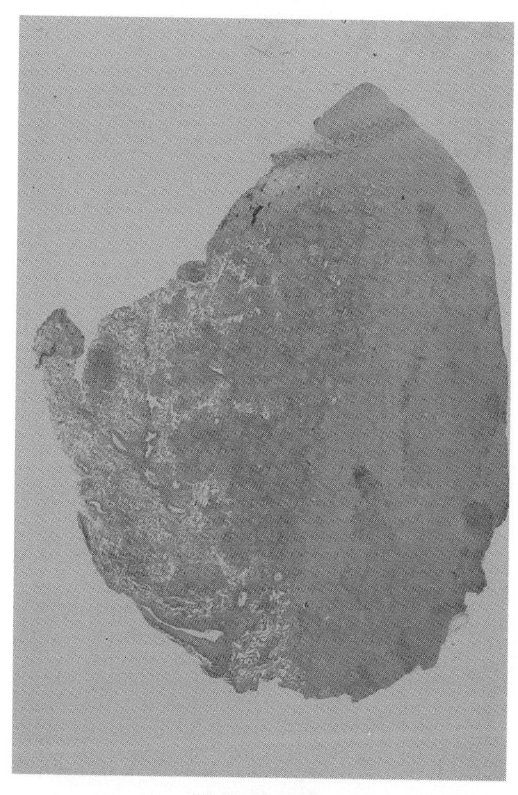

Figure 7–168.

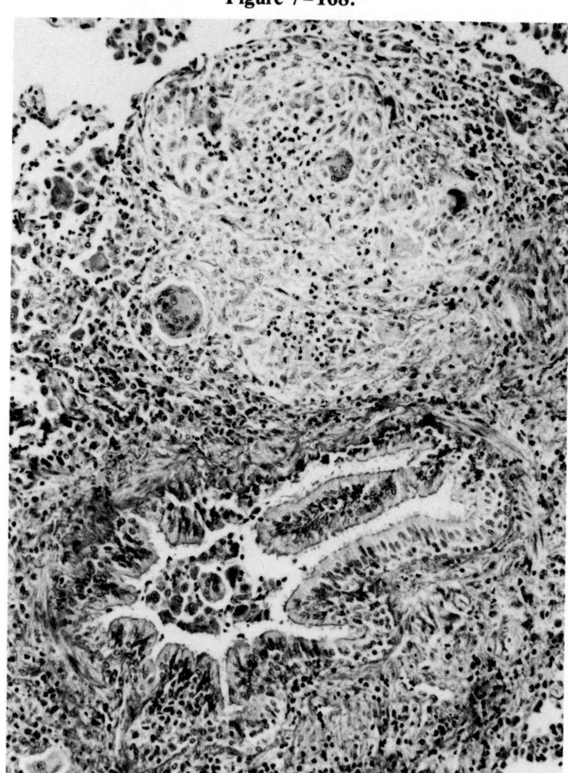

Figure 7–169.

Figures 7–168, 7–169. Necrotizing sarcoid. There is a large nodule composed of a confluent mass of granulomas with extensive central necrosis at the right. Airways at some distance from the main mass show typical peribronchiolar granulomas of sarcoid.

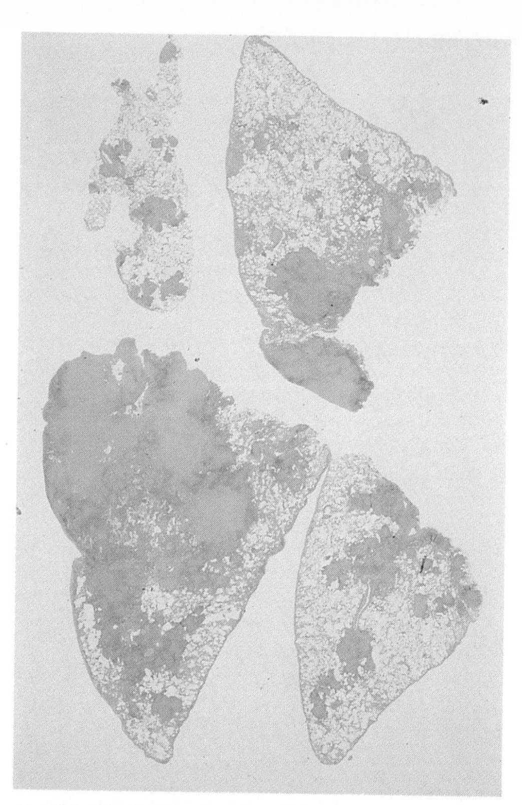

Figure 7–170. Necrotizing sarcoid. This whole-mount illustration shows nodules of varying sizes. The smallest lesions are non-necrotizing and perivascular granulomas, whereas the large nodules have extensive central necrosis.

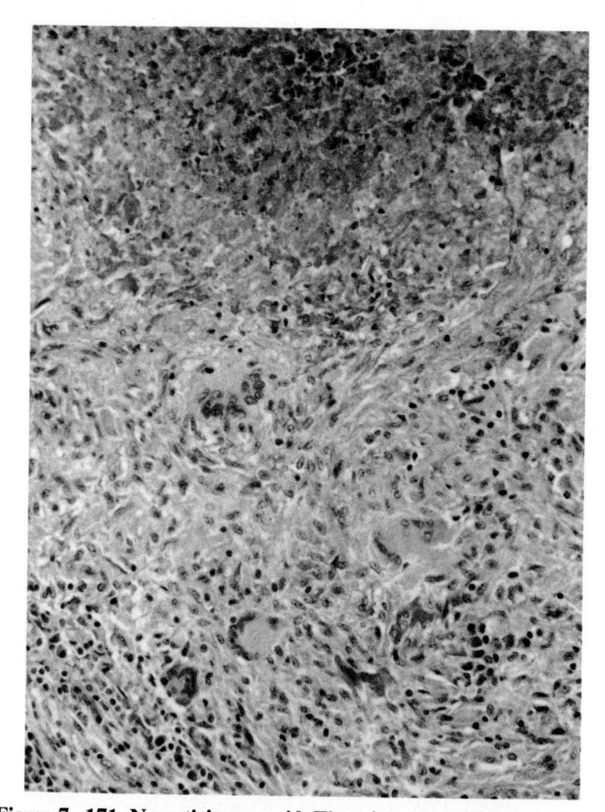

Figure 7–171. Necrotizing sarcoid. There is a necrotizing granuloma with central granular coagulative necrosis surrounded by a granulomatous reaction. The diagnosis in a case such as this should not be accepted until infection has been excluded by special stains *and* cultures.

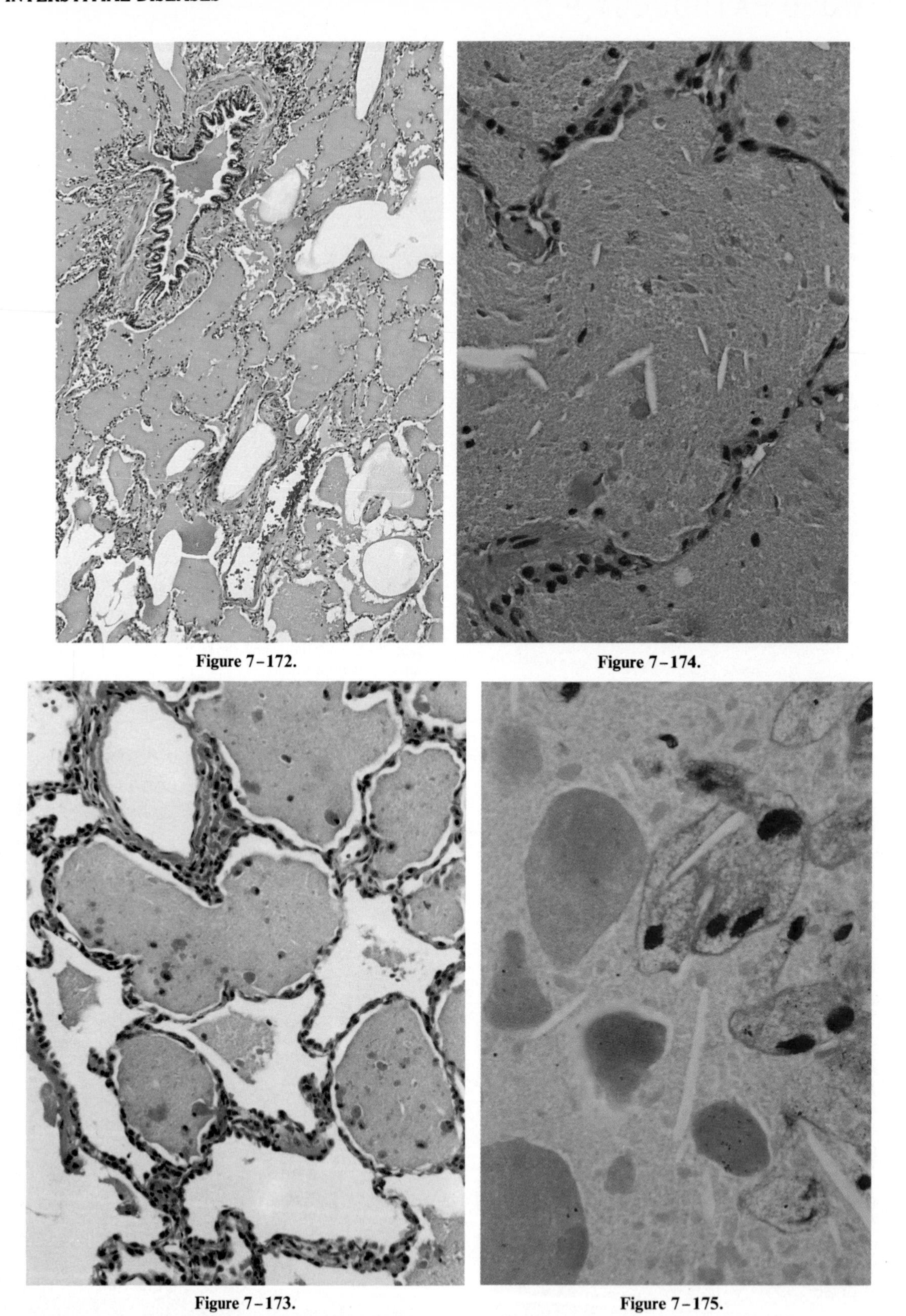

Figure 7–172.

Figure 7–174.

Figure 7–173.

Figure 7–175.

Figures 7–172, 7–173, 7–174, 7–175, 7–176. Classic pulmonary alveolar proteinosis with granular eosinophilic material filling airspaces and extending into small airways. Cellular debris, eosinophilic blobs, and small cholesterol clefts can be seen. Type II cell metaplasia and mild interstitial widening are present.

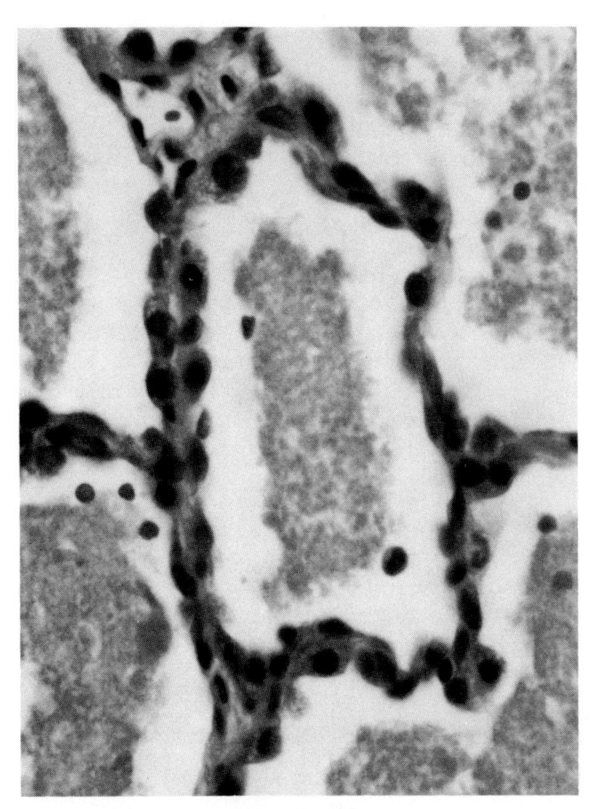

Figure 7-176.

■ Pulmonary Alveolar Proteinosis (Figs. 7-172 to 7-178)

Pulmonary alveolar proteinosis is a progressive bilateral alveolar filling process associated with progressive dyspnea and pulmonary infiltrates. A perihilar, "ground-glass" chest radiograph is a typical finding. A few cases are unilateral or localized.

The alveoli are stuffed with granular eosinophilic (periodic acid-Schiff [PAS]-positive) debris (corresponding to the lipoproteinaceous material), cholesterol (acicular) clefts, eosinophilic bodies, and a few histiocytes and cellular fragments. Interstitial reactions and inflammation are minimal. The presence of neutrophils, organization, or both should raise the possibility of secondary infection (*Nocardia* is sometimes implicated).

Diagnosis is possible by transbronchial biopsy *in the appropriate setting.* Differential diagnosis includes infections, acute silicosis, "dense edema" and fibrinous exudates, and pseudoproteinosis reactions.

References

Prakash UBS, Barham SS, Carpenter HA, Dines DE, Marsh HM. Pulmonary alveolar phospholipoproteinosis: experience with 34 cases and a review. Mayo Clin Proc 62:499-518, 1987.

Thurlbeck WM (ed). Pathology of the Lung. New York, Thieme, 1988.

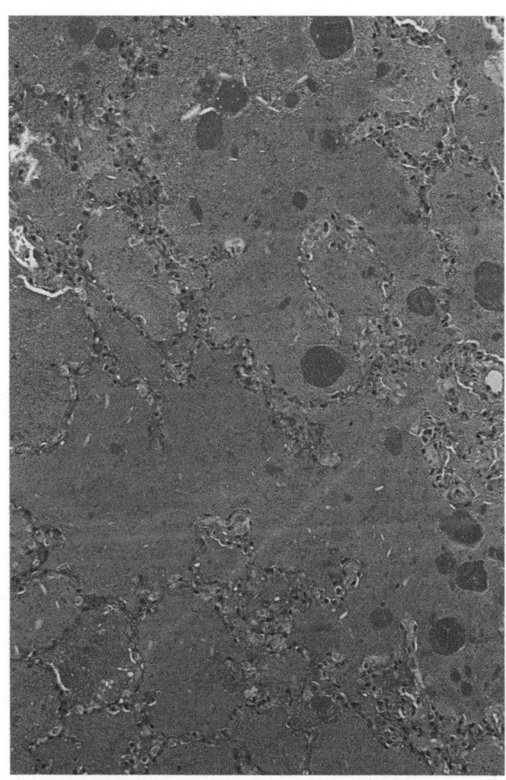

Figure 7-177. Pulmonary alveolar proteinosis. Periodic acid-Schiff (PAS) stain shows positivity in both the granular acellular material and the eosinophilic hyaline blobs.

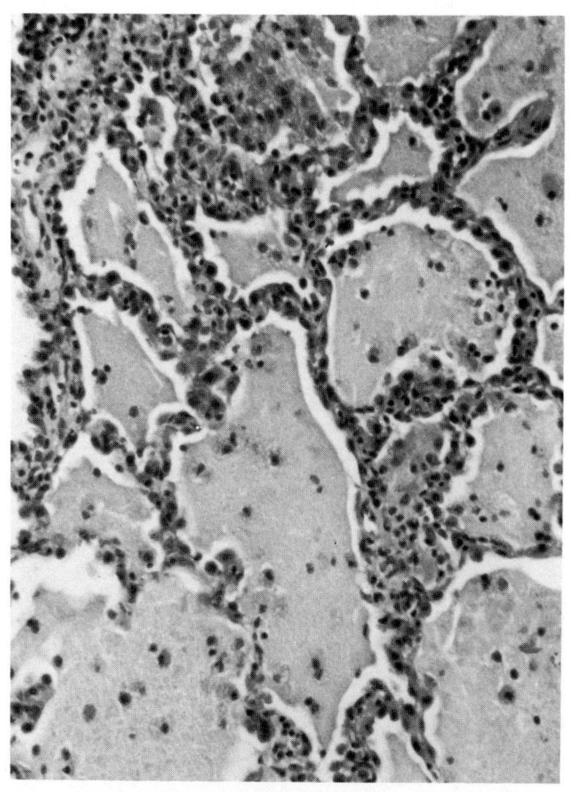

Figure 7-178. Pulmonary alveolar proteinosis. Prominent interstitial reaction and type II cell metaplasia are evident in this case.

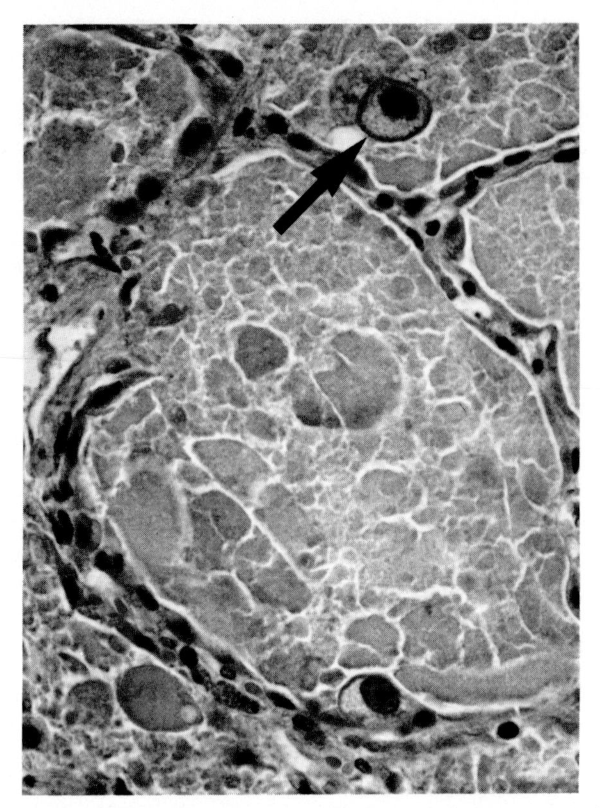

Figure 7–179. Pseudoproteinosis reaction in congenital cytomegalovirus infection. There is eosinophilic material filling airspaces. The appearance is very similar to that seen in classic pulmonary alveolar proteinosis. An alveolar macrophage contains an intranuclear inclusion characteristic of cytomegalovirus (arrow).

■ Pseudoproteinosis Reactions (Figs. 7–179 to 7–181)

A number of pathologic states are associated with eosinophilic airspace material that mimics pulmonary alveolar proteinosis. Such a reaction may be seen as a *focal change* adjacent to masses or associated with tumors. Acute silicosis and rarely other pneumoconioses may resemble pulmonary alveolar proteinosis. The largest group, however, is probably immunosuppressed individuals with infections that are associated with an extensive pseudoproteinosis reaction. A large number of agents have been implicated, especially *Pneumocystis,* viruses, and fungal infections.

A proteinosis-like reaction in an immunosuppressed patient should be considered to be an infection until proven otherwise.

References

Churg A, Green FHY. Pathology of Occupational Lung Disease. New York, Igaku-Shoin Medical Publishers, 1988.
Colby TV, Weiss RL. Current concepts in the surgical pathology of pulmonary infections. Am J Surg Pathol 11:25–37, 1987.
Dail DH, Hammer SP (eds). Pulmonary Pathology. New York, Springer-Verlag, 1988.
Thurlbeck WM (ed). Pathology of the Lung. New York, Thieme, 1988.

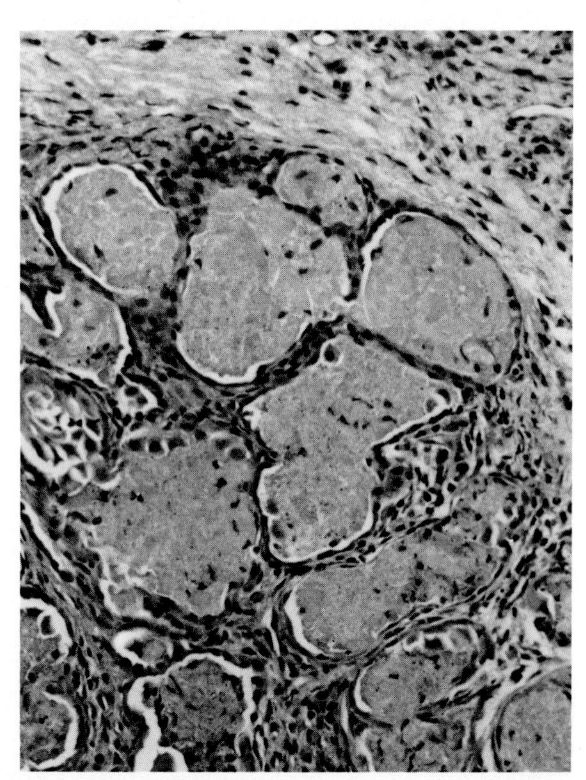

Figure 7–180. Pseudoproteinosis reaction associated with chronic respiratory syncytial virus infection in severe combined immunodeficiency syndrome.

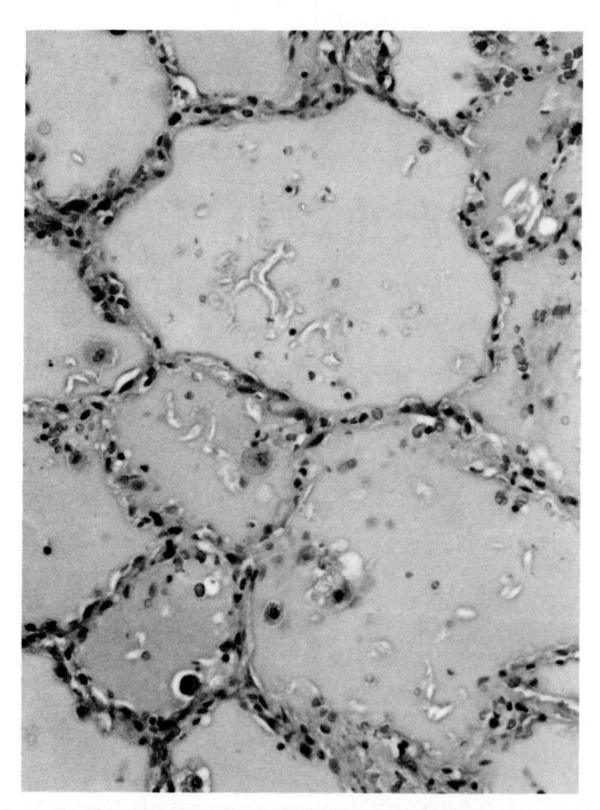

Figure 7–181. Alveolar edema. There is glassy, brightly eosinophilic material filling airspaces, simulating proteinosis; however, the granular character typical of proteinosis is absent. (From a case of diffuse alveolar damage.)

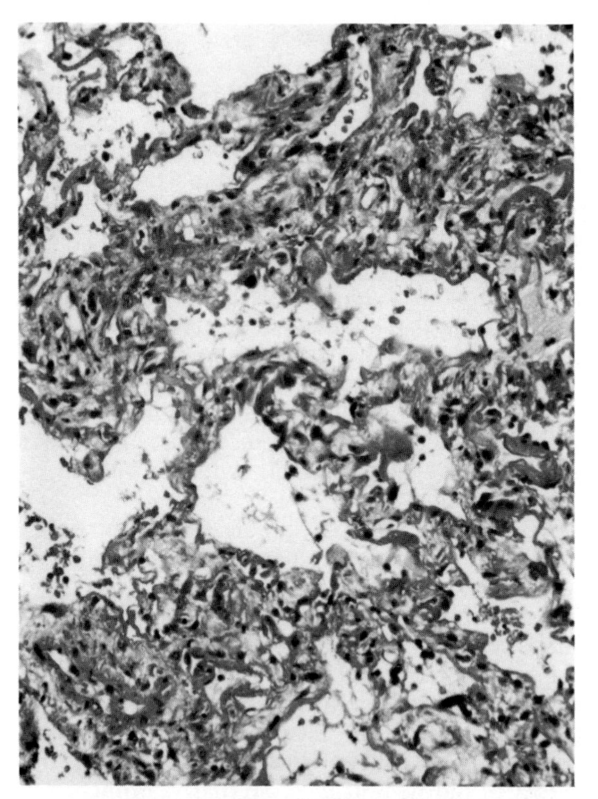

Figure 7-182.

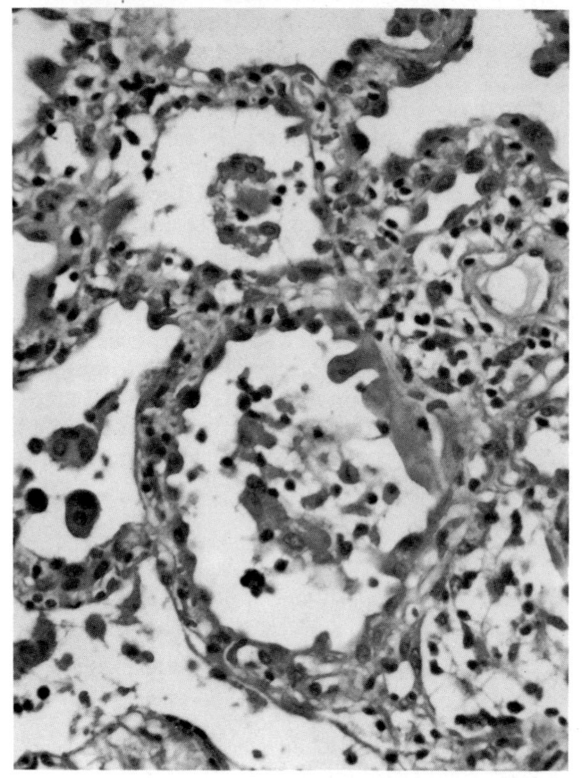

Figure 7-183.

■ Radiation Pneumonitis (Figs. 7-182 to 7-185)

In radiation pneumonitis, an acute or chronic (roughly dose-related) interstitial reaction in the lung is usually restricted to portions of the lung included in the radiation field, although there may be some extension beyond the radiation ports.

Early radiation damage has the appearance of DAD. Chronic radiation pneumonitis resembles UIP with interstitial fibrosis and foci of honeycombing. Vascular intimal thickening with atypical fibroblasts, foamy cells and bizarre endothelial cells, and atypical type II alveolar lining cells are characteristic of radiation damage. These changes are not specific, nor are they seen in all cases.

Note: History and location of the pathologic changes are extremely important in making a diagnosis of radiation pneumonitis. Usually, biopsy is not necessary for diagnosis unless it is performed to exclude some other lesion, mainly an infection. In such cases, the pathologist can rarely go further than a diagnosis of "consistent with" radiation reaction.

References

Dail DH, Hammer SP (eds). Pulmonary Pathology. New York, Springer-Verlag, 1988.

Fajardo LF. Pathology of Radiation Injury. New York, Masson Publishing USA, Inc, 1982.

Thurlbeck WM (ed). Pathology of the Lung. New York, Thieme, 1988.

Figures 7-182, 7-183. Acute radiation pneumonitis. There is acute diffuse alveolar damage characterized by edema of the alveolar walls and interstitial proliferation of fibroblastic cells. The alveoli are in part lined by the remnants of hyaline membranes and in part by metaplastic type II cells. Bizarre type II cells are frequent in this condition.

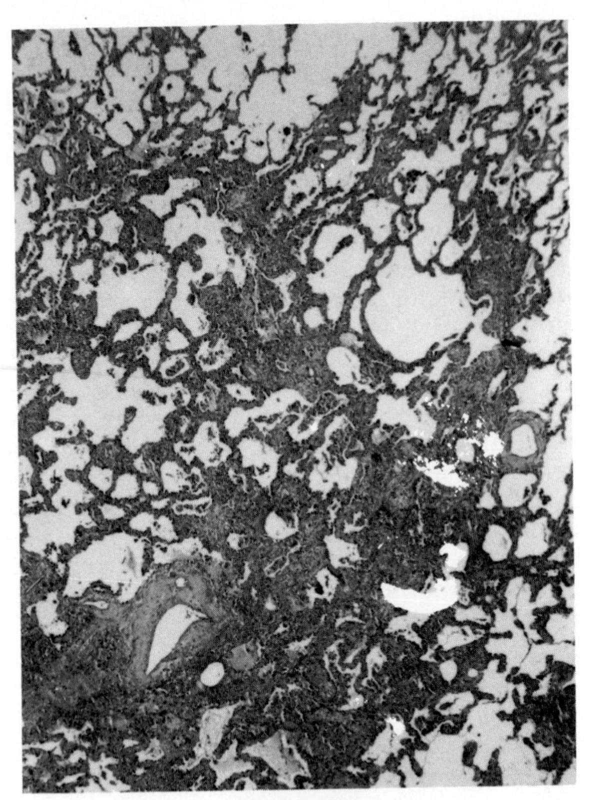

Figure 7-184.

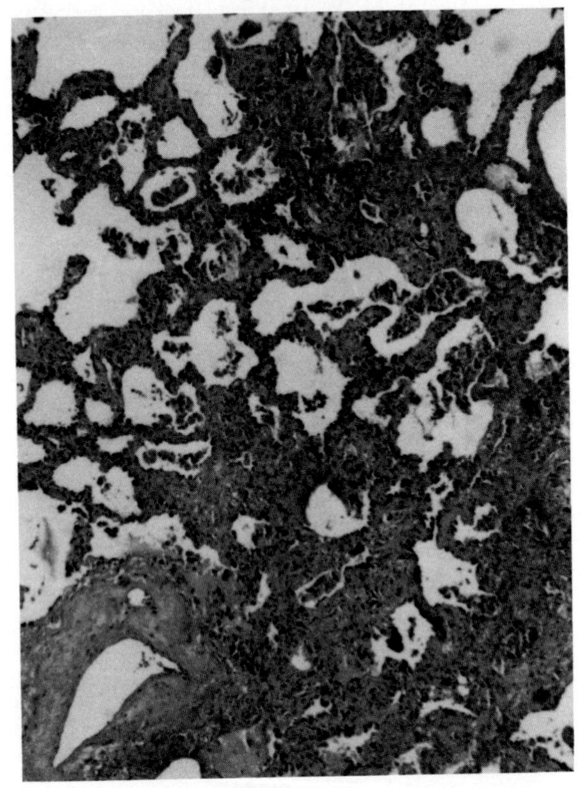

Figure 7-185.

Figures 7-184, 7-185. Chronic radiation pneumonitis. The histologic appearance is that of late organized diffuse alveolar damage with interstitial scarring, vascular thickening, and prominent, sometimes bizarre, metaplastic type II cells. The interstitium is thickened and fibrotic, and the architecture of the lung is distorted.

■ **Lymphangioleiomyomatosis** (Figs. 7-186 to 7-195)

Lymphangioleiomyomatosis (LAM) is an abnormal proliferation of immature smooth muscle found in young women who are nearly always in the childbearing years. Older patients receiving hormone therapy may rarely be affected. An identical histologic appearance is seen in a small percentage of women with tuberous sclerosis. Pelvic lymphangiomyomas, renal angiomyolipomas, and (in tuberous sclerosis) cutaneous angiofibromas and central nervous system changes occur as associated findings. In patients with LAM, progressive shortness of breath develops, often punctuated by recurrent pneumothoraces, chylous effusions, functional evidence of obstruction and decreased diffusion, and chest radiographs showing hyperinflation with progressive interstitial infiltrates.

There is a proliferation of spindle cells with special staining and ultrastructural characteristics of smooth muscle cells in the pulmonary interstitium, often along the septa and subpleural regions, and around bronchovascular structures. The typical low-power appearance is one of holes or subpleural emphysema, with irregular thickenings in the walls of the holes from the bundles of immature smooth muscle cells. The proliferation may involve pulmonary veins, and this is thought to cause the patchy foci of old hemorrhage. Similarly, bronchiolar and lymphatic obstruction lead to functional obstruction, pneumothoraces, and chylothoraces.

Note: Knowledge of the age and sex is critical in making the diagnosis of LAM. Most patients present in the third or fourth decade of life; one must be sure to distinguish the immature smooth muscle from fibrous tissue as well as from mature smooth muscle seen as a metaplastic change in honeycombing, and the nodules of benign metastasizing leiomyoma. Freezing tissue for estrogen and progesterone receptors is important. Transbronchial biopsy diagnosis is quite feasible (if one considers the diagnosis of LAM) because the proliferation typically occurs along airways and is accessible to bronchoscopic biopsy and the histologic appearance is specific. The most common mistake is to interpret LAM as emphysema but the holes in emphysema (Fig. 7-196) are more ragged in appearance and lack the mural bundles of smooth muscle.

References

Banner AS, Carrington CB, Emory WB, et al. Efficacy of oophorectomy in lymphangioleiomyomatosis and benign metastasizing leiomyoma. N Engl J Med 305:204-209, 1981.

Carrington CB, Cugell DW, Gaensler EA, et al. Lymphangioleiomyomatosis: physiologic-pathologic-radiologic correlations. Am Rev Respir Dis 116:977-995, 1977.

Corrin B, Liebow AA, Friedman PJ. Pulmonary lymphangiomyomatosis: a review. Am J Pathol 79:348-367, 1975.

Dail DH, Hammer SP (eds). Pulmonary Pathology. New York, Springer-Verlag, 1988.

Sinclair W, Wright JL, Churg A. Lymphangioleiomyomatosis presenting in a postmenopausal woman. Thorax 40:475-476, 1985.

Thurlbeck WM (ed). Pathology of the Lung. New York, Thieme, 1988.

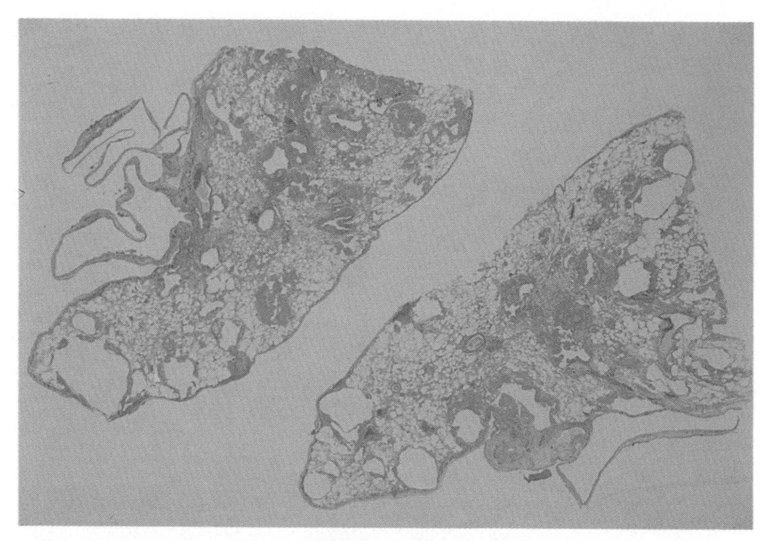

Figure 7–186.

Figures 7–186, 7–187, 7–188. Lymphangioleiomyomatosis (LAM). In this well-inflated biopsy, the parenchymal holes and pleural blebs that characterize lymphangioleiomyomatosis are clearly visible. The holes are the result of smooth muscle proliferation in airways and subsequent air trapping. Bullae and pleural blebs also develop. These frequently rupture and lead to pneumothorax, a history of which is extremely common in patients with lymphangioleiomyomatosis. The walls of the holes are lined in part by normal alveoli and in part by the bundles of abnormal smooth muscle. The lung architecture is otherwise intact.

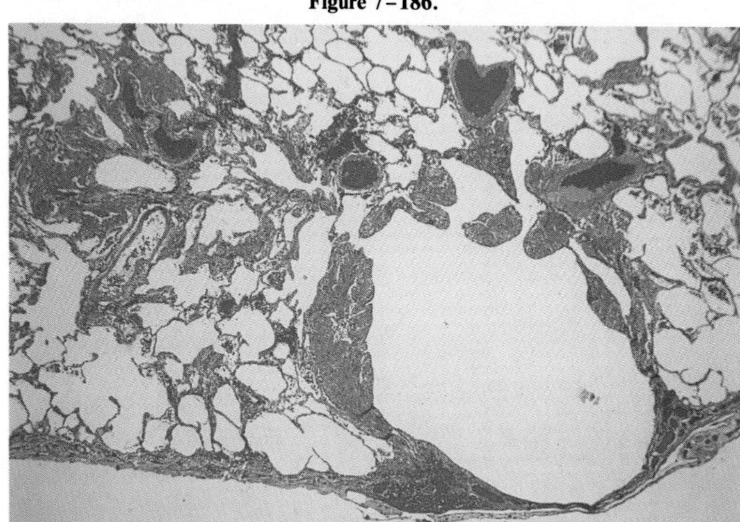

Figure 7–187.

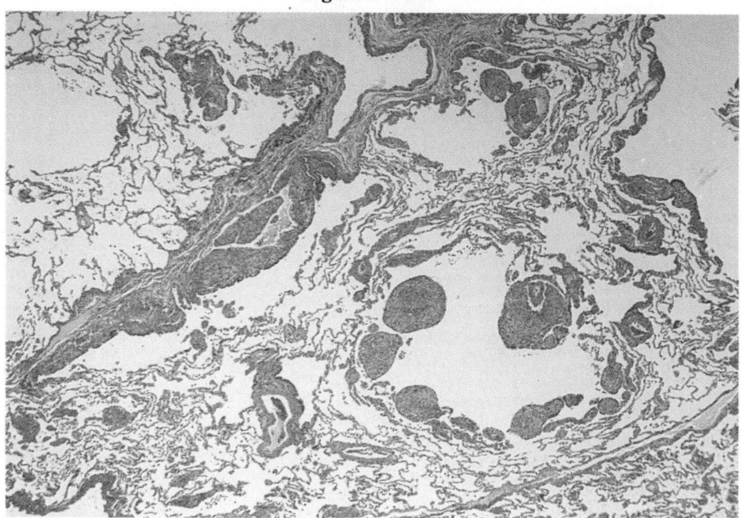

Figure 7–188.

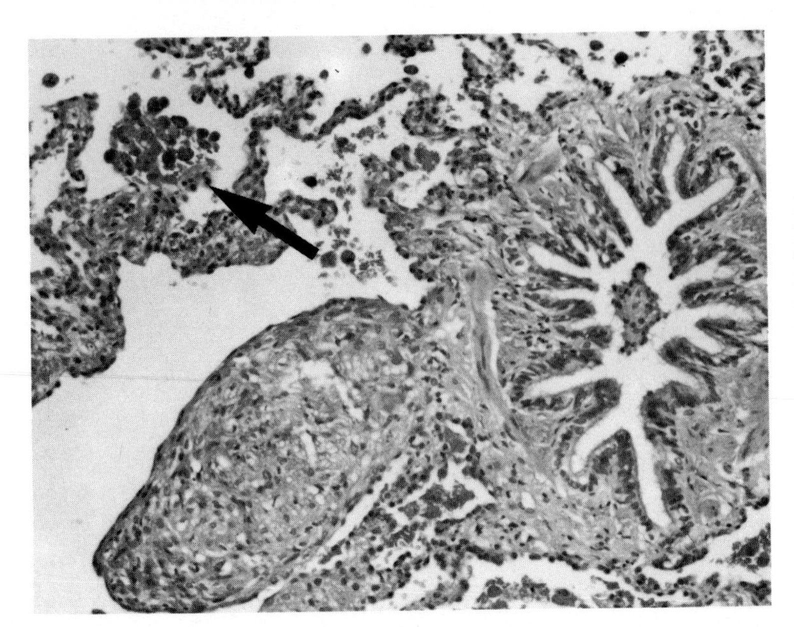

Figure 7-189. Lymphangioleiomyomatosis (LAM). A portion of an emphysematous hole with a bundle of smooth muscle in its wall is adjacent to a small airway. The smooth muscle proliferation may actually lead to small airway obstruction, and severe air trapping is common in lymphangioleiomyomatosis. The adjacent alveoli contain clusters of hemosiderin-filled macrophages (arrow), thought to be the result of venous involvement by lymphangioleiomyomatosis and secondary passive congestion.

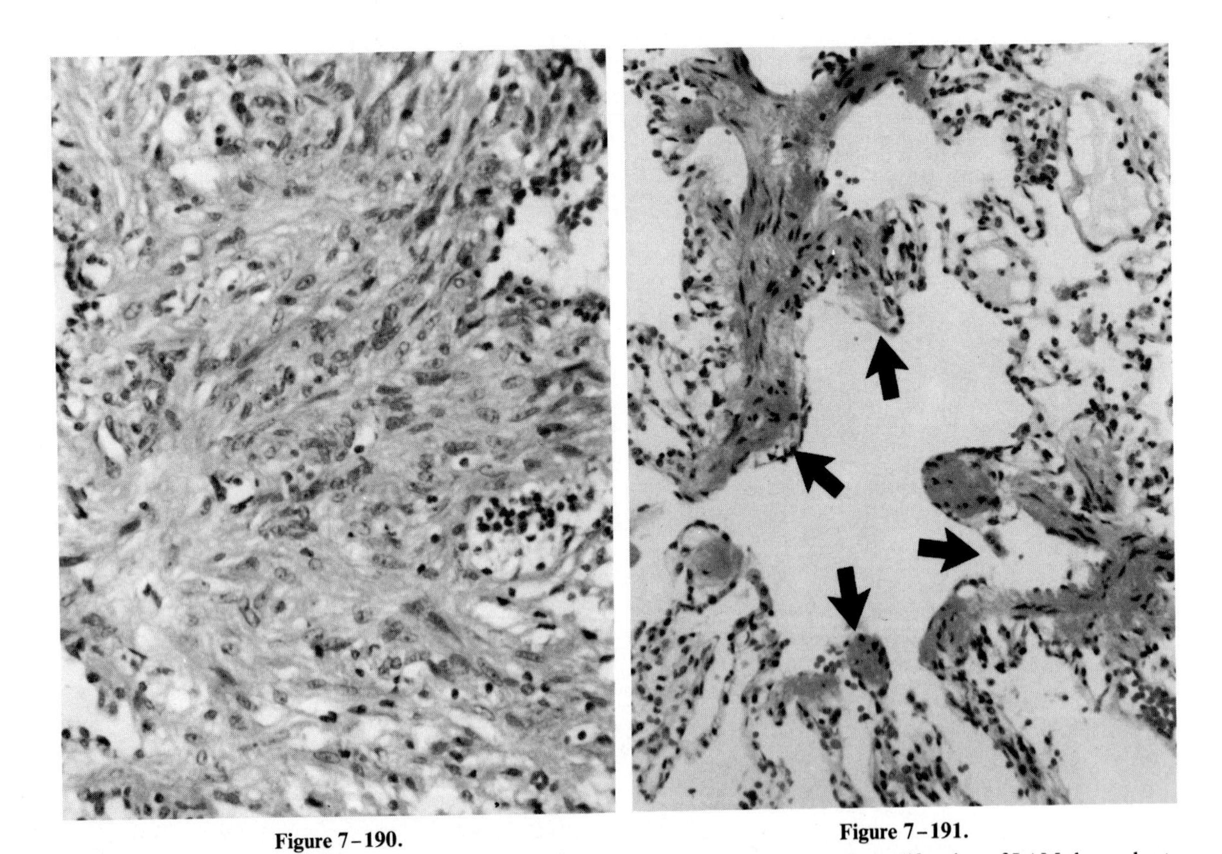

Figure 7-190. **Figure 7-191.**

Figures 7-190, 7-191. Lymphangioleiomyomatosis (LAM). Detail of the smooth muscle proliferation of LAM shows short, somewhat irregularly fasciculated cells with fibrillar cytoplasm typical of smooth muscle cells. The cells appear somewhat shorter and more immature (Fig. 7-190) than normal smooth muscle (Fig. 7-191), which is illustrated from around a respiratory bronchiole (arrows) in the same case. In general, the smooth muscle proliferation of LAM can be readily distinguished from normal mature smooth muscle.

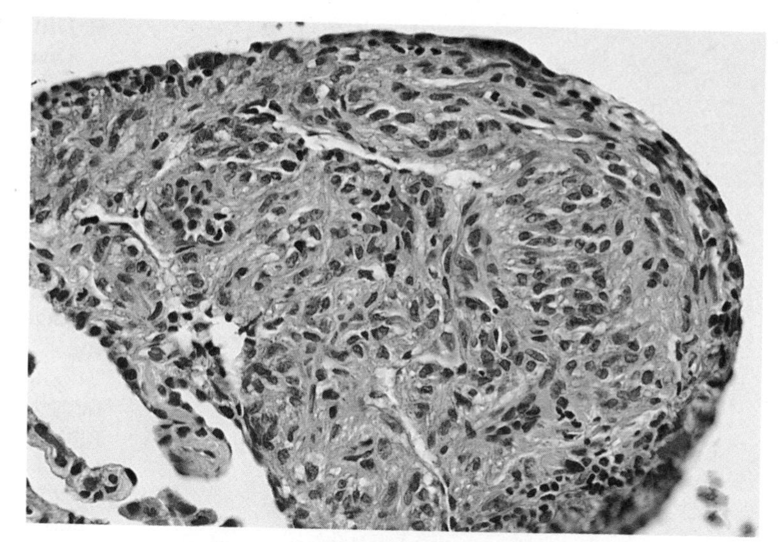

Figure 7-192.

Figures 7-192, 7-193, 7-194. Lymphangioleiomyomatosis (LAM). Detail of the smooth muscle proliferation from other cases shows a rounded and somewhat more epithelioid or "myoblastic" appearance to the proliferation. The clefts in between the small bundles are reminiscent of lymphatic spaces. The spindle cells stain reddish on a trichrome stain (Fig. 7-194).

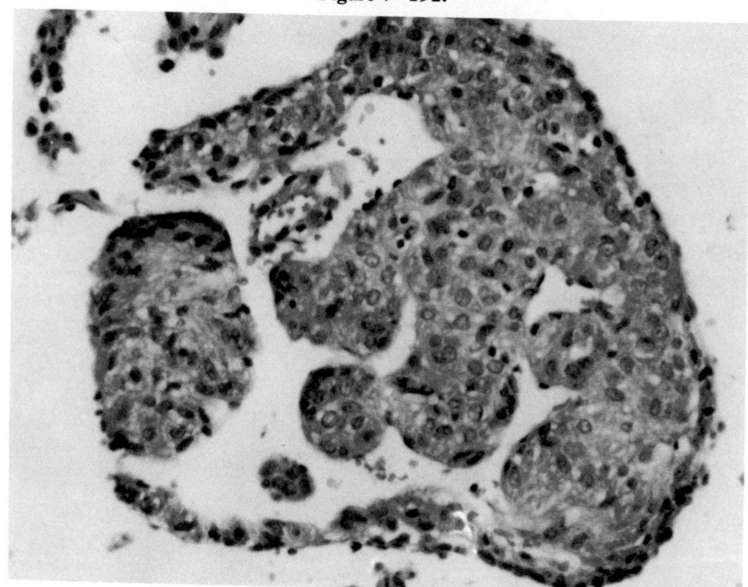

Figure 7-193.

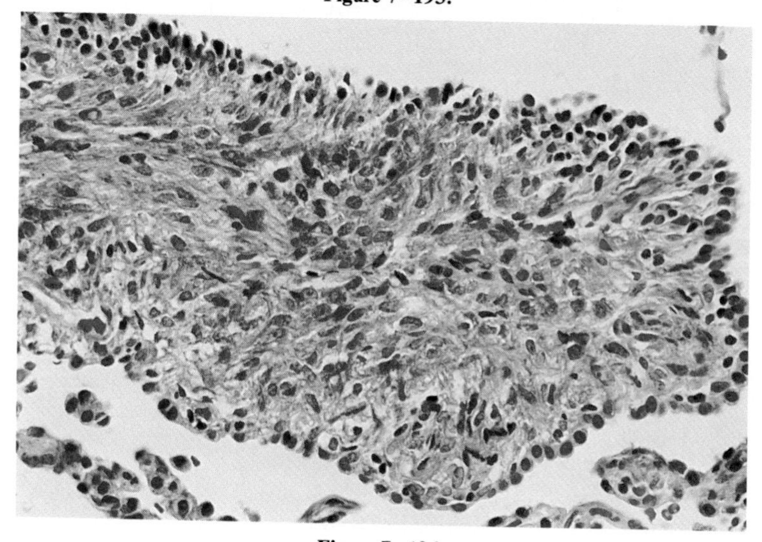

Figure 7-194.

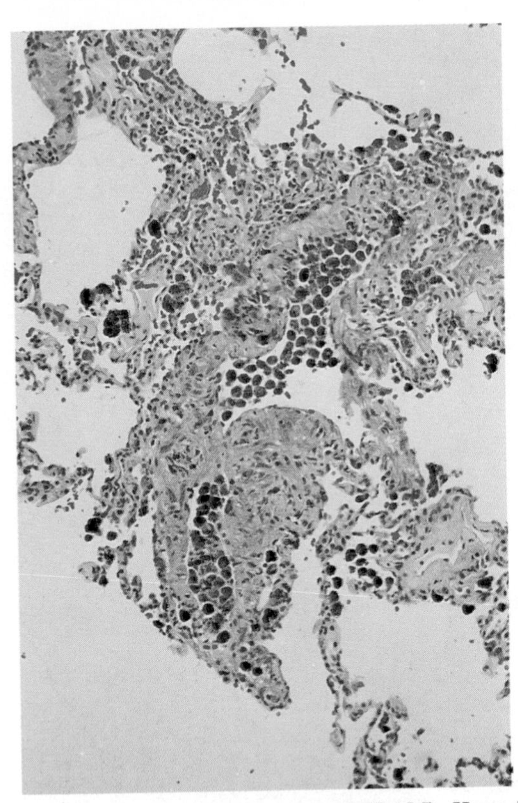

Figure 7-195. Lymphangioleiomyomatosis (LAM). Hemosiderin-filled macrophages are frequent in lymphangioleiomyomatosis, presumably owing to obstruction of small vessels by the smooth muscle proliferation with secondary hemorrhage.

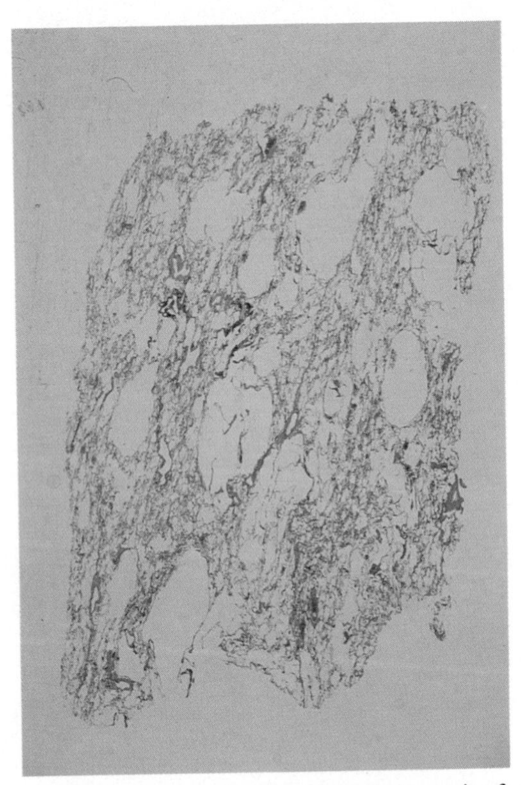

Figure 7-196. Emphysema of moderate histologic severity, for comparison with lymphangioleiomyomatosis (LAM). The bundles of proliferating cells seen in walls of the holes in LAM are absent.

■ Diffuse Malignancy Presenting As Interstitial Lung Disease

Many tumors, both primary and secondary, can produce interstitial lung disease by a variety of mechanisms:

1. Diffuse pulmonary arterial metastases. Thrombi are also present, as may be pulmonary hypertension clinically. Examples include metastatic carcinomas (especially adenocarcinoma) and angiosarcoma. Lymphangitic carcinoma is a frequent accompanying finding.
2. Diffuse intravascular (arterial, venous, lymphatic) neoplasm. This may be seen with intravascular lymphomatosis.
3. Lymphangitic carcinoma (either from the lung or an extrapulmonary site) filling the pulmonary lymphatics.
4. Infiltrates along lymphatic routes but often without obviously filling dilated lymphatics. This is characteristic of many lymphomas and leukemias, of Kaposi's sarcoma, and of some metastatic sarcomas and carcinomas.
5. Diffuse alveolar fillings as in bronchioloalveolar carcinoma and some metastatic carcinomas as well as lymphomas.

CHAPTER 8

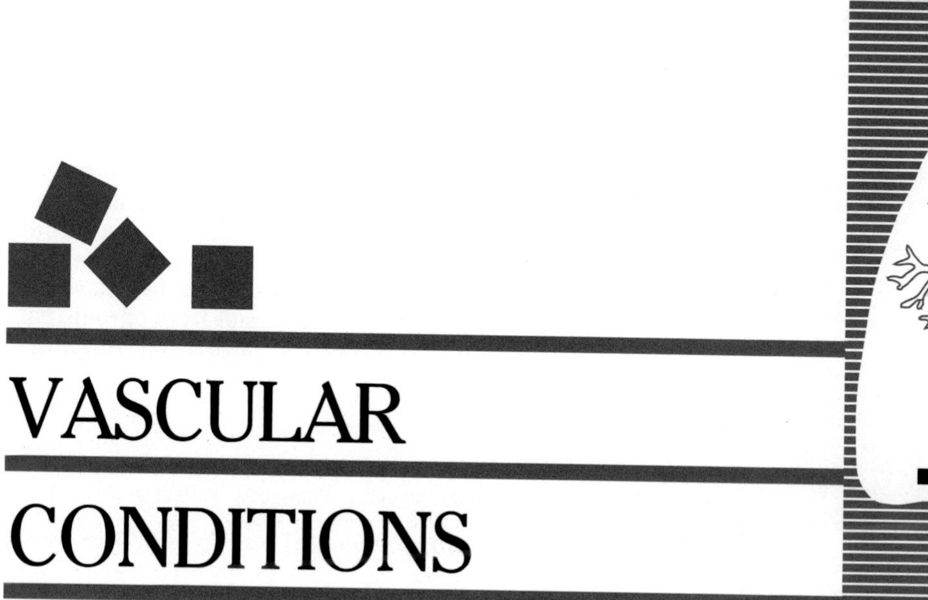

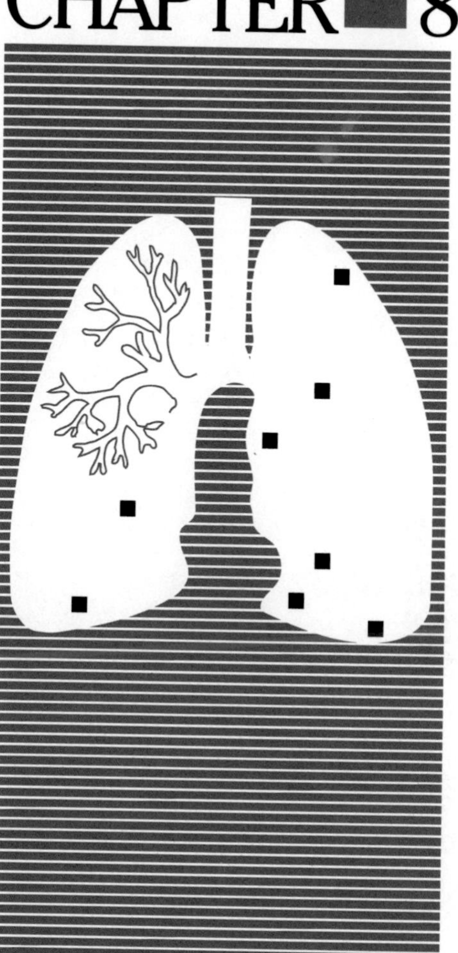

VASCULAR CONDITIONS

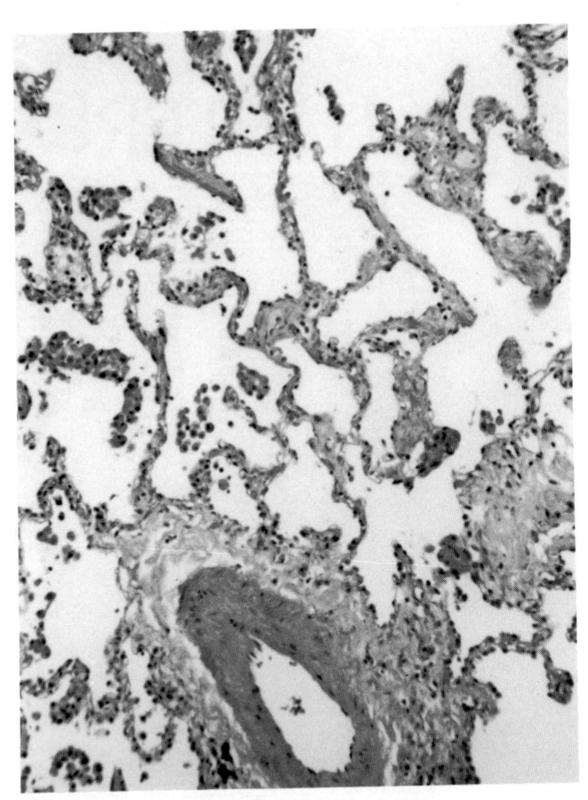

Figure 8-1.

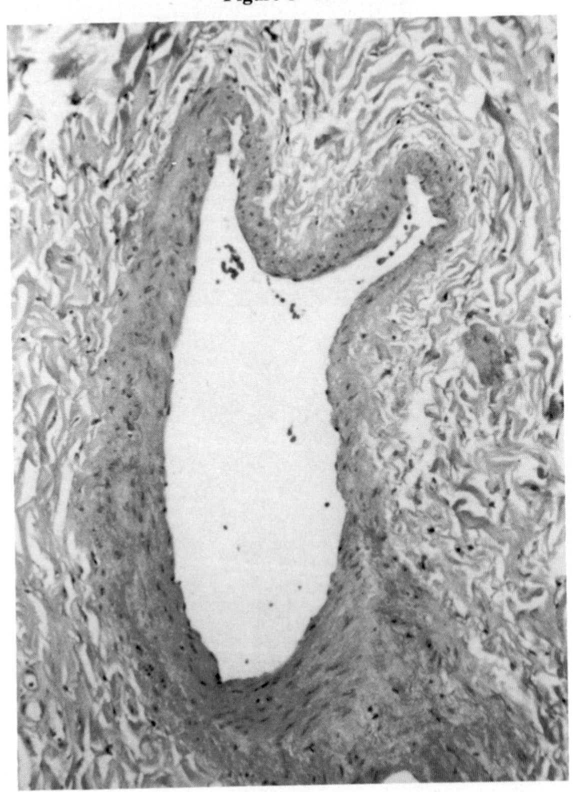

Figure 8-2.

Figures 8-1, 8-2. Severe long-standing chronic passive congestion. There is a slight increase in alveolar macrophages, but few contained much hemosiderin. The changes were manifested mainly in the vessels, with mural thickening of pulmonary arteries (Fig. 8-1) and veins (Fig. 8-2) as well as a slight diffuse thickening and fibrosis of alveolar walls.

■ Venous Obstruction and Chronic Passive Congestion (Figs. 8-1 to 8-3)

Venous obstruction, regardless of cause, may be associated with dramatic interstitial changes that are misinterpreted either as interstitial pneumonia or as pulmonary capillary hemangiomatosis. These changes may be localized or diffuse depending on the extent of venous involvement either locally or from cardiac causes.

Chronic venous obstruction results in engorgement of capillaries and in apparent increases in cellularity and in number of capillaries in the alveolar walls. Mild interstitial fibrosis with a scant, chronic inflammatory infiltrate may be an accompanying feature. The presence of hemosiderin-filled macrophages in the airspaces is also frequent. Another finding is the encrustation of interstitial elastic fibers by iron and calcium. Iron encrustation is quite nonspecific and is merely a reflection of a chronic venous obstruction (see Fig. 9-41). Sometimes a giant cell reaction to the iron-encrusted elastica develops. Intra-alveolar ossification may result from chronic passive congestion, and is classically associated with mitral stenosis.

References

Dail DH, Hammer SP (eds). Pulmonary Pathology. New York, Springer-Verlag, 1988.

Thurlbeck WM (ed). Pathology of the Lung. New York, Thieme, 1988.

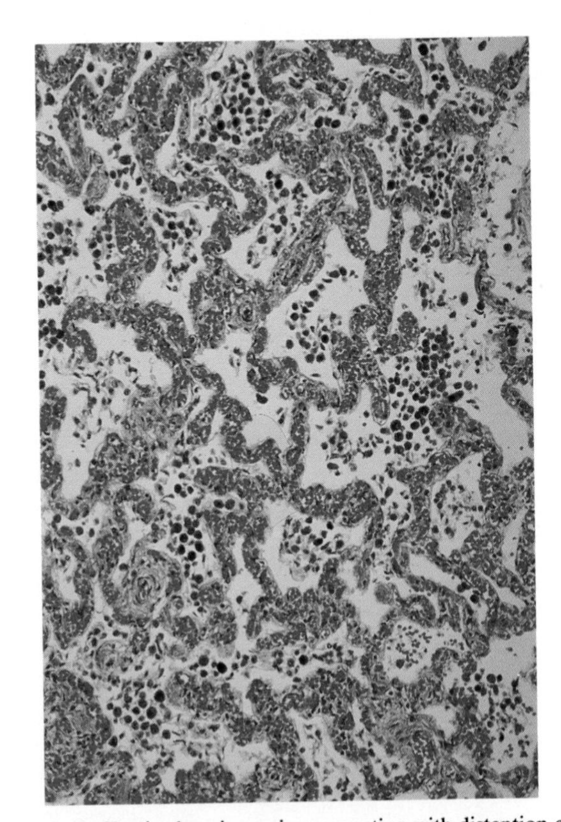

Figure 8-3. Classic chronic passive congestion with distention of alveolar walls by engorged capillaries and hemosiderin-filled macrophages in the alveoli.

■ Bone Marrow and Fat Emboli (Figs. 8–4 to 8–6)

An occasional bone marrow embolus is a common incidental finding at autopsy and is sometimes seen in biopsy material. Patients with massive fat emboli usually present with shortness of breath and with pulmonary infiltrates occurring after extensive tissue trauma, often accompanied by multiple broken bones. Biopsy is rarely performed in this setting. It has recently been reported that fat emboli may cause acute pulmonary infiltrates in patients receiving steroid therapy. Biopsy specimens show multiple fat emboli involving the pulmonary capillaries. The findings may be extremely subtle, unless one considers the diagnosis.

Histologically, many of the capillaries and small vessels appear dilated. If blood is present in the lumen, it appears to be displaced peripherally by a clear vacuole, which represents the fat vacuole dissolved during processing. Bone marrow elements may be admixed.

Fat emboli represent one of the conditions that should be considered in the lung biopsy specimen that appears histologically normal at first glance in a patient known to have pulmonary infiltrates.

References

Colby TV, Yousem SA. Pulmonary histology for the surgical pathologist. Am J Surg Pathol 12:223–239, 1988.

Pastore L, Kessler S. Pulmonary fat embolization in the immunocompromised patient. Am J Surg Pathol 6:315–322, 1982.

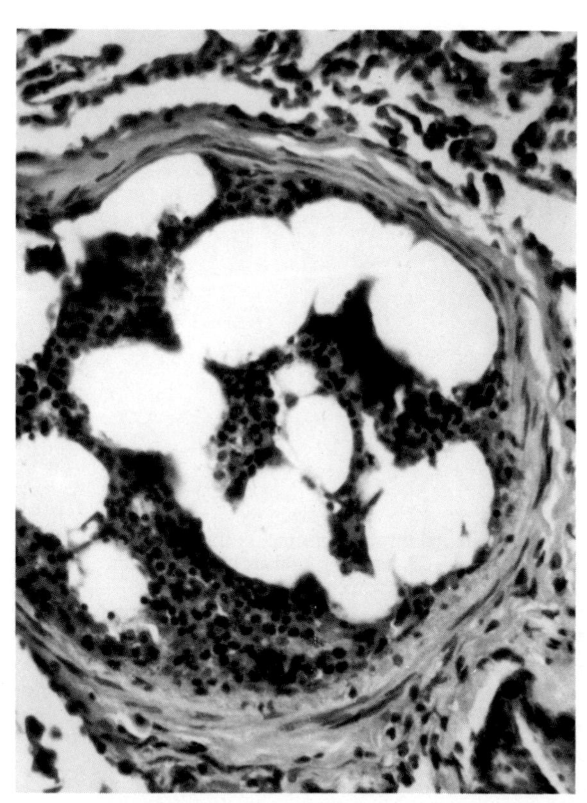

Figure 8–4. Incidental bone marrow embolus in a small pulmonary artery in a young woman with lymphangioleiomyomatosis. Bone marrow emboli are common incidental findings at autopsy and also are occasionally seen in lung biopsy specimens.

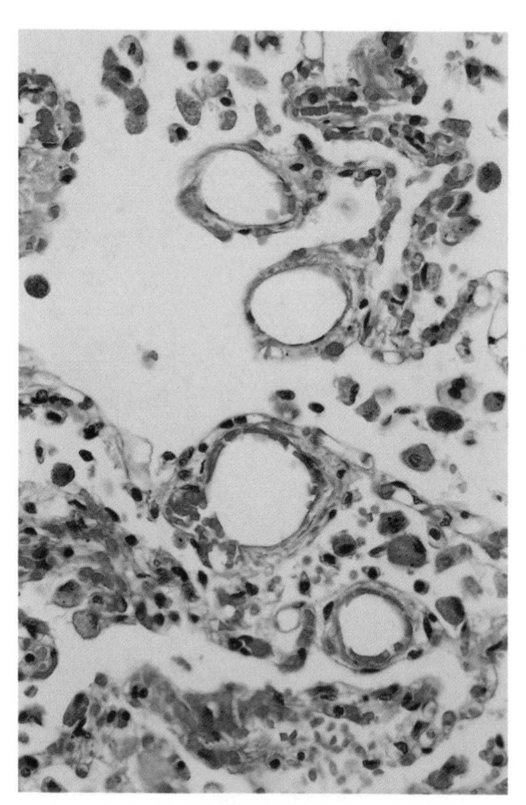

Figure 8–5.

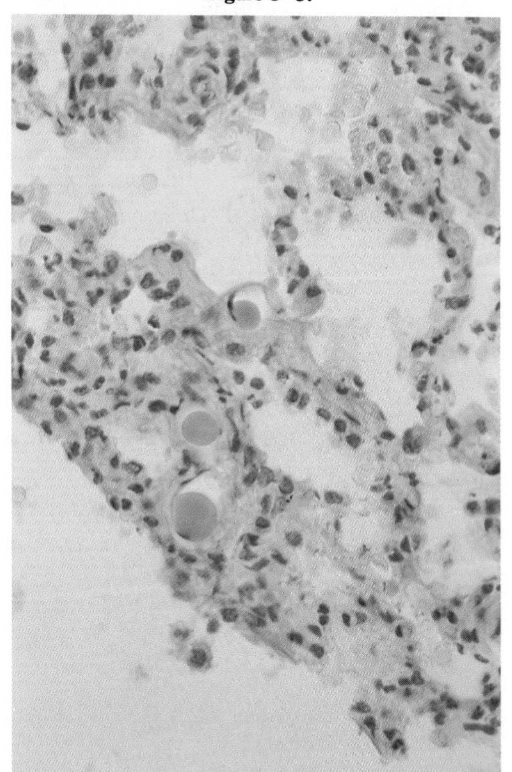

Figure 8–6.

Figures 8–5, 8–6. Pulmonary fat emboli. The hematoxylin and eosin (H & E) stain (Fig. 8–5) showed dilated vessels, with clear holes representing the fat that was dissolved during processing. The fat can be seen to have compressed red blood cells up against the capillary walls. In frozen sections, fat stains may be used to confirm the presence of fat emboli as illustrated in this oil red O stain (Fig. 8–6).

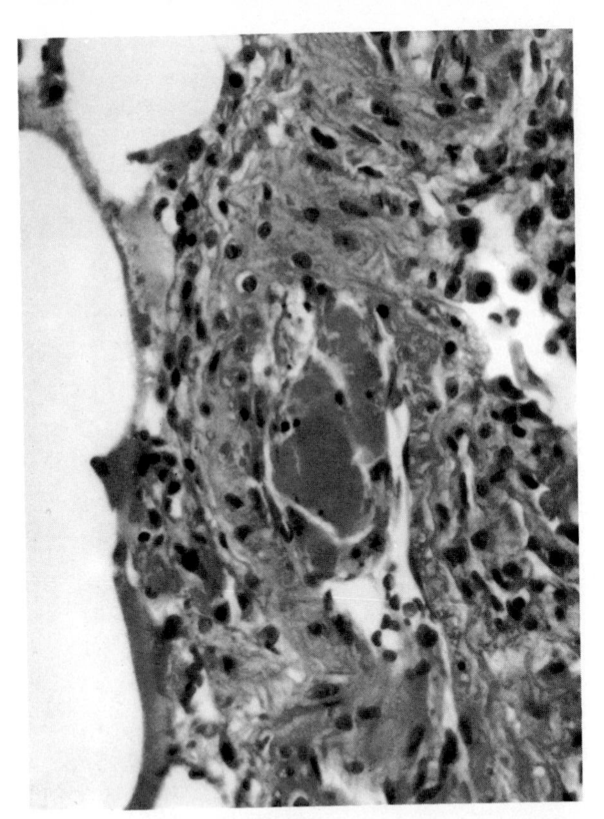

Figure 8–7.

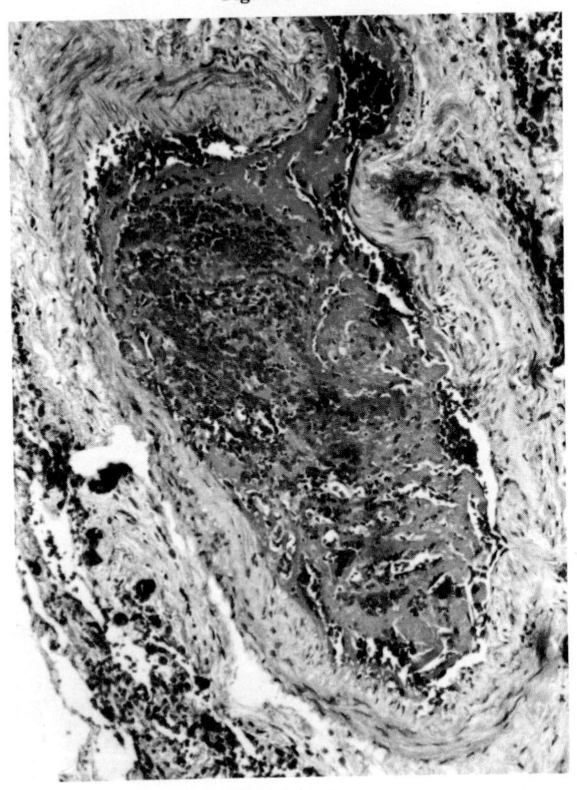

Figure 8–8.

■ Pulmonary Emboli and in Situ Pulmonary Arterial Thrombi (Figs. 8–7, 8–8)

Pulmonary emboli alone rarely lead to biopsy unless the emboli are chronic and diffuse in small vessels, leading to hypertension. Fat emboli and other embolic material are rarely seen in biopsy specimens with the exception of intravenous talcosis (p. 280).

Intravascular thrombi and emboli in varying stages of organization may be seen. Parenchymal hemorrhage and/or infarct may or may not be present.

Note: It is extremely common in any acute diffuse lung disease to see secondary thrombi in pulmonary arteries. These are usually of no clinical importance. If there is a question of their significance, they should be brought to the attention of the clinician with the knowledge that they might be *either* a significant *or* an incidental finding.

Figures 8–7, 8–8. Incidental thrombi in small pulmonary arteries from two cases of diffuse alveolar damage. Such thrombi are quite common and are only rarely associated with clinical evidence of pulmonary emboli. This finding in relatively normal lung tissue should lead one to consider pulmonary emboli. (Fig. 8–8 from Colby, TV, and Yousem, S.: Pulmonary histology for the surgical pathologist. Am. J. Surg. Pathol. 12:223, 1988, with permission of Raven Press.)

■ Pulmonary Leukostasis (Figs. 8-9 and 8-10)

Pulmonary leukostasis is a condition that is seen in patients with acute leukemia and extremely high peripheral blast counts. As a result of chemotherapy, necrotic leukemic blasts become lodged in the pulmonary vasculature and lead to secondary thrombosis, pulmonary edema, and hemorrhage. The pattern resembles diffuse alveolar damage.

Leukostasis has become quite well recognized clinically, and biopsy is rarely needed for diagnosis.

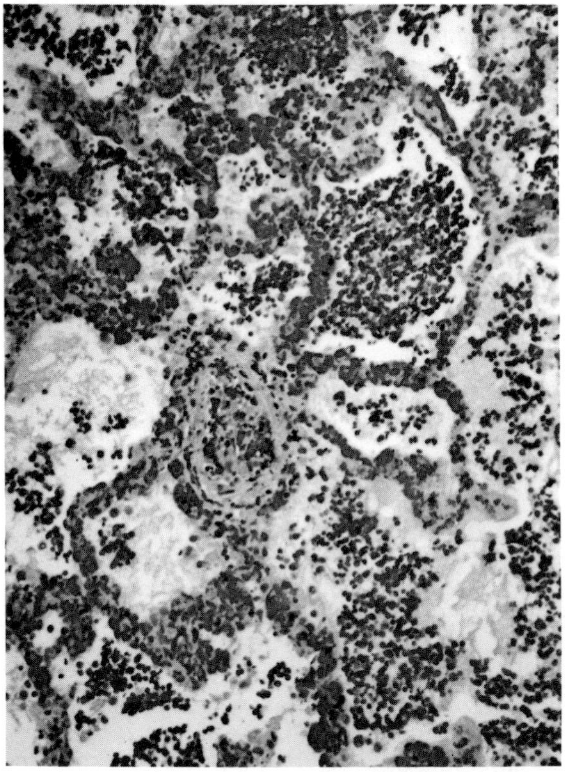

References

Myers TJ, Cole SR, Klatsky AU, Hild DH. Respiratory failure due to pulmonary leukostasis following chemotherapy of acute nonlymphocytic leukemia. Cancer 51:1808-1813, 1983.

■ Pulmonary Infarction

Single or multiple lesions are seen on chest radiographs. A lesion resected for diagnosis is the usual setting in which infarcts come to the attention of the surgical pathologist. Many patients have left-sided heart disease. The prior embolic event may or may not have been recognized, and most lesions are seen in later stages with some organization.

The classic peripheral, wedge-shaped character of a pulmonary infarct may not be all that obvious. Overlying fibrinous pleuritis is common.

Histologically there is coagulative necrosis in various stages of resorption and organization. Squamous metaplasia at the edge of lesions is common, which often have an interlobular septum at one border. The squamous metaplasia is sometimes confused with squamous carcinoma. The overlying pleura is usually viable, but may be fibrotic with adhesions. Old or late infarcts may be identical to an old granuloma, since they usually round up and form well-circumscribed nodules in which collapsed lung parenchyma and alveolar skeleton can be appreciated only with elastic tissue stains. An occluded vessel may sometimes be seen; occluded vessels, however, are common in any fibrotic pulmonary process.

Note: Infarcts may also be seen as a result of vascular occlusion by tumors that may be relatively inconspicuous themselves.

References

Thurlbeck WM (ed). Pathology of the Lung. New York, Thieme, 1988.

Figure 8-9.

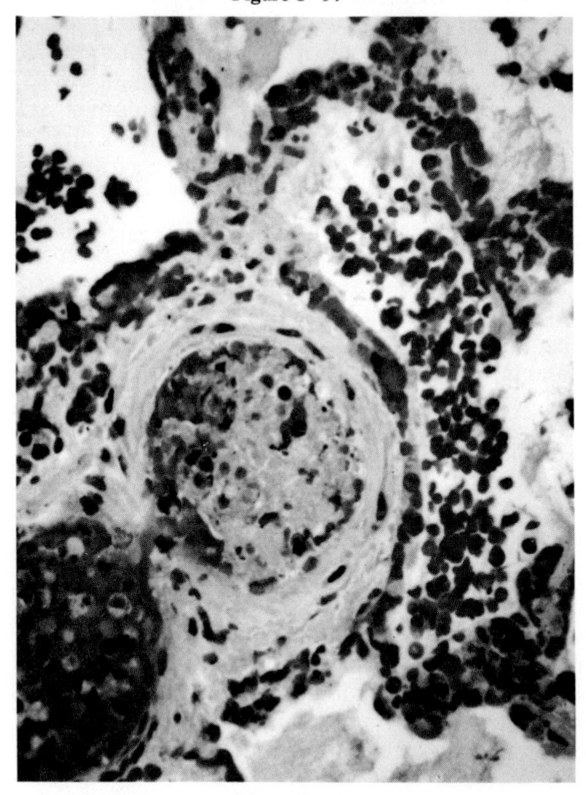

Figure 8-10.

Figures 8-9, 8-10. Leukostasis in acute myelogenous leukemia. In a patient with acute nonlymphocytic leukemia and high peripheral blast counts, acute pulmonary disease developed right after induction of chemotherapy. Biopsy shows necrotic tumor cells stuffing vessels with associated hemorrhage and exudate into the alveoli.

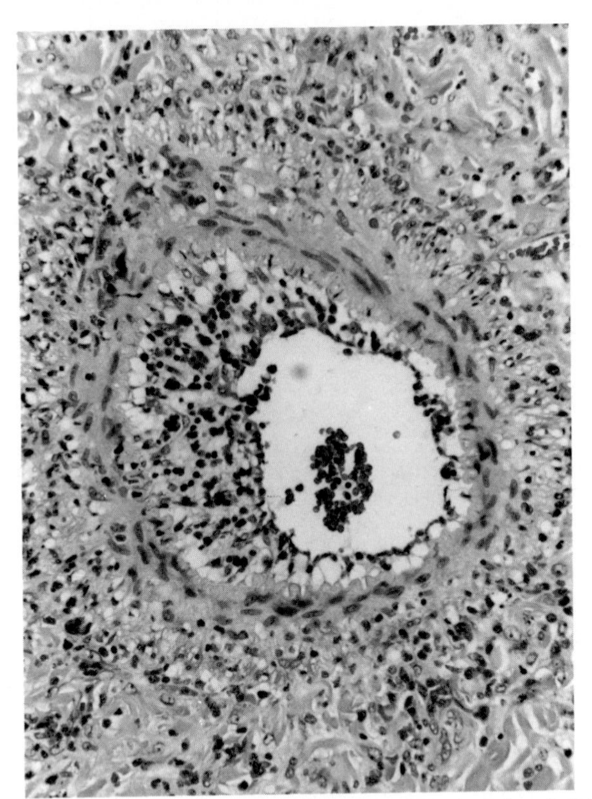

Figure 8–11. Wegener's granulomatosis. Early vascular lesions in Wegener's granulomatosis are endothelial and subendothelial accumulations of lymphocytes, monocytes, and a few eosinophils and neutrophils.

■ Wegener's Granulomatosis (Figs. 8–11 to 8–35)

This necrotizing granulomatous and vasculitic condition of unknown cause is classically associated with involvement of the upper airway, lungs, and kidneys. Practically any site or organ may be involved in individual cases. In some patients, features mimic collagen-vascular diseases. A significant percentage of patients with Wegener's granulomatosis have antibodies to neutrophil cytoplasm in their serum. Radiographic findings include bilateral infiltrates and/or nodules with or without cavitation.

The histologic appearance is best understood when one recognizes that Wegener's granulomatosis is *more than a vasculitis* but an inflammatory process with the following three components:

- Vasculitis
- Necrosis
- Inflammatory background

Vasculitis: Although vasculitis typically involves the arteries *and* veins, it may also involve the venules and capillaries (capillaritis). The vasculitis may be manifested simply as mural cellular infiltrates or rarely as fibrinoid necrosis. Typically, there is an intramural eccentric necrotizing granulomatous lesion dominated by monocytes with central neutrophils and neutrophilic debris. The capillaritis may be neutrophilic or, in rare instances, may be granulomatous. Capillaritis with hemorrhage may be the only finding in some cases of Wegener's granulomatosis.

Necrosis: The necrosis is granulomatous in character with central granular debris usually staining basophilic and containing neutrophil karyorrhectic debris, with surrounding palisaded histiocytic and giant cell reaction. Sarcoid-like non-necrotizing granulomas are very unusual and mitigate against the diagnosis of Wegener's granulomatosis. The necrosis appears to start as tiny interstitial clusters of neutrophils that enlarge to become microabscesses and finally large geographic zones of necrosis, which may breach the pleura. Necrosis may also start as degeneration of collagen. In some cases, necrosis may center on airways, mimicking bronchocentric granulomatosis.

Inflammatory Background: The vasculitis and necrosis of Wegener's granulomatosis are set in an inflammatory background that result in extensive parenchymal consolidation from abundant fibrinous exudate or organizing pneumonia, mixed infiltrates of lymphocytes and plasma cells, scattered individual giant cells, and variable numbers of eosinophils. Sarcoid-like non-necrotizing granulomas are generally lacking.

Clues to the diagnosis include (1) the absence of discrete sarcoid-like granulomas, which are typical of necrotizing infections; (2) necrosis originating as tiny clusters and microabscesses of neutrophils; (3) the presence of *both* acute and chronic inflammation with *scattered* giant cells; and (4) segmental monocyte-dominated vasculitis in medium-sized vessels.

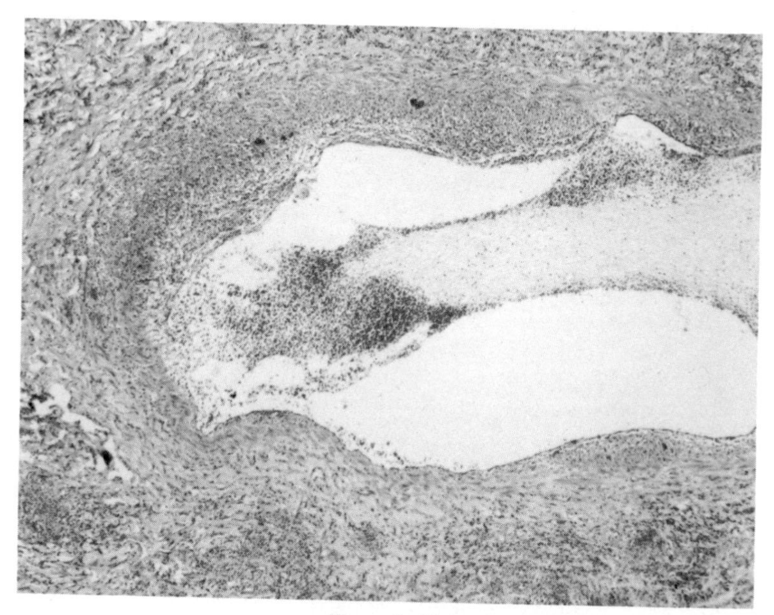

Figure 8–12.

Figures 8–12, 8–13, 8–14. Wegener's granulomatosis with more extensive involvement of the intima, with nodular infiltrates extending into the media. The infiltrates are composed of large numbers of cells resembling peripheral blood monocytes mixed with lymphocytes, neutrophils, and usually a few eosinophils. As the lesions expand, neutrophils tend to cluster into microabscesses (arrows), and this is the earliest intramural granuloma of Wegener's granulomatosis.

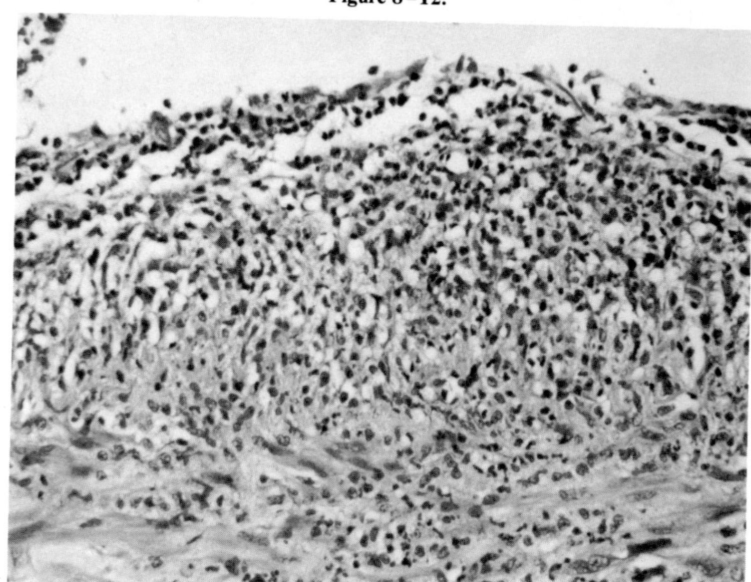

Figure 8–13.

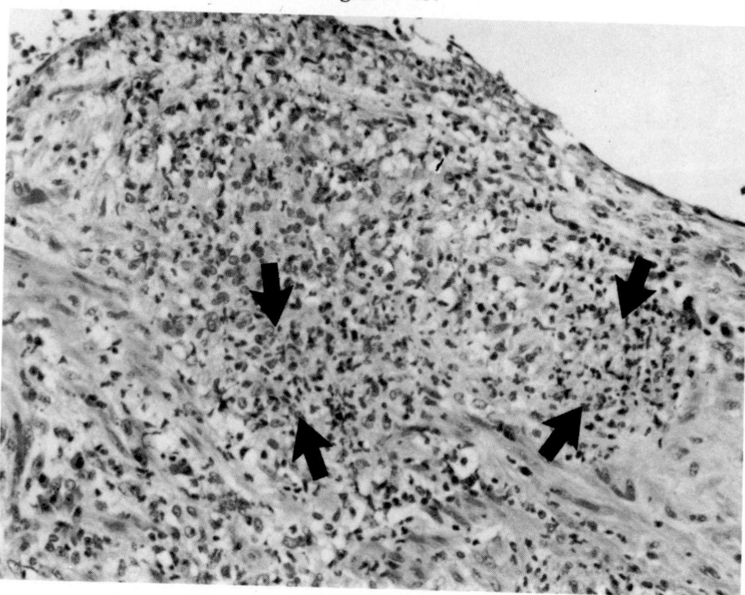

Figure 8–14.

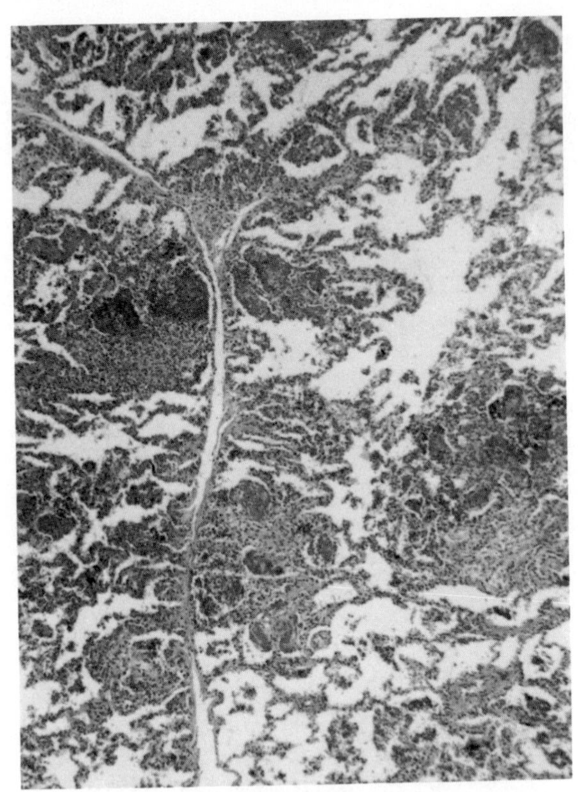

Figure 8–15.

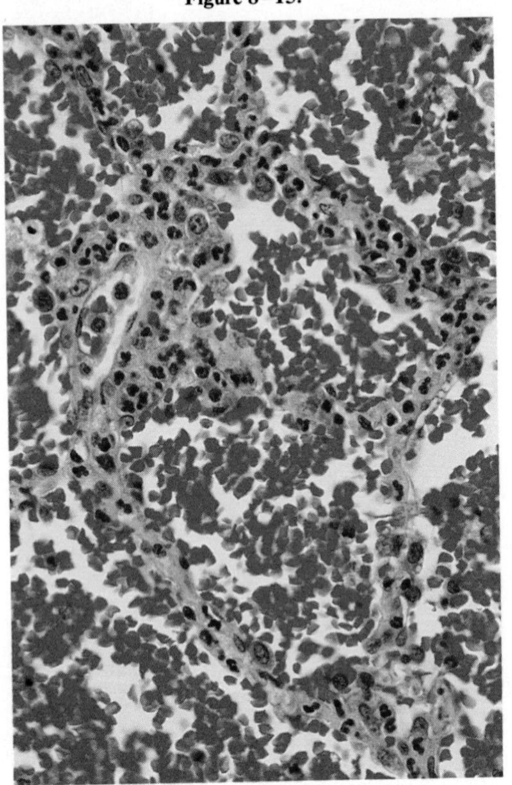

Figure 8–16.

Unusual patterns of Wegener's granulomatosis include:

1. Capillaritis and hemorrhage without necrosis or classic vasculitis.
2. Neutrophilic airspace infiltrates.
3. Pleural, septal, or bronchocentric prominence.
4. Focal intimal vasculitis only.
5. Fibrinoid necrotizing vasculitis.
6. Extensive organizing pneumonia.
7. Marked eosinophil infiltration.
8. Post-treatment with minimal diagnostic features.
9. Resemblance to an old healed granuloma.

The diagnosis of Wegener's granulomatosis depends on clinical and pathologic correlation and is one of exclusion of infection. A positive anti-neutrophil cytoplasmic antibody is a helpful supportive finding. Biopsy specimens from sites other than the lung, such as the upper airways, may be necessary to confirm a diagnosis in a case in which the pulmonary findings are nonspecific. Early diagnosis is important, since renal function can often be preserved.

References

Colby TV. Diffuse pulmonary hemorrhage in Wegener's granulomatosis. Semin Respir Med 10:136–140, 1989.

Fienberg R. The protracted superficial phenomenon in pathergic (Wegener's) granulomatosis. Hum Pathol 12:458–465, 1981.

Mark J, Matsubara O, Tau-Liu NS, Fienberg R. The pulmonary biopsy in the early diagnosis of Wegener's (pathergic) granulomatosis. Hum Pathol 19:1065–1071, 1988.

Figures 8–15, 8–16. Acute pulmonary hemorrhage with capillaritis (microvasculitis) in Wegener's granulomatosis. There are patchy infiltrates corresponding to hemorrhage and exudation into air spaces. Capillaritis is demonstrated by the presence of large numbers of neutrophils in the capillary wall associated with hemorrhage and relatively few neutrophils in the adjacent airspaces.

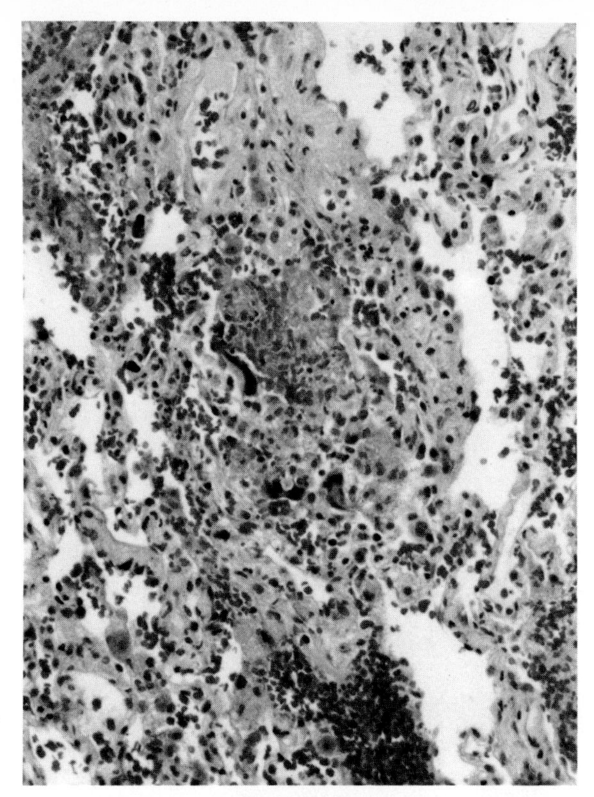

Figure 8-17.

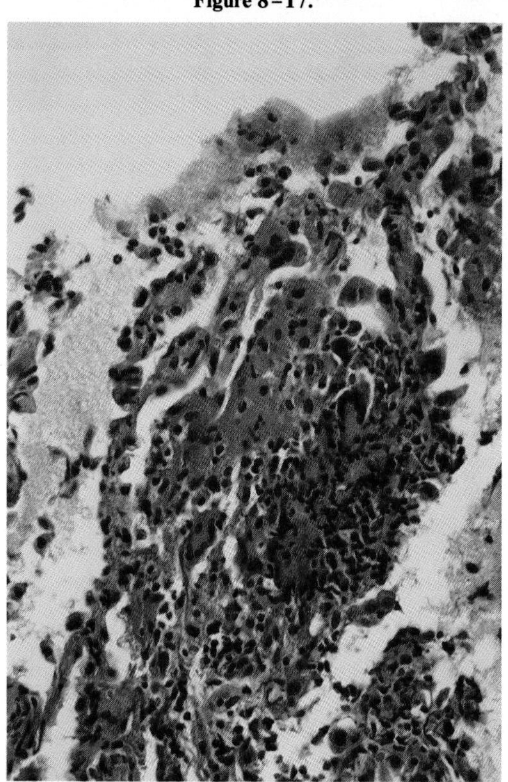

Figure 8-18.

Figures 8-17, 8-18. Granulomatous capillaritis in Wegener's granulomatosis. Two examples of granulomatous capillaritis in Wegener's granulomatosis. There is focal destruction of alveolar wall with hemorrhage and fibrinoid necrosis associated with scattered giant cells. Granulomatous capillaritis is an uncommon finding in Wegener's granulomatosis.

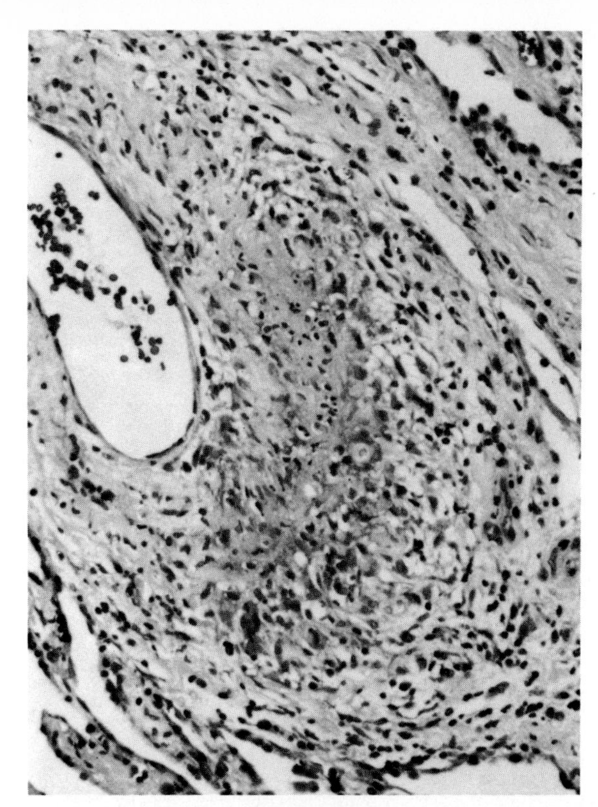

Figure 8-19.

Figure 8-19. Wegener's granulomatosis. There is an intramural necrotizing granuloma segmentally involving a small vein. Necrosis and a few neutrophils can be seen in the center.

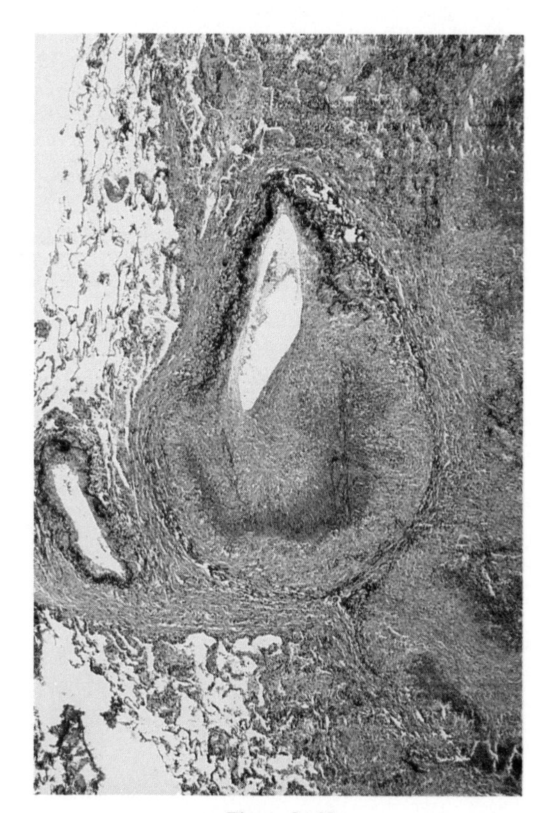

Figure 8-20.

Figure 8-20. Wegener's granulomatosis with the classic intramural necrotizing granuloma involving a medium-sized vessel highlighted with elastic tissue stain. The lesion is focal, segmental, and intramural in its location. It has a necrotic center with palisaded histiocytes and scattered giant cells surrounding the necrosis.

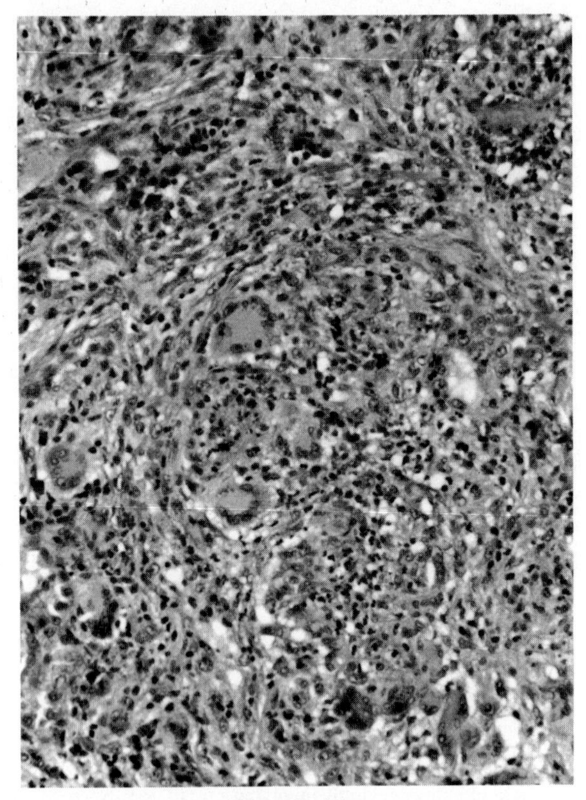

Figure 8–21.

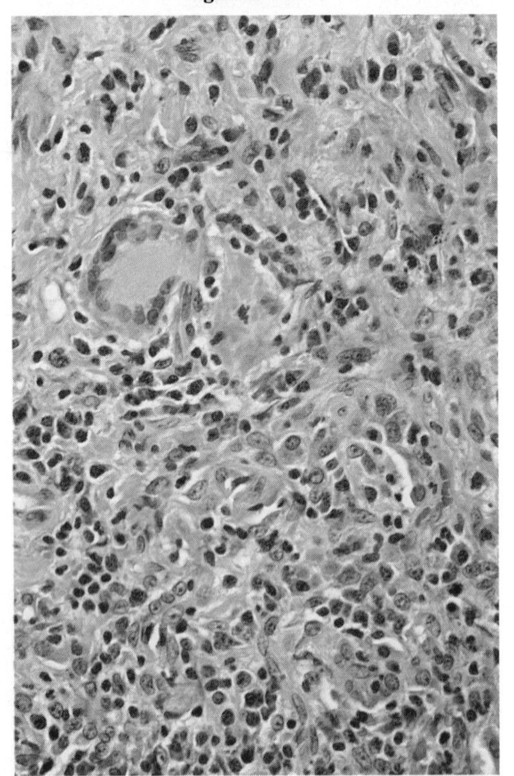

Figure 8–22.

Figures 8–21, 8–22. Wegener's granulomatosis. The inflammatory background in these cases is seen as parenchymal consolidation with fibroblast proliferation and a mixed infiltrate, including clusters of neutrophils, eosinophils, and giant cells.

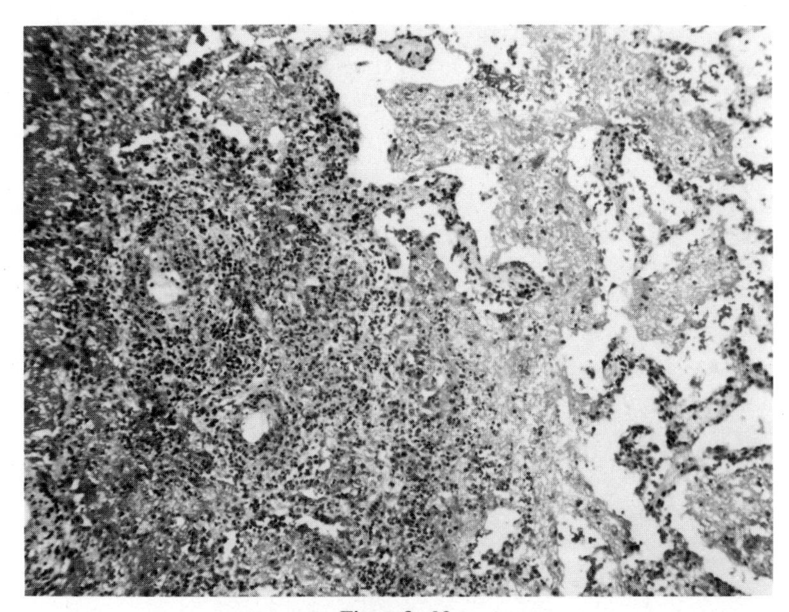

Figure 8-23.

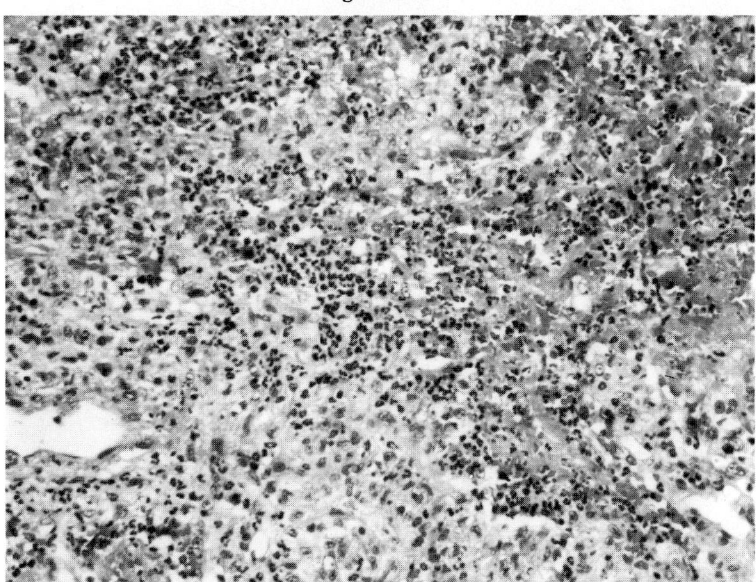

Figure 8-24.

Figures 8-23, 8-24, 8-25. Wegener's granulomatosis. The inflammatory background in Wegener's granulomatosis varies considerably. In this case, there is extensive airspace fibrinous exudate, consolidation, and marked infiltrates of neutrophils, which permeate the wall of the small vessel (Fig. 8-25).

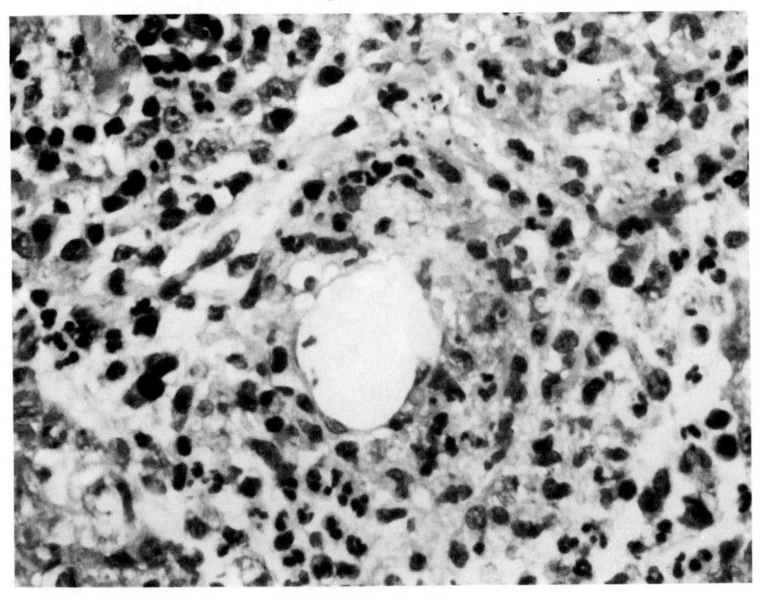

Figure 8-25.

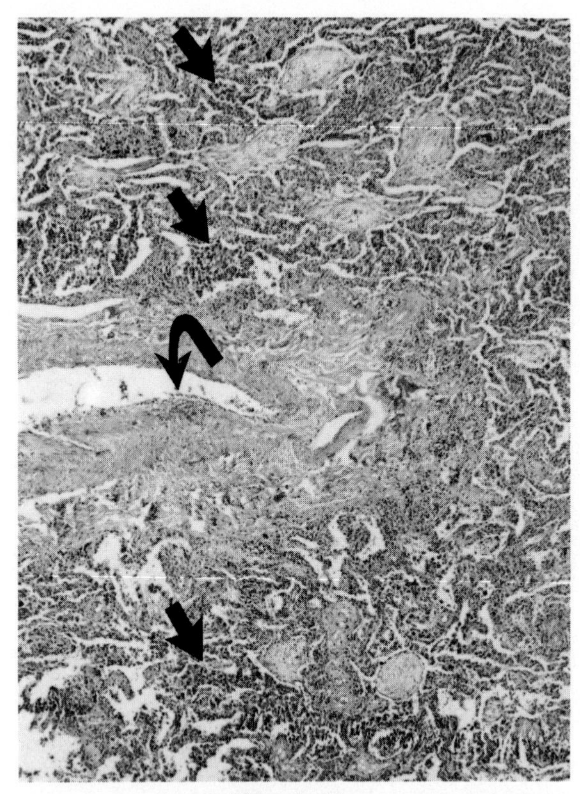

Figure 8-26.

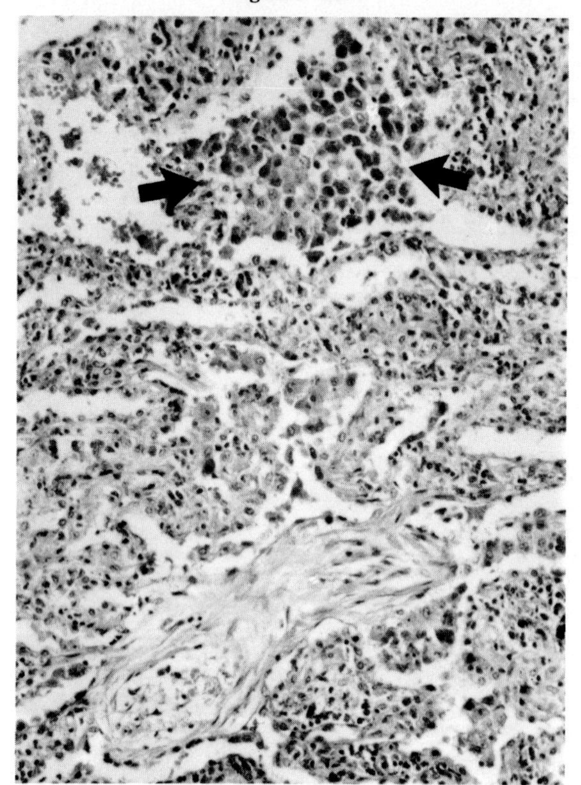

Figure 8-27.

Figures 8-26, 8-27. Wegener's granulomatosis. The inflammatory background resembles bronchiolitis obliterans organizing pneumonia (BOOP) with myxomatous connective tissue. The adjacent alveoli contain hemosiderin-filled macrophages (arrows) attesting to prior alveolar hemorrhage. An early vascular lesion (curved arrow) can be seen as an endothelial and subendothelial infiltrate.

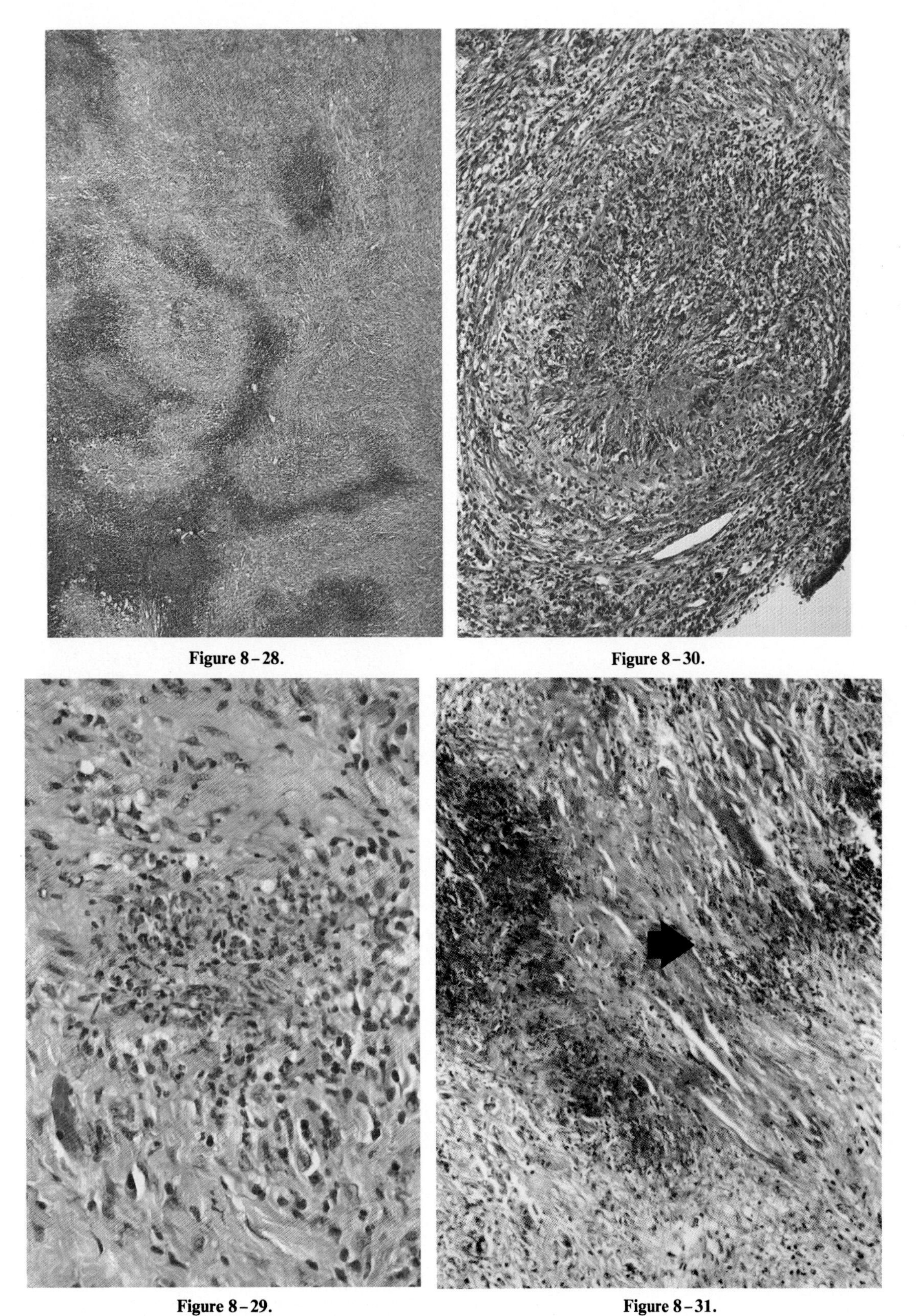

Figure 8-28.

Figure 8-30.

Figure 8-29.

Figure 8-31.

Figures 8-28, 8-29, 8-30, 8-31. Wegener's granulomatosis. The necrosis is characteristically geographic and basophilic in appearance (Fig 8-28). It appears to start as small microabscesses (Figs. 8-29, 8-30), which enlarge and coalesce. In some cases, necrosis of pre-existing collagenous bands (arrows) can be seen.

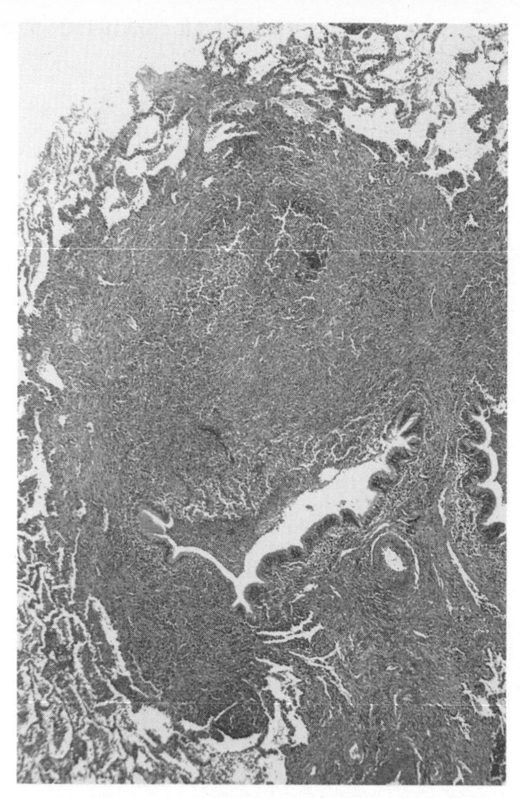

Figure 8-32. Wegener's granulomatosis. Necrosis is centered on a bronchiolar wall with the accompanying artery left unaffected.

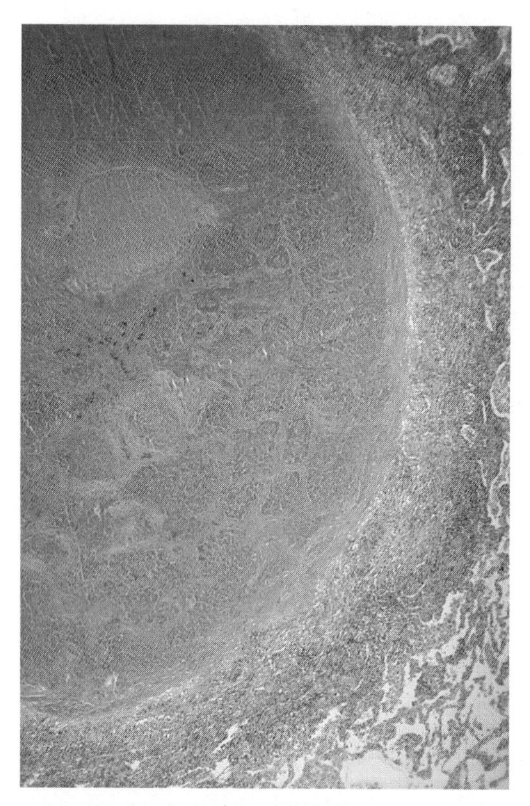

Figure 8-33. Wegener's granulomatosis. As the necrotic granulomas age, they round up and become less specific in their appearance. Late in their evolution, they may resemble an old, healing granuloma or infarct. There were no distinguishing features to the granuloma in this case, and the diagnosis was made on the basis of a history of biopsy-proven Wegener's granulomatosis in the upper airway and the subsequent development of multiple pulmonary nodules.

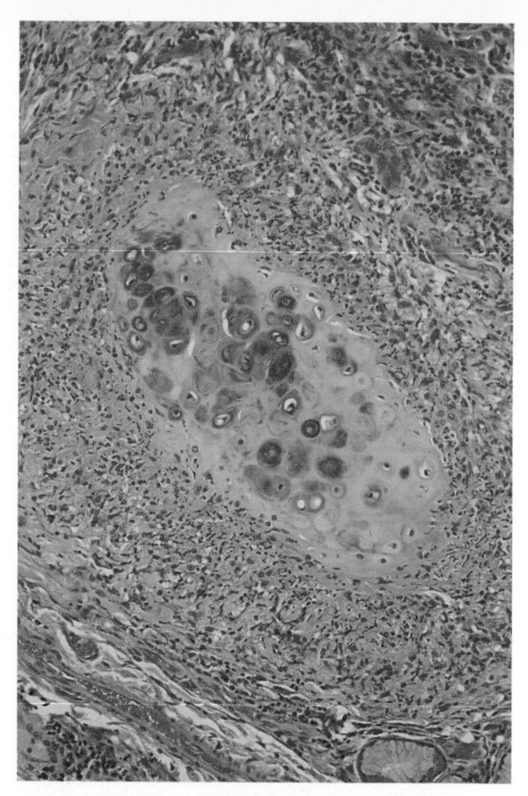

Figure 8-34.

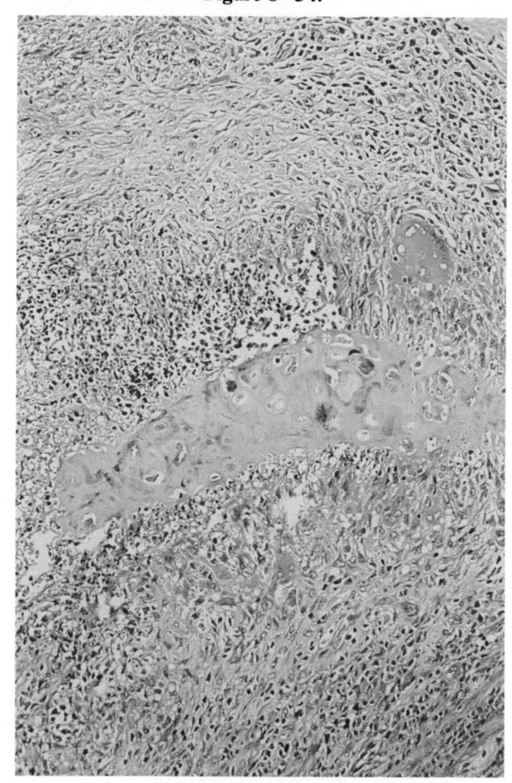

Figure 8-35.

Figures 8-34, 8-35. Wegener's granulomatosis. An inflammatory destructive perichondritis, occasionally with giant cells (Fig. 8-35), may be seen in cartilaginous airways in Wegener's granulomatosis.

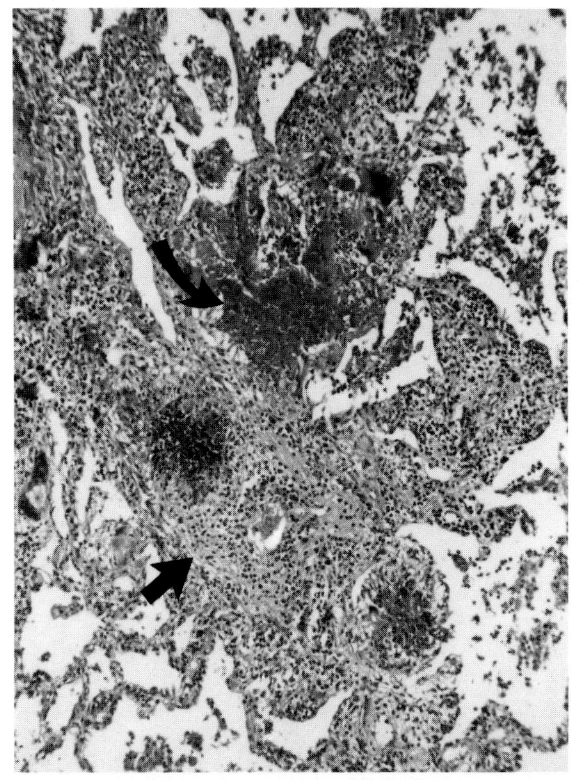

Figure 8–36. Churg-Strauss syndrome. Vasculitis (arrow) and an extravascular necrotizing granuloma (curved arrow) with surrounding inflammatory infiltrates, including scattered giant cells, are shown.

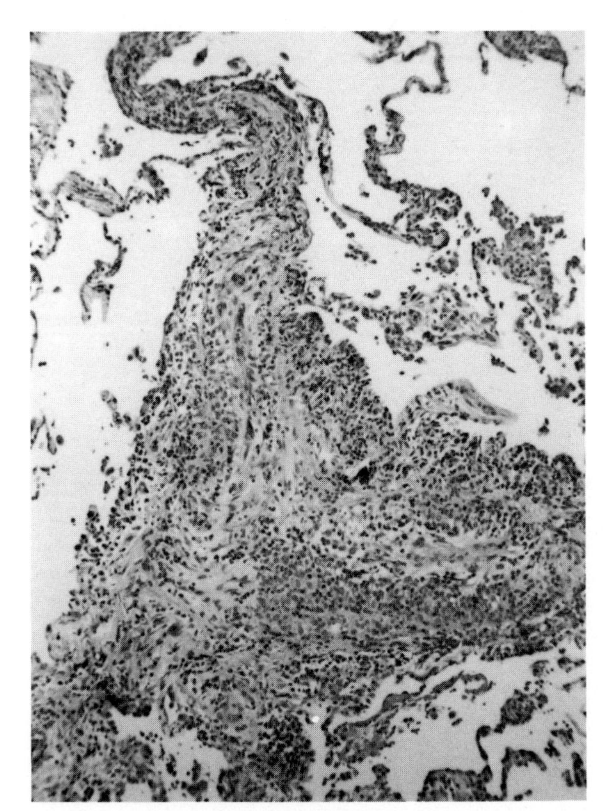

Figure 8–37. Churg-Strauss syndrome. A prominent venulitis is shown with inflammatory cells (which included numerous eosinophils) permeating the wall of a small vein.

■ Churg-Strauss Syndrome (Allergic Granulomatosis) (Figs. 8–36 to 8–40)

A systemic vasculitis and extravascular granulomatosis with necrosis that occurs in patients with a history of asthma; usually associated with peripheral eosinophilia and often allergic nasal polyps. This definition is relatively restrictive, and some authors have suggested a somewhat looser one.

There is vasculitis of medium-sized and small arteries and veins with inflammatory infiltration and necrosis of vessels walls, with numerous eosinophils. The parenchymal changes resemble those in eosinophilic pneumonia. Small epithelioid granulomas can be seen. Necrotizing granulomas that surround eosinophilic debris without parenchymal necrosis of lung also occur. In some cases, the vasculitis is nonspecific and lacks prominent eosinophils. The airways often show asthmatic changes.

Classic cases with *all* of the clinical and histologic features are extremely rare, and a significant number of patients must be assigned to an unclassified category. For this reason, a somewhat looser definition of Churg-Strauss syndrome may be appropriate. Diagnosis may be made from a biopsy specimen from any number of sites in the appropriate clinical setting. Some cases of Wegener's granulomatosis with massive numbers of eosinophils may mimic Churg-Strauss syndrome.

References

Dail DH, Hammer SP (eds). Pulmonary Pathology. New York, Springer-Verlag, 1988.

Lanham JG, Elkon KB, Pusey CD, Hughes GR. Systemic vasculitis with asthma and eosinophilia: a clinical approach to the Churg-Strauss syndrome. Medicine 62:142–158, 1983.

Thurlbeck WM (ed). Pathology of the Lung. New York, Thieme, 1988.

Yousem SA, Lombard CL. The eosinophilic variant of Wegener's granulomatosis. Hum Pathol 19:682–688, 1988.

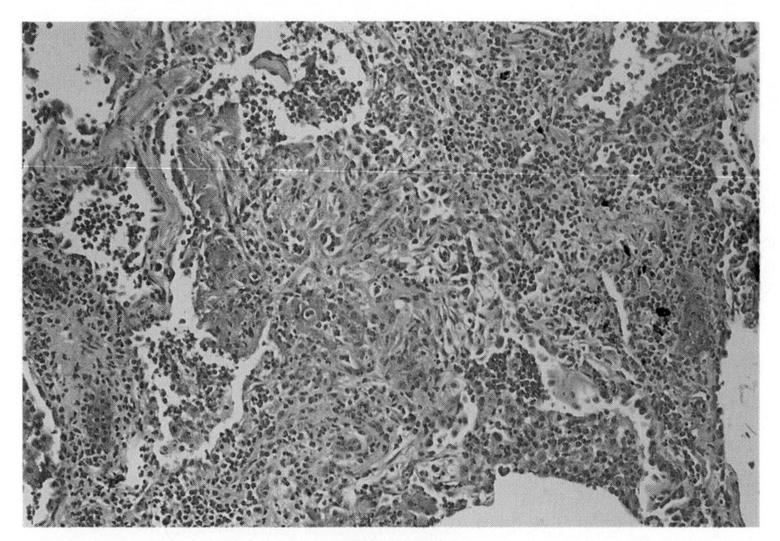

Figure 8–38.

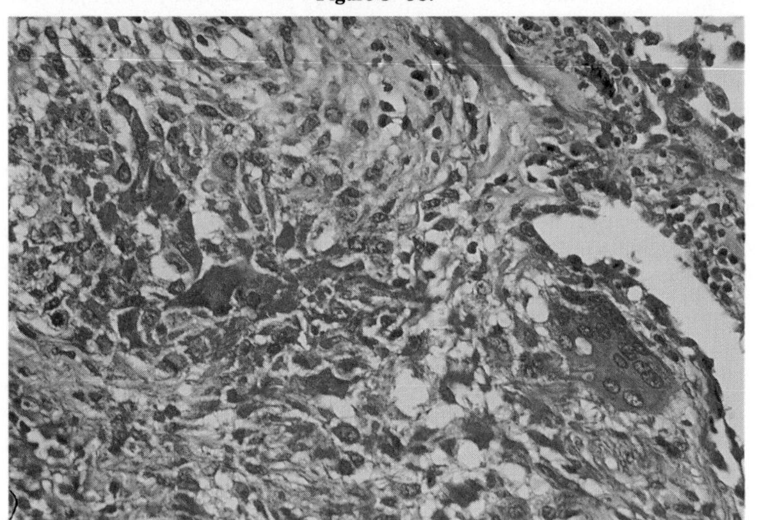

Figure 8–39.

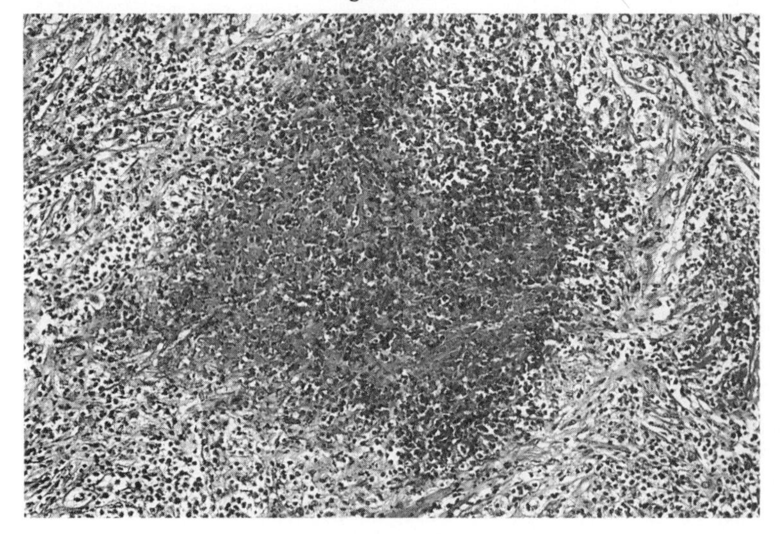

Figure 8–40.

Figures 8–38, 8–39, 8–40. Churg-Strauss syndrome. In some foci, there is eosinophilic pneumonia with airspace accumulations of eosinophils and histiocytes as well as eosinophilic necrosis.

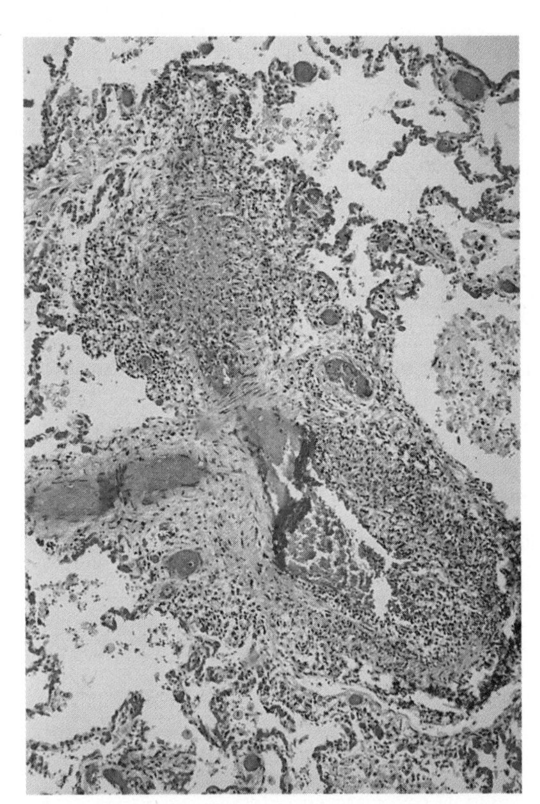

Figure 8–41. Polyarteritis nodosa. Polyarteritis nodosa rarely involves the lung; when this does occur, however, the pathologic changes are restricted to pulmonary arteries and show features typical of polyarteritis elsewhere, mainly fibrinoid necrosis with an infiltrate rich in neutrophils. (From an autopsy case of widespread polyarteritis nodosa.)

■ **Polyarteritis Nodosa** (Fig. 8–41)

This systemic necrotizing arteritis only rarely affects the lung. There is a necrotizing arteritis with fibrinoid necrosis and infiltrate of neutrophils restricted to pulmonary arteries, with sparing of veins and intervening lung parenchyma.

Note: This is a curiosity for the surgical pathologist.

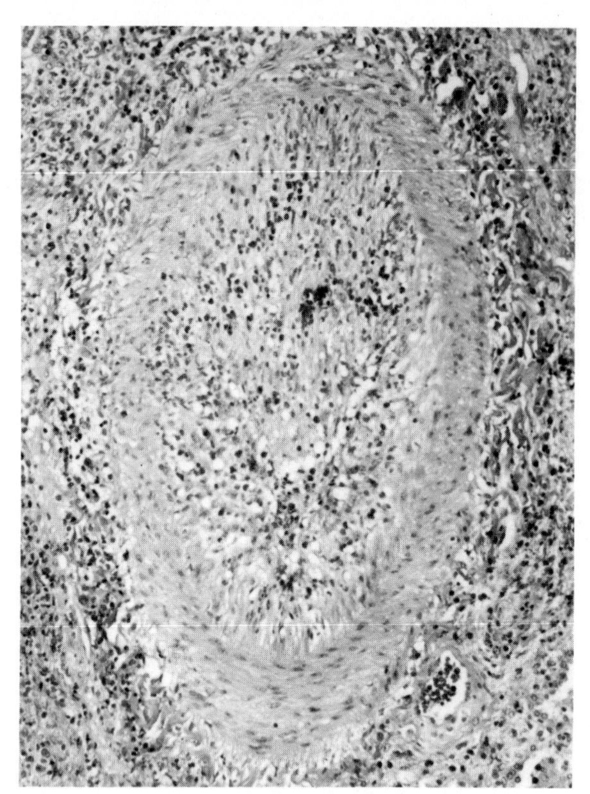

Figure 8-42.

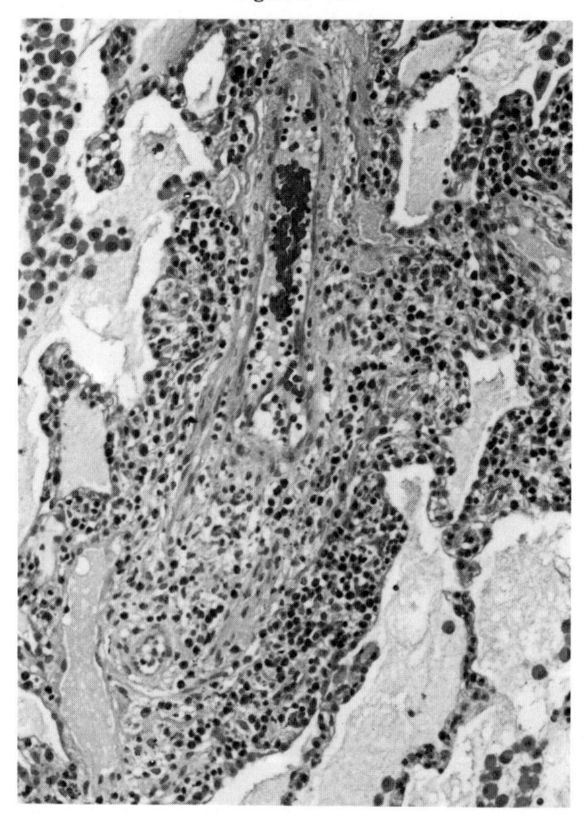

Figure 8-43.

■ Other Vasculitides (Figs. 8-42 to 8-47)

A number of other vasculitides may involve the lung, including giant cell arteritis, systemic hypersensitivity vasculitis (leukocytoclastic vasculitis), Behçet's syndrome, and others. Some cases are difficult to classify. It is important to remember that granulomatous involvement of vessels is extremely common in sarcoidosis and may also be seen in necrotizing sarcoid granulomatosis and granulomatous infections. In immunosuppressed patients and neonates, infections are sometimes the cause of a vasculitis. Capillaritis (including venulitis, which is a frequent concomitant) is discussed in the section on interstitial lung disease (see p. 236).

References

Thurlbeck WM (ed). Pathology of the Lung. New York, Thieme, 1988.

Figures 8-42, 8-43. Unclassified vasculitis. In a patient with a history of sarcoidosis (and granulomas elsewhere in the biopsy specimen), marked infiltration of both arteries (Fig. 8-42) and veins (Fig. 8-43) by massive numbers of eosinophils developed. The artery appears almost entirely occluded by intimal proliferation; yet vascular abnormalities were not apparent clinically. There was no history of asthma, there was no necrosis, and the case was considered an unclassified eosinophilic vasculitis. A reaction to an antibiotic was suggested but not proven.

Figures 8-44, 8-45, 8-46. Systemic eosinophilic microangiitis of unknown cause. A young woman presented with bilateral pulmonary infiltrates and skin lesions. Skin (Fig. 8-44) and lung (Fig. 8-45) biopsy specimens showed vascular and perivascular infiltrates of eosinophils, which in some foci in the lung spilled over into the airspaces, producing microscopic foci of eosinophilic pneumonia (Fig 8-46). A drug reaction was suspected, but none could be proven. The patient's disease cleared after steroid therapy. There was no history of asthma.

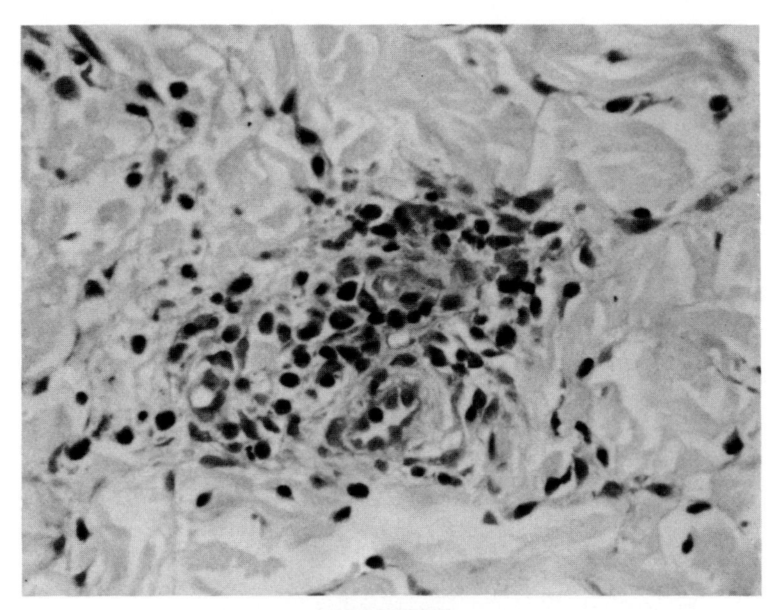

Figure 8-44.

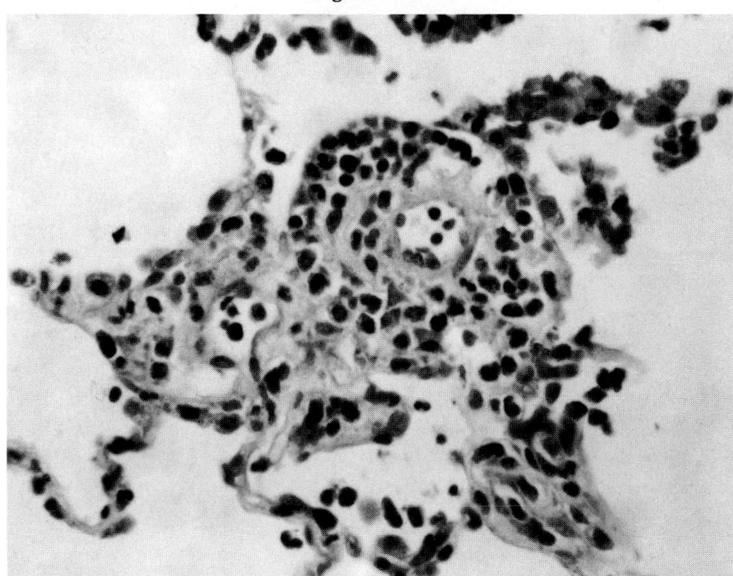

Figure 8-45.

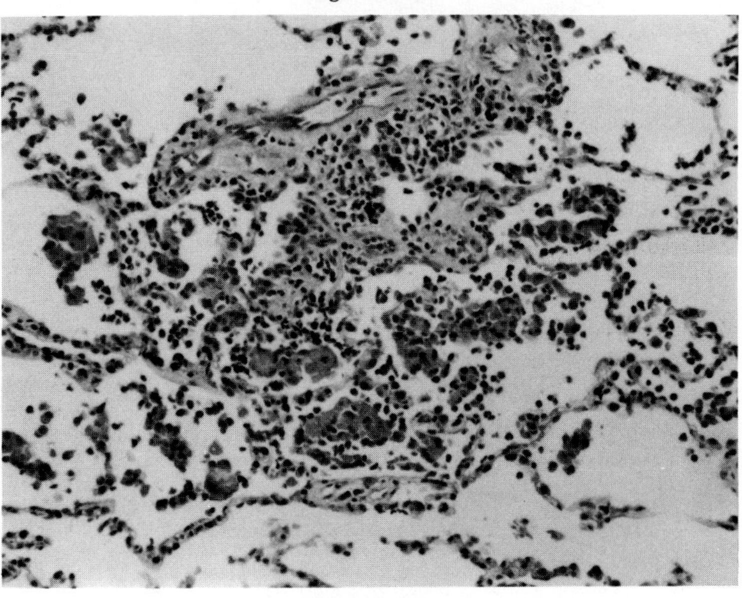

Figure 8-46.

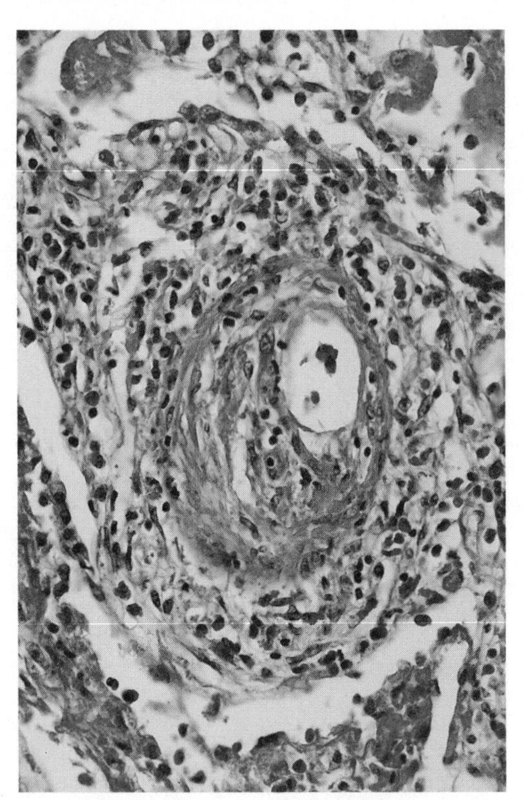

Figure 8–47. Hypersensitivity angiitis. In this case of pulmonary hypersensitivity angiitis, an infiltrate rich in eosinophils extends through the walls of a pulmonary vein. The lesion was related to the use of antibiotic therapy.

■ Pulmonary Hypertension (Figs. 8–48 to 8–63)

Only occasionally is pulmonary hypertension a surprise in a lung biopsy specimen. Biopsy may be performed to determine the type of pulmonary hypertension or to determine whether the changes present are reversible. In mild pulmonary hypertension, the vessels may be entirely normal; in such cases, the catheterization pressure studies should be trusted more than histologic interpretation of the vessels.

In established pulmonary hypertension, there is a progression of changes involving the media (muscular hypertrophy) and intima (fibroblastic and lamellar thickening); in severe cases, there is necrosis of the vessel wall and dilatation and plexiform lesions that are typical of, but not specific for, plexogenic arteriopathy.

Pulmonary hypertension may be caused by cardiac disease and may be secondary to hypoxia associated with a number of chronic lung diseases, especially chronic bronchitis and emphysema. Drugs (aminorex) and infections (e.g., schistosomiasis) are unusual causes. Unexplained or "primary" forms of pulmonary hypertension include the following:

1. Plexogenic arteriopathy.
2. Pulmonary veno-occlusive disease with secondary pulmonary arterial hypertension. This is caused by occlusive pulmonary venous lesions, which are best appreciated with elastic tissue stains. Interstitial edema, fibrosis, and hemosiderin-filled macrophages in the airspaces are typical of veno-occlusive disease, and a variable inflammatory infiltrate is common, *often mimicking a chronic interstitial pneumonia.*
3. Chronic thromboembolic pulmonary hypertension. This results in eccentric intimal plaques and webs in the pulmonary arteries and, rarely, fresh thromboemboli. Secondary thrombi in other forms of pulmonary hypertension should be considered and excluded.
4. Pulmonary capillary hemangiomatosis. This is an extremely rare cause of primary pulmonary hypertension caused by the proliferation of thin-walled capillaries in the pulmonary interstitium that produces a secondary veno-occlusive disease and that, in turn, leads to pulmonary arterial hypertension.

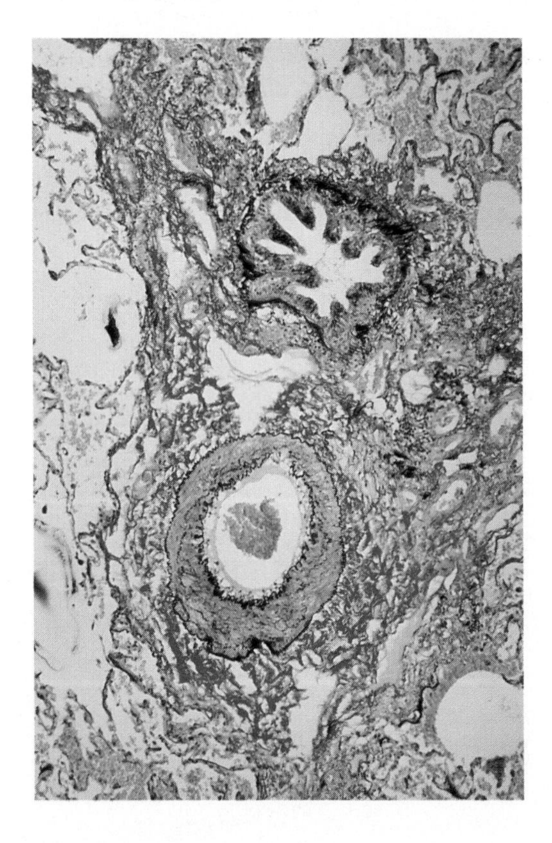

Figure 8–48. Pulmonary arterial hypertension. The earliest changes are subtle thickening of the media of the pulmonary arteries. In general, the study of histologic features (without using morphometry) is a relatively crude way of assessing the presence or absence of pulmonary hypertension, and one should trust the findings from catheterization pressure studies more than one's histologic findings in assessing the presence of and degree of pulmonary hypertension.

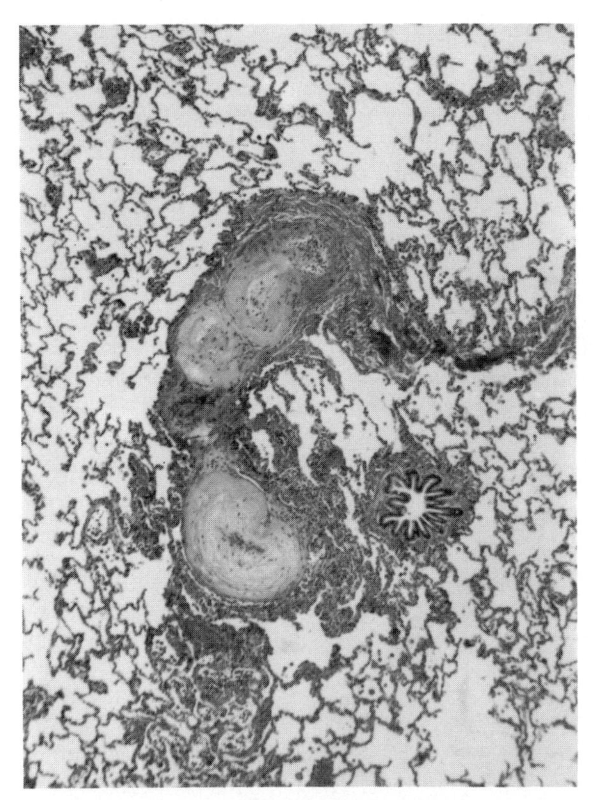

Figure 8-49.

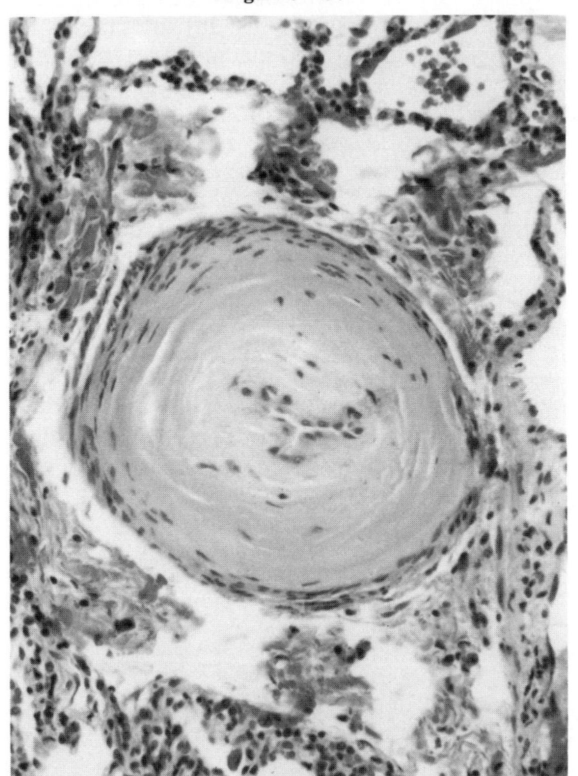

Figure 8-50.

Note: Pulmonary hypertension should always be considered in the differential diagnosis of a lung biopsy specimen that appears normal at first glance. Once pulmonary hypertension has developed, regardless of cause, pulmonary emboli or pulmonary arterial thrombosis may occur; therefore, the presence of a *few* healed emboli or thrombi in the pulmonary arterial tree is not specific for chronic thromboembolic hypertension. In chronic passive venous congestion, regardless of cause and especially when localized, an impressive degree of capillary proliferation can occur and can mimic pulmonary capillary hemangiomatosis.

Vascular changes in scarred lung tissue are often present and should be interpreted with caution. Parenchymal scarring per se may be accompanied by an impressive degree of myointimal proliferation in veins and arteries in the fibrotic zones.

References

Dail DH, Hammer SP (eds). Pulmonary Pathology. New York, Springer-Verlag, 1988.

Edwards WD. Pathology of pulmonary hypertension. Cardiovasc Clin 18:321-359, 1987.

Thurlbeck WM (ed). Pathology of the Lung. New York, Thieme, 1988.

Tron V, Magee F, Wright JL, Colby TV, Churg A. Pulmonary capillary hemangiomatosis. Hum Pathol 17:1144-1150, 1986.

Wagenvoort CA. Open lung biopsies in congenital heart disease for evaluation of pulmonary vascular disease: predictive value with regard to corrective operability. Histopathology 9:417-436, 1985.

Wagenvoort CA, Wagenvoort N. Pathology of Pulmonary Hypertension. New York, John Wiley & Sons, Inc, 1977.

Figures 8-49, 8-50. Pulmonary hypertension in scleroderma. In scleroderma, intimal proliferation may be very dramatic and may have an onion-skin appearance.

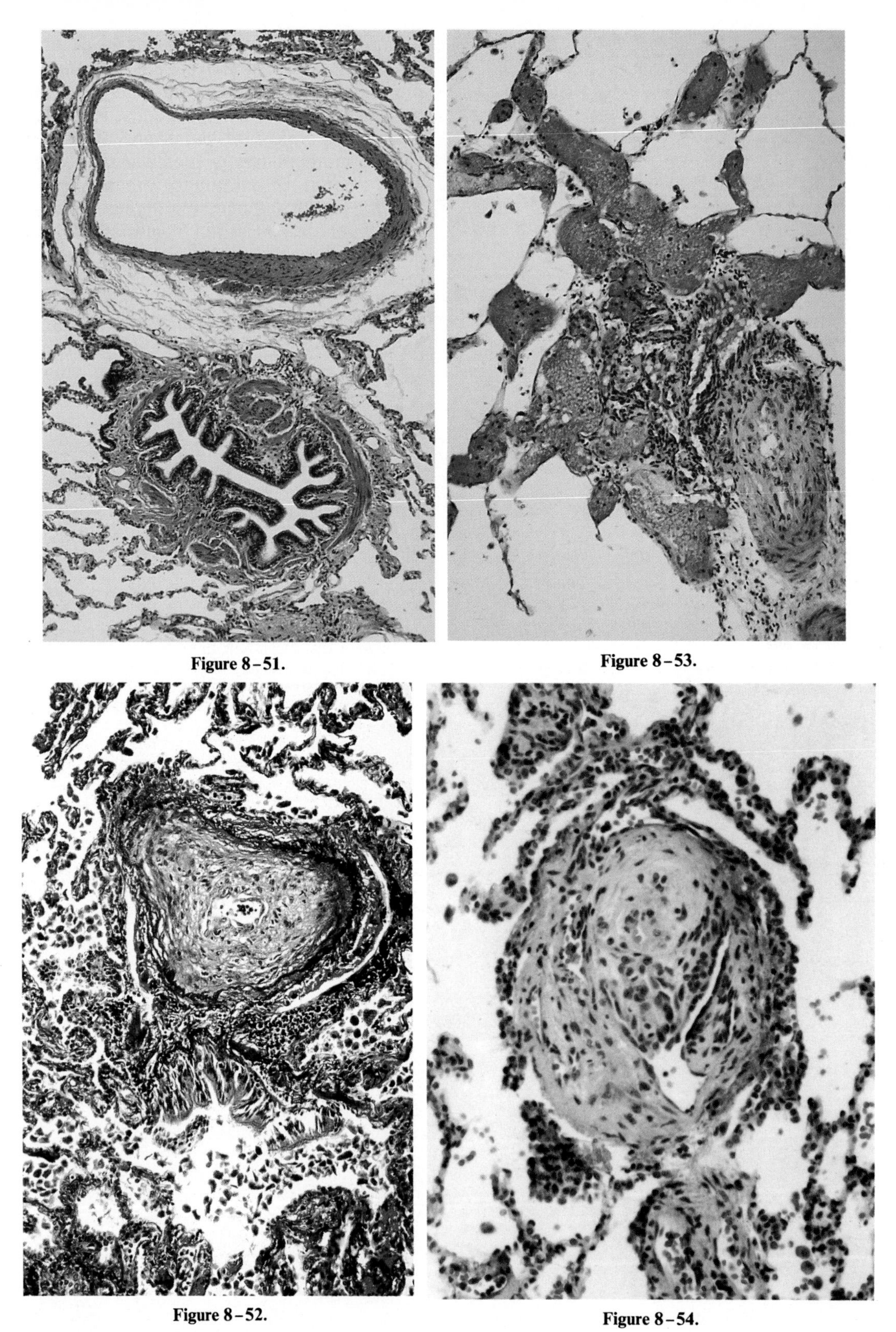

Figure 8-51.

Figure 8-53.

Figure 8-52.

Figure 8-54.

Figures 8-51, 8-52, 8-53, 8-54. Plexogenic arteriopathy. A variation in the appearance of one vessel to the next is common in plexogenic arteriopathy. One may encounter dilatation lesions (Fig. 8-51), arterioles showing marked intimal thickening (Fig. 8-52), and plexiform lesions that may be obvious (Fig. 8-53) or relatively subtle (Fig. 8-54).

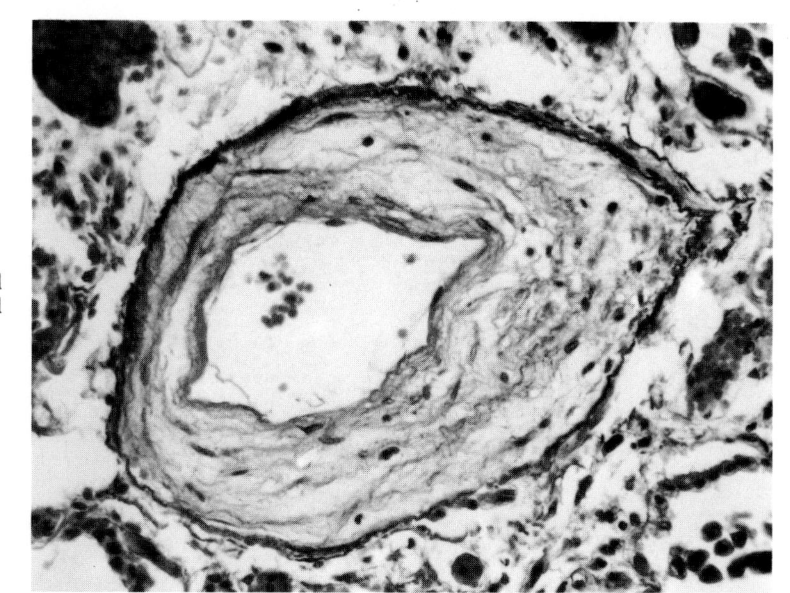

Figure 8-55. Pulmonary veno-occlusive disease. Partial venous occlusion by an intimal proliferation in a small septal vein is evident.

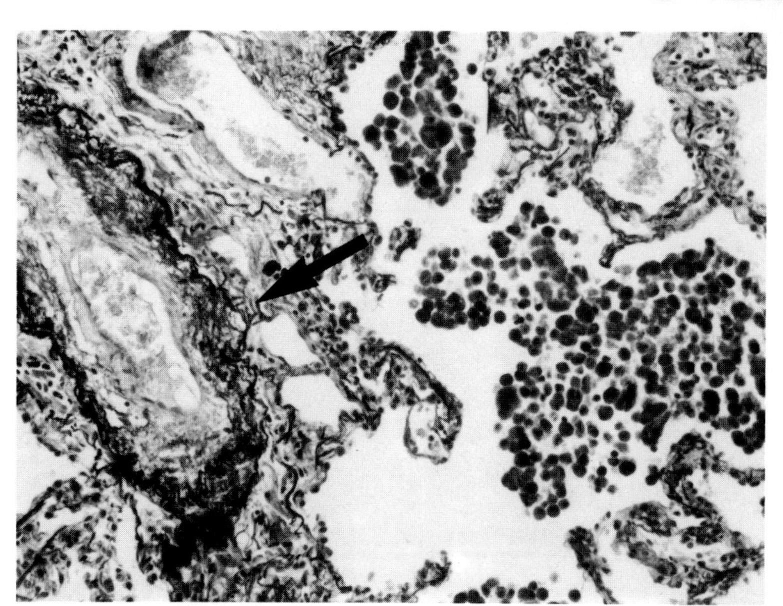

Figure 8-56. Pulmonary veno-occlusive disease. Partial occlusion of a septal vein (arrow) is shown: There is some duplication of the elastica. The adjacent alveolar spaces contain hemosiderin-filled macrophages, a characteristic finding in pulmonary veno-occlusive disease.

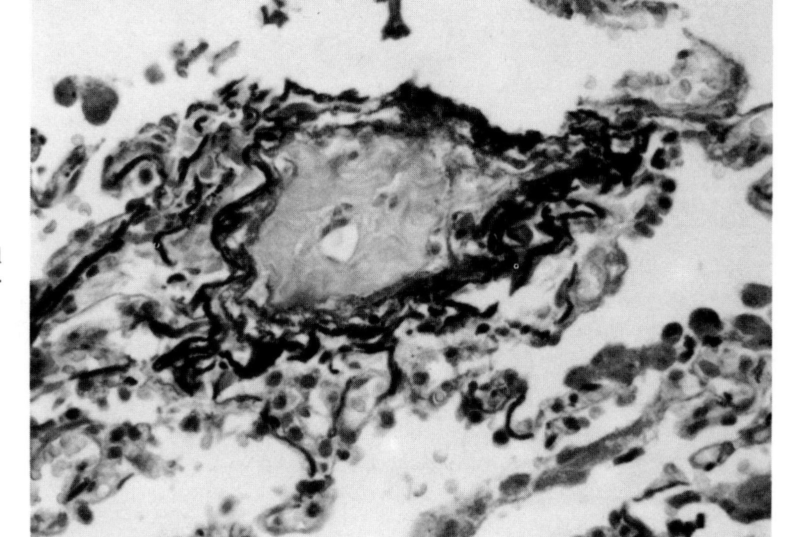

Figure 8-57. Pulmonary veno-occlusive disease. A small intraparenchymal vein is almost entirely occluded by intimal fibrosis.

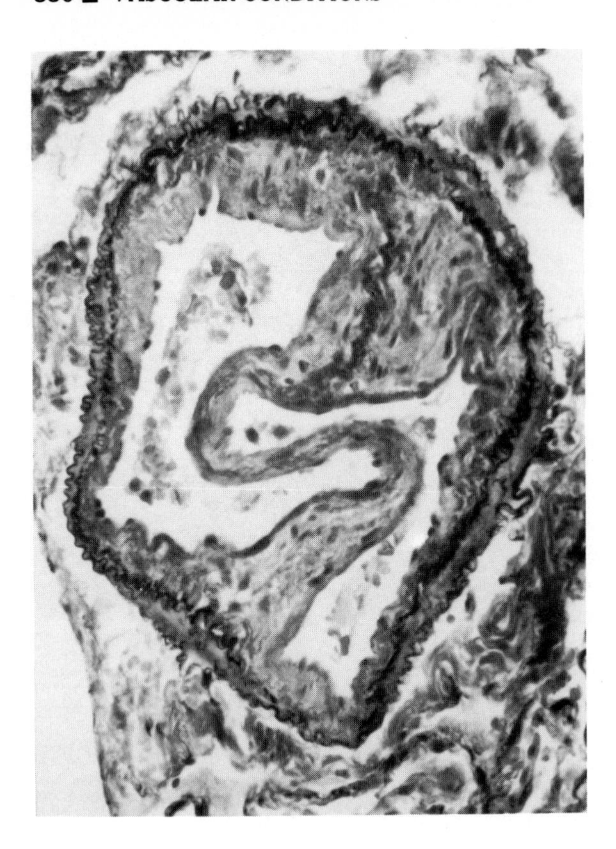

Figure 8–58. Pulmonary hypertension due to chronic thromboembolic disease. Most of the small arteries in this case contained healed thromboemboli. Healed thromboemboli with recanalization may occasionally resemble plexiform lesions, and it is useful to perform an elastic tissue stain (as in this case) to confirm the intravascular location of the changes and the maintenance of the elastica, which is disrupted in plexiform lesions.

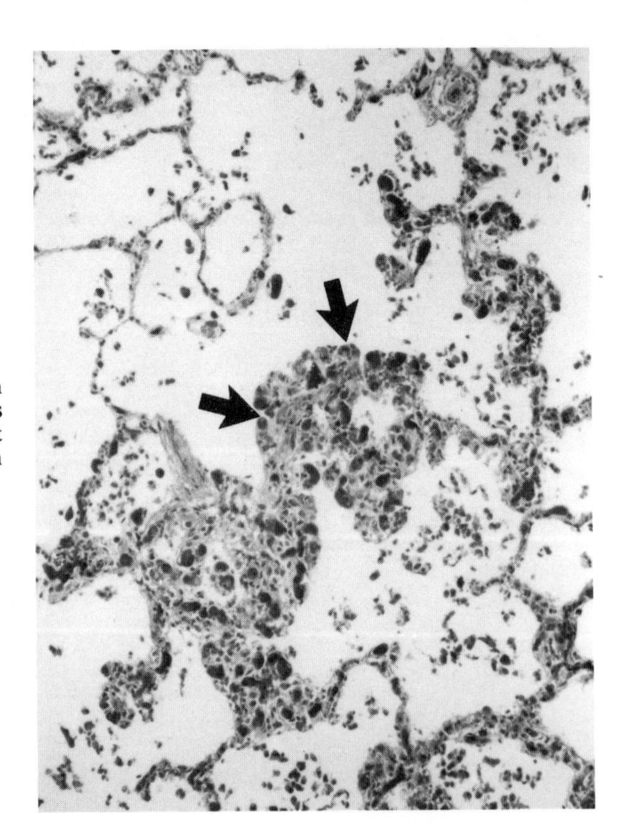

Figure 8–59. Pulmonary capillary hemangiomatosis. Capillary proliferation involving alveolar walls (arrows) adjacent to nearly normal alveolar walls is apparent. The pathogenesis of this condition is obscure; however, it is thought that capillary proliferation produces a secondary veno-occlusive disease that, in turn, causes secondary pulmonary hypertension.

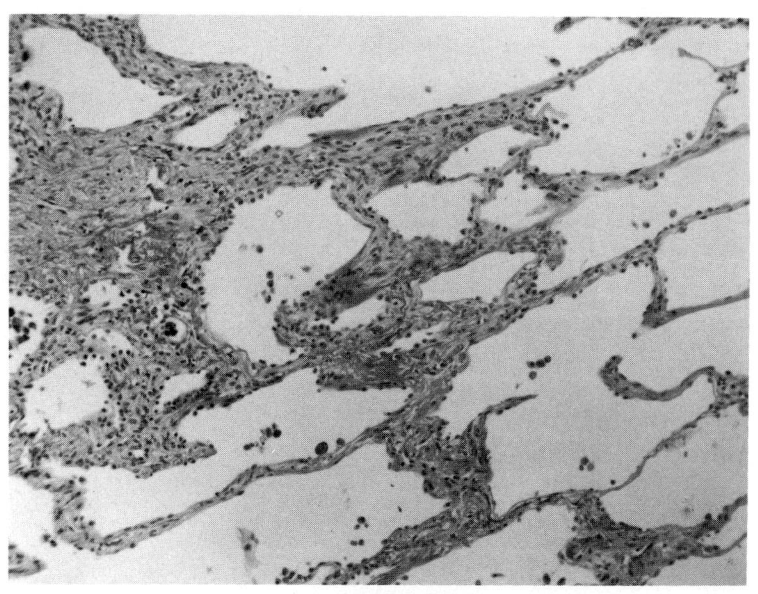

Figure 8-60.

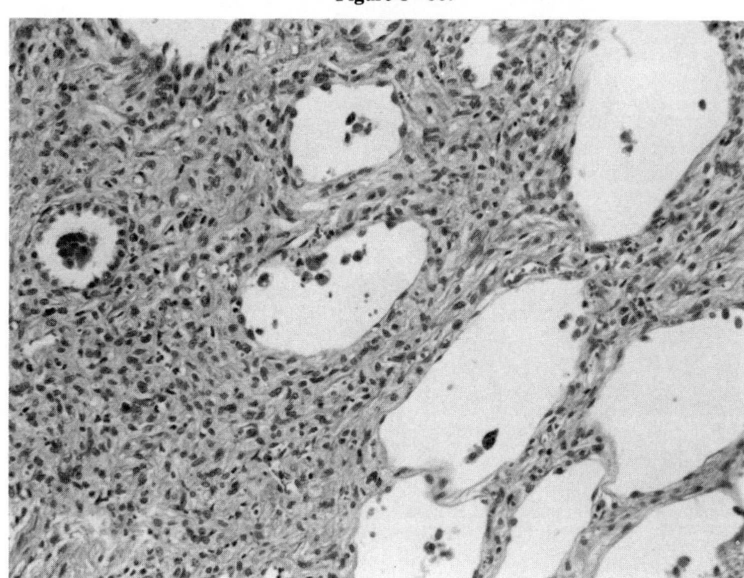

Figure 8-61.

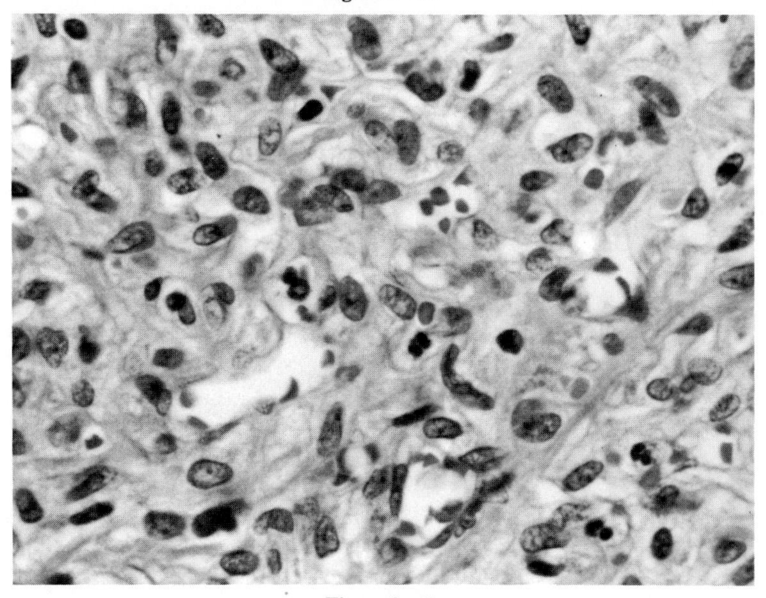

Figure 8-62.

Figures 8-60, 8-61, 8-62. Pulmonary capillary hemangiomatosis. Pulmonary capillary hemangiomatosis with interstitial hypercellularity caused by cells with nuclear features of endothelial cells and with the presence of numerous capillary lumens.

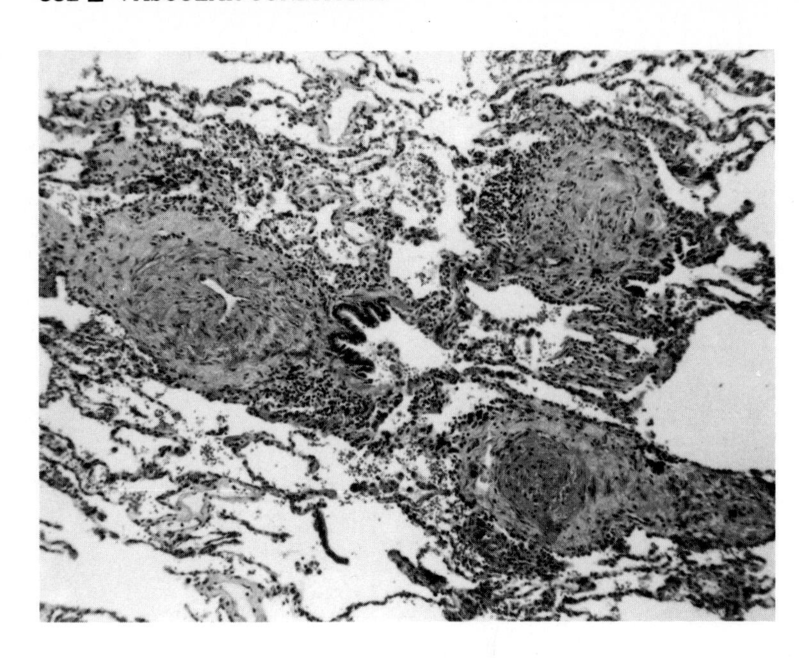

Figure 8–63. Intra-arterial metastatic carcinoma. Pulmonary hypertension associated with extensive intra-arterial metastatic carcinoma. This is the same case as the one illustrated in Figures 3–163 to 3–165. In many fields, only marked thickening of the pulmonary arteries and arterioles without obvious carcinoma cells could be appreciated.

CHAPTER 9

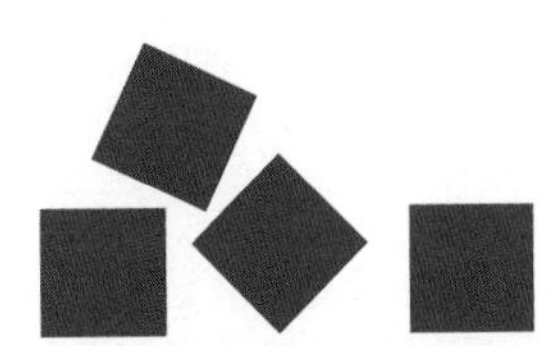

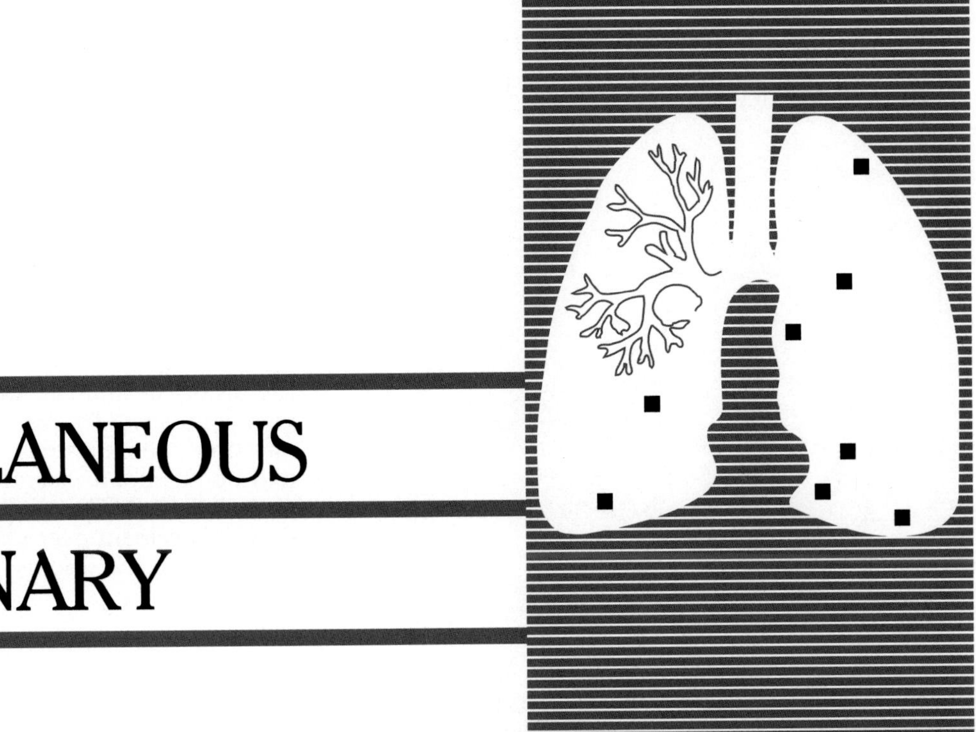

MISCELLANEOUS PULMONARY LESIONS

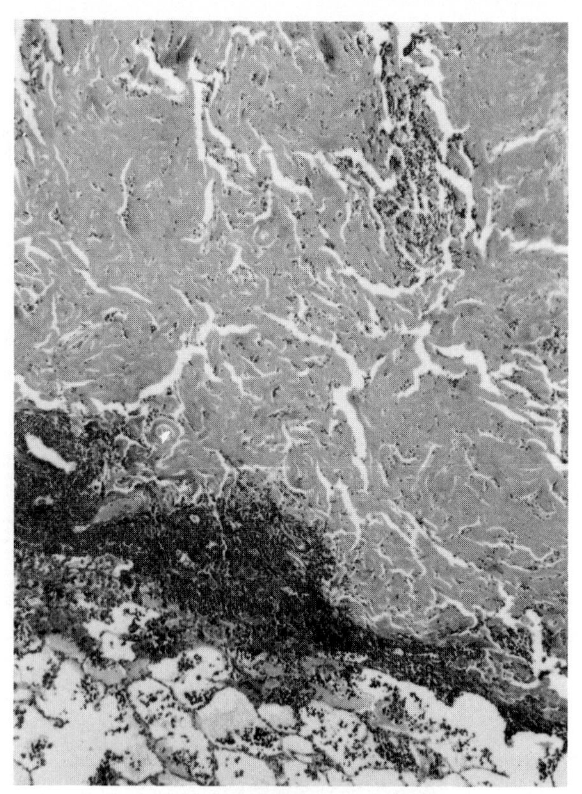

Figure 9-1.

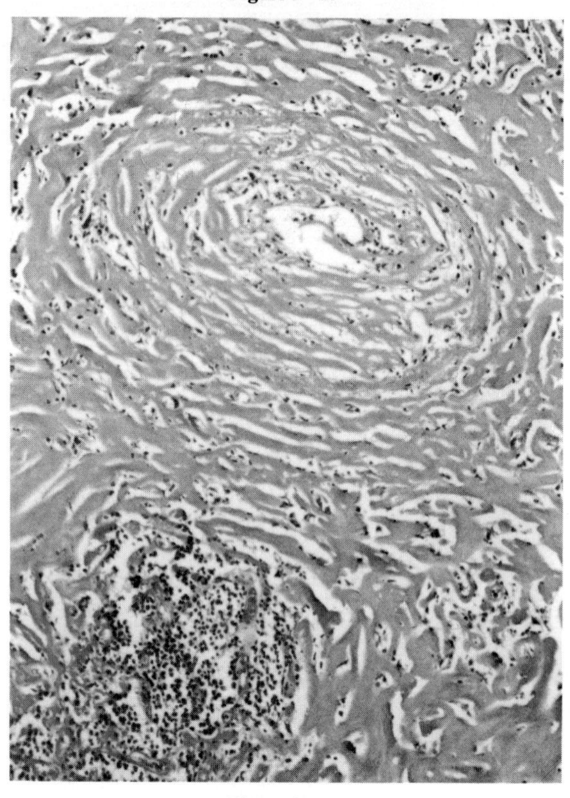

Figure 9-2.

■ Pulmonary Hyalinizing Granuloma (Figs. 9-1, 9-2)

Pulmonary hyalinizing granuloma is an uncommon condition that usually presents as multiple, bilateral slowly enlarging nodules. Single or unilateral nodules rarely occur. In many of the cases, the lesion is thought to be related to hyperimmunity to infection, particularly histoplasmosis, and is the pulmonary analog of sclerosing mediastinitis.

Histologically, dense, hyalinized connective tissue with thick lamellar bands of relatively acellular eosinophilic collagen is associated with a patchy lymphoid infiltrate, which can be quite dense focally and may be associated with a prominent perivasculitis and germinal center formation. An occasional noncaseating granuloma may be seen. Special stains do not show organisms. Caseous necrosis or microabscess formation is lacking, although degenerative necrosis may take place in the centers of large nodules.

The most distinctive features are the thick hyalinized collagen arranged in whorls and cartwheels and the clinical history of multiple lesions. Pulmonary hyalinizing granuloma should be distinguished from granulomatous infections; noninfectious granulomas, such as rheumatoid nodules; and pleural lesions, particularly hyaline pleural plaques. The condition is relatively benign, with slow enlargement over many years, and relatively few patients with this disorder experience problems.

References

Yousem SA, Hochholzer L. Pulmonary hyalinizing granuloma. Am J Clin Pathol 87:1-6, 1987.

Figures 9-1, 9-2. Pulmonary hyalinizing granuloma. There is a circumscribed densely fibrotic nodule with patchy chronic inflammation both around and within it. The nodule is composed of thick, hyalinized bands of collagen that stained negatively for amyloid.

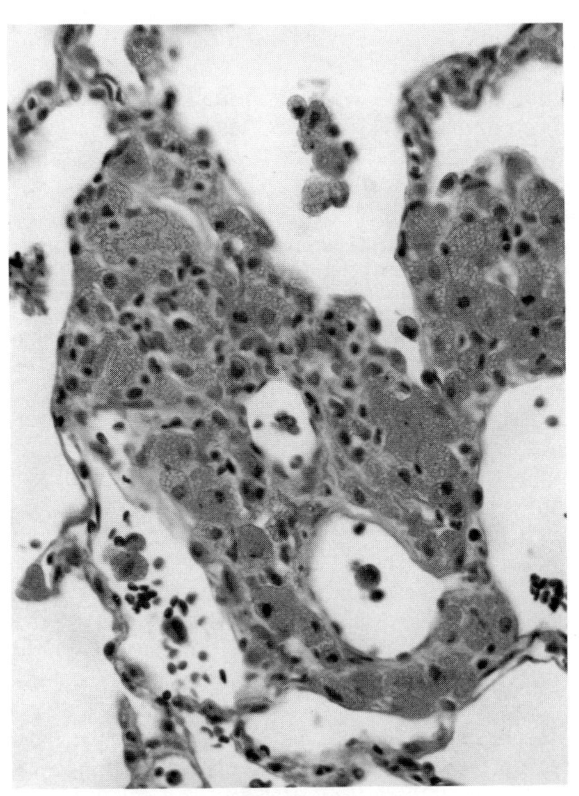

Figure 9-3.

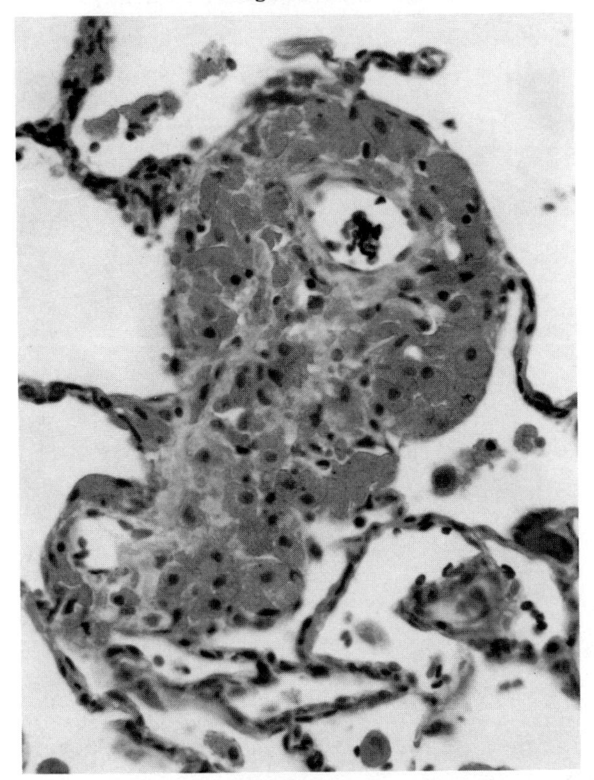

Figure 9-4.

Figures 9-3, 9-4. Barium aspiration. There is alveolar, alveolar septal, and perivascular accumulation of macrophages containing slightly refractile, tan-brown granular material. There is no significant inflammatory reaction.

■ Aspiration (Including Lipoid Pneumonia) (Figs. 9-3 to 9-14)

Aspiration of toxic substances may cause acute DAD, such as the acute chemical pneumonitis associated with gastric acid aspiration. Chronic aspiration from gastric reflux may mimic chronic bronchitis, chronic bronchiolitis, or an interstitial pneumonia such as usual interstitial pneumonia (UIP). Aspiration of infected material, resulting in bacterial pneumonia, is also discussed in the infection section (p. 158).

Barium may be aspirated during radiographic procedures and may be recognized histologically. Faintly birefringent gray to tan granular slightly refractile material is seen free in airspaces early on; later in intra-alveolar or perivascular histiocytes. There is little, if any, inflammatory reaction.

Lipoid pneumonia (exogenous lipid pneumonia) is a reaction to the aspiration of lipids. Relatively inert lipids, such as mineral and vegetable oils, cause little inflammatory reaction except in chronic aspiration. Oils with more free fatty acids, such as animal fats, produce a more intense inflammatory reaction. The lipid is taken up by alveolar macrophages, which contain small *and* large vacuoles in contrast to the uniform small vacuoles of endogenous lipid (obstructive) pneumonia. With chronicity there is scarring. Differential diagnosis includes amiodarone lung toxicity.

A pseudolipoid change (Figs. 9-8 to 9-10) occurs in atelectatic and crushed biopsy specimens with round spaces in the alveoli. This change can be distinguished from lipoid pneumonia by the paucity or absence of macrophages with vacuoles, and absence of the change in other parts of the biopsy specimen.

References

Dail DH, Hammer SP (eds). Pulmonary Pathology. New York, Springer-Verlag, 1988.

Thurlbeck WM (ed). Pathology of the Lung. New York, Thieme, 1988.

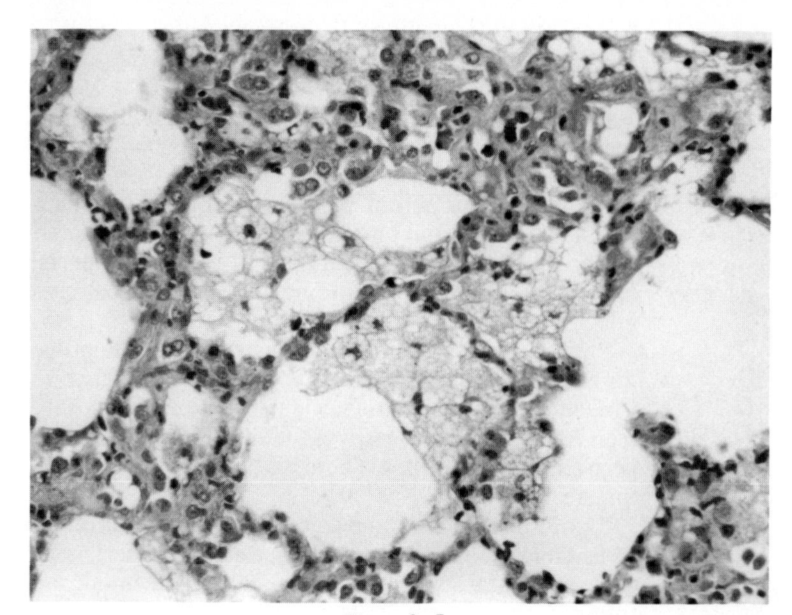

Figure 9–5.

Figure 9–5. Acute mineral oil aspiration. There is an accumulation of vacuolated macrophages within alveoli and a mild associated reaction in the alveolar walls manifesting as reactive type II cells and scattered chronic inflammatory cells. This open lung biopsy specimen was obtained from a patient who was knowingly aspirating mineral oil after aerosolizing it in an atomizer.

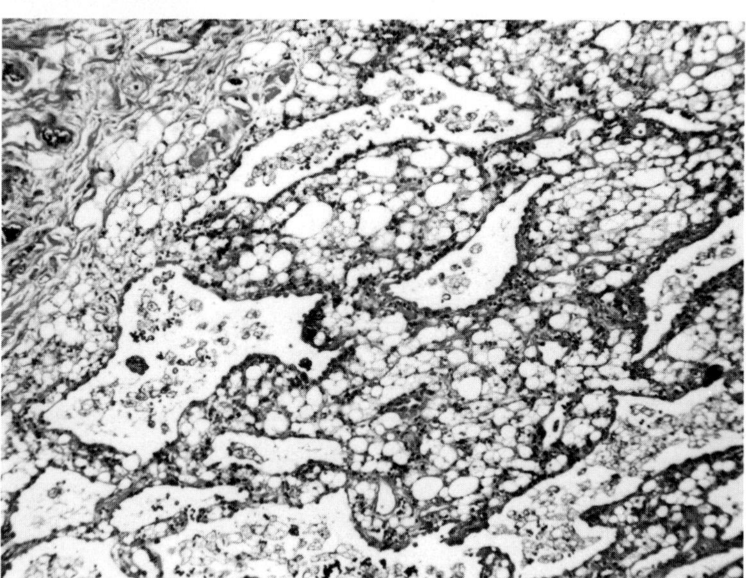

Figure 9–6.

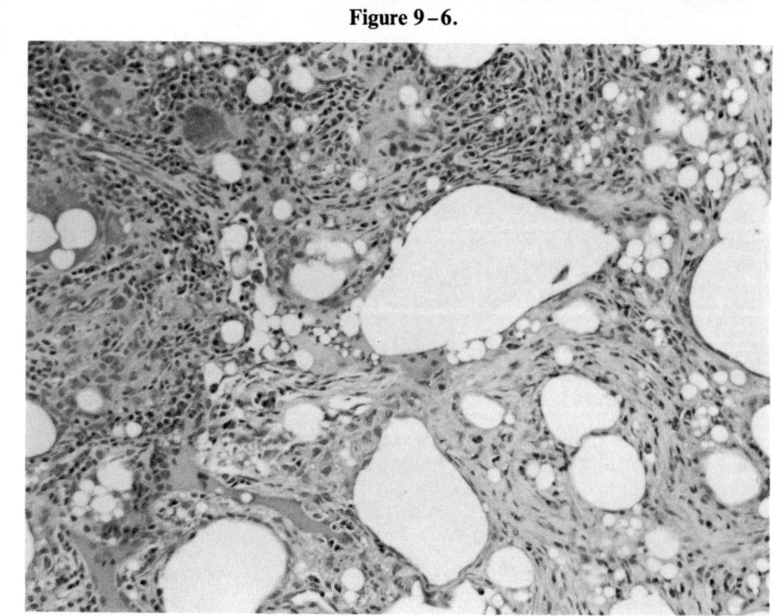

Figure 9–7.

Figures 9–6, 9–7. Chronic mineral oil aspiration. Chronic mineral oil aspiration (lipoid pneumonia). There are vacuoles of varying sizes located both within macrophages and extracellularly associated with fibrosis and chronic inflammation.

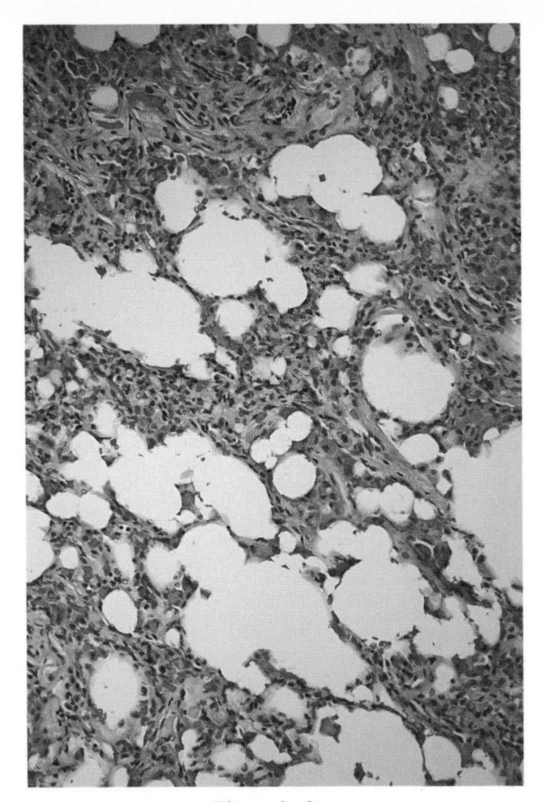

Figure 9-8.

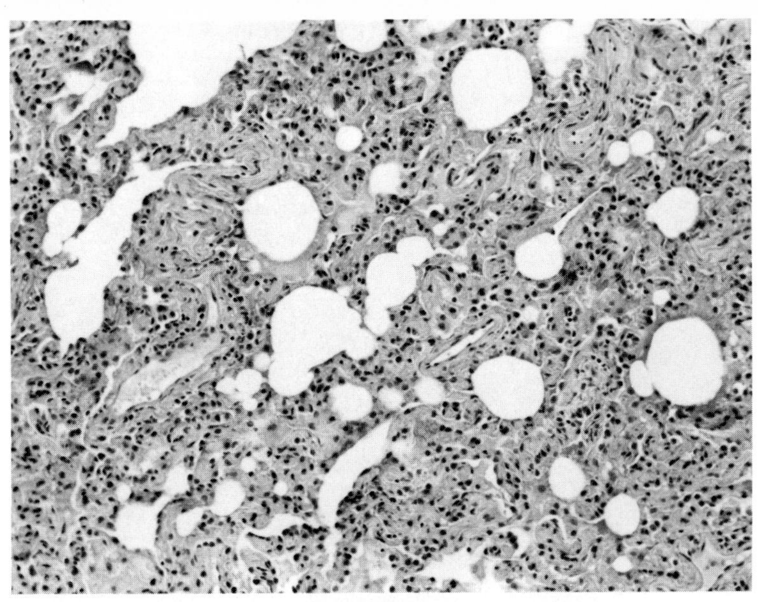

Figure 9-9.

Figures 9-8, 9-9, 9-10. Pseudolipoid artifact in a transbronchial biopsy specimen (Fig. 9-8). Partial crushing of the specimen produces rounded spaces that mimic lipoid pneumonia. The absence of macrophages containing small vacuoles is a helpful clue that this is an artifact. This change may be seen in open lung biopsy specimens as well (Fig. 9-9) and may be associated with traumatic hemorrhage (Fig. 9-10). (Figures 9-9 and 9-10 from Colby TV, Yousem S: Pulmonary histology for the surgical pathologist. Am J Surg Pathol, 12:223-239, 1988, with permission of Raven Press.)

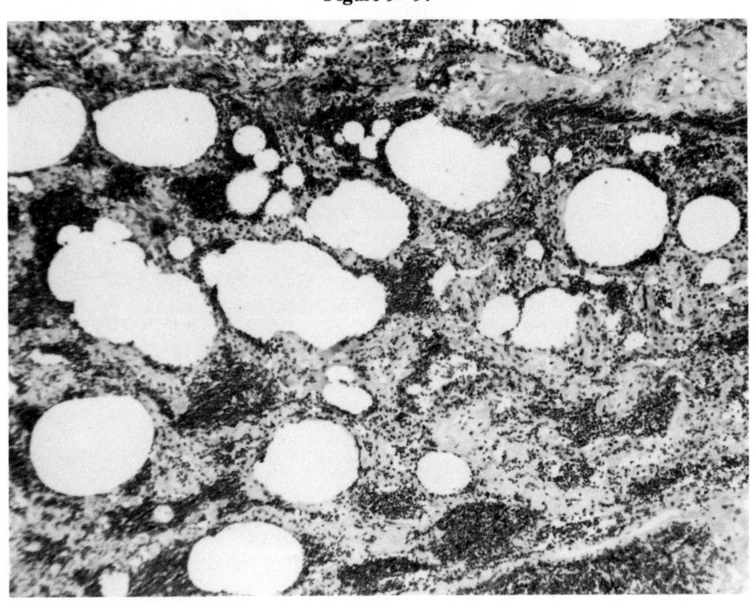

Figure 9-10.

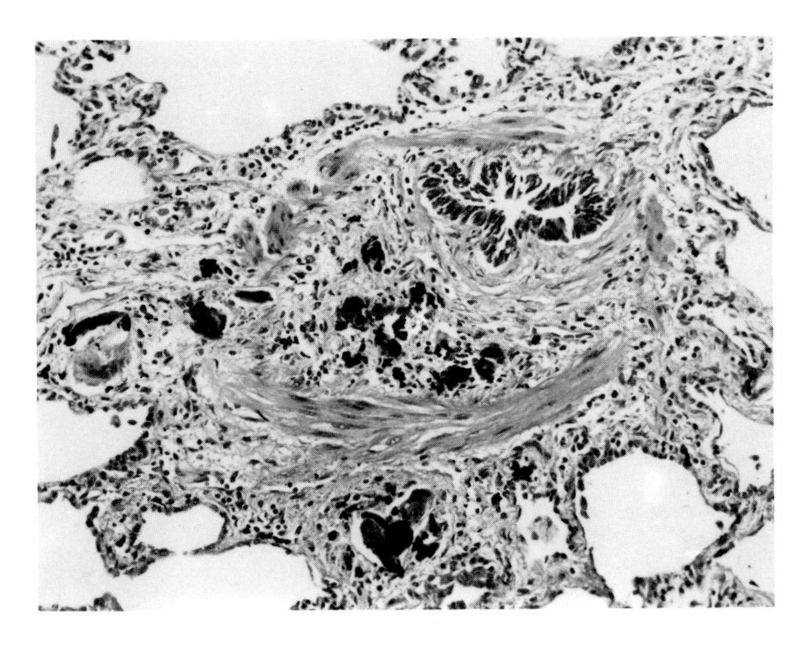

Figure 9-11. Charcoal aspiration. Charcoal aspiration associated with marked submucosal scarring in a small airway. Activated charcoal had been instilled into the patient's stomach after a drug overdose, but the material was aspirated. The black charcoal can be seen associated with an inflammatory reaction, including multinucleated giant cells.

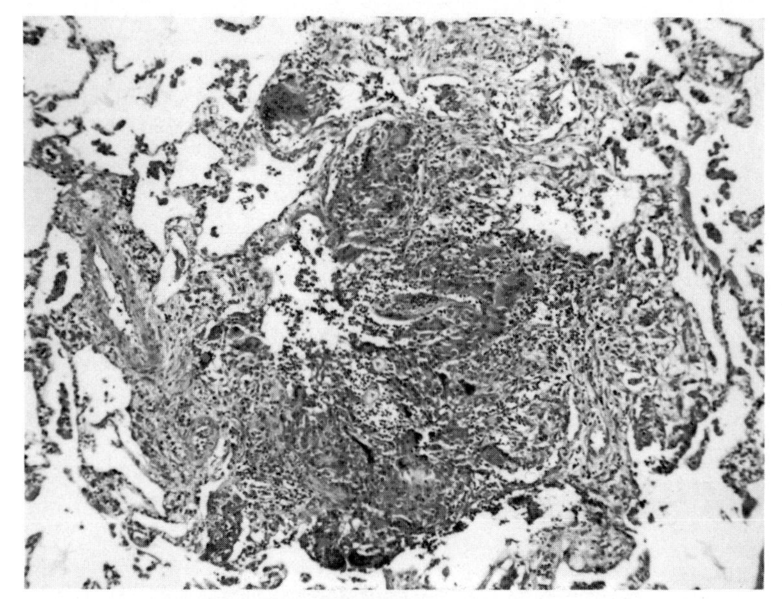

Figure 9-12.

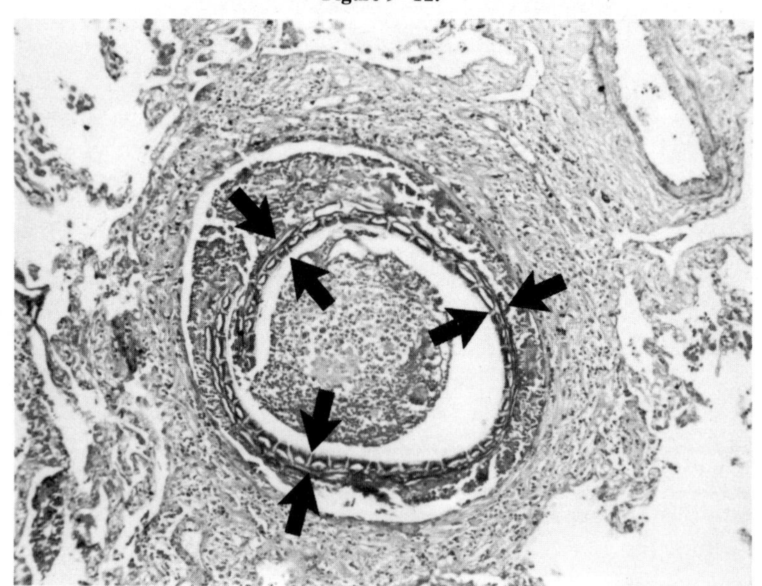

Figure 9-13.

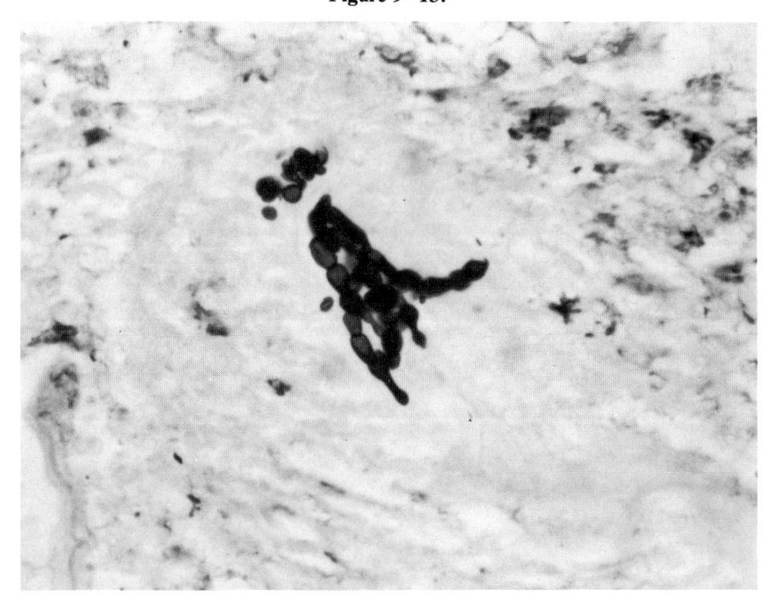

Figure 9-14.

Figures 9-12, 9-13, 9-14. Food aspiration. Granulomatous bronchiolitis caused by food aspiration. A chronic alcoholic presented with lower lobe infiltrates, and an open lung biopsy specimen showed a necrotizing granulomatous bronchiolitis with marked giant cell reaction in the wall of small airways. An occasional airway contained food material with identifiable cell walls (arrows), and secondary yeast growth (morphologically consistent with *Candida*) was found in the acute inflammatory exudate in some of the bronchioles (Fig. 9-14).

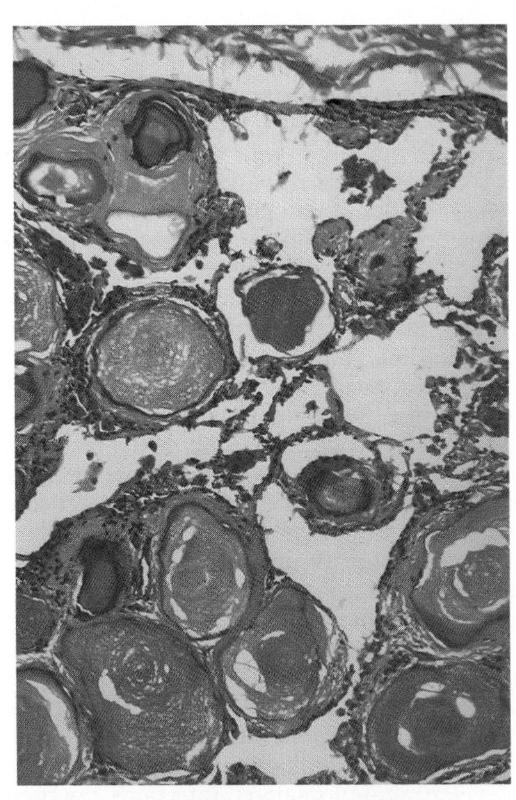

Figure 9-15.

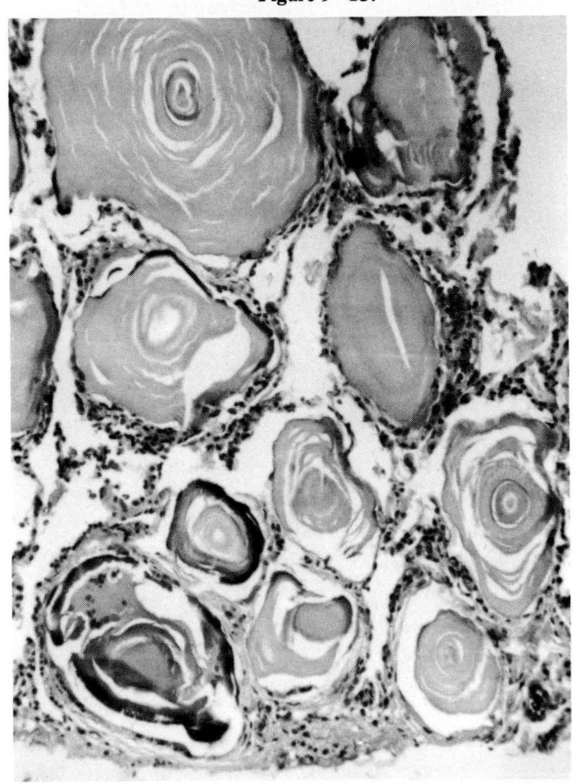

Figure 9-16.

■ Pulmonary Alveolar Microlithiasis (Figs. 9-15, 9-16)

Pulmonary alveolar microlithiasis (PAM) is an extremely rare condition with a nearly pathognomonic radiographic pattern. It is a slowly progressive interstitial disorder associated with restrictive pulmonary functions.

Histologically, there are eosinophilic balls and calcospherites somewhat resembling psammoma bodies filling many of the airspaces; sometimes, small forms can be seen in the interstitium. Interstitial fibrosis is a minor feature. Grossly, the cut surface of the lung is likened to sandpaper.

PAM is so rare that few pathologists will ever see a case. Nevertheless, the histologic features are unique. Diagnosis should be feasible on small biopsy specimens, such as in transbronchial biopsies, particularly if the diagnosis has already been suggested radiographically. By quantity and morphology (as illustrated), the structures can be readily separated from blue bodies, Schaumann's bodies, and copora amylacea.

References

Thurlbeck WM (ed). Pathology of the Lung. New York, Thieme, 1988.

Figures 9-15, 9-16. Pulmonary alveolar microlithiasis. There is extensive alveolar filling by laminated partially calcified bodies, some of which show an associated giant cell reaction.

■ Tracheobronchopathia Osteoplastica (Fig. 9–17)

This is a very rare condition associated with metaplastic bone and cartilage involving the trachea and large bronchi. Osteophyte-like spurs are seen to protrude into the airway by the bronchoscopist or at autopsy. The condition is usually unassociated with any clinical signs or symptoms and represents a rare clinical curiosity. Secondary changes of obstructive bronchiectasis, recurrent pneumonia, or both may occasionally dominate the clinical findings.

Histologically, nodules of metaplastic osteochondroid material are seen in the submucosa. The overlying mucosa is generally intact. This condition should be distinguished from bony metaplasia of tracheobronchial cartilages and tracheobronchial amyloidosis, which may also show ossification.

References

Thurlbeck WM (ed). Pathology of the Lung. New York, Thieme, 1988.
Young RH, Sandstrom RE, Mark EJ. Tracheopathia osteoplastica. J Thorac Cardiovasc Surg 79:537–541, 1980.

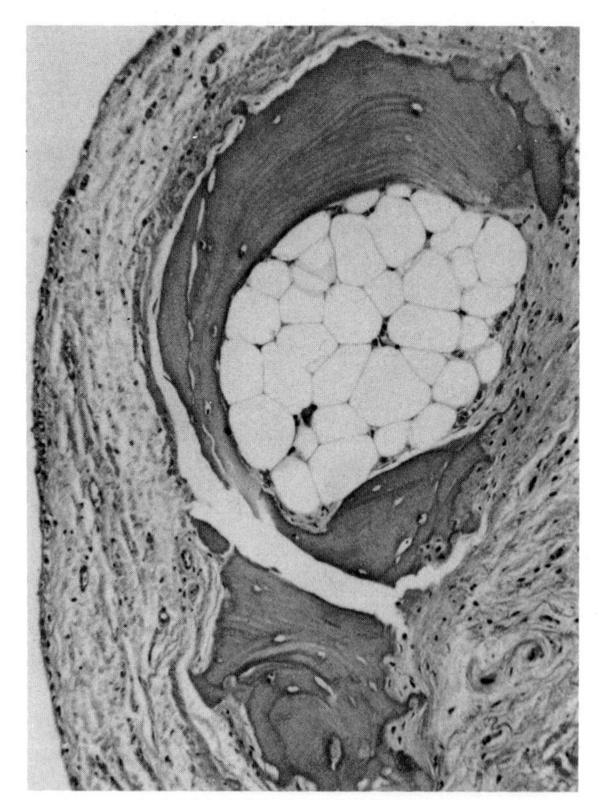

Figure 9–17. Tracheobronchopathia osteoplastica. Within the bronchial submucosa, there is mature lamellar bone with fatty marrow. The overlying mucosa was intact but was lost during processing.

■ Rheumatoid Nodules (Figs. 1–52, 1–53)

Rheumatoid nodules are usually multiple and bilateral, although occasionally they may be single. They occur more frequently in men with a long-standing history of rheumatoid arthritis and in individuals with subcutaneous nodules. Rheumatoid factor is frequently elevated. Rheumatoid nodules in the lung may precede the articular disease in rare instances.

Histologically, the nodules are usually pleural or septal in distribution, with central fibrinoid necrosis and with surrounding palisaded histiocytic reaction, which in turn is surrounded by fibrosis and a chronic inflammatory infiltrate. Occasionally, the necrotic center may contain neutrophils and neutrophilic debris, and a few giant cells and/or granulomas may be seen in the wall. The inflammatory reaction that is located away from the necrotic center is generally limited to the wall of the nodule and is not nearly as extensive or geographic as in Wegener's granulomatosis.

Some cases of rheumatoid nodules are extremely difficult to distinguish from Wegener's granulomatosis and infectious granulomas, and these cases are best solved by careful clinical correlation (i.e., knowledge of the history of rheumatoid arthritis) and/or follow-up. It should be remembered that patients with rheumatoid arthritis may also develop granulomatous infections, particularly those who have been undergoing steroid or immunosuppressant therapy, and patients with Wegener's granulomatosis may present with a clinical syndrome that early on may simulate rheumatoid arthritis. Special stains should be performed in all suspected cases of rheumatoid nodules, and cultures should be taken.

References

Yousem SA, Colby TV, Carrington CB. Lung biopsy in rheumatoid arthritis. Am Rev Respir Dis 131:770–777, 1985.

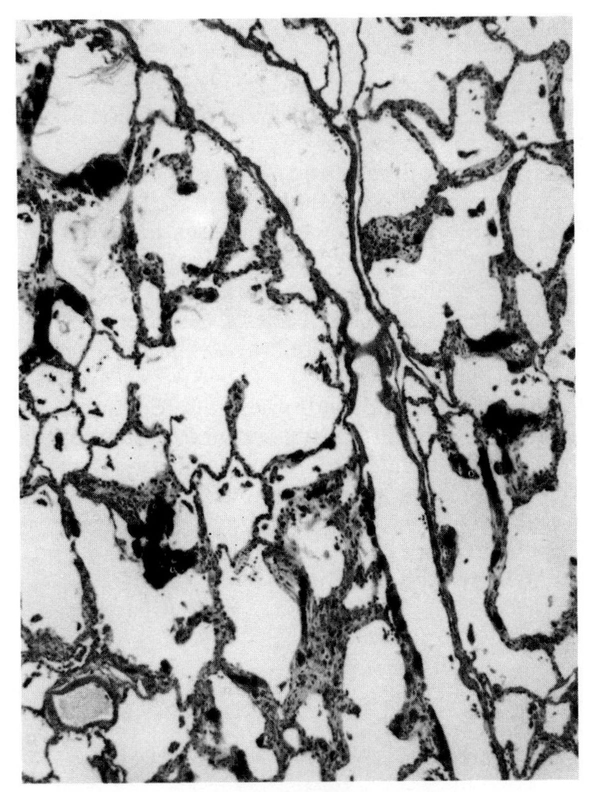

Figure 9-18.

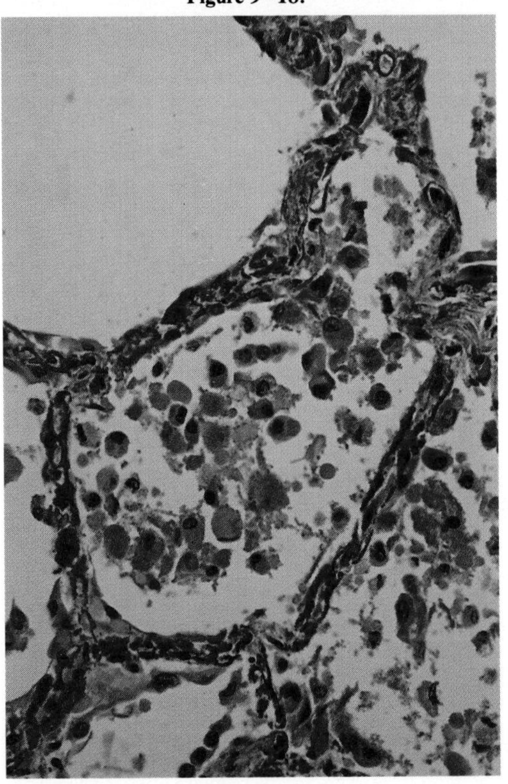

Figure 9-19.

■ Metastatic Calcification (Figs. 9-18, 9-19)

Metastatic calcification may produce localized or extensive interstitial infiltrates, apparent on radiographs and associated with findings of restrictive lung disease. Most patients have identifiable abnormalities in calcium or phosphate metabolism, especially chronic renal disease.

Histologically, there is diffuse deposition of calcium phosphate in alveolar walls as basophilic granular and platelike material. Encrustation of the elastica occurs, and a giant cell or granulomatous reaction is sometimes elicited.

Diagnosis is possible by means of transbronchial biopsy. The possibilities that more than one lesion is present and that the calcification is incidental should be kept in mind. Calcification of vessels sometimes is seen in chronic passive congestion or pulmonary veno-occlusive disease.

References

Thurlbeck WM (ed). Pathology of the Lung. New York, Thieme, 1988.

Figures 9-18, 9-19. Metastatic calcification in a patient with chronic renal disease. The alveolar architecture is intact; however, there is patchy thickening of alveolar walls and deposition of calcium as platelike basophilic material associated with a mild inflammatory and fibrotic reaction.

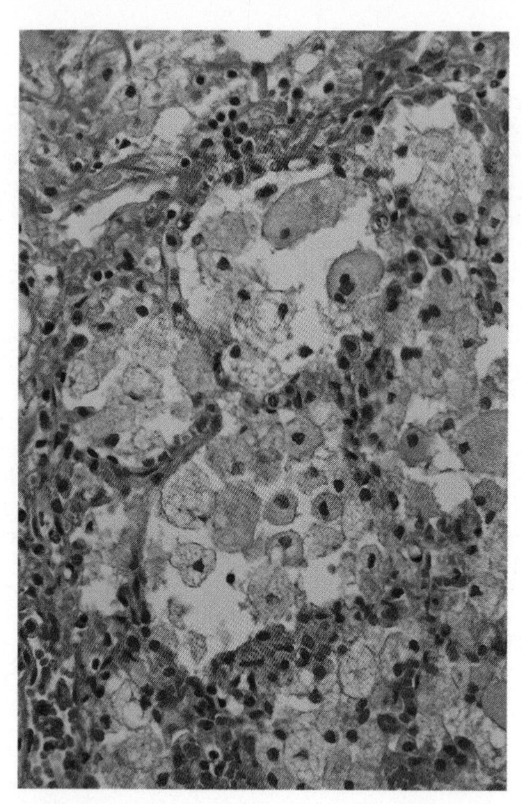

Figure 9–20. Pulmonary involvement in Niemann-Pick disease with accumulations of foamy histiocytes within the alveoli. In the absence of clinical history, a field such as this can easily be mistaken for simple obstructive pneumonia.

■ **Metabolic Diseases** (Fig. 9–20)

A number of metabolic and storage diseases may affect the lung; however, the surgical pathologist is rarely called upon for diagnosis.

Niemann-Pick disease and Gaucher's disease may be associated with histiocyte infiltrates in the lung and clinical evidence of pulmonary disease; however, lung biopsy is rarely performed.

Gaucher's disease may also be associated with pulmonary hypertension on the basis of Gaucher's cells impacted in the pulmonary microvasculature leading to secondary hypertension.

Hermansky-Pudlak syndrome is a rare familial form of oculocutaneous albinism associated with pulmonary involvement, resembling UIP. Histologically, there is patchy interstitial scarring and honeycombing. The feature that sets Hermansky-Pudlak syndrome apart from UIP is the presence of large numbers of ceroid pigment-laden histiocytes in the fibrotic foci.

References

Thurlbeck WM (ed). Pathology of the Lung. New York, Thieme, 1988.

■ Amyloidosis (Figs. 9-21 to 9-27)

Deposition of amyloid in the lung occurs in the following patterns: (1) localized nodule(s), (2) diffuse tracheobronchial deposition, (3) diffuse alveolar septal amyloid with deposition in the alveolar walls, and (4) senile amyloid, which is usually an incidental finding in vessel walls. Overlap among these forms does occur. Some patients, but not all, have an associated plasma cell dyscrasia or chronic inflammatory condition predisposing them to amyloidosis.

Localized amyloid nodules constitute the most common form seen in surgical pathology material.

Most localized amyloid tumors are isolated findings. Tracheobronchial amyloid is usually limited to the lungs and is associated with bronchiectasis and with recurrent infections. Diffuse alveolar septal amyloid may be restricted to the lungs, but more commonly is part of systemic amyloidosis, either primary or secondary.

In localized nodular amyloidosis the amyloid is usually associated with a mild plasma cell infiltrate. Giant cell reaction to the amyloid is typical. Secondary bone formation and fibrosis may be seen. Amyloid deposits in vessels, bronchi, and pleura are also apparent. Vascular involvement may be associated with infarction.

In tracheobronchial amyloidosis, the deposits are in the submucosa of the airways and should be distinguished from tracheobronchopathia osteoplastica.

In diffuse alveolar septal amyloidosis, deposits occur in all compartments of the lung parenchyma, including alveolar walls.

Some lung tumors, particularly lymphomas and myeloma, may be associated with amyloid production. The differential diagnosis also includes systemic light-chain deposition disease.

References

Cordier JF, Loire R, Brune J. Amyloidosis of the lower respiratory tract. Chest 90:827-831, 1986.
Dail DH, Hammer SP (eds). Pulmonary Pathology. New York, Springer-Verlag, 1988.
Gertz MA, Greipp PR. Clinical aspects of pulmonary amyloidosis (editorial). Chest 90:790-791, 1986.
Thurlbeck WM (ed). Pathology of the Lung. New York, Thieme, 1988.

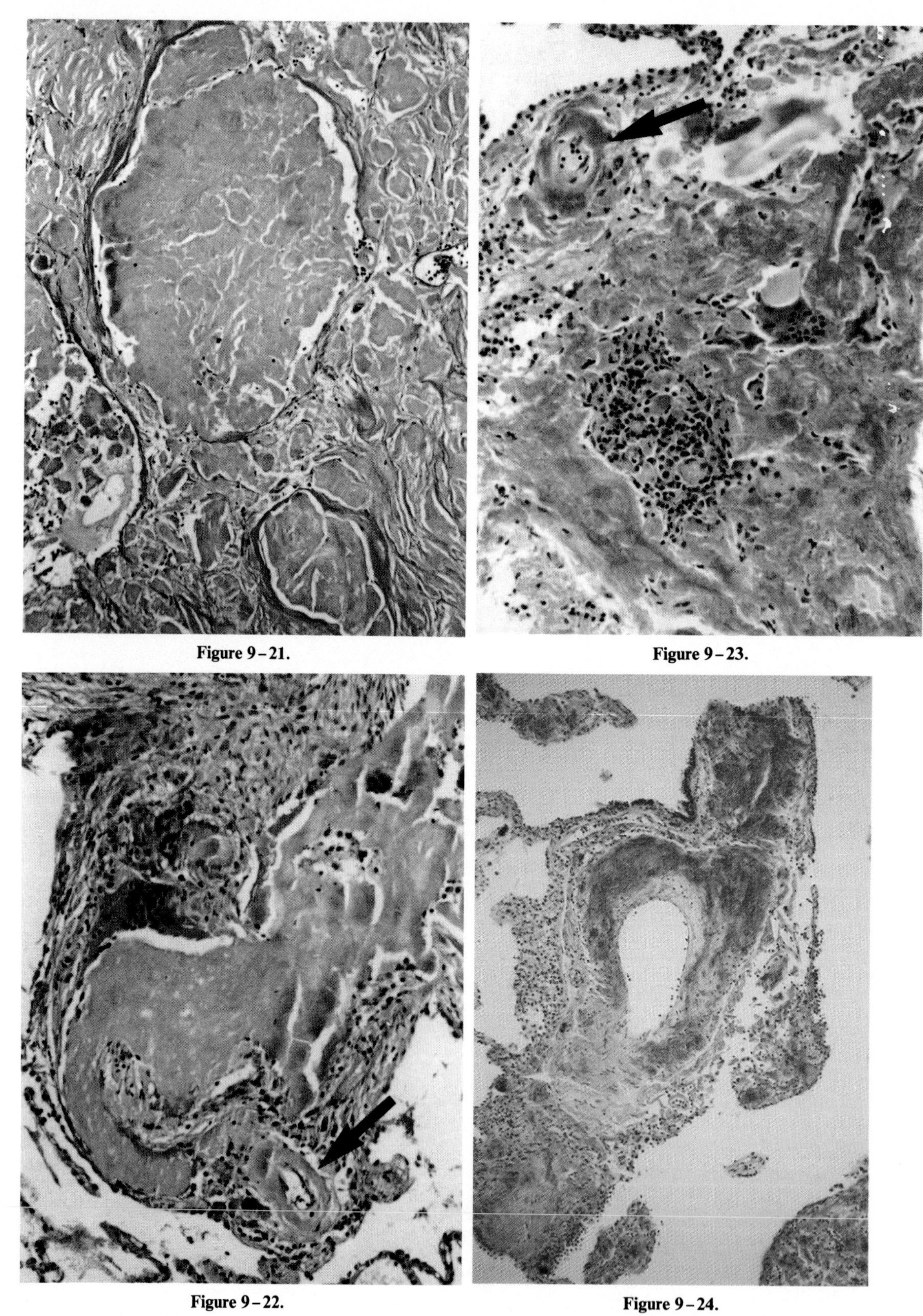

Figure 9–21.

Figure 9–23.

Figure 9–22.

Figure 9–24.

Figures 9–21, 9–22, 9–23, 9–24. Nodular amyloidosis. This well-circumscribed nodule was composed entirely of waxy eosinophilic material that stained positively with Congo red stain (Fig. 9–24). In some fields, there is a giant cell reaction and clusters of plasma cells (Fig. 9–23). Perivascular and mural vascular involvement is also apparent (arrows).

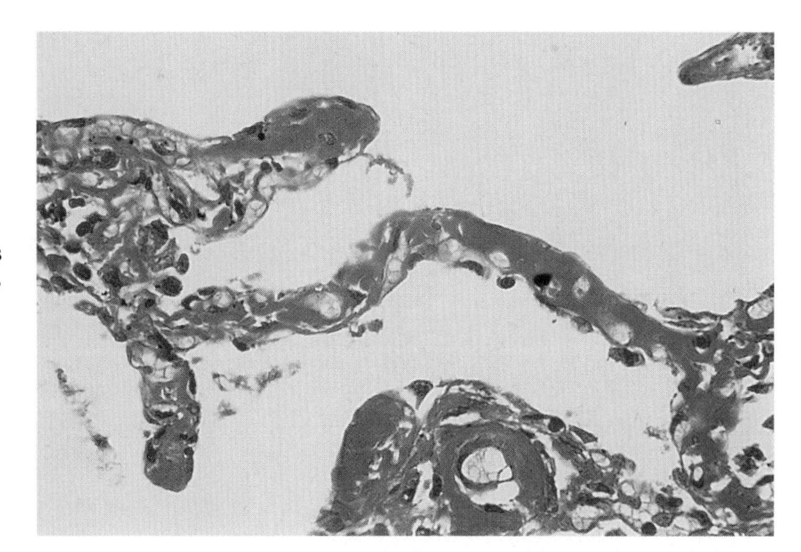

Figure 9–25. Diffuse alveolar septal amyloidosis. There is diffuse amyloid deposition within intact alveolar walls, and there is little associated inflammation.

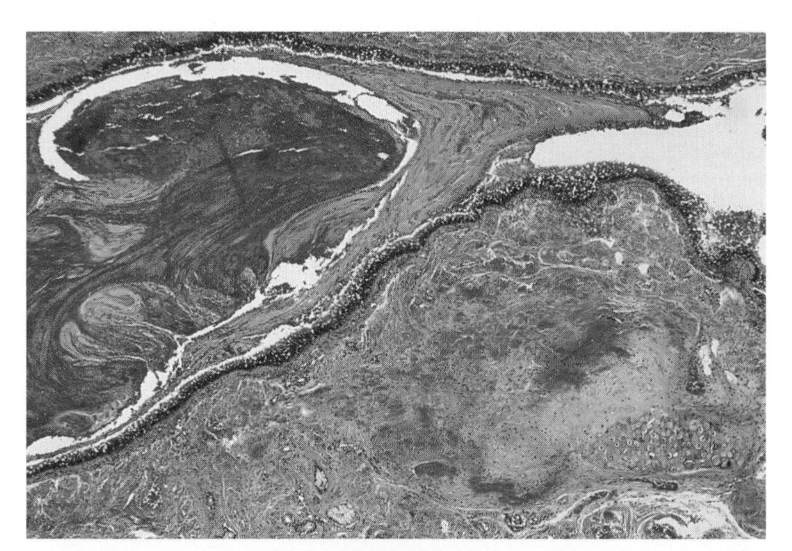

Figure 9–26.

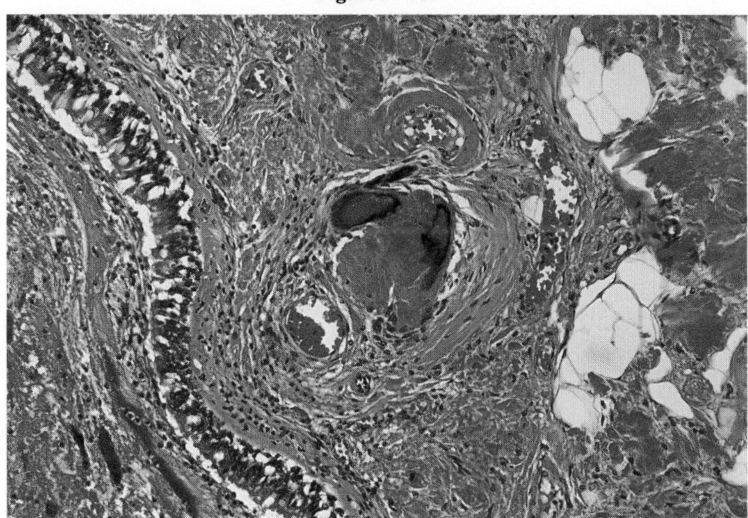

Figure 9–27.

Figures 9–26, 9–27. Tracheobronchial amyloidosis. There is a small bronchus containing a large plug of mucus (upper left). Within the wall of the bronchus, a nodular expansion, caused by eosinophilic material representing the amyloid, can be seen at the lower right. At higher-power microscopy, the interstitial and vascular amyloid deposition can be seen along with early ossification, which stains purplish.

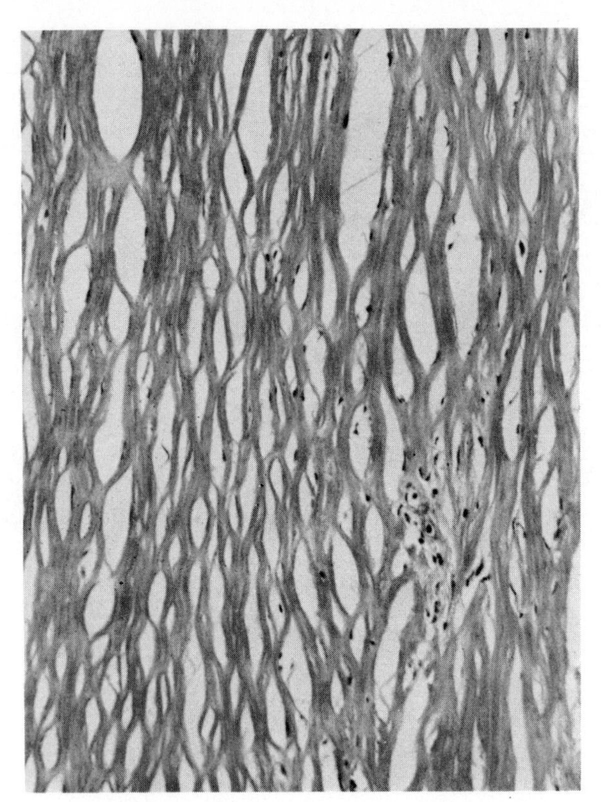

Figure 9–28. Hyaline pleural plaque. Hyaline pleural plaque with typical basket-weave pattern of fibrous lamellae from a patient with prior asbestos exposure.

■ Hyaline Pleural Plaques (Fig. 9–28)

Gray-white, elevated, dense, hyalinized fibrous pleural plaques may be seen in visceral or, more commonly, parietal pleura. When bilateral, the plaques are usually a marker of prior asbestos exposure. As a single lesion, they are quite nonspecific and may be the residue of a prior inflammatory process.

Histologically, there is a relatively acellular, basket-weave, dense, collagenous matrix. Foci of inflammation and more cellular fibrosis may be seen, as may an overlying organizing pleuritis, if an associated pleural effusion is present.

References

Churg A, Green FHY. Pathology of Occupational Lung Disease. New York, Igaku-Shoin, Medical Publishers, 1988.

■ Miscellaneous Structures and Findings

Schaumann's (Conchoidal) Bodies (Figs. 9–29 to 9–31) Calcific structures in giant cells formed by concentric calcific lamination are seen in a wide variety of granulomatous conditions. They may be birefringent.

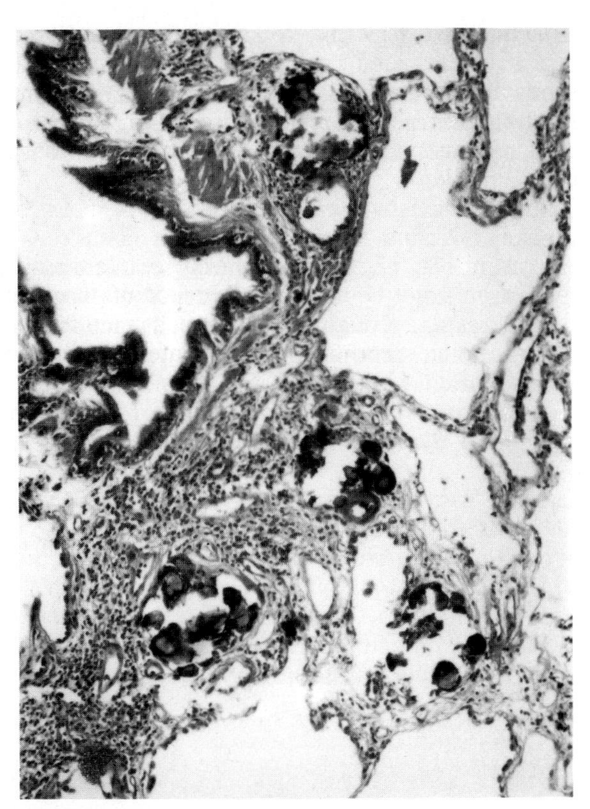

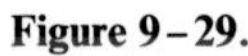

Figure 9–29.

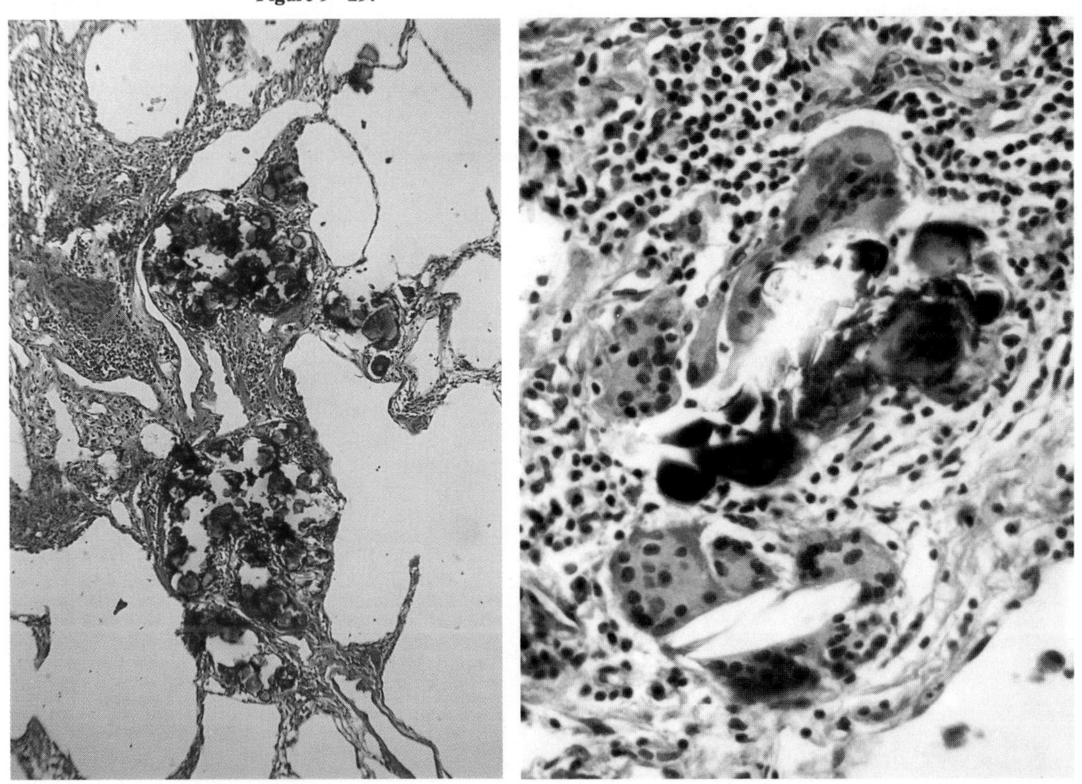

Figure 9–30. **Figure 9–31.**

Figures 9–29, 9–30, 9–31. Schaumann's bodies. Laminated basophilic calcified structures, which may attain hundreds of microns in size, are associated with a giant cell reaction. Small Schaumann's bodies are found within giant cells.

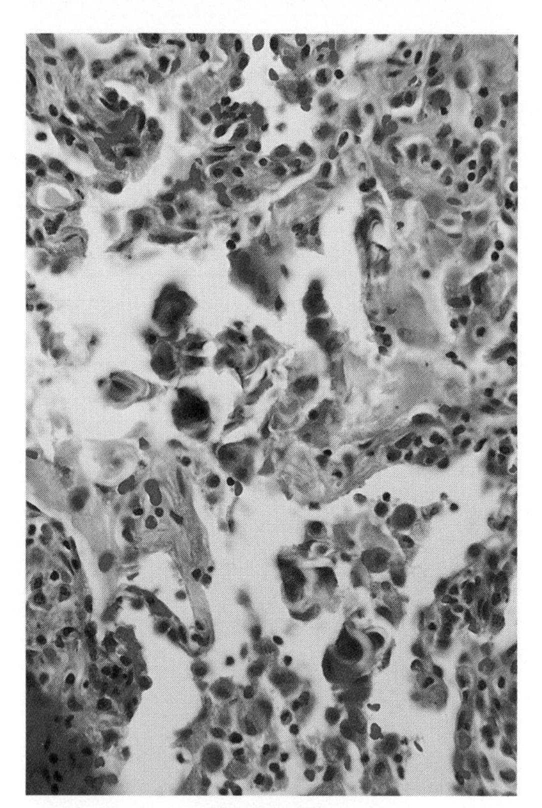

Figure 9–32.

Blue Bodies (Figs. 9–32, 9–33): Intra-alveolar, concentrically laminated, calcified (calcium carbonate) bodies within or around accumulations of alveolar macrophages seen in a number of conditions in which alveolar macrophages accumulate. Blue bodies are nonspecific.

Calcium Oxalate Crystals (Fig. 9–34): Lucent, plate-like, birefringent crystals seen in giant cells in many conditions. They are commonly seen in sarcoidosis and should not be taken as evidence of exogenous material causing a foreign-body giant cell reaction. They often accumulate around *Aspergillus* hyphae.

Asteroid Bodies (Figs. 9–35, 9–36): A proteinaceous, starlike, crystalloid body seen in giant cells (either interstitial or in airspaces) in disorders in which giant cells are formed, usually those that are granulomatous.

Corpora Amylacea (Figs. 9–37, 9–38): These are periodic acid–Schiff (PAS)–positive spheres, sometimes containing a bluish central nidus. They are noncalcified, and occasionally a giant cell or a macrophage is draped around them. Corpora amylacea represent clinically insignificant findings usually seen in older patients, perhaps as a reaction to some particulate material.

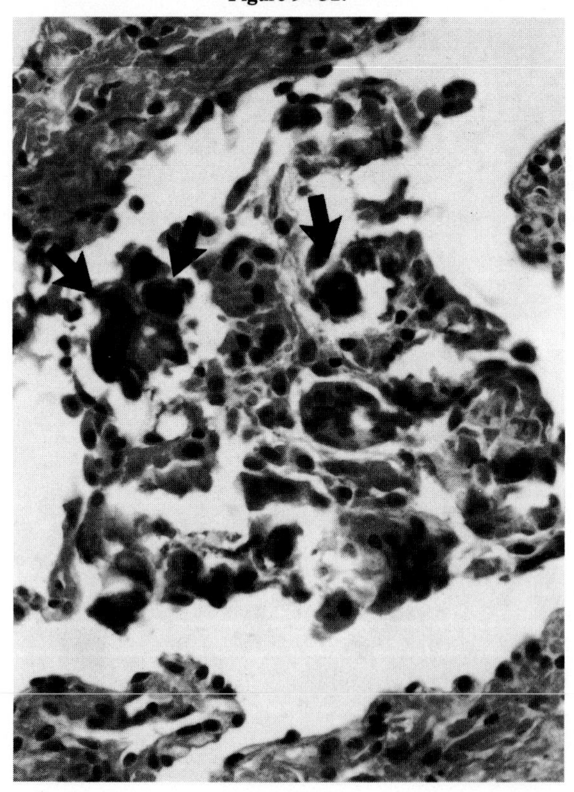

Figure 9–33.

Figures 9–32, 9–33. Blue bodies. Intra-alveolar laminated calcified bodies that appear bluish on hematoxylin and eosin (H & E) stains (Fig. 9–32) are seen within the alveolar spaces (arrows) associated with a macrophage and giant cell reaction. Blue bodies are seen in a large number of interstitial lung diseases and are nonspecific.

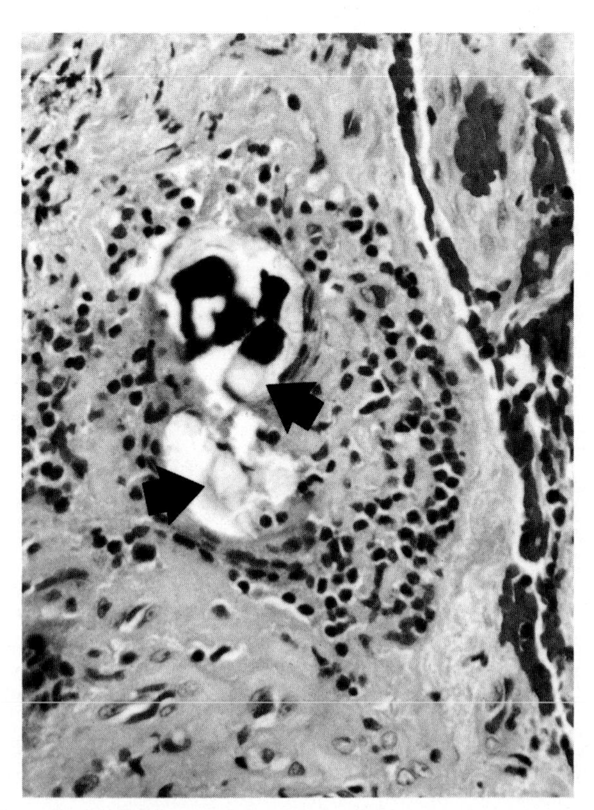

Figure 9–34. Calcium oxalate crystals. Calcium oxalate crystals are often seen in association with Schaumann's bodies. They are lucent and platelike (arrow) and best appreciated with polarization because they are brightly birefringent. (From Colby, TV and Yousem, S: Pulmonary histology for the surgical pathologist. Am J Surg Pathol 12:223–239, 1988, with permission of Raven Press.)

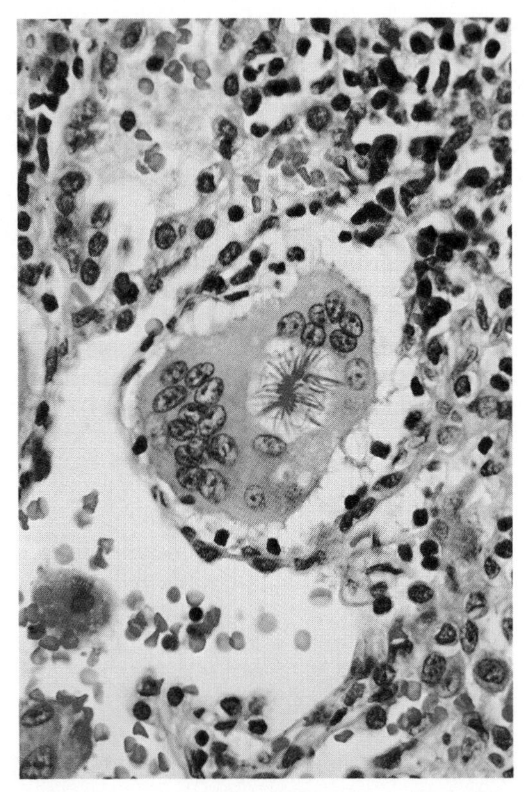

Figure 9-35.

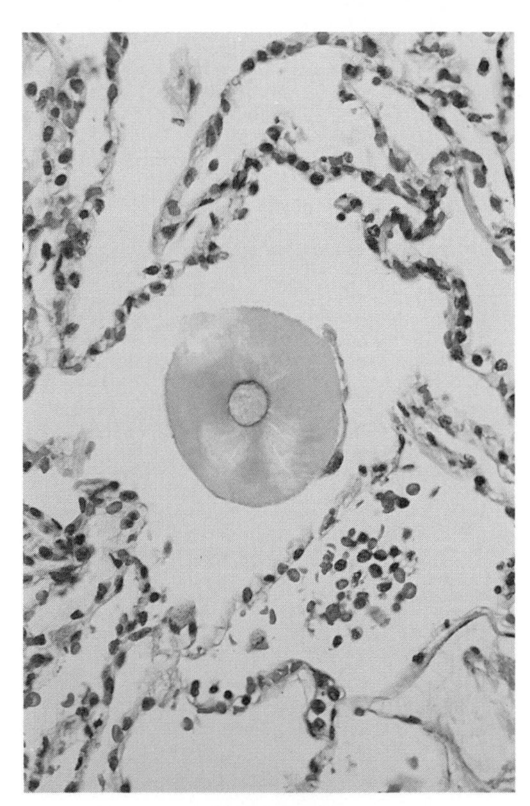

Figure 9-37.

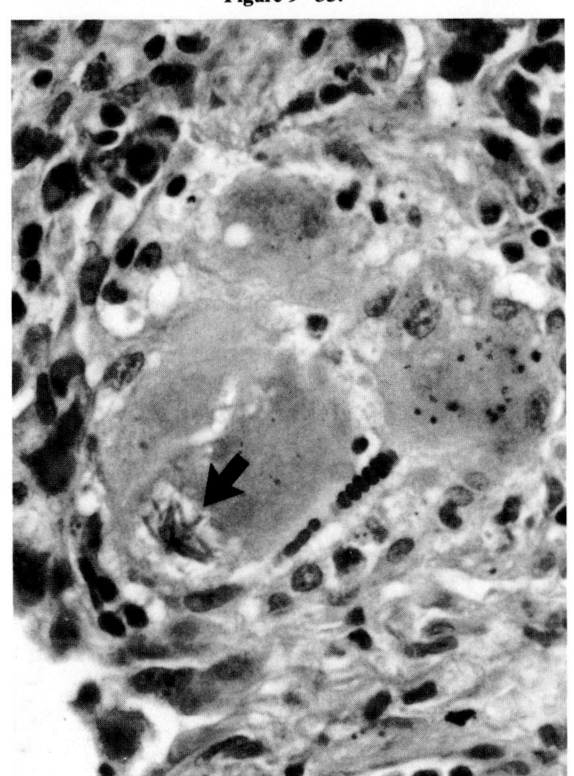

Figure 9-36.

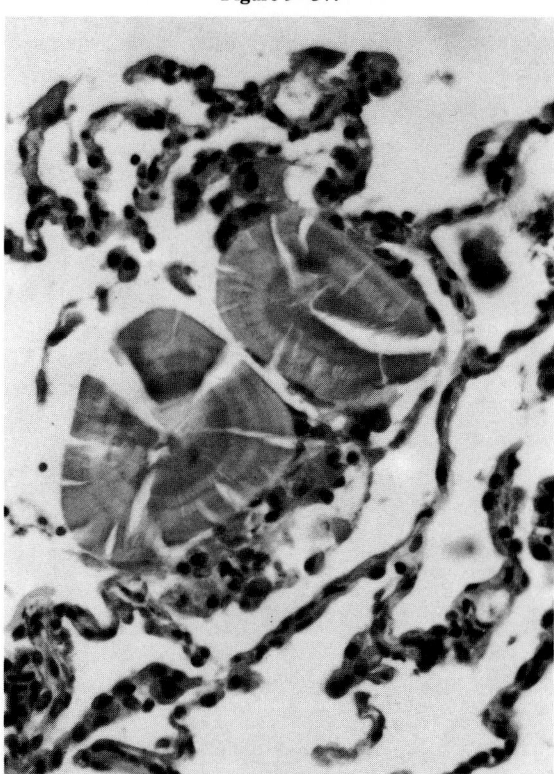

Figure 9-38.

Figures 9-35, 9-36. Asteroid bodies. These are peculiar starfish-like proteinaceous bodies (arrow) in giant cells. They are quite nonspecific and are seen in conditions associated with giant cells. In one of the cases shown, the giant cell reaction was associated with asbestos exposure as evidenced by the asbestos body (Fig. 9-36, center).

Figures 9-37, 9-38. Corpora amylacea. These proteinaceous intra-alveolar eosinophilic bodies sometimes have a central bluish nidus around which they are thought to form. Some show concentric layering, and they may appear cracked in routine sections.

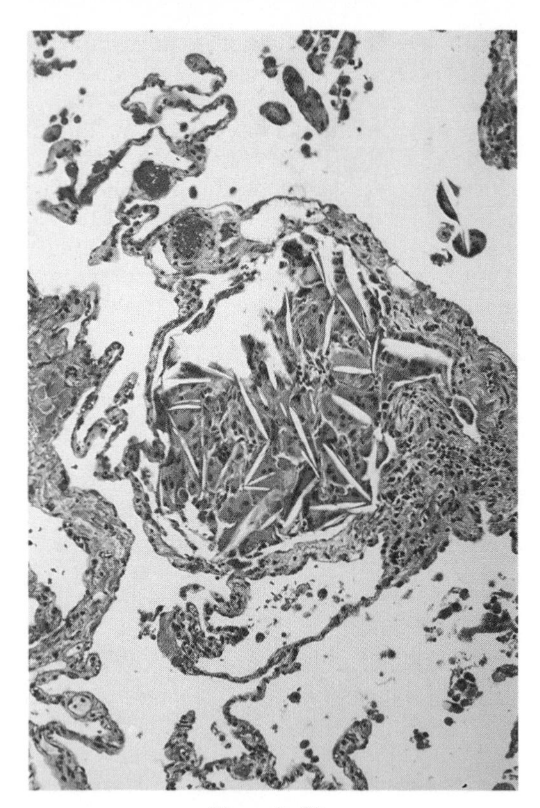

Figure 9–39.

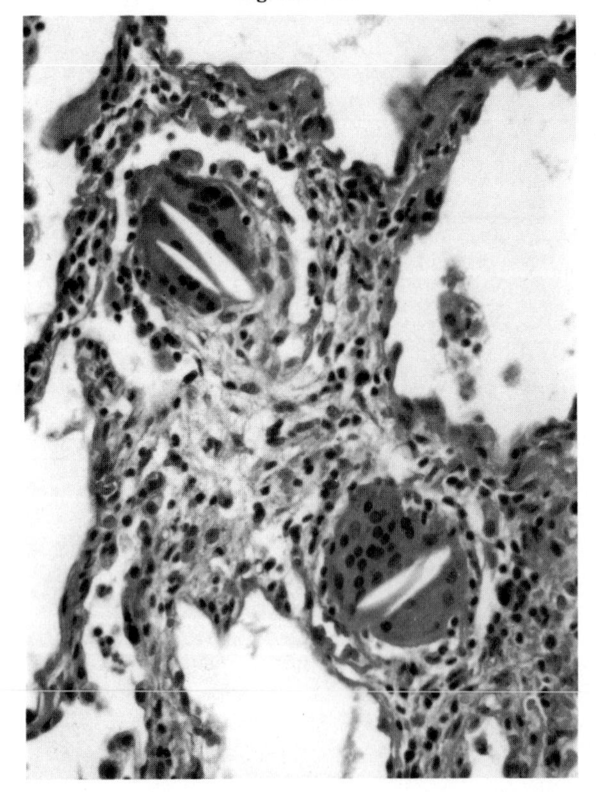

Figure 9–40.

Figures 9–39, 9–40. Giant cells containing cholesterol clefts. This finding is quite nonspecific.

Cholesterol Crystals and Granulomas (Figs. 9–39, 9–40): Giant cells and/or clusters of histiocytes and giant cells containing cholesterol clefts are a relatively common nonspecific finding that in some cases may represent the residue of prior hemorrhage. Perivascular xanthogranulomas are slightly more common in diabetics but also are nonspecific.

Hemosiderin: Hemosiderin in macrophages is seen as a result of prior alveolar hemorrhage from many causes. Alveolar macrophages in smokers are usually characterized by fine granular hemosiderin. When there is extensive hemosiderosis, usually from severe chronic passive congestion, interstitial encrustation of elastic fibers (sometimes with a giant cell reaction) can be seen (Fig. 9–41).

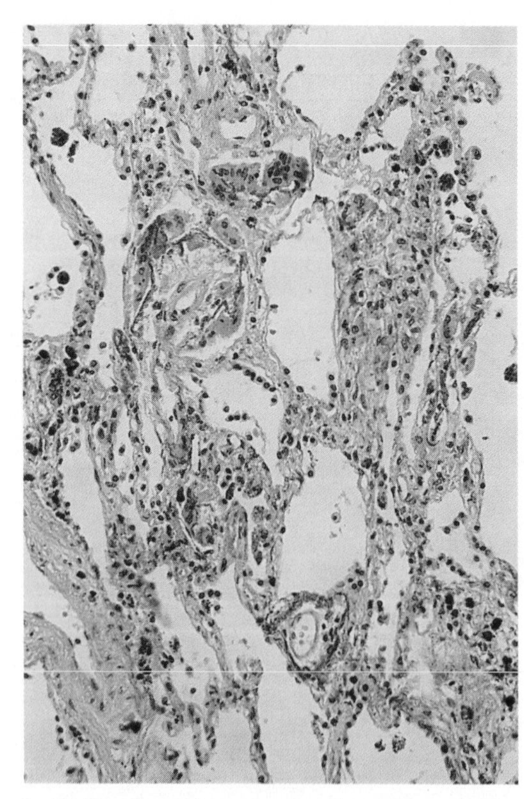

Figure 9–41. Chronic passive congestion. Somewhat grayish hemosiderin with an associated giant cell reaction encrusts elastic tissue fibers in this case of severe chronic passive congestion.

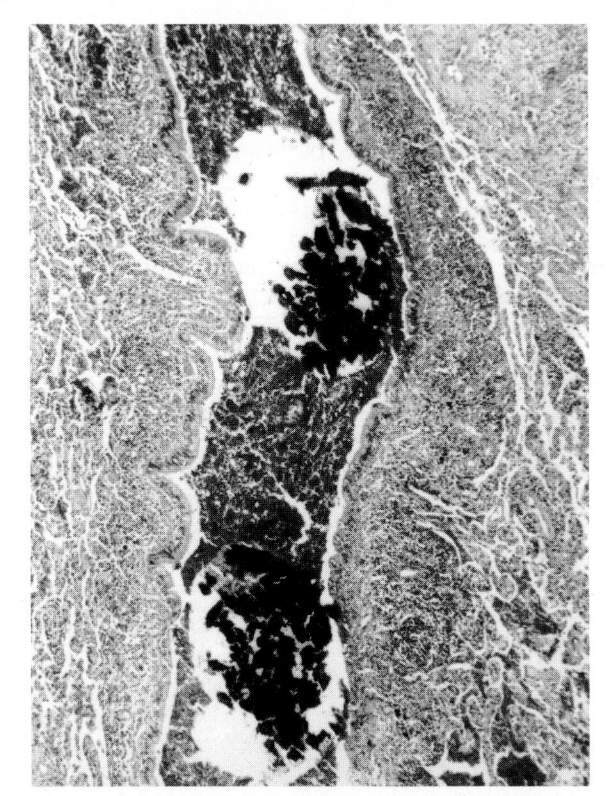

Figure 9-42. Broncholith. As aspirated calcified broncholith in a small airway is associated with acute and chronic inflammatory reaction.

Broncholiths and Broncholithiasis (Figs. 9-42, 9-43): Calcific debris gains access to the airways when a calcified peribronchial lymph node erodes through the airway wall and discharges its center. The material may be coughed up or aspirated, in which case it may be associated with a distal aspiration pneumonia containing calcific fragments with or without a granulomatous reaction.

Anthracosis: A deposition of carbonaceous pigment present along lymphatic routes. Deposition around small airways is common. Marked anthracosis characterizes coal-worker's pneumoconiosis (see Fig. 7-135) and anthracosis is more prominent in cigarette smokers than in nonsmokers.

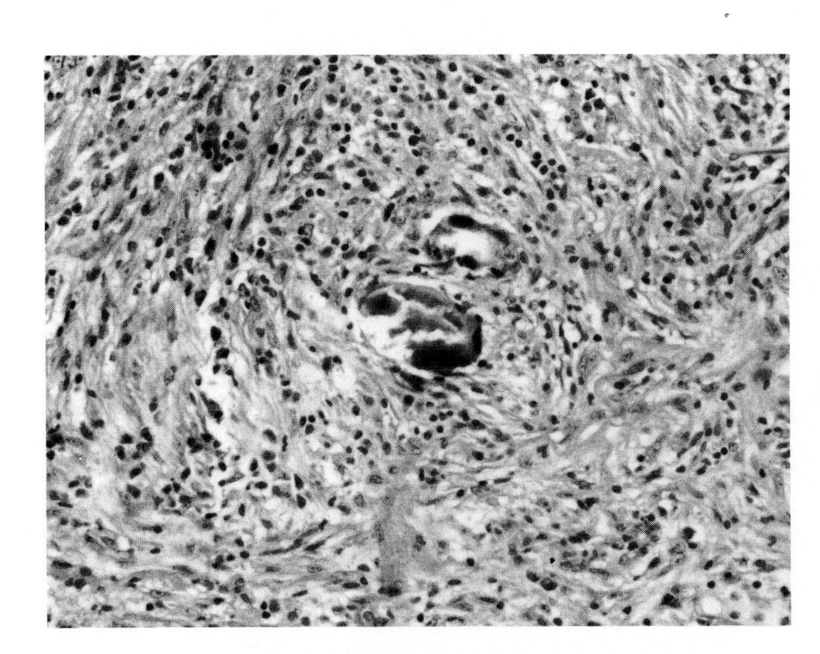

Figure 9-43. Broncholith aspiration pneumonia. In this case, the calcified fragments of the broncholith were relatively inconspicuous and were embedded in an acute and chronic organizing pneumonia. In some foci, there was a granulomatous reaction. The broncholiths were the result of calcified histoplasma granulomas in hilar nodes that had eroded into the airway. Antigens present in the calcified material probably provoked the granulomatous reaction. No organisms were identified by means of special stains.

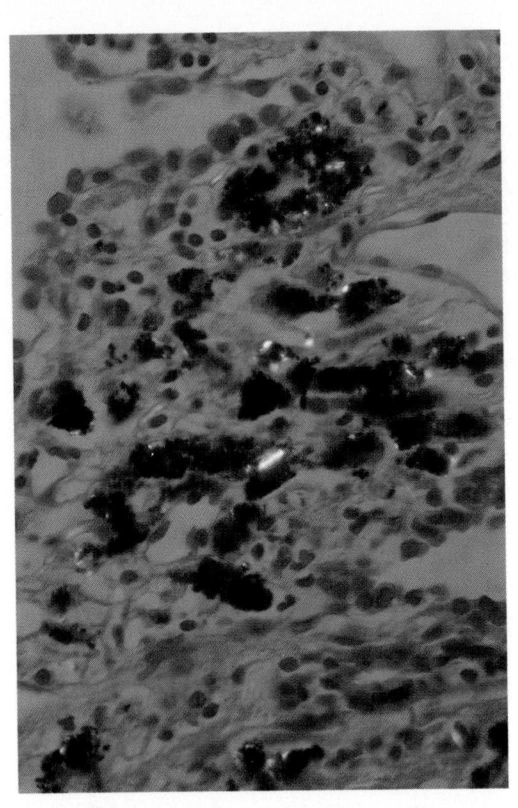

Figure 9–44. Birefringent silicates. Birefringent silicates seen as an incidental finding in a smoker who had undergone resection of a bronchioloalveolar carcinoma.

Silicates (Fig. 9–44): Brightly birefringent particles commonly found among the anthracotic pigment. These are normal findings in adults, particularly smokers and urban dwellers.

Silica: These weakly birefringent (less birefringent than the endogenous collagenous matrix of the lung) particles may also be associated with anthracotic pigment. Large amounts of silica are usually associated with an accumulation of macrophages along lymphatic routes, and silicotic nodules usually appear to arise in this setting of histiocytic infiltration. A small amount of silica particles in areas of anthracosis is a common nonspecific finding.

Megakaryocytes (Figs. 9–45, 9–46): These are extremely common in the lung and represent an incidental nonspecific finding. Megakaryocytes are usually seen in capillaries.

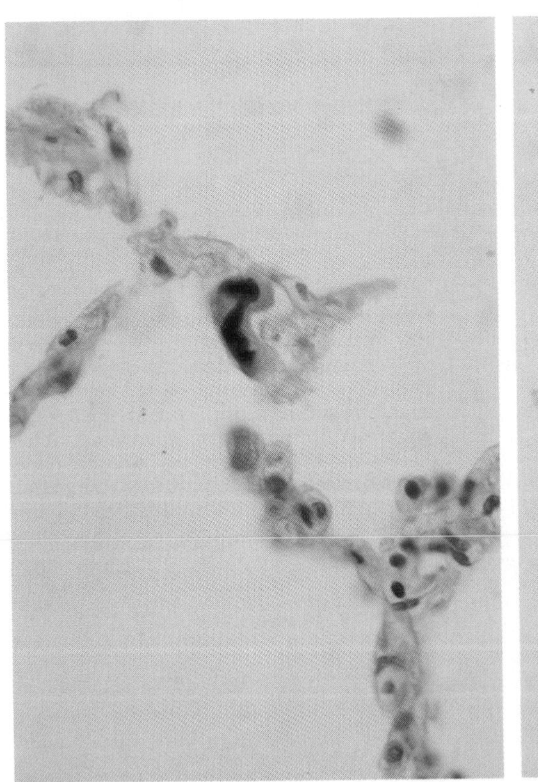

Figure 9–45. **Figure 9–46.**

Figures 9–45, 9–46. Megakaryocytes. Intracapillary megakaryocytes seen as an incidental finding.

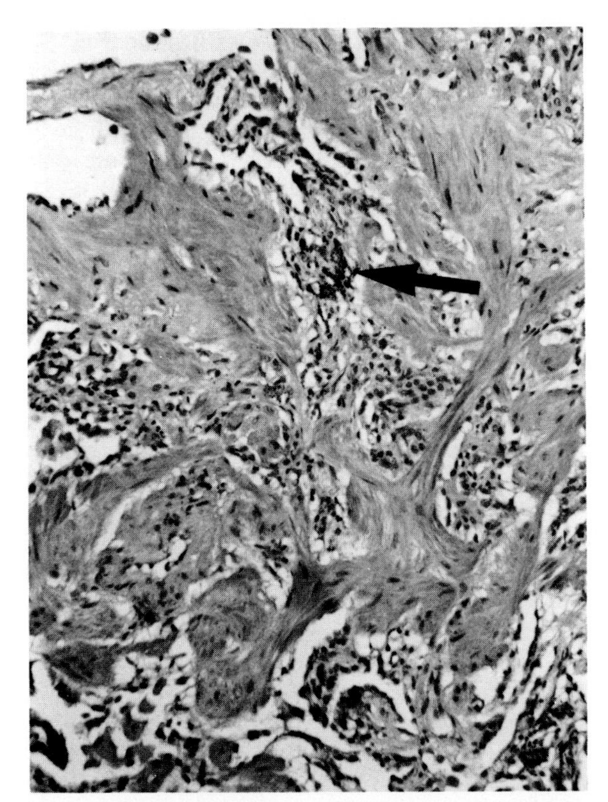

Figure 9–47. Focal nonspecific scar. A few tiny microscopic scars are relatively common in lung tissue showing some other pathologic problem. This example is from a patient who had a localized fibrous mesothelioma elsewhere. Focal scars may appear to center on alveolar ducts, and often they are associated with the accumulations of anthracotic pigment (arrow).

Nonspecific Focal Scars and Nodules (Figs. 9–47 to 9–49): With or without smooth muscle proliferation, incidental scars and nodules often center on small airways in patients with obstructive lung disease. Thickened vessels with intimal proliferation may be an accompanying finding. When involving the pleura (Figs. 9–48, 9–49), they may be associated with pleural blebs (Fig. 9–49).

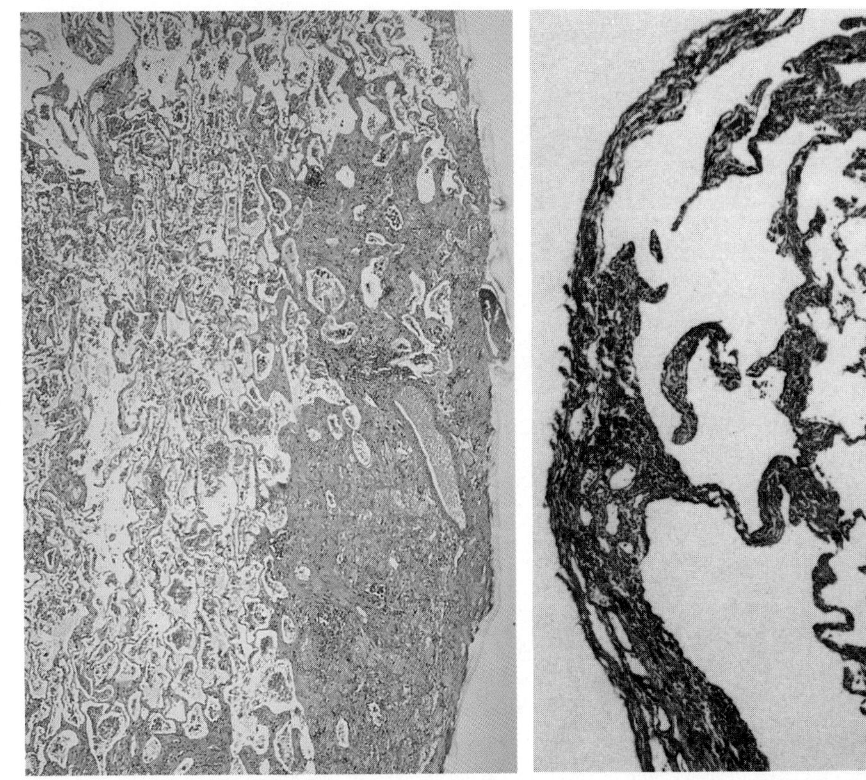

Figure 9–48. **Figure 9–49.**

Figures 9–48, 9–49. Nonspecific subpleural scarring. Nonspecific subpleural scarring and emphysema. These changes are often the only histologic correlate of pneumothoraces in otherwise healthy young adults.

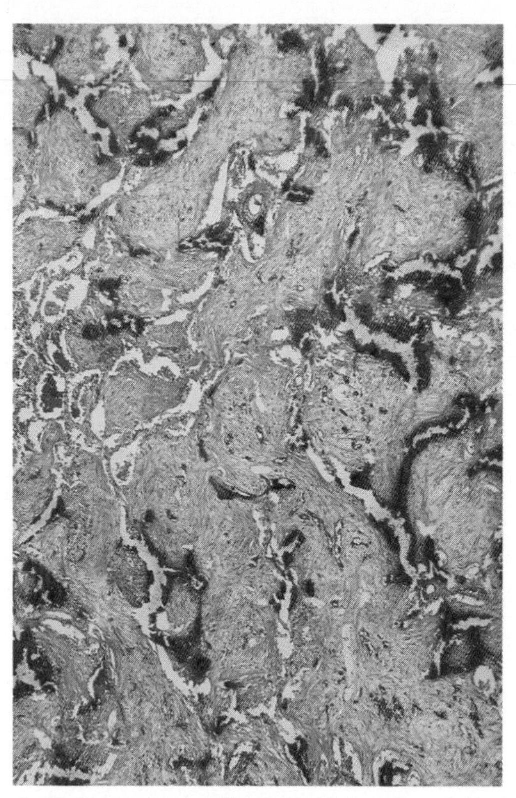

Figure 9-50. Dystrophic calcification with irregular calcified masses of connective tissue in a focal organizing pneumonia.

Dystrophic Calcification and Ossification (Figs. 9-50 to 9-52): Focal calcification or ossification is a common, incidental finding especially in scarred lungs. Extensive intra-alveolar nodular ossification with no associated fibrosis may be the result of chronic passive congestion from left-sided heart disease.

Ossified Tracheal Cartilages: With or without bone marrow, this condition is common in the elderly. The presence of tracheal or bronchial submucosal bone should lead to a consideration of tracheobronchopathia osteoplastica and tracheobronchial amyloid with secondary osseous metaplasia.

Interstitial Emphysema: Small pockets of interstitial air occur as an incidental finding in a variety of conditions, including lungs that are emphysematous or fibrotic as well as in tissue from individuals with prior pneumothorax. Histologically, one sees small holes or clefts lined by giant cells as a response to the interstitial air. Clefts lacking a giant cell or histiocytic reaction also occur but are easily overlooked.

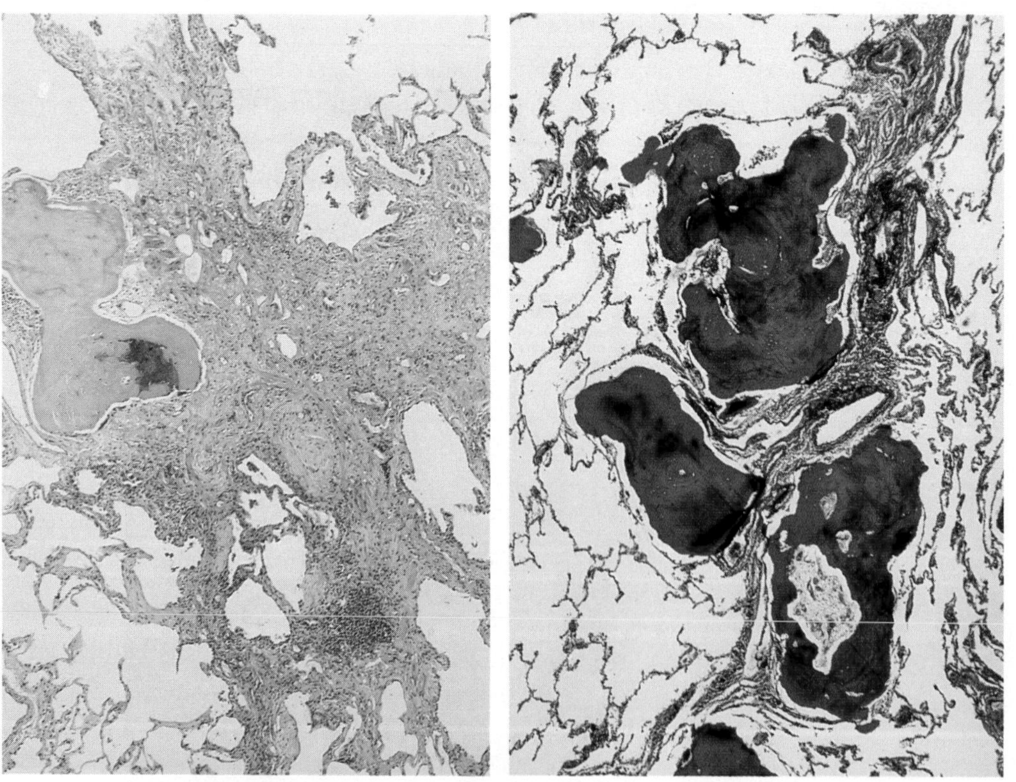

Figure 9-51. Figure 9-52.

Figures 9-51, 9-52. Dystrophic ossification. Two cases of dystrophic ossification are illustrated, one showing bony metaplasia within the scar in a patient with usual interstitial pneumonia (Fig. 9-51) and the other within airspaces in a patient with chronic passive congestion from mitral stenosis (Fig. 9-52).

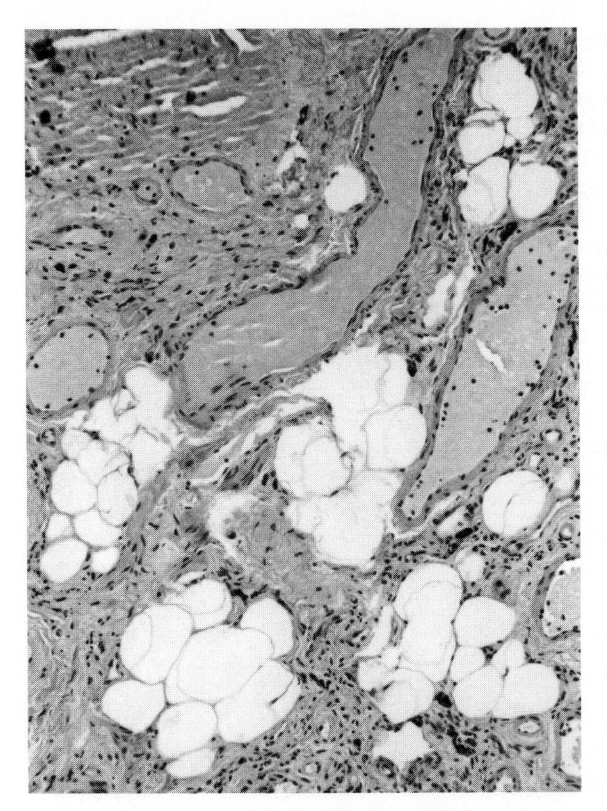

Fatty Metaplasia (Fig. 9-53): Fatty metaplasia in the visceral pleura occurs in foci of pleural scarring. Thickened visceral pleural vessels may be an accompanying finding.

Intrapulmonary Lymph Nodes (Fig. 9-54): Normal lymph nodes may be seen in the pleura and septa or along bronchovascular structures, especially in smokers. The nodes commonly show anthracosis.

Oncocytic Metaplasia (Fig. 9-55): This common aging change is seen in bronchial glands.

Mallory's Hyaline-like Material (Fig. 9-56 [arrows]): This material may be seen in reactive type II cells.

References

Colby TV, Yousem SA. Pulmonary histology for the surgical pathologist. Am J Surg Pathol 12:223-239, 1988.

Dail DH, Hammer SP (eds). Pulmonary Pathology. New York, Springer-Verlag, 1988.

Reinla A. Perivascular xanthogranulomatosis in the lungs of diabetic patients. Arch Pathol Lab Med 100:542-543, 1976.

Schaumann J. On the nature of certain peculiar corpuscles present in the tissue of lymphogranulomatosis benigna. Acta Med Scand 56:240-253, 1941.

Thurlbeck WM (ed). Pathology of the Lung. New York, Thieme, 1988.

Visscher D, Churg A, Katzenstein ALA. Significance of crystalline inclusions in lung granulomas. Mod Pathol 1:415-419, 1988.

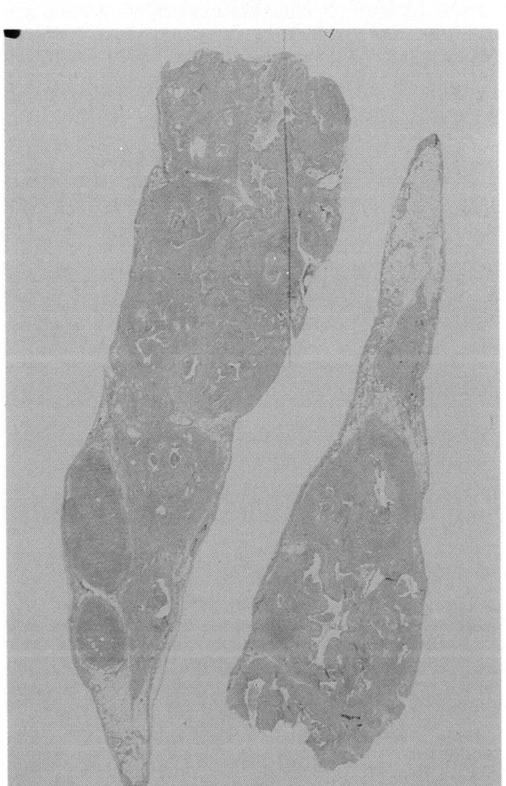

Figure 9-54.

Figures 9-53, 9-54. Pleural fatty metaplasia occurs in foci of pleural scarring and especially at lobar tips (Fig. 9-54). An intrapulmonary lymph node is also shown (Fig. 9-54).

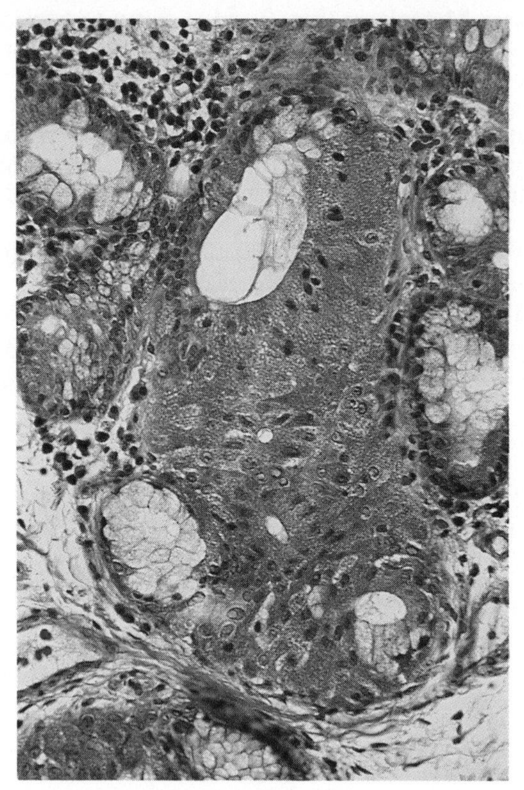

Figure 9–55. Oncocytic metaplasia involving a tracheal submucosal gland.

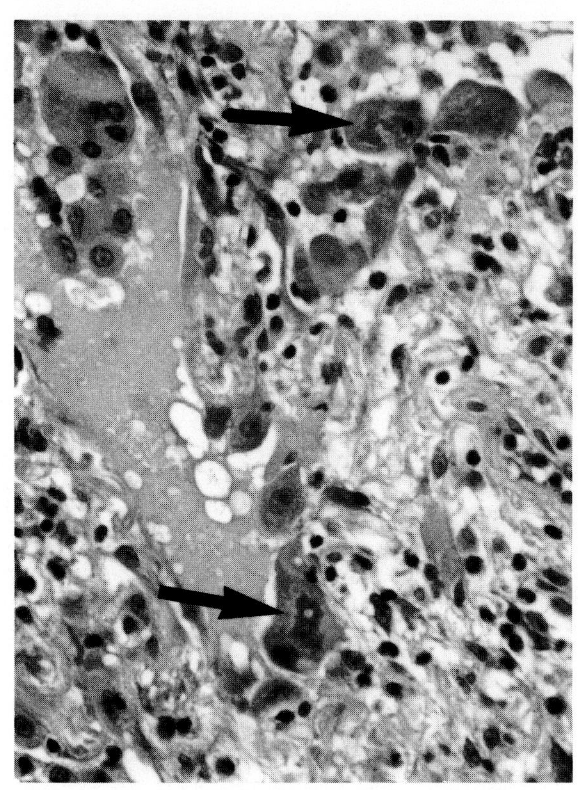

Figure 9–56. Mallory's hyaline-like material in reactive type II cells (arrows) from a case of asbestosis.

APPENDIX I

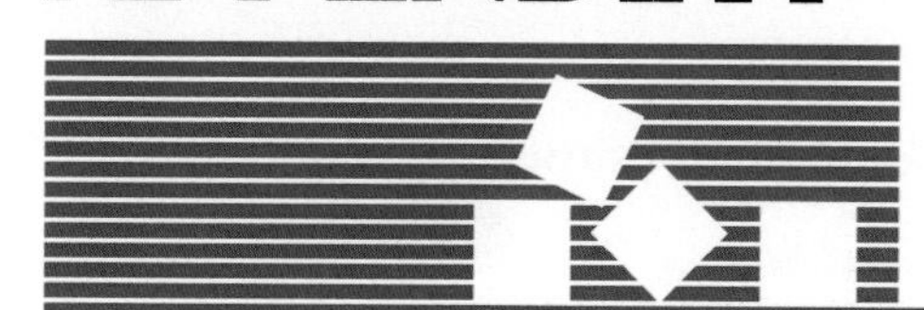

Masses and Localized Lesions: Diagnostic Considerations

■ Cysts and Anomalies

1. Cystic adenomatoid malformation
2. Bronchogenic cyst, bronchial atresia
3. Congenital lobar emphysema
4. Localized persistent interstitial emphysema
5. Cystic rhabdomyosarcoma
6. Lymphangioma and lymphangiectasis
7. Sequestration
8. Papillomatosis
9. Abscess
10. Bronchiectasis
11. Mycetoma
12. Pneumatocele
13. Echinococcal cyst
14. Apical fibrobullous change
15. Mesenchymal cystic hamartoma
16. Multiple cystic fibrohistiocytic tumors
17. Cavitary and cystic inflammatory lesions (e.g., Wegener's granulomatosis)
18. Cavitating malignant tumors
19. Localized honeycombing
20. Cystic metastatic sarcomas

The first eight lesions in this list represent those that are usually seen in children or young adults. Sequestrations often have extensive inflammation, but some may have only extensive mucin pooling within airspaces. Tracheobronchial involvement by papillomatosis in children may be associated with multiple cysts.

Honeycombing may be localized or diffuse and may or may not be associated with cystic change on a radiograph. Honeycombing can sometimes be recognized as such radiographically. Honeycombing may be the result of any number of previous inflammatory reactions.

Apical fibrobullous change is characteristic of ankylosing spondylitis, and the diagnosis is usually made radiographically when ankylosing spondylitis is known to be present.

■ Lesions with Prominent Vascular Components or Vascularity

1. Arteriovenous malformation
2. Sclerosing hemangioma
3. Epithelioid hemangioendothelioma (intravascular bronchioloalveolar tumor [IVBAT])
4. Hemangioma
5. Lymphangiomatosis
6. Castleman's disease
7. Pulmonary capillary hemangiomatosis
8. Localized venous obstruction
9. Pulmonary emboli (other emboli)
10. Incidental vascular changes (e.g., in scars in the lung or in scarred pleura)
11. Vasotropic carcinomas, both primary and metastatic
12. Sarcomas, primary and metastatic (e.g., hemangiopericytomas, angiosarcomas)

Pulmonary capillary hemangiomatosis is generally diffuse; however, a similar proliferation of capillaries may occur in chronic venous hypertension, including localized venous obstruction.

Vasotropic malignancies, including primary and metastatic tumors (particularly angiosarcoma), may be subtle and/or overshadowed by the effects of vascular occlusion and secondary infarction.

Any localized fibrosing lesion in the lung may be associated with vascular obstruction. A form of endarteritis obliterans is common in pulmonary scars and is not necessarily indicative of primary vascular disease. Similar changes also occur in the scarred pleura, where muscular hypertrophy of vessels may be very prominent.

■ Distribution

Angiocentric or Vasculitic Lesions

1. Angioinvasive infection (especially fungal)
2. Primary vasculitis
   a. Wegener's granulomatosis
   b. Polyarteritis nodosa
   c. Necrotizing sarcoid granulomatosis
   d. Allergic granulomatosis (Churg-Strauss syndrome)
   e. Other vasculitides
3. Emboli and infarcts
4. Tumors (especially angiocentric lymphomas, angioinvasive carcinomas, primary and metastatic, and sarcomas including metastatic angiosarcoma, pulmonary artery sarcoma, and Kaposi's sarcoma)

Airway-Centered (Bronchocentric and Bronchiolocentric) Lesions

1. Bronchiectasis and nonspecific focal chronic bronchitis (with or without organizing pneumonia; includes right middle lobe syndrome and its lingular counterpart)
2. Cystic fibrosis
3. Aspiration
4. Mucoid impaction
5. Bronchocentric granulomatosis
6. Infections (especially coccidioidomycosis, tuberculosis, viral infections, mycoplasma)
7. Wegener's granulomatosis (rarely)
8. Airway obstruction by proximal endobronchial mass
9. Mycetoma

Pleural and Subpleural Lesions

1. Apical cap (often bilateral)
2. Old infarct, granuloma, scar
3. Rounded atelectasis
4. Hyaline pleural plaque
5. Pleural blebs, subpleural scarring
6. Eosinophilic pleuritis
7. Tumors obscured by scarring, necrosis, from vascular invasion with secondary infarction

Hyaline pleural plaques with a basket-weave pattern are characteristically associated with asbestos exposure and occur in the parietal pleura. Similar localized plaques may be the residue of prior inflammatory disorders, but when bilateral and extensive, prior asbestos exposure is likely.

Subpleural scarring, blebs, and small bullae are the usual histologic correlates of pneumothorax in young adults.

■ Cellular Components

Epithelial (Epithelioid) Masses

1. Histologically benign
   a. Clear cell tumor (sugar tumor)
   b. Sclerosing hemangioma
   c. Carcinoid tumorlet(s)
   d. Minute pulmonary chemodectomas (meningothelioma-like nodules)
   e. Alveolar adenoma
   f. Papillary adenoma of type II cells
   g. Focal honeycombing with prominent epithelial metaplasia
   h. Mucous gland adenoma
   i. Pleomorphic adenoma
   j. Squamous papilloma or papillomatosis, papillomas of other histologic types
   k. Granular cell tumor
   l. Peribronchiolar squamoid or squamous metaplasia in organizing pneumonia or infarct
   m. Miscellaneous rare tumors (e.g., intrapulmonary thymoma)
   n. Bronchioloalveolar carcinoma with very bland cytologic features ("pulmonary adenomatosis") and other low-grade carcinomas

It is a quite arbitrary point at which one separates a small carcinoid tumor (which should always be considered of low-grade malignancy) from a large tumorlet.

Some endobronchial papillomas are mixed in composition with squamoid cells, columnar cells, mucous cells, or mixtures. Rarely, deceptively bland endobronchial tumors can be associated with metastases.

Sclerosing hemangiomas have a prominent papillary configuration, may appear epithelial, and even resemble bronchioloalveolar carcinoma.

2. Low-grade malignancies
   a. Carcinoid tumors and their histologic variants
   b. Mucoepidermoid tumors (low-grade)
   c. Adenoid cystic carcinoma
   d. Epithelioid hemangioendothelioma (IVBAT)

A number of histologic variants of carcinoid tumors occur.

When considering carcinoid tumor, also consider metastatic breast or prostatic carcinoma.

The vast majority of mucoepidermoid tumors are low grade and resemble their salivary gland counterparts. High-grade mucoepidermoid carcinoma should not be diagnosed unless there is a concomitant low-grade tumor associated with it.

3. Frank malignancies, both primary and metastatic
   a. Squamous cell carcinomas: keratinizing, nonkeratinizing, basaloid, spindled, papillary
   b. Adenocarcinomas, including bronchioloalveolar carcinoma, papillary, and endobronchial (Sclerosing hemangioma may be mistaken for a bronchioloalveolar carcinoma.)

c. Large cell undifferentiated carcinomas, including spindled and giant cell carcinomas
d. Small cell undifferentiated carcinomas
e. Mixed carcinomas
f. Other bronchogenic carcinomas
g. High-grade mucoepidermoid carcinoma
h. Epithelioid hemangioendothelioma (IVBAT)
i. Blastoma with prominent epithelial component
j. Carcinosarcoma with prominent epithelial component
k. Metastatic carcinomas
l. Primary sarcomas with epithelioid appearance such as rhabdomyosarcoma
m. Metastatic sarcomas with epithelioid appearances such as epithelioid sarcoma, angiosarcoma, and alveolar soft part sarcoma
n. Metastatic or primary melanoma
o. Pleural mesothelioma

There are numerous histologic variants of bronchogenic carcinomas, and heterogeneity is becoming increasingly accepted with up to one third of tumors showing multidirectional differentiation.

In some carcinosarcomas and blastomas, the stromal component is inconspicuous, especially in blastomas, in which the epithelial component may resemble endometrial carcinoma or fetal lung.

Not uncommonly, one is faced with determining whether a mass in the lung is a metastasis from some other site or a primary carcinoma. This is particularly true in a patient with a previously discovered tumor. In general, one must individualize each case and use all available data. The most important first step is to compare the two tumors; this solves the majority of the problems.

Mesenchymal and/or Spindle Cell Lesions

1. Histologically benign
   a. Hamartomas
   b. Mesenchymal cystic hamartoma
   c. Granular cell tumor
   d. Leiomyoma (parenchymal or endobronchial)
   e. Benign metastasizing leiomyoma
   f. Sclerosing hemangioma
   g. Plasma cell granuloma, organizing pneumonia, inflammatory pseudotumor, fibrous histiocytoma, hyalinizing granuloma
   h. Neurofibroma
   i. Schwannoma
   j. Intrapulmonary fibrous mesothelioma ("fibroma")
   k. Minute pulmonary chemodectoma
   l. Chondroma
   m. Spindle cell carcinoid
   n. Nonspecific old scar
   o. Miscellaneous rare tumors

Benign metastasizing leiomyoma probably represents metastasis from a low-grade smooth muscle tumor found elsewhere in the body, usually the uterus, but the cytologic features may be so bland as to appear histologically benign.

The variants of hamartomas are numerous, and many contain no cartilage and have varying amounts of fat, smooth muscle cells, myxoid tissue, or myofibroblastic-like cells.

In some sclerosing hemangiomas, the interstitial component is prominent with fibroblastic or fibrotic tissue.

2. Malignant
   a. Primary lung sarcomas, including leiomyosarcoma, hemangiopericytoma, fibrosarcoma, malignant fibrous histiocytoma, chondrosarcoma, rhabdomyosarcoma, osteosarcoma
   b. Mesenchymomas and mixed sarcomas
   c. Carcinosarcoma or blastoma with prominent sarcomatous elements
   d. Pulmonary artery sarcoma
   e. Epithelioid hemangioendothelioma (IVBAT)
   f. Spindled or metaplastic carcinomas, primary and metastatic
   g. Spindled carcinomas, primary and metastatic
   h. Kaposi's sarcoma
   i. Metastatic sarcomas
   j. Metastatic melanoma
   k. Sarcomatous mesothelioma

Mixed Epithelial and Mesenchymal Lesions or Epithelioid and Spindled Lesions

1. Histologically benign
   a. Mixed tumor (primary or metastatic)
   b. Fibroepithelial polyp
   c. Alveolar adenoma
   d. Sclerosing hemangioma
2. Malignant
   a. Mesothelioma
   b. Blastoma
   c. Carcinosarcoma
   d. Metastatic carcinosarcoma, cystosarcoma, mixed Müllerian tumor and so forth.
   e. Primary and metastatic teratomas
   f. Metastatic synovial sarcoma
   g. Metastatic sarcomas with epithelial trapping
   h. Metastatic stromal sarcomas of uterus or ovary with sex cord differentiation

Benign and malignant spindle cell lesions in the lung, both primary and metastatic, commonly grow within the interstitium, entrap airspaces, and produce a pseudobiphasic appearance. Recognition of this phenomenon is facilitated by the finding of partially entrapped airspaces at the edge of the lesion and of a uniform bland cytologic appearance to the epithelial component.

Neutrophils and Necrosis

1. Acute infections
   a. Bacterial
   b. Mycobacterial
   c. Fungal
   d. Viral (rarely)
   e. Protozoan (rarely)
2. Abscess
3. Localized bronchiectasis, bronchitis, or bronchiolitis
4. Aspiration
5. Infected infarct
6. Wegener's granulomatosis, other vasculitides
7. Bronchocentric granulomatosis
8. Sequestration with secondary inflammation
9. Malignant tumors obscured by inflammation and necrosis

Granulomatous Inflammation With or Without Necrosis

1. Infectious agents
   a. Bacterial (actinomycosis, botryomycosis, *Nocardia*)
   b. Mycobacterial
   c. Fungal
   d. Protozoan (rarely pneumocystosis)
   e. Parasitic (especially *Dirofilaria*)
   f. Aspiration pneumonia
2. Noninfectious agents
   a. Wegener's granulomatosis
   b. Rheumatoid nodule(s)
   c. Bronchocentric granulomatosis
   d. Churg-Strauss syndrome (allergic granulomatosis)
   e. Nodular sarcoid
   f. Necrotizing sarcoid granulomatosis
   g. Pulmonary hyalinizing granuloma
   h. Drug reaction
   i. Nodular amyloid
   j. Foreign body reaction
   k. Exogenous lipoid pneumonia
   l. Localized bronchiectasis with granulomatous reaction
   m. Lymphomas and other tumors with granulomatous component (especially Hodgkin's disease)

The amount of granulomatous reaction with the above lesions varies enormously.

Lesions, such as Wegener's granulomatosis and rheumatoid nodules, typically have palisaded histiocytes around foci of necrosis, and thus they are granulomatous; however, only rarely do these lesions have discrete, non-necrotizing, "sarcoid-like" granulomas.

Occasionally, there are only a few scattered small granulomas associated with hyalinizing granulomas, amyloidosis, and bronchiectasis.

The degree of granulomatous reaction associated with some lymphomas, particularly Hodgkin's disease, may be marked.

A significant percentage of necrotic granulomas have uncertain etiologies after all special stain and culture results are back. In most of these, one can adopt a wait-and-see attitude, and a diagnosis may be forthcoming with follow-up.

Eosinophilic Infiltrates

1. Localized idiopathic eosinophilic pneumonia
2. Infections
   a. Fungal (especially coccidioidomycosis)
   b. Mycobacterial
   c. Parasitic *(Dirofilaria, Echinococcus)*
3. Churg-Strauss syndrome (allergic granulomatous angiitis)
4. Bronchocentric granulomatosis
5. Mucoid impaction (allergic bronchopulmonary aspergillosis)
6. Wegener's granulomatosis
7. Tumors with eosinophilia (especially lymphomas, including Hodgkin's disease)
8. Drug reactions

A few eosinophils are extremely common in a large number of localized and diffuse lung lesions.

Other than *Dirofilaria* and the occasional echinococcal cyst, parasitic lung diseases are uncommon in the United States.

Some cases of Wegener's granulomatosis show dramatic eosinophilic infiltrates, and a few eosinophils are almost the rule in active Wegener's granulomatosis.

Some infections may exactly mimic bronchocentric granulomatosis with necrotic eosinophilic debris surrounded by palisaded histiocytes replacing small airways; careful sampling and cultures are necessary in such cases.

Lymphocytes and/or Plasma Cells

See also Lymphoid Tissue below.

1. Focal organizing pneumonia
2. Plasma cell granuloma
3. Pseudolymphoma
4. Benign fibrous histiocytoma
5. Pulmonary hyalinizing granuloma
6. Inflammatory pseudotumor
7. Sequestration
8. Pneumoconiosis (cases with zones of progressive massive fibrosis where a localized lesion appears dominant)
9. Aspiration
10. Chronic abscess (a central necrotic nidus may be quite small)

11. Localized bronchiectasis and nonspecific localized chronic bronchitis
12. Healing infections
13. Nodular amyloid
14. Nonspecific old healed scar tissue, granuloma, infarct
15. Tumors with mononuclear cell infiltrate (especially some lymphomas, some adenocarcinomas, nasopharyngeal-type carcinomas)

There is considerable overlap among the categories labeled as focal organizing pneumonia, plasma cell granuloma, pseudolymphoma, benign fibrous histiocytoma, and inflammatory pseudotumor.

Infections rarely produce masses dominated by mononuclear cells, although one notable example is Q fever pneumonia, which may appear as slowly resolving nodules on a chest radiograph.

In amyloid tumors, the amyloid deposits dominate, with plasma cells being relatively inconspicuous. In hyalinizing granulomas, the degree of infiltrate and lymphoid hyperplasia with germinal centers may be prominent.

A number of localized lesions composed predominantly of chronic inflammatory cells with varying degrees of organization and fibrosis are never specifically diagnosed. Those that appear bronchocentric are probably the residue of some prior airway inflammatory reaction, and the terms "nonspecific localized chronic bronchitis" or "chronic organizing pneumonia" may be appropriate. Aspiration should be considered in such cases.

Histiocytes (With or Without Foamy Cytoplasm), Airspace or Interstitial

1. Granulomatous infections (especially with poorly formed granulomas)
2. Actinomycosis, botryomycosis
3. Abscess and xanthogranulomatous reaction in localized acute and chronic bronchitis, bronchiectasis
4. Aspiration, chronic
5. Proximal obstruction
6. Focal organizing pneumonia
7. Benign fibrous histiocytoma
8. Plasma cell granuloma
9. Granular cell tumor, other rare tumors
10. Malakoplakia, Whipple's disease
11. Focal eosinophilic pneumonia
12. Localized pseudo-desquamative interstitial pneumonia ("pseudo-DIP") reaction around another lesion
13. Nonspecific accumulation of dust and anthracotic pigment-laden histiocytes in foci of scarring
14. *Pneumoconiosis* (especially silicosis) with dominant nodule

A few airspace histiocytes are extremely common in localized lung disease and are quite nonspecific.

Among localized lesions, foamy histiocytes are often a marker of obstruction.

Dust-filled histiocytes tend to accumulate in foci of fibrosis, possibly from interruption of normal lymphatic drainage.

Lymphoid Tissue

1. Polymorphous in composition
   a. Pseudolymphoma, hyalinizing granuloma, plasma cell granuloma, focal organizing pneumonia, fibrous histiocytoma
   b. Non-Hodgkin's lymphomas of mixed cell composition, including those lesions classified as angiocentric lymphoma and angio-immunoblastic lymphadenopathy
   c. Hodgkin's disease
   d. Mycosis fungoides
   e. Carcinomas with prominent lymphoid stroma, both primary and secondary
   f. Noninfectious inflammatory processes (e.g., Wegener's granulomatosis)
   g. Chronic infections with prominent lymphoid tissue
2. Monomorphous in composition
   a. Non-Hodgkin's lymphomas of all histologic subtypes, primary or secondary
   b. Other lymphoreticular infiltrates including leukemias, mycosis fungoides, plasmacytoma, myeloma

Any lymphoreticular infiltrate in the lung often has a polymorphous appearance at its edge, whereas monomorphism is best appreciated centrally. The presence of germinal centers within a lesion is not necessarily evidence of a benign lesion.

Lymphoepithelioma-like carcinoma primary in the lung and metastatic nasopharyngeal lymphoepitheliomas may have abundant lymphoid stroma and may be mistaken for lymphomas.

Inflammatory lesions, both infectious and noninfectious, may suggest a primary lymphoreticular proliferation.

Secondary involvement of the lung by myocosis fungoides, leukemias, and myeloma may be associated with masses or localized infiltrates on dust radiographs.

Fibrosis and Organizing Pneumonia (With or Without Necrosis)

1. Focal organizing pneumonia, including right middle lobe syndrome and its lingular counterpart
2. Plasma cell granuloma, pseudolymphoma
3. Chronic, healing, or resolved infections
4. Hyalinizing granuloma, sclerosing mediastinitis
5. Abscess, aspiration
6. Wegener's granulomatosis

7. Old healed scar, granuloma, infarct
8. Apical cap
9. Rounded atelectasis
10. Pneumoconiosis (especially with localized foci of progressive massive fibrosis)
11. Nodular amyloid
12. Organization and scarring in a sequestration
13. Primary or metastatic spindle cell tumors
14. Other tumors with extensive organization

Fibrosis and organization are extremely common in a wide variety of lesions.

The lingula and right middle lobe appear to be predisposed by their anatomic characters to bouts of pneumonitis that may eventually require resection, and the histologic appearance is that of a nonspecific organizing pneumonia. Other than excluding the presence of an obstructing airway lesion, pathologists often cannot discern much more than the presence of organizing pneumonia and chronic bronchiolitis.

In hyalinizing granulomas, the fibrosis is of a dense hyaline nature, which also characterizes the fibrosis in old granulomas, particularly those due to histoplasmosis and sclerosing mediastinitis.

As the name would imply, apical caps are seen in the apex of the lung as fibrous tissue convexities of the visceral pleural and subpleural parenchyma, rich in elastic fibers, in which background alveolar architecture of the lung can sometimes be discerned.

Rounded atelectasis is a result of focal pleural scarring and puckering, which produce a localized zone of atelectasis and a coin lesion on the chest radiograph. The lesions are removed because of the suspicion of malignancy, and surgeons are often incredulous that no tumor is present. A history of asbestos exposure is common.

APPENDIX II

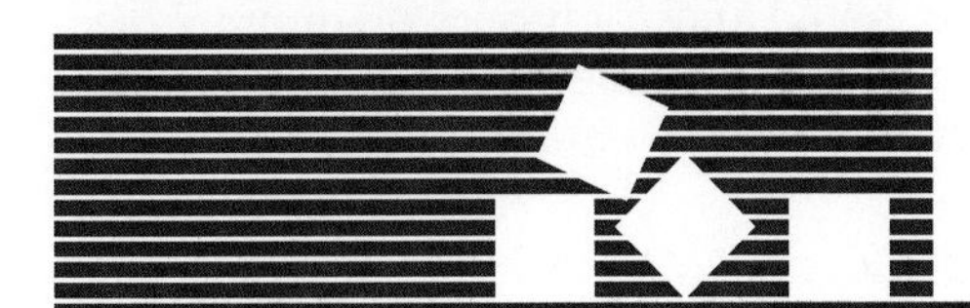

Diffuse and Multifocal Processes of Acute or Recent Onset: Diagnostic Considerations

■ Distribution

Angiocentric Lesions

1. Emboli (exclude the possibility of secondary emboli in a diffuse inflammatory process)
2. Vasculitis, including hypersensitivity, Wegener's granulomatosis, drug reactions, other vasculitides
3. Sepsis and toxic shock
4. Capillaritis (infectious and noninfectious causes; see text)
5. Rapidly progressive malignancy (especially lymphoreticular or massive vascular involvement by metastatic carcinoma)
6. Intravenous drug abuse

Airway-Centered (Bronchocentric and Bronchiolocentric) Lesions

1. Acute exacerbation of chronic bronchitis, bronchiolitis, bronchiectasis, cystic fibrosis, and so on
2. Viral and mycoplasmal infections, including respiratory syncytial virus (RSV), adenovirus in children
3. Toxic inhalations
4. Eosinophilic granuloma
5. Collagen vascular diseases
6. Extrinsic allergic alveolitis, acute
7. Bronchocentric granulomatosis (BCG)
8. Bronchocentric infection

Cellular bronchiolitis with or without bronchiolitis obliterans and/or organizing pneumonia is often a prominent feature.

Many of these lesions are dominated by a cellular bronchitis or bronchiolitis; however, the defining feature of bronchocentric granulomatosis is a necrotizing bronchocentric or bronchiolocentric lesion with palisaded histiocytes. Mycobacterial and fungal infections may mimic BCG almost exactly.

Lymphatic Distribution

1. Sarcoidosis presenting as an acute process
2. Malignancy (especially lymphoma, leukemia, lymphangitic carcinoma)
3. Viral pneumonia with lymphoid hyperplasia

Miliary Nodules

1. Infections (viral, fungal, bacterial, mycobacterial, protozoan [e.g., toxoplasmosis])
2. Sarcoidosis
3. Eosinophilic granuloma
4. Tumors (lymphoreticular, lymphangitic carcinoma)

The distribution of miliary nodules often appears random. In most miliary infections, there is usually some acute exudate or necrosis associated with the nodules.

■ Cellular or Histologic Components

Interstitial or Alveolar Edema (With or Without Hyaline Membranes)

1. Early diffuse alveolar damage (DAD), including acute interstitial pneumonia (AIP)
2. Collagen-vascular diseases (especially systemic lupus)
3. Pulmonary edema
4. Acute allergic reaction or toxic exposure
5. Acute infection (especially viral)

One must exclude the possibility of an unrecognized immunosuppressed state. The clinician is usually worried about infection; therefore, cultures and special stains should always be performed.

Noninfectious causes of diffuse alveolar damage, such as acute interstitial pneumonia, are diagnoses of exclusion. Patients with an acute allergic or toxic reaction may have a history supportive of these diagnoses.

The diagnosis of an acute viral infection may be retrospective after appropriate serologic findings or cultures are known.

Alveolar Hemorrhage and/or Hemosiderin Deposition With or Without Capillaritis

1. Wegener's granulomatosis (other vasculitides)
2. Goodpasture's disease (antiglomerular basement membrane disease)
3. Collagen-vascular diseases (especially systemic lupus erythematosus)
4. Idiopathic pulmonary hemosiderosis
5. Drug and toxic reactions (especially paraquat)
6. Acute infection (especially viral but also *Pneumocystis*)
7. Diffuse alveolar damage with marked hemorrhage
8. Coagulopathies
9. Early infarcts
10. Pulmonary leukostasis
11. Malignancy (e.g., metastatic angiosarcoma)
12. Unclassified hemorrhage syndromes

One must carefully exclude the possibility that "acute hemorrhage" may be an artifact. A helpful feature is the presence of hemosiderin-filled macrophages; however, these are not always present, and they may be the result of some other process, such as chronic passive congestion.

In the setting of diffuse alveolar hemorrhage, freezing lung tissue for immunofluorescent studies is appropriate.

A significant number of patients who present with alveolar hemorrhage syndromes remain unclassified despite extensive clinical evaluation.

In cases of local hemorrhage treated by surgical resection, the airways should be examined carefully for foci of ulceration and the vessels carefully assessed with elastic stains. A cause of hemorrhage is often not found in this setting, but one should look for bronchitis or bronchiectasis and for evidence of abnormal vessels, especially changes of localized venous obstruction.

Alveolar Fibrinous Exudate

1. Diffuse alveolar damage (see text for the many causes)
2. Infections (especially *Pneumocystis carinii*)
3. Pulmonary alveolar proteinosis
4. Pseudoproteinosis reactions
5. "Dense" edema (see below)
6. Pneumoconiosis (especially acute silicosis)
7. Mucus pooling from obstruction, bronchioloalveolar carcinoma, or in honeycombing
8. Eosinophilic pneumonia
9. Reaction associated with lymphomatous infiltrates, other tumors, and non-infectious inflammatory processes (e.g., Wegener's).

Pseudoproteinosis includes reactions that resemble alveolar proteinosis but have some recognizable cause; these are usually seen in immunosuppressed patients and are associated with an infection.

Dense edema is a descriptive term for dense eosinophilic airspace material, which is probably just a chronic proteinaceous exudate. It is quite nonspecific.

Some pneumoconioses, particularly acute silicosis, may result in a proteinosis-like appearance.

Prominent mucostasis suggests obstruction or proximity to mucinous bronchioloalveolar carcinoma. It is also often marked in foci of honeycombing with bronchiolar metaplasia.

Some lymphomas presenting as diffuse lung disease have prominent eosinophilic alveolar exudates.

Acute Neutrophilic Inflammation (Interstitial, Perivascular, and/or Within Airspaces)

1. Acute infection and sepsis (especially bacterial)
2. Capillaritis
3. Wegener's granulomatosis (other vasculitides)
4. Acute allergic alveolitis
5. Eosinophilic pneumonia
6. Eosinophilic granuloma
7. Drug reaction and other allergic reactions
8. Artifactual

Acute inflammation is usually a component in cases showing several histologic features but may be the dominant finding in capillaritis. Occasional cases of Wegener's granulomatosis have extensive acute neutrophilic airspace consolidation for which no infectious cause can be found.

Variable numbers of neutrophils are common in eosinophilic pneumonia. Neutrophils may also be prominent in eosinophilic granuloma and extrinsic allergic alveolitis.

Operative trauma may result in the artifactual presence of neutrophils, especially marginating in small vessels.

Eosinophilic Inflammation (Airspace, Vascular, or Interstitial)

1. Asthma and related syndromes
2. Eosinophilic pneumonia (both acute and chronic, with or without organization)
3. Allergic granulomatosis (Churg-Strauss syndrome)
4. Wegener's granulomatosis
5. Bronchocentric granulomatosis
6. Some acute infections (e.g., parasites)
7. Eosinophilic granuloma
8. Hypereosinophilic syndromes
9. Tumor-associated (especially Hodgkin's disease and T-cell lymphomas)
10. Drug reactions

A few eosinophils are present in many conditions; they are nonspecific and may even be misleading.

Churg-Strauss disease is extremely rare, and clinical correlation is required for diagnosis.

Some cases of Wegener's granulomatosis are dominated by eosinophil infiltrates.

In BCG, there are bronchocentric and bronchiolocentric foci of necrosis with eosinophilic debris.

Some infections, notably coccidioidomycosis, may be associated with significant eosinophilia, sometimes mimicking BCG.

Interstitial Chronic Inflammatory Infiltrate

1. Healing or organizing diffuse alveolar damage, including infectious and noninfectious causes; includes acute interstitial pneumonia
2. Infections (especially viral and mycoplasmal)
3. Extrinsic allergic alveolitis
4. Drug reactions
5. Wegener's granulomatosis (vasculitis, giant cells, and/or microabscesses are usually also present)
6. Lymphoma and leukemia
7. Chronic interstitial pneumonias with superimposed DAD (especially usual interstitial pneumonia [UIP])
8. Nonspecific cellular interstitial infiltrates

The presence of chronic inflammatory cells should not be considered to be indicative of a chronic lesion.

Lymphomas and leukemias may be relatively subtle cytologically when they involve the lung diffusely, and they may or may not be overtly malignant on cytologic grounds.

A significant portion of chronic interstitial pneumonias (mainly UIP) may present in an acute exacerbation phase with DAD superimposed. Background chronic scarring and honeycombing are present.

A portion of cases in this category remain unclassified and may be descriptively termed nonspecific cellular interstitial infiltrates. Some of these may be indicative of a slowly healing diffuse alveolar damage or resolving viral infections, or they are very early stages of a lesion that may be recognized with follow-up.

Granulomas and Giant Cells

1. Infections (especially mycobacterial, fungal)
2. Extrinsic allergic alveolitis
3. Drug reactions
4. Eosinophilic pneumonia
5. Sarcoidosis with acute clinical presentation
6. Intravenous drug abuse
7. Wegener's granulomatosis
8. Bronchocentric granulomatosis

In some cases of extensive allergic alveolitis, giant cells and/or granulomas may be quite inconspicuous.

In Wegener's granulomatosis, a few scattered giant cells may be the only clue to suggest the diagnosis. In intravenous drug abusers, the perivascular giant cells with foreign material may be the most apparent lesion even though another process may actually causing clinical symptoms.

Extensive Airspace Organization or Interstitial Fibroblast Proliferation

1. Organizing infections
2. Organizing DAD including acute interstitial pneumonia
3. Organizing allergic reactions, including extrinsic allergic alveolitis and eosinophilic pneumonia
4. Bronchiolitis obliterans organizing pneumonia (BOOP)
5. Wegener's granulomatosis
6. Hodgkin's disease and other lymphomas
7. DAD superimposed on chronic interstitial pneumonia

Organization is generally seen within airspaces as tufts of granulation tissue; its counterpart in the interstitium is an edematous fibroblastic proliferation, which contrasts with mature interstitial fibrosis with abundant collagen.

APPENDIX III

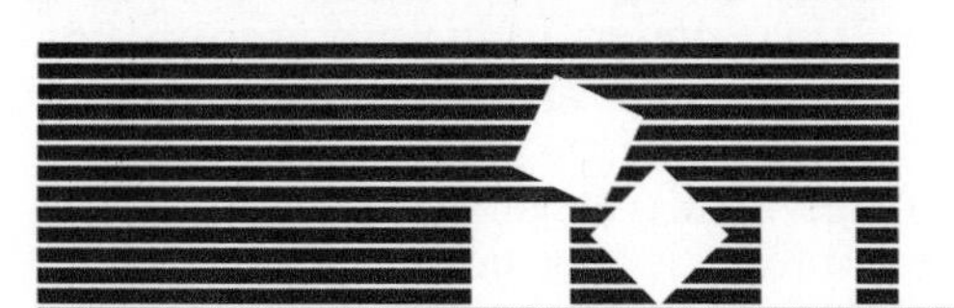

Diffuse and Multifocal Processes with Subacute and Chronic Clinical History: Diagnostic Considerations

■ Distribution

Angiocentricity

1. Pulmonary hypertension
   a. Primary forms, including plexogenic arteriopathy, chronic thromboembolic disease, and pulmonary veno-occlusive disease
   b. Hypertension secondary to cardiac or chronic lung disease
2. Pulmonary emboli, acute and chronic
3. Intravenous drug abuse
4. Vasculitis: Wegener's, Churg-Strauss, polyarteritis nodosa, others
5. Sarcoidosis
6. Amyloidosis
7. Infection: sepsis, perivenular infiltrates of a miliary viral infection, angioinvasive fungal infections
8. Capillaritis
9. Pneumoconioses: dust accumulation along the lymphatic routes around the vessels
10. Tumors, particularly lymphomas, lymphangitic carcinoma, carcinomatous arteriopathy, Kaposi's sarcoma, angiosarcoma, pulmonary artery sarcoma, and IVBAT (intravascular bronchioloalveolar tumor) either within lymphatic vessels or within arteries and veins themselves
11. Collagen vascular diseases causing vasculitis or pulmonary hypertension
12. Drug reaction with vasculitis (usually small vessel: "hypersensitivity angiitis")
13. Lung transplant rejection
14. Post-inflammatory scarring from numerous causes
15. Bronchocentric lesions affecting bronchovascular structures may sometimes suggest angiocentricity
16. Any lesion along lymphatic routes

The lesions in this group reflect those with the changes of pulmonary hypertension, inflammatory lesions in the vessel walls (i.e., vasculitis), or conditions that follow structures adjacent to the vessels, such as the lymphatics or the airways.

Airway-Centered (Bronchocentric and Bronchiolocentric) Lesions

1. Lesions with proliferative bronchiolitis and organizing pneumonia (see p. 213)
2. Healed diffuse alveolar damage, particularly after respiratory distress syndrome in neonates
3. Extrinsic allergic alveolitis
4. Eosinophilic granuloma, particularly early cellular lesions
5. Bronchiolitis obliterans organizing pneumonia
6. Collagen vascular diseases
7. Pneumoconioses: silicosis, hard metal disease, anthracosis, any pneumoconiosis with dust macules
8. Drug reactions
9. Respiratory bronchiolitis-associated interstitial lung disease
10. Bronchocentric granulomatosis (BCG)
11. Infections mimicking BCG
12. Sarcoidosis

13. Diffuse panbronchiolitis
14. Follicular bronchiolitis
15. Fume exposure
16. Aspiration
17. Bronchiolitis obliterans in transplant patients (bone marrow or heart-lung transplants)
18. Chronic infection, chronic bronchitis, bronchiectasis, constrictive bronchiolitis (see p. 216), cystic fibrosis
19. Asthma
20. Idiopathic small airways injury
21. Lymphoma and leukemia (e.g., chronic lymphocytic leukemia)

The lesions listed include those in which there are cellular infiltrates along airways as well as those in which there is organization and/or fibrosis centering on the airways.

A significant number of cases that show mild inflammation and scarring of airways remain unresolved and are included in the idiopathic small airways injury group.

Many early pneumoconioses manifest as dust macules with dust-filled macrophages centered on the bronchioles.

Bronchiolocentricity of eosinophilic granuloma is best seen in the early lesions and is less commonly appreciated in larger fibrotic lesions.

Lymphatic Distribution

1. Sarcoidosis
2. Pneumoconioses: berylliosis, silicosis
3. Lymphangioleiomyomatosis
4. Lymphoid hyperplasia: immunodeficiency states, hypersensitivity or reactive condition such as viral infection (e.g., mononucleosis), collagen-vascular diseases
5. Diffuse malignancy: lymphoma, Kaposi's sarcoma, lymphangitic carcinoma

Pleural Fibrosis and Pleural Inflammation

1. Usual interstitial pneumonia (primarily when associated with prominent subpleural fibrosis)
2. Pneumoconiosis, especially asbestosis
3. Collagen vascular diseases
4. Amyloidosis
5. Incidental finding in a biopsy showing other parenchymal features
6. Eosinophilic pneumonia with pleuritis

Many chronic interstitial pneumonias may appear more severe in the subpleural regions. That is particularly true in some cases of UIP with a peripheral acinar pattern.

The pleura is often quite markedly thicker in collagen vascular diseases because of fibrosis of the subpleural parenchyma and because of chronic pleuritis and fibrosis.

Amyloid occasionally presents with massive pleural involvement mimicking pleural fibrosis.

■ Cellular or Histologic Components

Fibrinous Exudates or Eosinophilic Intra-alveolar Material

1. Diffuse alveolar damage
2. Infections (especially *P. carinii,* mycobacterial, viral)
3. Pulmonary alveolar proteinosis, including pseudoproteinosis reactions
4. Eosinophilic pneumonia
5. Bronchiolitis obliterans organizing pneumonia (BOOP)
6. Radiation reaction
7. Drug reactions
8. Wegener's granulomatosis

Many of these present as diffuse alveolar damage and may be clinically acute (see Appendix II).

The material in alveolar proteinosis is granular and often contains degenerating cells, eosinophilic bodies, and cholesterol clefts. This material is lipoproteinaceous in contrast to the fibrinous exudate that characterizes most of the other lesions.

A small amount of glassy, dense eosinophilic material ("dense edema") can be seen as a focal reaction in a large number of pulmonary conditions and is not helpful diagnostically.

In some cases of Wegener's granulomatosis, there are large zones of airspace fibrinous exudate.

Pseudoproteinosis reactions—lesions mimicking proteinosis—are usually seen in immunosuppressed individuals who have a pulmonary infection. In such cases, infections should be carefully excluded.

Chronic Inflammatory Infiltrate

A large number of lesions show this feature. The following is only a partial list.

1. An acute process with chronic inflammatory infiltrate with or without organizing pneumonia
2. Idiopathic chronic interstitial lung disease: UIP, DIP, LIP, BOOP, eosinophilic granuloma, sarcoidosis, eosinophilic pneumonia
3. Respiratory bronchiolitis-associated interstitial lung disease
4. Pneumoconioses, especially asbestosis, berylliosis, hard metal disease (giant cell interstitial pneumonia [GIP])
5. Drug reactions
6. Radiation therapy
7. Chronic airway lesions (see below)
8. Healing and chronic infections (e.g., healing viral pneumonia)
9. Chronic aspiration
10. Chronic granulomatous infections

11. Extrinsic allergic alveolitis
12. Wegener's granulomatosis and other vasculitides
13. Pulmonary veno-occlusive disease and chronic passive congestion
14. Nonspecific, miscellaneous and unclassified lesions
15. A reaction around some other lesion that has not been sampled (i.e., sampling error)

Numerous lesions in the lung are associated with a chronic inflammatory interstitial infiltrate, and this finding by itself is rarely specific. Generally, one looks for other features to help make a diagnosis, such as Langerhans cells in eosinophilic granuloma, fibrosis and honeycombing in UIP, and so on.

A number of cases remain unclassified—interstitial pneumonias that do not fit into a recognized clinicopathologic entity.

With small biopsy specimens, sampling error and the possibility that one is seeing a reaction around some other process should always be kept in mind.

Lymphoid Hyperplasia and Dense Interstitial Infiltrates

1. Lymphocytic interstitial pneumonia
2. Diffuse lymphoid hyperplasia
3. Follicular bronchitis and bronchiolitis
4. Extrinsic allergic alveolitis
5. Collagen vascular diseases
6. Immunodeficiency states
7. Hypersensitivity reactions (inhaled antigens, drug reactions)
8. Chronic airway inflammation and infection from chronic bronchitis, bronchiectasis, cystic fibrosis
9. Tumors, especially lymphomas, Kaposi's sarcoma
10. Diffuse panbronchiolitis

The presence of a dense lymphoid infiltrate in the interstitium is evidence against the diagnosis of UIP.

Technically, one can separate lymphoid hyperplasia with lymphoid follicles along the lymphatic routes of the lung from diffuse interstitial lymphoid infiltrates; however, the term lymphocytic interstitial pneumonia has often been used for both.

Extrinsic allergic alveolitis may produce a pattern that is identical to that of LIP. The distinction between follicular bronchiolitis and diffuse lymphoid hyperplasia is somewhat arbitrary, and the two carry similar implications.

Some lymphomas may mimic inflammatory processes, particularly well-differentiated lymphocytic lymphomas presenting diffusely in the lung, and diffuse mixed cell lymphomas with large numbers of histiocytes.

Histiocytes (Airspace or Interstitial With or Without "Foamy" Changes)

1. Obstructive pneumonia, regardless of cause
2. Desquamative interstitial pneumonia (DIP)
3. Respiratory bronchiolitis-associated interstitial lung disease
4. Eosinophilic granuloma
5. Pseudo-DIP reactions
6. Barium or lipid aspiration, lipoid pneumonia
7. Pneumoconioses: silicosis, hard metal lung disease, reactions to aluminum
8. Eosinophilic pneumonia
9. Chronic and recurrent pulmonary hemorrhage or chronic passive congestion
10. Intravenous drug abuse
11. Drug reactions, especially amiodarone
12. Tumors with histiocytic differentiation and/or appearance (for example, acute myelomonocytic leukemia); bronchioloalveolar carcinoma with alveolar filling by histiocyte-like carcinoma cells
13. Metabolic defects, such as Niemann-Pick disease, Gaucher's disease, Hermansky-Pudlak syndrome
14. Whipple's disease, malakoplakia, mycobacterial infections
15. Diffuse panbronchiolitis
16. BOOP, extrinsic allergic alveolitis, and UIP; all may have foci with large numbers of foamy histiocytes

In eosinophilic granuloma, the Langerhans histiocytes are generally interstitial in location; however, they may be associated with large numbers of airspace histiocytes around the lesions, producing a pseudo-DIP reaction.

Any mass lesion, whether small or large, may have a pseudo-DIP reaction in the surrounding airspaces.

Hemosiderin-Filled Macrophages

1. Lesion with acute hemorrhage (See Appendix II)
2. Idiopathic pulmonary hemosiderosis
3. Collagen-vascular disease
4. Chronic passive congestion
5. Pulmonary veno-occlusive disease
6. Occupational exposures: asbestos, welding, hematite mining
7. Respiratory (smoker's) bronchiolitis
8. Eosinophilic granuloma
9. Organizing hemorrhagic pneumonias
10. Lymphangioleiomyomatosis
11. Incidental finding (e.g., chronic passive congestion or smoker's bronchiolitis in a patient with an unrelated condition)

The staining character of the Prussian blue–positive material may be helpful: it is pale blue and finely granular in smokers' macrophages, and it is coarse and dark brown in the macrophages of welders.

Eosinophil Infiltrates

1. Eosinophilic pneumonia
2. Eosinophilic granuloma
3. Wegener's granulomatosis and Churg-Strauss syndrome
4. Hypereosinophilic syndromes
5. Drug reactions
6. Collagen vascular diseases (especially rheumatoid arthritis)
7. Asthma and related syndromes
8. Infections
9. Unclassified (allergic) reactions
10. Tumors with eosinophilic infiltrates (especially Hodgkin's disease and non-Hodgkin's lymphomas)

Some cases of Wegener's granulomatosis are characterized by numerous eosinophils and are distinguished from Churg-Strauss syndrome only by the clinical features.

Drug reactions may mimic eosinophilic pneumonia; a hypersensitivity vasculitis of veins dominated by eosinophilic infiltrate is also often present.

A few eosinophils are common in many diseases and are quite nonspecific. Eosinophilic infiltrates are not often seen in extrinsic allergic alveolitis (hypersensitivity pneumonitis) despite the "allergic" etiology of this condition.

Granulomas With or Without Necrosis

1. Sarcoidosis, nodular sarcoid
2. Extrinsic allergic alveolitis
3. Drug reaction
4. Miliary infection (especially mycobacterial, fungal)
5. Pneumoconioses: especially berylliosis
6. Noninfectious necrotizing granulomatous processes
   a. Wegener's granulomatosis
   b. Bronchocentric granulomatosis
   c. Churg-Strauss syndrome
   d. Necrotizing sarcoid granulomatosis
7. Intravenous drug abuse
8. Pulmonary veno-occlusive disease

Rare granulomas or occasional giant cells are not uncommon incidental findings in lung biopsy findings, and sometimes one should overlook their presence.

The lesions included above generally have significant granulomatous character to them, except for extrinsic allergic alveolitis, in which the granulomas may be small or poorly formed and few in number.

Giant Cells (Singly or in Clusters)

1. Any lesion with numerous alveolar macrophages
2. Part of granulomatous processes
3. Extrinsic allergic alveolitis
4. Reaction to iron-encrusted elastic fibers in chronic passive congestion, veno-occlusive lesions
5. Intravenous drug abuse
6. Reaction to chronic interstitial air (interstitial emphysema)
7. Asbestos exposure with giant cell reaction to asbestos bodies
8. Associated with blue bodies, Schaumann's bodies, calcium oxalate crystals, amyloid, corpora amylacea
9. Foreign material (may or may not be polarizable)
10. Hard metal pneumoconiosis (GIP)
11. Wegener's granulomatosis
12. Giant cell pneumonias (measles, parainfluenza, RSV)
13. Aspiration

In intravenous drug abusers, a giant cell reaction to polarizable foreign material is seen along vessels.

The giant cells in GIP are within airspaces and often show cannibalism of histiocytes.

One lesion with numerous histiocytes, which is often interpreted as a granulomatous reaction, is early silicosis.

In any lesion with numerous histiocytes, relatively numerous giant cells (presumably by cell fusion) may be present.

Pulmonary veno-occlusive disease is sometimes associated with a giant cell or granulomatous reaction, probably caused by chronic passive congestion.

Organizing Pneumonia (Proliferative Bronchiolitis Obliterans Often Present)

1. Bronchiolitis obliterans organizing pneumonia (BOOP)
2. Organizing diffuse alveolar damage
3. Collagen vascular diseases
4. Organizing infections: mycoplasma, viral, *Pneumocystis,* bacterial
5. Drug reactions
6. Allergic alveolitis and eosinophilic pneumonia
7. Fume exposure
8. Aspiration
9. Distal to obstruction

10. Chronic bronchitis, bronchiectasis with distal organizing pneumonia
11. As a nonspecific part of a large number of other reactions (e.g., Wegener's granulomatosis)

In aspiration and fume exposures, there is bronchocentricity that can be appreciated at low power.

Interstitial Fibrosis (With or Without Honeycombing)

1. Usual interstitial pneumonia
2. Desquamative interstitial pneumonia
3. Respiratory (smoker's) bronchiolitis
4. Lymphocytic interstitial pneumonia
5. Collagen vascular diseases
6. Drug reactions
7. Pneumoconioses: asbestosis, berylliosis, silicosis, hard metal disease
8. Sarcoidosis
9. Eosinophilic granuloma
10. Chronic granulomatous infections
11. Chronic aspiration
12. Chronic extrinsic allergic alveolitis
13. Late organizing chronic eosinophilic pneumonia
14. Organized and organizing diffuse alveolar damage
15. Chronic interstitial pulmonary edema, passive congestion
16. Radiation
17. Healed pneumonias
18. Pulmonary veno-occlusive disease
19. Late organizing pneumonia (e.g., BOOP)
20. Lesions with spindle cells, neoplastic and nonneoplastic (e.g., lymphangioleiomyomatosis, spindle cell tumors, either primary or metastatic)
21. Small airway injury
22. Unclassified interstitial pneumonias

For accurate diagnosis (e.g., radiation reaction), a medical history is often required.

Careful assessment of the distribution will help in making the diagnosis, such as airway centering in respiratory (smoker's) bronchiolitis.

Burned-out granulomatous reactions may leave fibrosis in which Schaumann's bodies are embedded. Late cases of sarcoidosis may show fibrosis distributed along lymphatic routes.

Organized chronic eosinophilic pneumonia may be characterized by an absence of eosinophils and tends to be subpleural in location.

In pulmonary veno-occlusive disease, interstitial fibrosis is minimal.

Nodular Fibrosis

1. Eosinophilic granuloma
2. Sarcoidosis, nodular sarcoid
3. Pneumoconioses: silicosis, berylliosis, hard metal disease
4. Lesions mimicking fibrosis, including minute pulmonary chemodectomas, lymphangioleiomyomatosis, benign metastasizing leiomyomas, metastatic or primary spindle cell tumors
5. Nonspecific old healed scars

The character of the fibrosis may be helpful, with rounded nodules being typical of silicosis and stellate or irregular nodules being characteristic of eosinophilic granuloma.

In hard metal disease, there is marked scarring centered on airways.

Any biopsy specimen may contain a focal nonspecific scar or a minute pulmonary chemodectoma, and the possibility that these lesions may be incidental should always be kept in mind. Old scars sometimes contain abundant mature smooth muscle.

Smooth Muscle Proliferation

1. Asthma and other chronic airway diseases.
2. Metaplastic smooth muscle in any chronic fibrosing interstitial pneumonia or scarring reaction
3. Lymphangioleiomyomatosis (LAM)
4. Benign metastasizing leiomyoma
5. Diffuse primary or metastatic spindle cell malignancy

Metaplastic smooth muscle has the appearance of mature smooth muscle and is in contrast to LAM, in which the cells are shorter and stubbier and appear immature.

Benign metastasizing leiomyoma usually is associated with nodular lesions both radiographically and pathologically.

APPENDIX IV

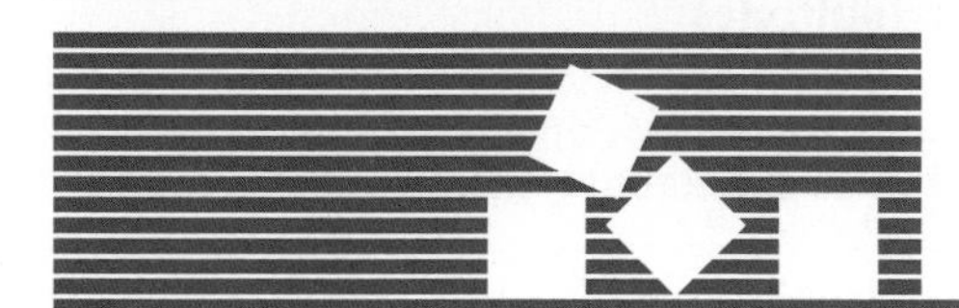

Biopsy Specimens from Immunosuppressed Patients: Diagnostic Considerations

■ Apparently Normal Lung Biopsy

1. Edema and early diffuse alveolar damage (DAD)
2. Fat emboli
3. Infection with minimal reaction (e.g., *P. carinii*)
4. Subtle miliary infection (look for tiny inflammatory nodules, often perivenular)

■ Diffuse Alveolar Damage (DAD)

1. Idiopathic DAD (so-called idiopathic interstitial pneumonia in bone marrow transplants, nonspecific interstitial pneumonia in AIDS)
2. Drug reactions, including delayed reaction after drugs have been stopped (usually chemotherapeutic agents; many have been implicated)
3. Viral infection: CMV, HSV, adenovirus, respiratory synctial virus (RSV), measles
4. Other infection: bacterial, toxoplasmosis, pneumocystosis, and others
5. Radiation reaction (if history appropriate)
6. Leukostasis in patients with treated leukemia

This is probably the most common pattern seen in open biopsy specimens from immunosuppressed patients with acute pulmonary infiltrates. Many cases remain unresolved and should be given the descriptive diagnosis of diffuse alveolar damage of unknown etiology. In fact, the majority of these are probably drug reactions, although proof is difficult to obtain.

If necrosis is present, one should redouble efforts to find an organism. It is not inappropriate to spend 10 to 15 minutes looking for viral inclusions and to study step sections with special stains. Two lesions may be present, one causing the necrosis and the other the diffuse alveolar damage, e.g., diffuse CMV pneumonia with foci of necrosis caused by another agent. A lack of inclusions does not exclude a viral infection, and the clinician should be apprised of this. Drug reactions very rarely, if ever, are associated with necrosis, and the diagnosis of a drug reaction should depend on careful clinicopathologic correlation.

■ Nodular Lesions

This category includes gross and/or microscopic nodules.

1. Miliary viral infection: CMV, HSV, others
2. Fungal infection (with or without miliary pattern): *Candida, Aspergillus,* mucormycosis, many others on rare occasions (confirm specific diagnosis by culture)
3. Nocardiosis (with or without miliary pattern)
4. Mycobacterial infection
5. *P. carinii* (especially in AIDS)
6. Bacterial pneumonia (rarely)
7. Other unusual infections (protozoal, parasitic)
8. De novo lymphoproliferative diseases
9. Kaposi's sarcoma
10. Recurrent and metastatic types of lymphoma, leukemia, carcinoma, or sarcoma
11. Lesions as in non-immunosuppressed patients

Infarction is characteristic of invasive fungal infection, and one should look in the vessels for organisms. Miliary viral infections typically show a perivenular distribution. Necrosis in any nodule in an immunosuppressed patient should be considered infection until proven otherwise. *Nocardia* may be difficult to see with special stains and may necessitate careful examination to identify organisms. Some fungi, particularly *Candida,* may have only a focal microscopic nidus of organisms with extensive surrounding reaction that is nonspecific and lacking in organisms.

■ Pulmonary Alveolar Proteinosis–like Reactions

Rigorously rule out infection before accepting a diagnosis of pulmonary alveolar proteinosis in an immunosuppressed patient. This type of reaction may be seen with:

1. Viral infections
2. Bacterial infections (e.g., *Nocardia*)
3. Mycobacterial infections
4. Fungal infections (a nidus of organisms may be very tiny)
5. *P. carinii*

■ Capillaritis

1. Infection and sepsis (viral, bacterial, fungal)
2. Primary disease process (e.g., pulmonary capillaritis with hemorrhage in systemic lupus erythematosus)
3. As in non-immunosuppressed patients

■ Neutrophilic Infiltrates

These infiltrates should be considered infection until proven otherwise. The different types include the following:

1. Bacterial
2. Mycobacterial
3. Viral
4. Fungal
5. Others, including parasitic

■ Histiocytic Infiltrates

1. Rule out infection with poorly formed granulomas (mycobacterial, fungal)
2. Malakoplakia
3. As in non-immunosuppressed patients

■ Pulmonary Hemorrhage

1. Traumatic hemorrhage from biopsy procedure
2. Severe diffuse alveolar damage with hemorrhage
3. Disseminated intravascular coagulation
4. Leukostasis in leukemics on chemotherapy
5. Sepsis
6. As in non-immunosuppressed patients

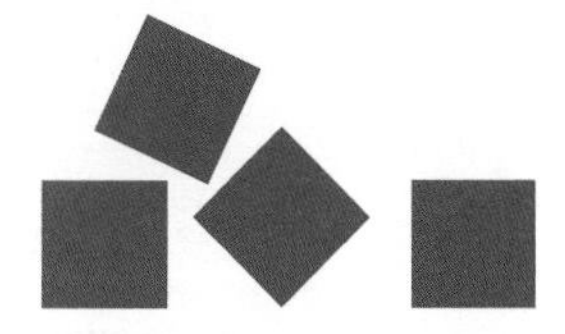

INDEX

Note: Page numbers in *italics* refer to illustrations; page numbers followed by *t* refer to tables.